Tumors of the Thyroid and Parathyroid Glands

AFIP Atlas
of
Tumor Pathology

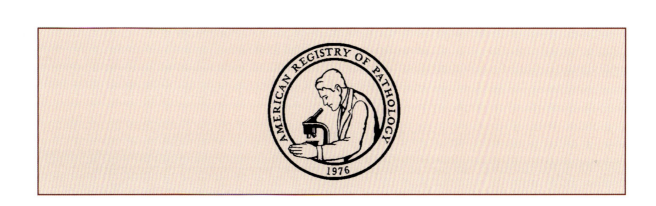

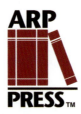

ARP PRESS

Silver Spring, Maryland

Editorial Director: Mirlinda Q. Caton
Production Editor: Dian S. Thomas
Editorial Assistant: Magdalena C. Silva
Editorial Assistant: Alana N. Black

Available from the American Registry of Pathology
Silver Spring, Maryland 20910
www.arppress.org
ISBN 1-933477-32-6
978-1-933477-32-9

AFIP ATLAS OF TUMOR PATHOLOGY

Fourth Series
Fascicle 21

TUMORS OF THE THYROID AND PARATHYROID GLANDS

by

Juan Rosai, MD

Centro Diagnostico Italiano (CDI), Milan, Italy
Adjunct Professor of Pathology
University of Utah and ARUP Laboratories
Salt Lake City, Utah
Adjunct Professor, Department of Pathology and Laboratory Medicine
Weill Cornell Medical College, Cornell University
New York, New York

Ronald A. DeLellis, MD

Department of Pathology and Laboratory Medicine
Warren Alpert Medical School of Brown University
Providence, Rhode Island
Consultant, Department of Pathology
Rhode Island Hospital and The Miriam Hospital
Providence, Rhode Island

Maria Luisa Carcangiu, MD

Director, Anatomic Pathology 1
Fondazione IRCCS
Istituto Nazionale dei Tumori
Milan, Italy

William J. Frable, MD

Professor of Pathology (Emeritus)
Medical College of Virginia
Virginia Commonwealth University
Richmond, Virginia

Giovanni Tallini, MD

Professor of Anatomic Pathology
University of Bologna School of Medicine
Bologna, Italy

Published by the
American Registry of Pathology
Silver Spring, Maryland
2014

AFIP ATLAS OF TUMOR PATHOLOGY

EDITORS' NOTE

The Atlas of Tumor Pathology has a long and distinguished history. It was first conceived at a cancer research meeting held in St. Louis in September 1947 as an attempt to standardize the nomenclature of neoplastic diseases. The first series was sponsored by the National Academy of Sciences-National Research Council. The organization of this formidable effort was entrusted to the Subcommittee on Oncology of the Committee on Pathology, and Dr. Arthur Purdy Stout was the first editor-in-chief. Many of the illustrations were provided by the Medical Illustration Service of the Armed Forces Institute of Pathology (AFIP), the type was set by the Government Printing Office, and the final printing was done at the Armed Forces Institute of Pathology (hence the colloquial appellation "AFIP Fascicles"). The American Registry of Pathology (ARP) purchased the Fascicles from the Government Printing Office and sold them virtually at cost. Over a period of 20 years, approximately 15,000 copies each of nearly 40 Fascicles were produced. The worldwide impact of these publications over the years has largely surpassed the original goal. They quickly became among the most influential publications on tumor pathology, primarily because of their overall high quality, but also because their low cost made them easily accessible the world over to pathologists and other students of oncology.

Upon completion of the first series, the National Academy of Sciences-National Research Council handed further pursuit of the project over to the newly created Universities Associated for Research and Education in Pathology (UAREP). A second series was started, generously supported by grants from the AFIP, the National Cancer Institute, and the American Cancer Society. Dr. Harlan I. Firminger became the editor-in-chief and was succeeded by Dr. William H. Hartmann. The second series' Fascicles were produced as bound volumes instead of loose leaflets. They featured a more comprehensive coverage of the subjects, to the extent that the Fascicles could no longer be regarded as "atlases" but rather as monographs describing and illustrating in detail the tumors and tumor-like conditions of the various organs and systems.

Once the second series was completed, with a success that matched that of the first, ARP, UAREP, and AFIP decided to embark on a third series. Dr. Juan Rosai was appointed as editor-in-chief, and Dr. Leslie Sobin became associate editor. A distinguished Editorial Advisory Board was also convened, and these outstanding pathologists and educators played a major role in the success of this series, the first publication of which appeared in 1991 and the last (number 32) in 2003.

The same organizational framework applies to the current fourth series, but with UAREP and AFIP no longer functioning, ARP is now the responsible organization. New features include a hardbound cover and illustrations almost exclusively in color. There is also an increased emphasis on the cytopathologic (intraoperative, exfoliative, or fine needle aspiration) and molecular genetic features that are important in diagnosis and prognosis. What does not change from the three previous series, however, is the goal of providing the practicing pathologist with thorough, concise, and up-to-date information on the nomenclature and classification; epidemiologic, clinical, and pathogenetic features; and, most importantly, guidance in the diagnosis of the tumors and tumorlike lesions of all major organ systems and body sites.

As in the third series, a continuous attempt is made to correlate, whenever possible, the nomenclature used in the Fascicles with that proposed by the World Health Organization's Classification of Tumors, as well as to ensure a consistency of style. Close cooperation between the various authors and their respective liaisons from the Editorial Board will continue to be emphasized in order to minimize unnecessary repetition and discrepancies in the text and illustrations.

Particular thanks are due to the members of the Editorial Advisory Board, the reviewers (at least two for each Fascicle), the editorial and production staff, and the individual Fascicle authors for their ongoing efforts to ensure that this series is a worthy successor to the previous three.

Steven G. Silverberg, MD
Ronald A. DeLellis, MD
Leslie H. Sobin, MD

PREFACE

Many years have elapsed since the publication of the Third Series AFIP Fascicles Tumors of the Thyroid Gland, by J. Rosai, M. L. Carcangiu and R. A. DeLellis (1992), and Tumors of the Parathyroid Gland, by R. A. DeLellis (1993). During this period, awareness of the remarkable morphologic diversity of thyroid carcinoma has notably expanded, and great advances have been made in unraveling the molecular genetic features of thyroid and parathyroid tumors. There has also been an increased interest in the use of the fine-needle aspiration technique for the diagnosis and management of thyroid tumors, and in the role of the pathologist in the operative handling of the hyperfunctioning parathyroid gland. In this Fascicle, we document the most significant advances that have taken place in these areas, emphasizing those with a practical application at the clinical level. The format remains similar to that of the previous versions, but the two Fascicles have been merged into one, and most of the black and white gross photographs and photomicrographs have been replaced with color images. We have tried to include the most recent references, but have not ignored the classic works in the field, many of which have descriptions, illustrations, and insights that cannot be bettered.

Dr. Ronald A. DeLellis wrote the chapter on medullary thyroid carcinoma and C-cell hyperplasia, and all the chapters on tumors of the parathyroid gland; Dr. William J. Frable wrote the chapter on cytopathology of thyroid tumors and the cytopathology portion of the chapters dealing with the major thyroid tumors; Dr. Giovanni Tallini wrote the chapters on genes involved in thyroid tumorigenesis and on the molecular genetic alterations of specific tumor types; and Drs. Juan Rosai and Maria Luisa Carcangiu wrote the remaining portions on thyroid tumors. These various components were circulated among the five authors in order to produce a uniform style and philosophy throughout this Fascicle.

We are grateful to Dr. Steven G. Silverberg for his gentle guidance of this effort and for his admirable restraint and patience; to Mrs. Mirlinda Q. Caton and her staff for their expert editorial assistance, and to the many pathologists with whom we interacted over the years in a variety of venues. Some of these esteemed colleagues will recognize their thoughts and opinions in these pages. Among these experts, we owe special thanks to Drs. Virginia LiVolsi, Manuel Sobrinho-Simões, and E. D. Williams.

We hope that this Fascicle will fulfill the original goal of this series, which is that of helping the pathologist diagnose and anticipate the behavior of tumors and tumor-like lesions included in this publication.

Juan Rosai, MD
Ronald A. DeLellis, MD
Maria Luisa Carcangiu, MD
William J. Frable, MD
Giovanni Tallini, MD

ACKNOWLEDGMENTS

Dr. R. A. DeLellis would like to thank the following individuals for having generously contributed photographic and other material: Medullary Carcinoma and C-cell hyperplasia chapter: V. Eusebi, O Ljungberg, X. Matias-Guiu, and M. Papotti; Parathyroid chapters: M. Beland, M. DePaepe, A. Gill, L. Grimelius, P. Mazzaglia, J. Monchik, L. Pisharodi, G. Randolph, S.I. Roth, P. Sadow, M. Stolte, and C. Wang.

CONTENTS

1. Normal Thyroid Gland 1
   Embryology 1
   Anatomy 3
   Histology 4
   The Follicular Cell 8
      Thyroid Hormones 10
   The C-Cell 11
      Calcitonin and Calcitonin Gene-Related Peptide 14
   Solid Cell Nests 15
2. Genes Involved in Thyroid Tumorigenesis 23
   TSH Receptor/cAMP Pathway 25
   MAPK Pathway 31
      Tyrosine Kinase Receptors (RET, NTK1, MET) 31
      RAS 36
      BRAF 37
   P13K/PTEN/AKT Pathway 39
   PPARγ Rearrangement 41
   ß-Catenin/APC/Wnt Signaling 42
   TERT 43
   Tumor Protein p53 45
3. General Features of Thyroid Tumors 57
   Incidence of Thyroid Carcinoma 57
   Thyroid Tumors and Iodine Deficiency 57
   Thyroid Tumors and Radiation Exposure 57
   Thyroid Tumors in Childhood 58
4. Classification of Thyroid Tumors 61
   Primary Tumors 62
   Secondary Tumors and Tumor-Like Lesions 62
5. Follicular Thyroid Adenoma and Variants 65
   Follicular Adenoma 65
   Adenoma Variants 73
      Adenoma with Bizarre Nuclei 73
      Hyalinizing Trabecular Adenoma 73
      Adenolipoma and Adenochondroma 78
      Atypical Adenoma (Including Spindle Cell Adenoma) 78
      Adenoma with Papillary Features 79
      "Toxic" Adenoma 81

6. Follicular Thyroid Carcinoma 85
    Minimally Invasive (Encapsulated) Type 86
    Widely Invasive Type... 97

7. Papillary Thyroid Carcinoma and Variants... 103
    Papillary Carcinoma 103
    Papillary Carcinoma Variants 127
        Papillary Microcarcinoma 127
        Encapsulated Variant.. 130
        Follicular Variant... 131
        Encapsulated Follicular Variant of PTC and the "Uncertain Malignant
            Potential (UMP)" Concept.. 135
        Solid/Trabecular Variant... 139
        Diffuse Sclerosing Variant 141
        Oncocytic and Warthin-Like Variants 143
        Tall and Columnar Cell Variants.. 146
        Cribriform/Morular Variant 149

8. Poorly Differentiated Thyroid Carcinoma 165
    Insular Carcinoma 165
    Other Poorly Differentiated Carcinomas.. 172

9. Undifferentiated (Anaplastic) Thyroid Carcinoma 177

10. Thyroid Tumors with Oncocytic (Hürthle Cell) Features 199
    General Considerations 199
    Oncocytic Adenoma (Hürthle Cell Adenoma)...................................... 203
    Oncocytic Carcinoma (Hürthle Cell Carcinoma).................................. 209
    Papillary Oncocytic Neoplasms.. 215

11. Thyroid Tumors with Clear Cell, Squamous, and Mucinous Features 221
    Tumors with Clear Cell Features.. 221
        General Considerations... 221
        Tumor Types.. 222
        Other Conditions 227
    Tumors with Squamous Features 228
    Tumors with Mucinous Features 233

12. Medullary Thyroid Carcinoma and C-Cell Hyperplasia 241
    Medullary Thyroid Carcinoma 241
    Medullary Carcinoma Variants.. 261
        Papillary Variant.. 261
        Follicular (Tubular) Variant 261
        Small Cell Variant.. 261
        Giant Cell Variant.. 261

        Clear Cell Variant 262

        Melanotic Variant 262

        Oncocytic Variant 262

        Squamous Cell Variant 264

        Amphicrine Cell Variant 264

        Paraganglioma-Like Variant 264

        Angiosarcoma-Like Variant 265

        Encapsulated Variant 265

        Medullary Microcarcinoma 265

        Heritable Forms of Medullary Carcinoma 266

     Mixed Medullary and Follicular Cell Carcinoma 266

     C-Cell Hyperplasia 272

13. Sarcomas of the Thyroid Gland 289

     General Considerations 289

     Angiosarcoma 291

14. Malignant Lymphoma of the Thyroid Gland and Related Lesions 299

     Malignant Lymphoma 299

     Other Lymphoid Tumors and Tumor-Like Conditions 305

        Hodgkin Lymphoma 305

        Plasmacytoma 307

        Plasma Cell Granuloma and Related Lesions 307

15. Miscellaneous Thyroid-Related Tumors 311

     Parathyroid Tumors 311

     Paraganglioma 311

     Teratoma 313

     Solitary Fibrous Tumor 314

     Other Benign Soft Tissue-Type Tumors 314

     Tumors with Thymic or Related Branchial Pouch Differentiation 315

        Ectopic Cervical Thymoma 315

        Ectopic Hamartomatous Thymoma 316

        Spindle Epithelial Tumor with Thymus-Like Differentiation 316

        Carcinoma Showing Thymus-Like Differentiation 319

        Salivary Gland-Type Tumors 320

16. Secondary Tumors of the Thyroid Gland 325

17. Tumor-Like Conditions of the Thyroid Gland 331

     Nodular Hyperplasia 331

     Diffuse Hyperplasia 335

     Dyshormonogenetic Goiter 336

     Thyroiditis 339

        Hashimoto Thyroiditis 339

Subacute Granulomatous (DeQuervain) Thyroiditis 342

Fibrosing (Riedel) Thyroiditis 342

Multifocal Fibrosing (Sclerosing) Thyroiditis 345

Malakoplakia 347

Other Forms of Thyroiditis 347

Miscellaneous Lesions 347

Langerhans Cell Histiocytosis 347

Rosai-Dorfman Disease 347

Radiation Changes 348

Amyloid Goiter 349

18. Benign Thyroid Tissue in Abnormal Locations 355

Ectopia 355

Mechanical Implantation 357

Parasitic Nodule 358

Thyroid Inclusions in Lymph Nodes 360

Thyroid as a Component of Teratoma (Including Struma Ovarii) 361

19. Molecular Genetic Alterations of Specific Thyroid Tumors of Follicular Cells 365

Follicular Adenoma and Variants 365

Follicular Carcinoma 367

Papillary Carcinoma and Variants 371

Poorly Differentiated Carcinoma 379

Undifferentiated (Anaplastic) Carcinoma 380

Other Tumors 382

20. Cytopathology of Thyroid Tumors 395

The Normal Thyroid Gland 397

Cytology of Thyroid Tumors and Tumor-Like Conditions 400

Nodular Hyperplasia 400

Diffuse Hyperplasia 404

Hashimoto Thyroiditis 404

Follicular Neoplasms 406

Papillary Carcinoma 416

Variants of Papillary Thyroid Carcinoma 427

Insular Carcinoma 431

Undifferentiated (Anaplastic) Carcinoma 433

Tumors with Oncocytic Features 433

Tumors with Clear Cell Features 439

Tumors with Squamous Features 440

Medullary Carcinoma 441

Malignant Lymphoma 445

Secondary/Metastatic Tumors 447

Diagnostic Molecular Genetics of FNAB 450

Accuracy of Cytology: What Can be Expected.. 452

Pitfalls of Thyroid FNAB 455

Histologic Alterations Following FNAB 456

Complications of FNAB 456

21. Clinical Aspects of Thyroid Tumors 465

Clinical and Laboratory Evaluation of Thyroid Nodules.. 465

Demographics 465

Family History 465

History of Hashimoto Thyroiditis.. 465

Rate of Growth 465

Palpation 465

Isotopic Imaging Study 465

Ultrasonography (Ultrasound).. 466

Computerized Tomography (CT) and Magnetic Resonance Imaging (MRI).......... 466

Serum Thyroglobulin Levels 466

Serum Calcitonin Levels.. 466

Frozen Section Examination 466

Cytologic Evaluation.. 467

Pathologic Evaluation and Reporting.. 467

Handling.. 467

Description 467

Sections for Histology 467

Example of Gross Description 468

Standardized Reporting.. 468

ADASP Recommended Protocol.. 468

CAP Recommended Protocol/Checklist.. 468

Microscopic Grading 468

Staging of Thyroid Carcinoma 469

Ancillary Testing 471

Treatment of Thyroid Tumors 472

Prognostic Factors 474

22. Immunohistochemical Markers of the Normal and Neoplastic Thyroid Gland 481

23. The Normal Parathyroid Gland.. 493

Embryology.. 493

Anatomy 494

Gross and Microscopic Findings 494

Immunohistochemical Findings.. 499

Ultrastructural Findings 501

24. Physiology and Pathophysiology of Parathyroid Glands 505
    Calcium Homeostasis 505
    Parathyroid Hormone and Parathyroid Hormone-Related Protein 505
    Hypercalcemia 506
    Hyperparathyroidism... 506
        General Considerations... 506
        Primary Hyperparathyroidism 506
        Bone Manifestations... 507
        Renal and Other Manifestations 509
    Hypercalcemia of Malignancy 509
25. Parathyroid Adenoma and Variants 513
    Parathyroid Adenoma.. 513
    Adenoma Variants 531
        Oncocytic Adenoma.. 531
        Lipoadenoma... 532
        Water Clear Cell Adenoma 532
        Atypical Adenoma 532
        Adenoma-Associated Parathyroid Glands.. 537
26. Parathyroid Carcinoma 543
    General Features 543
    Clinical Features 543
    Gross Findings 544
    Microscopic Findings.. 544
    Cytologic Findings.. 552
    Immunohistochemical Findings 552
    Ultrastructural Findings.. 553
    Molecular Genetic Findings.. 553
    Differential Diagnosis 554
    Treatment and Prognosis 554
    Staging of Parathyroid Carcinoma 556
27. Primary Chief Cell Hyperplasia, Clear Cell Hyperplasia, and Heritable
    Hyperparathyroidism Syndromes.. 561
    Primary Chief Cell Hyperplasia 561
    Clear Cell Hyperplasia 566
    Heritable Hyperparathyroidism Syndromes.. 568
        Multiple Endocrine Neoplasia Type 1 568
        Multiple Endocrine Neoplasia Type 2 570
        Multiple Endocrine Neoplasia Type 4 571
        Hyperparathyroidism-Jaw Tumor Syndrome.. 571

Familial Hypocalciuric Hypercalcemia and Neonatal Severe Primary
Hyperparathyroidism.. 571
Familial Isolated Hyperparathyroidism 572

28. Secondary and Tertiary Hyperparathyroidism, and Parathyroid Grafts 575
Secondary Hyperparathyroidism... 575
Tertiary Hyperparathyroidism 579
Parathyroid Grafts... 580

29. Miscellaneous Parathyroid Lesions 583
Parathyroid Cysts... 583
Parathyromatosis 583
Secondary Tumors 585

30. Diagnostic Approaches to Parathyroid Lesions............................. 589
Intraoperative Diagnosis... 589
Fat Stains... 590
Density Gradients 591
DNA Cytometry 591
Preoperative Localization and Intraoperative Parathyroid Hormone Assays 591
Index 597

1 THE NORMAL THYROID GLAND

EMBRYOLOGY

The thyroid *anlage* appears as a bilobate vesicular structure at the foramen cecum of the tongue. It then descends as a component of the thyroglossal duct to reach its definitive position in the neck (fig. 1-1). After involution of the thyroglossal duct, the thyroid anlage begins to expand laterally to form the thyroid lobes (1–3).

Microscopically, the initially solid thyroid anlage begins to form cords and plates of follicular cells during the 9th gestational week. A small lumen appears within the follicles by the 10th week, with colloid secretion becoming evident by the 12th week. By the 14th week, the gland already consists of well-developed follicles lined by follicular cells and containing thyroglobulin-positive colloid in their lumens (figs. 1-2–1-3). Labeled amino acid studies have shown that thyroglobulin synthesis begins at a very early stage, when the thyroid gland is still a solid mass at the base of the tongue, and long

before lumen formation and colloid secretion can be detected (4,5).

It has recently become clear that thyroid gland organogenesis and the differentiation of follicular cells are directed by the concerted action of a series of transcription factors, while thyroid-stimulating hormone (TSH) influences thyroid differentiation only after the anatomic outline of the gland is well established. The most important of these transcription factors are thyroid transcription factor (TTF)-1 (Nkx2-1), TTF-2 (Foxe1), PAX8, and Hhex (6). Although these factors are also expressed and influence differentiation in other developing tissues, all four are coexpressed only in the thyroid anlage (6). Since they regulate the expression of thyroid-specific genes (e.g., those responsible for the production of thyroid peroxidase and thyroglobulin) they are important not only for organogenesis but for the functional differentiation of the gland in later stages of prenatal development and postnatally (6,7).

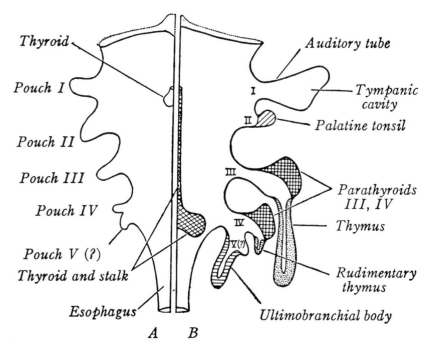

Figure 1-1

BRANCHIAL ARCHES AND THEIR DERIVATES

The branchial arches (A) and the adult organs that arise from them (B) are illustrated schematically. Note the thyroid anlage in the midline, attached to the thyroglossal duct.

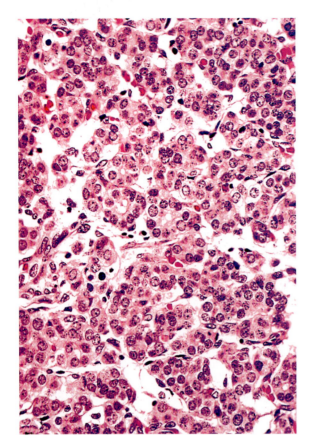

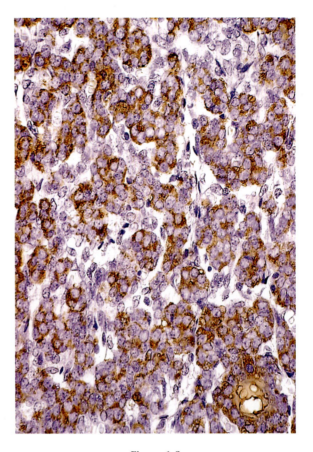

Figure 1-2

FETAL THYROID GLAND

A small lumen appears in the minute follicles of a 10-week fetal thyroid gland.

Figure 1-3

FETAL THYROID GLAND

Well-developed small follicles have small lumens that contain colloid in a 12-week fetal thyroid gland (thyroglobulin immunostain).

Figure 1-4

FETAL THYROID GLAND

Calcitonin is demonstrable immunohistochemically in the fetal thyroid gland.

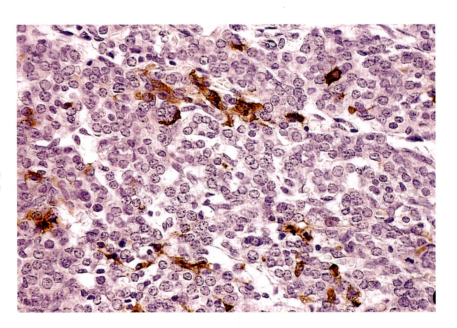

Embryologic, histochemical, and immuno-histochemical studies have led to the conclusion that the C-cells (the primary site of synthesis and storage of calcitonin) are derived from the neural crest and that they migrate to the ultimobranchial bodies before their incorporation into the thyroid gland (fig. 1-4) (8–12). The ultimobranchial bodies, in turn, are derived from branchial pouch complex IV-V (13). In some species, such as birds, the thyroid gland and the ultimobranchial bodies are separate structures in the adult, and the C-cells are confined to the latter.

The development of the ultimobranchial body is divisible into four stages: 1) branchial pouch stage (3 to 12 mm, 5 to 7 weeks); 2) separation stage (13 to 17 mm, 7 to 8 weeks); 3) incorporation stage (18 to 27 mm, 8 to 9 weeks); and 4) dissolution stage (28 to 520 mm, 9 weeks to term) (3). In the branchial pouch stage, the ultimobranchial body is a thick-walled stratified epithelial cyst that is in continuity with the primitive pharyngeal cavity. At the beginning of the separation stage, pouch complex IV-V separates into the parathyroid IV and the ultimobranchial component, the latter of which ultimately divides into central and peripheral portions in the dissolution phase. The central portion is represented by a stratified epithelial-lined cyst, whereas the peripheral portion is dispersed into a few cell groups that eventually become cystic.

Additional support for the ultimobranchial origin of the C-cells is provided by studies of patients with the DiGeorge syndrome (14,15). Affected individuals typically have complete or partial absence of derivatives of pouch complexes III and IV-V. In studies reported by Burke et al. (14), only 27 percent of patients with DiGeorge syndrome had C-cells within their thyroid gland. In contrast, the number of bronchopulmonary calcitonin-containing cells was within normal limits. These observations support the interpretation that the bronchopulmonary calcitonin-containing cells develop independently of derivatives of branchial pouches III and IV-V.

ANATOMY

The normal adult thyroid gland is a bilobate structure located in the midportion of the neck, immediately in front of the larynx and trachea. It wraps itself around these two structures and firmly adheres to them. The two lobes extend along either side of the larynx to the midportion of the thyroid cartilage. Their upper and lower extremities are referred to as the upper and lower poles of the gland, respectively. The two lobes are joined by the isthmus, which lies across the trachea anteriorly, below the level of the cricoid cartilage. Sometimes one lobe (particularly the right) is larger than the other. In some individuals, the isthmus is unusually wide.

A pyramidal lobe is a vestige of the thyroglossal duct and is found in about 40 percent of normal individuals. It is a narrow projection of thyroid tissue extending upward from the isthmus and lying on the surface of the thyroid cartilage. Any diffuse pathologic process (such as diffuse hyperplasia or Hashimoto thyroiditis) can result in gross enlargement of the pyramidal lobe.

The normal weight of the thyroid gland in a middle-aged adult is 15 to 25 g in areas without endemic goiter. As an average, each lobe measures 4.0 x 1.5–2.0 x 2.0–4.0 cm, and the isthmus measures 2.0 x 2.0 x 0.2-0.6 cm. There are, however, marked variations related to functional activity, gender, hormonal status, size of the individual, and amount of iodine intake. The thyroid gland is larger and heavier in women than in men, and it becomes even larger during pregnancy.

The thyroid gland is completely enveloped by a continuous fibrous capsule, with septa that divide the gland incompletely into lobules. The parathyroid glands are usually located adjacent to the posterior surface of the thyroid lobes (see chapter 23). The recurrent laryngeal nerves run in the cleft between the trachea and esophagus, just medial to the thyroid lobes.

The thyroid blood supply derives from the right and left superior thyroid arteries (which arise from the external carotid artery) and the right and left inferior thyroid arteries (which arise from the thyrocervical trunk of the subclavian arteries). The thyroid veins drain into the internal jugular, the brachycephalic, and, occasionally, the anterior jugular veins.

The thyroid gland is endowed with a rich lymphatic network that encircles the follicles and connects both lobes through the isthmus. In neonates and children, some of these lymph vessels appear as empty, elongated, tortuous spaces that simulate a retraction artifact but which are lined by D2-40–positive lymphatic endothelial cells (16). This network coalesces in

Table 1-1

REGIONAL LYMPH NODES OF THE THYROID GLAND[a]

The *pericapsular* nodes: whole organ sections of the thyroid have shown that the intraglandular lymph vessels penetrate the capsule and merge with the pericapsular lymph nodes forming a plexus around the gland (17)

The *internal jugular chain* nodes (including the *subdigastric* nodes)

The *pretracheal*, *paratracheal*, and *prelaryngeal* nodes: the pretracheal node located near the thyroid isthmus is sometimes referred to as the *Delphian* node

The *recurrent laryngeal nerve chain* nodes

The *retropharyngeal* and *retroesophageal* nodes

[a]The *anterosuperior mediastinal* nodes are secondary to the recurrent laryngeal nerve chain and pretracheal groups; however, studies have shown that dye injected into the thyroid isthmus can also drain directly into them (18).

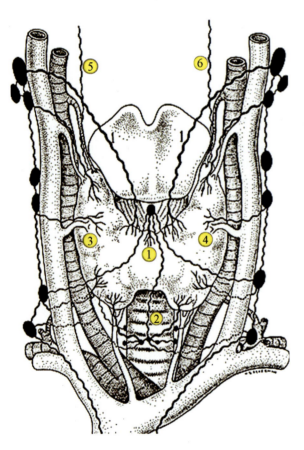

Figure 1-5

LYMPHATIC DRAINAGE OF THE THYROID GLAND

This figure illustrates the medial superior trunk (1), the median inferior trunk (2), the right and left lateral trunks (3,4), and the posterosuperior trunks (5,6). All of these drain to the regional lymph nodes listed in the Table 1-1. The pericapsular lymph nodes are not illustrated. (Figure 340 from Del Regato JA, Spjut HJ. Ackerman and Del Regato's Cancer. Diagnosis, treatment and prognosis; 5th ed. St. Louis: CV Mosby; 1977:411.)

the subcapsular region to give rise to the median superior, median inferior, right and left lateral, and posterosuperior trunks. These collecting trunks leave the organ in close proximity to the veins to empty into the regional lymph nodes, which are shown in Table 1-1 and figure 1-5.

Some correlation exists between the site of a thyroid carcinoma within the gland and the location of the initial lymph node metastasis. For instance, involvement of the subdigastric nodes of the internal jugular chain is common with upper pole lesions. However, the degree of anastomosis between these various nodal groups is such that any may be the site of disease regardless of the precise location of the primary tumor. Even the nodes of the posterior triangle group are affected with some frequency. Conversely, submandibular triangle involvement is rare and usually limited to cases with extensive metastases in other cervical nodal groups. Similarly, involvement of antero-superior mediastinal nodes is rarely seen in the absence of widespread cervical disease.

HISTOLOGY

The functional unit of the thyroid gland is the *follicle*, a closed sac lined by a single layer of epithelial glandular cells known as *follicular cells*. The average diameter of the follicle is 200 nm, but there is considerable variation in size, depending on the degree of activity of the gland. The shape of the normal follicle varies from round to oval. Markedly elongated tubular and branching follicles are regarded as abnormal and often indicative of a hyperplastic or neoplastic disorder. A characteristic structure, present in the normal gland but accentuated in hyperplastic

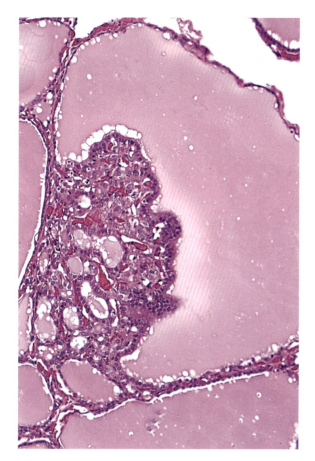

Figure 1-6

SO-CALLED SANDERSON POLSTER

A conglomerate of follicles protrudes into the lumen of a cystically dilated follicle.

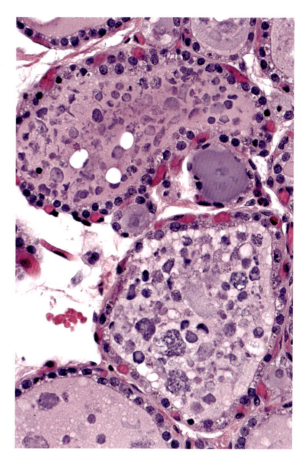

Figure 1-7

COLLOID ARTIFACT IN NORMAL FOLLICLES

The colloid in the lumens of these thyroid follicles is flocculent and strongly basophilic. This change is probably of an artifactual nature and of no pathologic significance.

conditions, is the *Sanderson polster* (cushion) (fig. 1-6). The term refers to an architectural arrangement in which a collection of small follicles bulges into the lumen of a large one. The lining epithelium of the follicle is columnar in the area of the bulge but flattened elsewhere.

The lumen of thyroid follicles contains a viscous material known as *colloid*, in which concentrated thyroglobulin is present. This material is strongly periodic acid–Schiff (PAS) positive, and sometimes focally mucicarminophilic. Its staining quality in hematoxylin-eosin (H&E) sections is somewhat dependent on the degree of activity of the follicles: weakly eosinophilic and flocculent in active follicles and strongly eosinophilic and homogeneous when stored in large inactive follicles (19). Often, darkly staining and elongated clumps appear within the colloid,

suggesting an artifactual coagulation-type phenomenon (fig. 1-7). Anisotropic (birefringent) crystals of calcium oxalate may be present in the follicular lumens, particularly in older or less active glands (fig. 1-8) (20). Their highest prevalence is in inactive follicles, as supported by the fact that there seems to be an inverse relationship between their presence and the degree of immunoreactivity for thyroglobulin. Katoh et al. (21) found them in 88 percent of nodular goiters, 60 percent of follicular adenomas, 33 percent of follicular carcinomas, and only 5 percent of papillary carcinomas. The overall prevalence was 69.4 percent in benign nodules and 7.6 percent in malignant nodules. A heavy deposit of these crystals was seen almost exclusively in benign conditions.

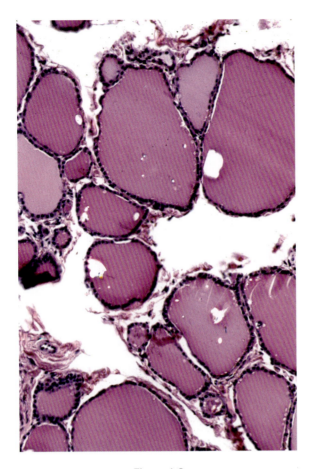

Figure 1-8

**CALCIUM OXALATE CRYSTALS
IN NORMAL THYROID FOLLICLES**

The calcium oxalate crystals in the lumens of normal thyroid follicles are associated with decreased function of the gland, such as that induced by exogenous suppression.

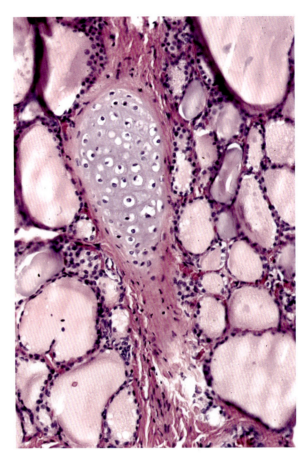

Figure 1-9

ECTOPIC CARTILAGE IN THYROID GLAND

This finding, which is of no clinical significance, probably represents a remnant of the branchial cleft pouch apparatus.

Each follicle is surrounded by a richly vascularized stroma. A group of 20 to 40 follicles compartmentalized by connective tissue and supplied by a single branch of one of the thyroid arteries constitutes a *thyroid lobule*, a structure that becomes more apparent in pathologic conditions such as hyperplasia or fibrosis. As already indicated, an intricate lymphatic network between the follicles empties into subcapsular channels, which in turn lead to numerous collecting trunks. Many cross communications exist between the lymph vessels within the thyroid gland, some of which cross the midline to connect one lobe to the other.

There are a number of variations in the microscopic appearance of the thyroid gland that have no pathologic significance but that are important to the pathologist because some of them may be confused with lesions of greater import. They include: 1) intrathyroidal islands of mature cartilage (fig. 1-9) (22); 2) intrathyroidal islands of ectopic thymus (fig. 1-10) (23); 3) intrathyroidal parathyroid gland (fig. 1-11); 4) solid cell nests; 5) intrathyroidal salivary gland tissue (24); 6) pancreatic tissue in perithyroidal cervical cyst (25); 7) diffuse or focal adipose metaplasia of the interfollicular stroma (fig. 1-12) (26); 8) intrathyroidal bundles of skeletal muscle (fig. 1-13); and 9) accumulation of melanin-like pigment in the cytoplasm of follicular cells in old age, a process that may become massive after the administration of some

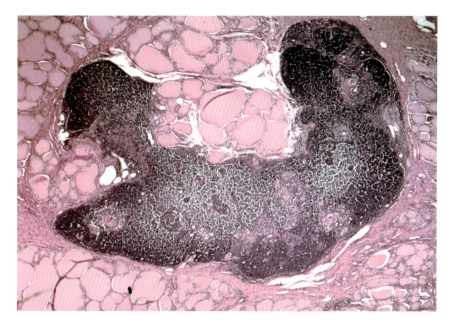

Figure 1-10

ECTOPIC THYMUS IN THYROID GLAND

A well-developed island of thymic tissue is entirely surrounded by thyroid follicles. Note the Hassall corpuscles.

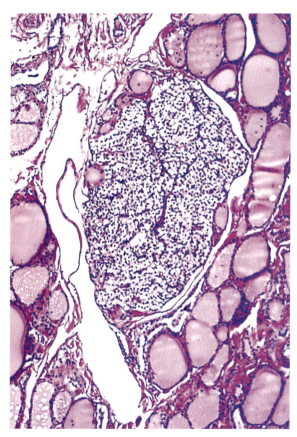

Figure 1-11

ECTOPIC PARATHYROID IN THYROID GLAND

A histologically normal parathyroid gland is seen entirely surrounded by thyroid parenchyma.

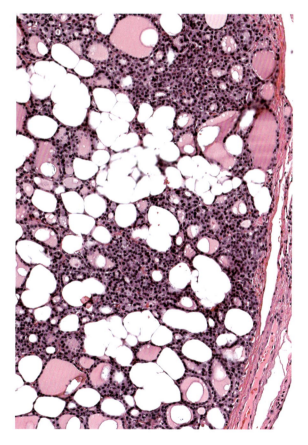

Figure 1-12

ADIPOSE METAPLASIA IN THYROID GLAND

Islands of mature fat are intermingled with normal thyroid follicles.

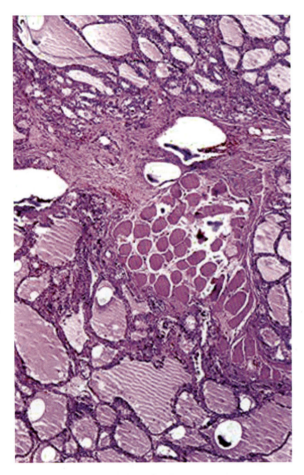

Figure 1-13

**NORMAL SKELETAL MUSCLE
WITHIN THYROID GLAND**

This should not be misinterpreted as invasion of skeletal muscle by a thyroid neoplasm.

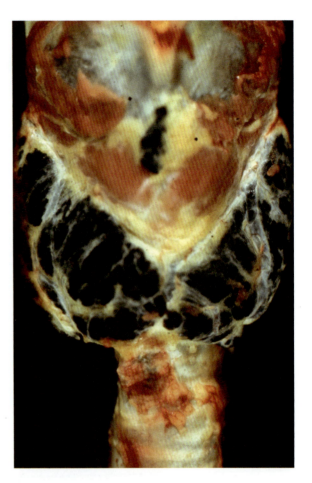

Figure 1-14

SO-CALLED BLACK THYROID

This impressive gross appearance of the thyroid gland can occur spontaneously, but is more commonly seen following minocycline therapy.

medications, such as minocycline (27). When intense, it is appreciable grossly and referred to as melanosis thyroidi, or black thyroid (fig. 1-14). At the ultrastructural level, the granules contain a mixture of lipofuscin and colloid, and therefore may belong to the category of ambilysosomes (28).

The first five of the variations described above are thought to be of branchial pouch or related derivation, and the sixth to represent a foregut remnant (see fig. 1-1). Also, microscopically normal thyroid tissue can be found outside the anatomic confines of the gland. In a study of 56 thyroid glands obtained at autopsy from normal individuals between 20 and 40 years old, Hanson et al. (29) found thyroid tissue

outside the recognizable capsule of the gland in 40 cases and in the skeletal muscles of the neck in 6 cases. This ectopic thyroid tissue can be involved by any of the diseases affecting the main organ, particularly hyperplasia and thyroiditis (see chapter 18).

THE FOLLICULAR CELL

The nucleus of the *follicular cell* is round to oval. Its chromatin may be finely granular or clumped, and there is usually a single nucleolus. In actively secreting cells, the nucleus enlarges and the chromatin undergoes dispersion; this is accompanied by cytoplasmic enlargement, predominantly in the apical half, so that the nucleus acquires a basal position. The cytoplasm

Functional Status	Very slow secretion	Slow secretion	Rapid secretion	Rapid excretion	End of excretion
Cell Shape	Endothelioid	Cuboidal	Cuboidal	Cylindrical	Cylindrical
Mitochondria	Lateral	Lateral, basal, and apical, without orientation	Long, predominantly subnuclear, absent in apical pole	Two groups, oriented along the longest side of cell	Two groups, less clearly oriented
Nucleus	Spindle	Spherical	Ovoid or spherical	Median	Ovoid or spherical
Other Features		Apical secretion vacuole		Apical cuticle (inconstant), fine lipid droplets and vacuoles, vacuole of Bensley	Large lipid droplets, no basal vacuoles
Schematic Drawing	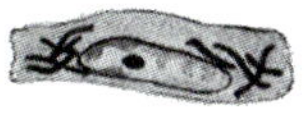	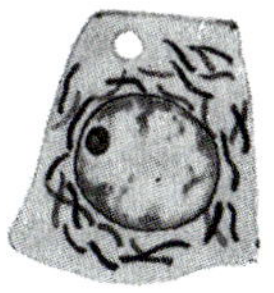	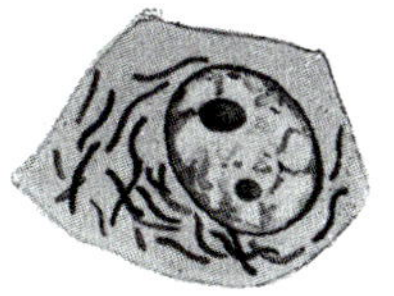	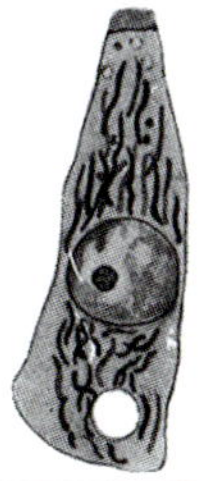	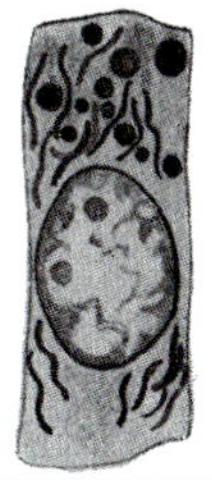

Figure 1-15

THYROID FOLLICULAR CELL

This schematic illustrates the morphology of the thyroid follicular cell depending on its functional status and is adapted from the classic study of Feyer and Varangot (30).

may appear pale eosinophilic or amphophilic in H&E-stained preparations. In contrast to parathyroid cells, the PAS stain shows little or no glycogen in the cytoplasm of normal follicular cells; however, this is not necessarily true in neoplastic conditions (see chapter 11).

The amount, shape, and appearance of the follicular cell cytoplasm vary depending on its functional status (fig. 1-15) (30). Three major cell types are described, with the understanding that they are part of a continuous morphologic spectrum: flattened (endothelioid), cuboidal, and columnar (cylindrical). The flattened cells are relatively inactive. The cuboidal cells secrete colloid into the follicular lumen and may contain apical secretory vacuoles. The columnar cells resorb the thyroglobulin-containing colloid, liberate the active hormones, and excrete them into blood vessels; they may feature an apical cuticle, apical lipid droplets, and one or more basilar vacuoles (vacuoles of Bensley).

Ultrastructurally, the thyroid follicular cell exhibits numerous microvilli on its luminal surface, particularly during active resorption (31). The cell membranes of adjacent cells interdigitate in a complex fashion and are joined by a junctional complex toward the apex. At the base, a continuous basal lamina separates the follicular cell from the stroma. The cytoplasm contains an abundant granular endoplasmic reticulum and a well-developed Golgi apparatus. The latter is located between the nucleus and the luminal surface, and becomes prominent in actively secreting cells. Mitochondria are well represented; their length and cytoplasmic location vary according to the functional status of the cell. When mitochondria are unduly numerous, the cell acquires oncocytic features at the light microscopic level, an abnormality described in chapter 10. Lysosomes are numerous in actively secreting cells; most are located toward the apical side (fig. 1-16).

Immunohistochemically, the most useful markers of follicular epithelium are thyroglobulin and thyroid transcription factor-1 (TTF-1) (fig. 1-17), the former having a degree of specificity rarely matched in the entire immunohistochemistry repertory. As a matter of fact, thyroglobulin may be the only marker that is absolutely specific for a cell type, i.e, the thyroid follicular cell and the tumors derived from it. Very different is the situation for a large number

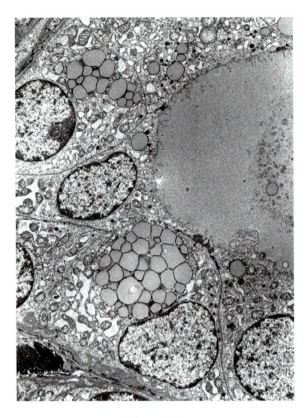

Figure 1-16

NORMAL THYROID FOLLICLE

The follicular cells in this electron micrograph exhibit microvilli on the luminal surface and are joined by junctional complexes toward the apex. The cytoplasm contains mitochondria, a moderate amount of dilated endoplasmic reticulum, and clusters of large lysosomes. The small darker granules are also probably of a lysosomal nature. (Courtesy of Dr. R. Erlandson, New York, NY.)

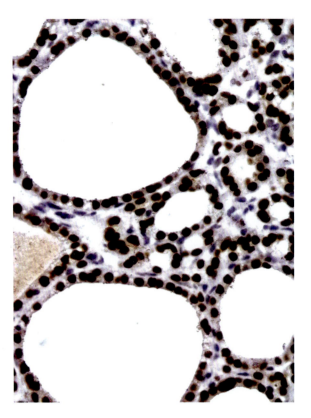

Figure 1-17

TTF-1 IMMUNOREACTIVITY IN NORMAL THYROID FOLLICLES

Almost all the nuclei of the follicular cells react to this marker.

of molecules that are expressed in the normal follicular cells, many of which play a role in thyroid metabolism. These molecules have been evaluated at the immunohistochemical level in a variety of hyperplastic and neoplastic conditions of the thyroid gland. A listing of those molecules is given in chapter 22, with a short description of their main features (32,33).

Thyroid Hormones

The functions of the thyroid follicular cell are expressed through the secretion of (iodinated) thyroid hormones. Biosynthesis of these hormones begins by absorption of ingested iodine into the bloodstream, its transport as iodide into the extracellular fluid compartment, and its energy-dependent concentration in the thyroid gland. This results in intracellular levels at least 30 times higher than in the peripheral blood. The intrathyroidal iodide is then oxidized to iodine by a peroxidase and bound organically to tyrosine radicals of thyroglobulin to form monoiodotyrosine and diiodotyrosine. Oxidative coupling of diiodotyrosine gives rise to *thyroxine (T4, tetraiodothyronine)*, whereas a similar coupling of monoiodotyrosine and diiodotyrosine gives rise to *triiodothyronine (T3)* (fig. 1-18). All of these iodothyronines are then incorporated into *thyroglobulin*, which plays an essential role as a carrier protein of these hormones.

Thyroglobulin is a large glycoprotein with a 19S sedimentation coefficient and a molecular weight of 670,000. It is formed by two identical subunits with a 12S sedimentation coefficient to which many oligosaccharides are linked. Thyroglobulin is encoded by a gene spreading over more than 200 kilobases in the bovine genome

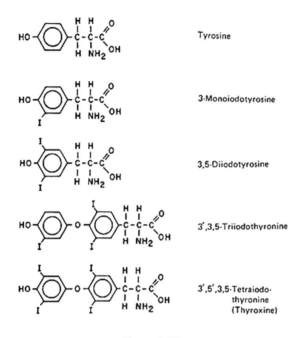

Figure 1-18

THYROID HORMONES

The molecular structure of major iodoamino acids found in thyroglobulin and their precursors.

(34). The molecular mechanisms involved in the tissue-specific and hormone-dependent expression of the thyroglobulin gene have been studied in follicular cells in primary cultures and cell lines (35,36).

The synthesis of thyroglobulin begins in the endoplasmic reticulum of the follicular cell and continues in the Golgi apparatus, where the end sugars of the carbohydrate site are incorporated. It is then packaged into small apical microvesicles, the contents of which are discharged into the follicular lumen after fusion of the vesicle membranes with the luminal side of the plasma membrane.

Resorption of thyroglobulin takes place through cytoplasmic streamers, which engulf minute portions of colloid that are then drawn into the cell in the form of membrane-bound colloid droplets. These subsequently fuse with lysosomes, and their content is digested by the lysosomal enzymes. The breakdown products, including thyroxine and triiodothyronine, diffuse through the cell membrane and the basement membrane into the adjacent capillar-

ies, and most of the molecules become bound to a specific carrier protein known as thyroxine-binding globulin (37–39).

Thyroid hormone acts by binding to specific thyroid hormone receptors present in nearly all tissues. It stimulates metabolism, increases oxygen consumption, and causes a rise in heat production, cardiac output, and heart rate. It is essential for normal development, growth, and maturation. The acceleration of growth may result from a direct action on the cells to increase their rate of division, by acting permissively for other hormones, or by inducing the synthesis of a variety of growth-promoting hormones (38,40–46).

Thyroid secretory activity is controlled by the level of *thyrotropin (thyroid-stimulating hormone)* in the blood. This hormone operates through thyrotropin receptors located on the basolateral surface of the follicular cell membrane and the adenylate cyclase system (47,48). Stimulation of the thyroid gland by thyrotropin increases its secretory activity and vascularity, and results in both hypertrophy and hyperplasia of follicular cells, accompanied by reduction of colloid storage. At the functional level, this is reflected by an increase in iodide concentration and organic binding, hormone synthesis, and hormone secretion (39,49,50). In turn, the release of thyrotropin by the pituitary gland is regulated by *thyrotropin-releasing hormone*, which is produced by the neurons of the medial-basal hypothalamus and carried into the pituitary gland via the hypophyseal-portal vessels.

THE C-CELL

The *C-cell* is difficult to identify in routinely stained formalin-fixed, paraffin-embedded sections (51,52). The nuclei are somewhat larger and paler than those of the follicular cells while the cytoplasm often appears clear. Prior to the advent of immunohistochemistry, a number of histochemical stains, including argyrophil staining sequences (53), lead hematoxylin (54), toluidine blue or coriophosphine O for masked metachromasia (54), and Ulex europaeus agglutinin I (55) were used for the demonstration of C-cells. These methods are now primarily of historical interest.

At present, immunostains for calcitonin are the most accurate and reproducible methods for the demonstration of C-cells (fig. 1-19) (53,

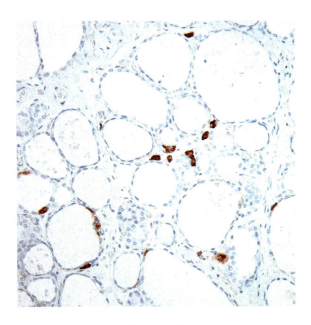

Figure 1-19

NORMAL C-CELL DISTRIBUTION

C-cells are present in small groups around the follicles (immunoperoxidase stain for calcitonin).

56,57). C-cells predominate at the junctions of the upper and middle thirds of the lateral lobes along a hypothetical central axis (58,59). They tend to be most prominent in the vicinity of solid cell nests, as discussed below. The extreme upper and lower poles as well as the isthmus are generally devoid of C-cells. C-cells occur singly or in clusters of up to four cells. They are present at the bases of the follicular cells, and are separated from the interstitium by the follicular basement membrane. Individual C-cells are round, ovoid, or spindle shaped, and some have processes that extend beneath the adjacent follicular cells.

Early studies of the distribution of C-cells in adult thyroid glands revealed fewer than 10 C-cells per single low-power microscopic field (100X) (59). Subsequent studies, however, revealed that 50 or more C-cells per low-power field are present in some normal adult glands (60,61). Rather than being present as single cells or small cell clusters, in some instances C-cells completely encircle a single thyroid follicle. Gibson et al. (60) demonstrated that occasional normal adult thyroid glands contain large C-cell nodules, particularly in patients over 50 years, either as evidence of age-related hyperplasia or

as a normal variation in C-cell ontogeny. An alternative explanation is that some of the nodules could represent microscopic foci of medullary thyroid carcinoma. O'Toole et al. (61) studied the influence of age on C-cell distribution and noted fairly constant numbers of C-cells up to the age of 59 years. After that, the numbers of C-cells were extremely variable, with a suggestion of an age-related increase, which did not differ significantly from the number observed in younger individuals.

In a computer quantitative image analysis study of adult thyroid glands, Guyetant et al. (62) reported that the maximum C-cell surface area ranged from 28×10^3 to 470×10^3 μm^2 (mean, 167×10^3 μm^2). Interestingly, the maximum C-cell surface area was twice as high in men (201×10^3 μm^2) as in women (91×10^3 μm^2). This study demonstrated that 15 percent of women and 41 percent of men had evidence of C-cell hyperplasia, as defined by having three microscopic fields (100x) with more than 50 C-cells. These findings suggest that either a substantial portion of the population has C-cell hyperplasia or that the criteria for the definition of this entity are inaccurate (fig. 1-20). Abnormal pentagastrin stimulation tests, however, are found in only 5 percent of the normal population as compared to the 30 percent frequency of C-cell hyperplasia, as defined histologically. These observations suggest that there may be considerable variation in normal C-cell distribution and that these variations may not be accompanied by hypercalcitoninemia. Although only a small number of infant thyroid glands were examined in this study, the maximum C-cell surface area was considerably lower than in adults, in contrast to the higher density of C-cells reported in earlier studies.

Normal C-cells are positive for low molecular weight cytokeratins and are variably positive for vimentin (56,63,64). Neurofilaments are generally absent from normal C-cells although medullary thyroid carcinomas are frequently positive for these proteins. C-cells are also positive for generic neuroendocrine markers, including chromogranin A, synaptophysin, synaptic vesicle protein 2 (SV2), the synaptosomal protein of 25 kDa (SNAP-25), and the prohormone convertases, peptidylglycine alpha-amidating monooxygenase and peptidylamidoglycolate lyase (56,63,64). In clinical practice, the most

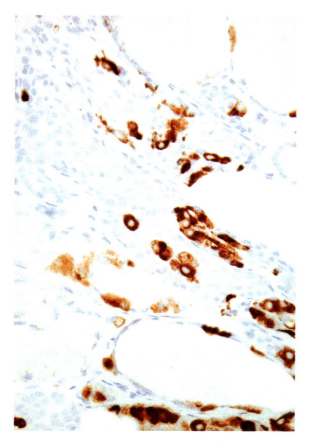

Figure 1-20

VARIATIONS IN NORMAL C-CELL DISTRIBUTION

In some normal individuals, C-cells may be present in increased numbers, particularly in areas adjacent to solid cell nests (immunoperoxidase stain for calcitonin.)

useful generic neuroendocrine markers are chromogranin A and synaptophysin.

In addition to calcitonin, C-cells contain katacalcin and the calcitonin gene-related peptide (CGRP) (65). Messenger RNAs encoding both calcitonin and CGRP have been demonstrated in normal C-cells with in situ hybridization techniques (66). Somatostatin is present in the C-cells of most species, but in humans only a few calcitonin-positive cells contain somatostatin (53,67). Gastrin-releasing peptide (GRP) and its corresponding mRNA have been identified in most C-cells in the human fetus and neonate, whereas studies of adult thyroid glands show GRP in less than 20 percent of the C-cells (68). Pancreatic polypeptide is another peptide that is present in normal C-cells (69). Although

pro-opiomelanocortin-derived peptides have been found in medullary thyroid carcinomas, their occurrence in normal C-cells is a matter of debate. Similarly, a variety of other peptides, including substance P, vasoactive intestinal peptide, gastrin/cholecystokinin, neurotensin, and ghrelin (70), which are present in some cases of medullary thyroid carcinoma, have not been demonstrated in normal C-cells. Some of these peptides may be present within intrathyroidal nerves, however (71). Helodermin, a peptide that shows considerable homology with vasoactive intestinal peptide, has been demonstrated in normal C-cells, where it is co-localized with calcitonin. In addition to regulatory peptide products, C-cells also contain a variety of biologically active amines, including serotonin (72).

Thyrotropin-releasing hormone is present in the C-cells of some species (73) while thyrotropin receptor protein is expressed heterogeneously in normal, hyperplastic, and neoplastic C-cells (74). Somatostatin receptors are commonly expressed in medullary thyroid carcinomas (75). Estrogen receptor-beta is commonly expressed in hyperplastic and neoplastic C-cells while estrogen receptor-alpha is negative (76). Androgen receptor protein is present in approximately 50 percent of cases of C-cell hyperplasia but less than 10 percent of medullary carcinomas (76).

Normal, hyperplastic, and neoplastic C-cells are variably positive for TTF-1 (77,78) in contrast to follicular cells, which are more uniformly positive. Carcinoembryonic antigen is expressed in normal C-cells and in all phases of C-cell proliferation (79,80). Polysialic acid of NCAM, on the other hand, is absent from normal C-cells and cases of secondary C-cell hyperplasia, while it is expressed in medullary thyroid carcinoma and cases of C-cell hyperplasia associated with medullary thyroid carcinoma (81). Tenascin C, a matrix glycoprotein, is expressed in the stroma of medullary microcarcinomas and in the stroma next to foci of C-cell hyperplasia (82). This marker is expressed more commonly in cases of C-cell hyperplasia with concomitant medullary thyroid carcinoma than in isolated C-cell hyperplasia of both hereditary and nonhereditary types. Galectin-3 is present in medullary thyroid carcinomas but is reportedly absent from cases of C-cell hyperplasia (83). Hector Battifora Mesothelial Epitope-1 (HBME-1) antibody (84),

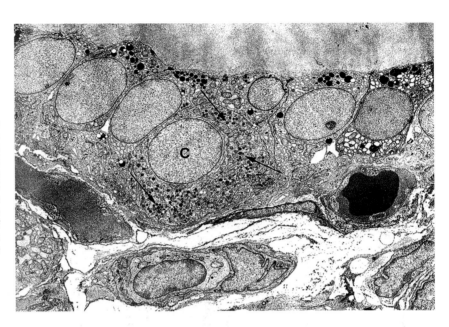

Figure 1-21

**ELECTRON MICROGRAPH
OF A C-CELL**

This photograph was taken from a patient with mild C-cell hyperplasia. This C-cell is identical to a normal adult C-cell with respect to its intrafollicular location and its content of secretory granules (arrows). The C-cell is separated from the colloid by the cytoplasm of adjacent follicular cells and from the interstitium by the follicular basal lamina.

cyclooxygenase-2, and matrix metalloproteinases (85) are variably expressed in medullary thyroid carcinomas, but there are no detailed studies of these markers in normal or hyperplastic C-cells. BCL-2 is variably expressed in advanced medullary thyroid carcinoma while multiple endocrine neoplasia (MEN) 2-associated C-cell hyperplasia and small medullary thyroid carcinoma are strongly positive (86). There is some suggestion that downregulation of BCL-2 may identify a subset of tumors with a more aggressive clinical course (87).

Ultrastructurally, C-cells contain variable numbers of secretory granules that range from 60 to 550 nm in diameter (fig. 1-21) (53). Type I granules have an average diameter of 280 nm, with moderately electron-dense, finely granular contents that are closely applied to the limiting membranes. Type II granules have an average diameter of 130 nm, with more electron-dense contents that are separated from their limiting membranes by a small but distinct electron-lucent space. In general, normal C-cells are filled with type I granules. Ultrastructural immunocytochemical studies have demonstrated that both granule types contain calcitonin (88).

Calcitonin and Calcitonin Gene-Related Peptide

Calcitonin is a 32-amino acid peptide that is secreted by the thyroid C-cells when plasma calcium levels are increased. The calcium sensing receptor cloned from parathyroid cells is also

expressed in C-cells and contributes to the regulation of calcitonin secretion (89). Calcitonin administration to experimental animals with high bone turnover or to patients with Paget disease results in a fall of plasma calcium levels. This effect is mediated by inhibition of osteoclastic activity (90). When calcitonin is administered chronically, as in patients with Paget disease, the number of osteoclasts diminishes progressively.

Calcitonin also acts on the kidney to enhance the production of vitamin D. The major physiologic role of calcitonin most likely relates to the protection of the skeleton during periods of calcium stress (e.g., growth, pregnancy, lactation). An absence of calcitonin is not associated with hypercalcemia, and a marked excess of this hormone, such as is found in patients with medullary thyroid carcinoma, is not associated with hypocalcemia. Gastrin and cholecystokinin also induce the secretion of calcitonin, as does the chronic administration of estrogenic hormones (90). The secretion of calcitonin is inhibited by somatostatin, which is synthesized by a subset of C-cells. In addition to the thyroid gland, calcitonin is present in many other tissues including lung, adrenal medulla, hypothalamus, pituitary gland, and parathyroid gland (91). Non-neuroendocrine cells may also produce low levels of the hormone (92).

Calcitonin is synthesized as a 141-amino acid precursor (preprocalcitonin) within the C-cells (90,93). Preprocalcitonin first undergoes cleavage of a signal peptide to form procalcitonin, which consists of 116 amino acids. There is a 57-amino acid peptide at the amino terminus and a 21-amino acid peptide at the carboxy terminus (katacalcin). The immature calcitonin peptide consists of 33 amino acids and is converted to mature calcitonin by the enzyme peptidylglycine-amidating monooxidase.

The calcitonin-related alpha gene (*CALCA*), previously known as *CALC1*, is present on chromosome 11p15.2. It consists of 6 exons that are alternatively spliced in a tissue-specific manner to yield the mRNAs encoding calcitonin and the calcitonin gene-related peptide (CGRP) (90,93). The mRNA encoding calcitonin results from splicing of the first 4 exons and represents more than 95 percent of the mature transcripts in the thyroid gland. Splicing of the first 3 exons to exons 5 and 6 results in a mRNA that encodes alpha-CGRP. Alpha-CGRP is expressed in many tissues and is the only mature transcript of the calcitonin gene detected in neural tissues. A second CGRP gene encodes the closely related beta-CGRP. The tissue distribution of beta-CGRP is similar to that of alpha-CGRP.

The levels of serum calcitonin vary widely since different assays use antibodies that recognize different epitopes of the hormone (94, 95). Generally, two-site immunometric assays provide the most accurate and reproducible results. The reference range for calcitonin with these assays is less than 10 ng/L (10 pg/mL) and are somewhat higher in healthy adult males than in females. Calcitonin levels are high during the first 6 months of life but gradually decline to adult levels by the third year of life. Patients with early C-cell disease (C-cell hyperplasia and microscopic foci of medullary thyroid carcinoma) generally have increased levels of the hormone, which increase further with the course of the disease.

Increased levels of calcitonin have also been identified in patients with chronic renal failure, sepsis, neuroendocrine tumors of the lung and other sites, hypergastrinemia, mastocytosis, autoimmune thyroid disease, and type 1A pseudohyperparathyroidism (95). False positive increases occur in association with the presence of heterophil antibodies.

Occasional patients with early C-cell disease may have normal calcitonin levels; measurements of serum calcitonin following the administration of secretagogues (pentagastrin, calcium) can be used to detect such cases (95). Peak-stimulated levels of less than 30 ng/L are present in 95 percent of normal individuals; stimulated levels of greater than 100 ng/L are suggestive of C-cell disease; and moderate elevations (less than 100 ng/L) may occur in adults with other thyroid diseases.

SOLID CELL NESTS

Solid cell nests (SCNs) were first recognized as remnants of the ultimobranchial bodies more than a century ago (96,97). They are found most commonly along the central axis of the middle and upper thirds of the lateral lobes. Most SCNs measure 0.1 mm in diameter, but occasional nests measure 2 mm or more (98). They are present in 3 percent of routinely examined thyroid glands and in more than 60 percent of glands that are blocked serially at 2-3 mm intervals. On occasion, SCNs are found in association with cartilage, salivary gland tissue, or fat (99).

SCNs appear as cellular clusters with a lobulated configuration within the interstitium of the thyroid gland and are composed of two cell types (figs. 1-22–1-24). The main cells are polygonal to ovoid, with round to ovoid nuclei containing finely granular chromatin and frequent grooves. Occasional main cells exhibit squamous metaplasia. Ultrastructurally, these cells have tonofilaments, desmosomes, and intraluminal cytoplasmic projections. Microfollicular structures lined by ciliated cells are also seen (100). The second component of the SCN is the calcitonin-containing clear cell (figs. 1-25, 1-26) (101). Typically, SCNs are present in areas of the thyroid gland that contain the highest concentration of C-cells, as is expected based on their common origins from the ultimobranchial bodies. Occasional SCNs are connected to thyroid follicular cells to form mixed follicles.

The SCNs may contain small cysts with intraluminal accumulations of acidic mucins demonstrable with the Alcian blue stain. Cystic ultimobranchial remnants are present in 55 percent of neonatal thyroid glands, and occasional cysts contain papillary structures (102). Approximately 20 percent of the cysts are lined by ciliated columnar cells. Cysts of similar morphology may also be present in the soft tissues of the neck.

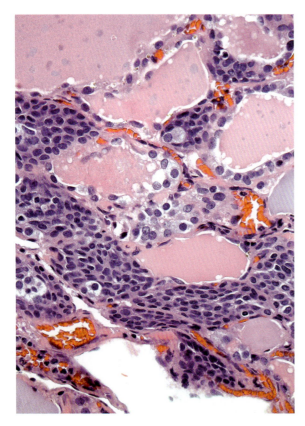

Figure 1-22

SOLID CELL NEST

C-cells have clear to amphophilic cytoplasm and are present within the solid cell nest and the adjacent follicles.

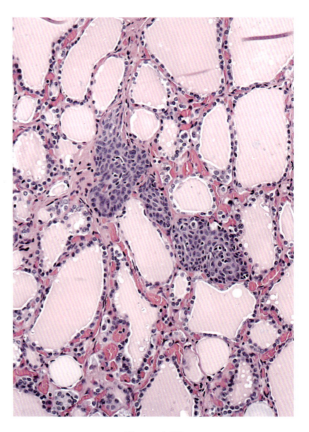

Figure 1-23

SOLID CELL NEST

At low power, this insignificant vestigial structure can be misinterpreted as a papillary microcarcinoma.

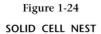

Figure 1-24

SOLID CELL NEST

Lobular configuration of a solid cell nest composed of predominantly solid areas and small cystic foci.

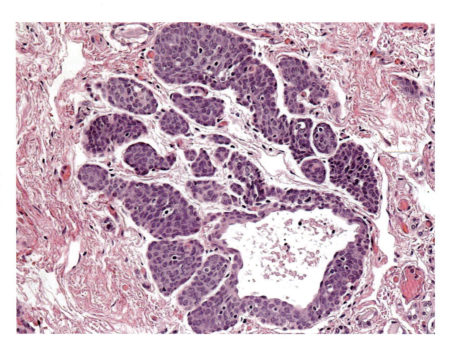

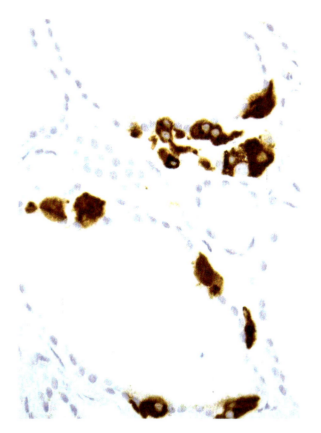

Figure 1-25

C-CELLS IN REGION OF SOLID CELL NEST

C-cells have a polyhedral shape, with occasional cell processes (immunoperoxidase stain for calcitonin).

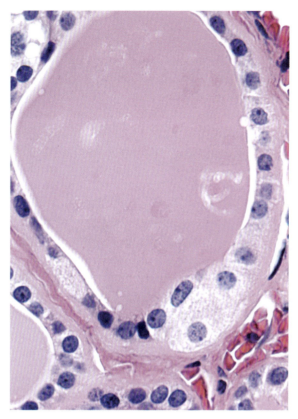

Figure 1-26

C-CELLS IN REGION OF SOLID CELL NEST

The C-cells have an intrafollicular distribution and are characterized by the presence of slightly enlarged nuclei and abundant granular cytoplasm.

The main cells of the SCNs are positive for high and low molecular weight keratins and carcinoembryonic antigen but are negative for thyroglobulin (99). Most main cells are negative for TTF-1, although some degree of positivity has been observed in a few cells forming mixed follicles (103). Positivity for p63, telomerase, and BCL-2 has suggested the possibility of a thyroid stem cell role for SCNs (fig. 1-27) (104,105). Both galectin-3 and cytokeratin 19 are present in the main cells of SCNs; this pattern of staining should not be interpreted as indicating the presence of a papillary thyroid carcinoma (103).

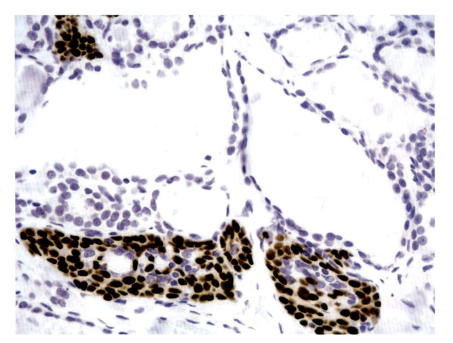

Figure 1-27

**p63 POSITIVITY
IN SOLID CELL NEST**

The nuclei of the cells of a solid cell nest are strongly immunoreactive for p63.

REFERENCES

1. Hoyes AD, Kershaw DR. Anatomy and development of the thyroid gland. Ear Nose Throat J 1985;64:318-33.
2. Norris EH. The early morphogenesis of the human thyroid gland. Am J Anat 1918;24:443-65.
3. Sugiyama S. The embryology of the human thyroid gland including ultimobranchial body and others related. Ergeb Anat Entwicklungsgesch 1971;44:3-111.
4. Gitlin D, Biasucci A. Ontogenesis of immunoreactive thyroglobulin in the human conceptus. J Clin Endocrinol Metab 1969;29:849-53.
5. Shepard TH. Onset of function in the human fetal thyroid: biochemical and radioautographic studies from organ culture. J Clin Endocrinol Metab 1967;27:945-58.
6. De Felice M, Di Lauro R. Thyroid development and its disorders: genetics and molecular mechanisms. Endocr Rev 2004;25:722-46.
7. Fagman H, Nilsson M. Morphogenesis of the thyroid gland. Mol Cell Endocrinol 2010;8:35-54.
8. Ito M, Kameda Y, Tagawa T. An ultrastructural study of the cysts in chicken ultimobranchial glands, with special reference to C-cells. Cell Tissue Res 1986;246:39-44.
9. Le Douarin N, Fontain J, LeLievre C. New studies on the neural crest origin of the avian ultimobranchial glandular cells—interspecific combinations and cytochemical characterization of C cells based on the uptake of biogenic amine precursors. Histochemistry 1974;38:297-305.
10. Le Douarin NM, Teillet MA. The migration of neural crest cells to the wall of the digestive tract in avian embryo. J Embryol Exp Morphol 1973;30:31-48.
11. Nadig J, Weber E, Hedinger CH. C-cell in vestiges of the ultimobranchial body in human thyroid glands. Virchows Arch B Cell Pathol 1978;27:189-91.
12. Pearse AG, Polak JM. Cytochemical evidence for the neural crest origin of mammalian ultimobranchial C cells. Histochemie 1971;27:96-102.
13. Williams ED, Toyn CE, Harach HR. The ultimobranchial gland and congenital thyroid abnormalities in man. J Pathol 1989;159:135-41.
14. Burke BA, Johnson D, Gilbert EF, Drut RM, Ludwig J, Wick MR. Thyrocalcitonin-containing cells in the DiGeorge anomaly. Hum Pathol 1987;18:355-60.
15. Conley ME, Beckwith JB, Mancer JF, Tenckhoff L. The spectrum of the DiGeorge syndrome. J Pediatr 1979;94:883-90.
16. Drut R, Altamirano E, Ollano AM. Lymphatic vessels in the thyroid gland of children. Rev Esp Patol 2009;42,159-60.

17. Russell WO, Ibanez ML, Clark RL, White EC. Thyroid carcinoma. Classification, intraglandular dissemination, and clinicopathological study based upon whole organ sections of 80 glands. Cancer 1963;16:1425-60.
18. Crile G Jr. The fallacy of the conventional radical neck dissection for papillary carcinoma of the thyroid. Ann Surg 1957;145:317-20.
19. Rigaud C, Bogomoletz WV. "Mucin secreting" and "mucinous" primary thyroid carcinomas: pitfalls in mucin histochemistry applied to thyroid tumors. Am J Clin Pathol 1987;40:890-5.
20. Reid JD, Choi CH, Oldroyd NO. Calcium oxalate crystals in the thyroid. Their identification, prevalence, origin, and possible significance. Am J Clin Pathol 1987;87:443-54.
21. Katoh R, Kawaoi A, Murtamatsu A, Hemmi A, Suzuki K. Birefringent (calcium oxalate) crystals in thyroid diseases. A clinicopathologic study with possible implications for differential diagnosis. Am J Surg Pathol 1993;17:698-705.
22. Finkle HI, Goldman RL. Heterotopic cartilage in the thyroid. Arch Pathol 1973;95:48-9.
23. Scopa CD, Petrohilos J, Spiliotis J, Melachrinou M. Autopsy findings in clinically normal thyroids. Int J Surg Pathol 1993;1:25-32.
24. Cameselle-Teijeiro J, Varela-Durán J. Intrathyroid salivary gland-type tissue in multinodular goiter. Virchows Arch 1994;425:331-4.
25. Langlois NE, Krukowski ZH, Miller ID. Pancreatic tissue in a lateral cervical cyst attached to the thyroid gland—a presumed foregut remnant. Histopathology 1997;31:378-80.
26. Morizumi H, Sano T, Tsuyuguchi M, Yoshinari T, Morimoto S. Localized adiposity of the thyroid, clinically mimicking an adenoma. Endocr Pathol 1991;2:226-9.
27. Bell CD, Kovacs K, Horvath E, Rotondo F. Histologic, immunohistochemical, and ultrastructural findings in a case of minocycline-associated "black thyroid." Endocr Pathol 2001;12:443-51.
28. Veinot JP, Ghadially FN. Melanosis thyroidi. Ultrastruct Pathol 1998;22:401-6.
29. Hanson GA, Komorowski RA, Cerletty JM, Wilson SD. Thyroid gland morphology in young adults: normal subjects versus those with prior low-dose neck irradiation in childhood. Surgery 1983;94:984-8.
30. Feyel P, Varangot J. Recherches cytologiques sur la glande thyroide normale et pathologique (Maladie de Basedow). Ann d'Anat Path 1938;15:135.
31. Klinck GH, Oertel JE, Winship T. Ultrastructure of normal human thyroid. Lab Invest 1970;22:2-22.
32. Raphael SJ. The meanings of markers: ancillary techniques in diagnosis of thyroid neoplasia. Endocr Pathol 2002;13:301-11.
33. Fischer S, Asa SL. Application of immunohistochemistry to thyroid neoplasms. Arch Pathol Lab Med 2008;132:359-72.
34. De Martynoff G, Pohl V, Mercken L, Van Ommen GJ, Vassart G. Structural organization of the bovine thyroglobulin gene and of its 5'-flaking region. Eur J Biochem 1987;164:591-9.
35. Christophe D, Gerard C, Juvenal G, et al. Identification of a cAMP-responsive region in thyroglobulin gene promoter. Mol Cell Endocrinol 1989;64:5-18.
36. Lee NT, Nayfeh SN, Chae CB. Induction of nuclear protein factors specific for hormone-responsive region during activation of thyroglobulin gene by thyrotropin in rat thyroid FRTL-5 cells. J Biol Chem 1989;264:7523-30.
37. Deiss WP, Peake RL. The mechanism of thyroid hormone secretion. Ann Intern Med 1968;69:881-90.
38. Green WL. The physiology of the thyroid gland and its hormones. In: Green WL, ed. The thyroid. New York:Elsevier,1987:1-46.
39. Liddle GW, Liddle RA,. Endocrinology. In: Smith LH, Their SO, eds. Pathophysiology. Philadelphia: WB Saunders, 1981:653-754.
40. Bernal J, Liewendhal K, Lamberg BA. Thyroid hormone receptors in fetal and hormone resistant tissues. Scand J Clin Lab Invest 1985;45:577-83.
41. Muller MJ, Seitz HJ. Thyroid hormone action on intermediary metabolism. I. Respiration, thermogenesis and carbohydrate metabolism. Klin Wochenschr 1984;62:11-8.
42. Muller MJ, Seitz HJ. Thyroid hormone action on intermediary metabolism. II. Lipid metabolism in hyper and hypothyroidism. Klin Wochenschr 1984;62:49-55.
43. Muller MJ, Seitz HJ. Thyroid hormone action on intermediary metabolism. III. Protein metabolism in hyper and hypothyroidism. Klin Wochenschr 1984;62:97-102.
44. Oppenheimer JH. Thyroid hormone action at the nuclear level. Ann Intern Med 1985;102:374-84.
45. Oppenheimer JH, Samuels HH, Apriletti JW. Molecular basis of thyroid hormone action. New York: Academic Press, 1983.
46. Sterling K. Thyroid hormone action at the cell level. N. Engl J Med 1979;300:117-23; 173-7.
47. Atassi MZ, Manshouri T, Sakata S. Localization and synthesis of the hormone-binding regions of the human thyrotropin receptor. Proc Natl Acad Sci USA 1991;88:3613-7.
48. Parmentier M, Libert F, Maenhaut C, et al. Molecular cloning of the thyrotropin receptor. Science 1989;246:1620-2.
49. Pittman JA Jr. Thyrotropin-releasing hormone. Adv Intern Med 1974;19:303-25

50. Wilber JF. Thyrotropin releasing hormone: secretion and actions. Annu Rev Med 1973;24:353-64.

51. Braunstein H, Stephens CL. Parafollicular cells of human thyroid. Arch Pathol 1968;86:659-66.

52. Teitelbaum SL, Moore KE, Shieber W. Parafollicular cells in the normal human thyroid. Nature 1971; 230:334-45.

53. DeLellis RA, Wolfe HJ. The pathobiology of the human calcitonin C-cell: a review. Pathol Annu 1981;16:25-52.

54. Pearse AG. Common cytochemical and ultrastructural characteristics of cells producing polypeptide hormones (the APUD series) and their relevance to thyroid and ultimobranchial C cells and calcitonin. Proc R Soc Lond B 1968;170:71-80.

55. González-Cámpora R, Sanchez Gallego F, Martín Lacave I, Mora Marín J, Montero Linares C, Galera-Davidson H. Lectin histochemistry of the thyroid gland. Cancer 1988;62:2354-62.

56. DeLellis RA. Endocrine tumors. In: Colvin RB, Bhan AK, McCluskey RT, eds. Diagnostic immunopathology, 2nd ed. New York, Raven Press, 1995.

57. McMillan PJ, Hooker WM, Deftos LJ. Distribution of calcitonin-containing cells in the human thyroid. Am J Anat 1974;140:73-80.

58. Wolfe HJ, DeLellis RA, Voelkel EF, Tashjian AH Jr. Distribution of calcitonin-containing cells in the normal neonatal human thyroid gland: a correlation of morphology with peptide content. J Clin Endocrinol Metab 1975;41:1076-81.

59. Wolfe HJ, Voelkel EF, Tashjian AH Jr. Distribution of calcitonin-containing cells in the normal adult human thyroid gland: a correlation of morphology with peptide content. J Clin Endocrinol Metab 1974;38:688-94.

60. Gibson WC, Peng TC, Croker BP. C-cell nodules in adult human thyroid. A common autopsy finding. Am J Clin Pathol 1981;75:347-50.

61. O'Toole K, Fenoglio-Preiser C, Pushparaj N. Endocrine changes associated with human aging process: III. Effect of age on the number of calcitonin immunoreactive cells in the thyroid gland. Hum Pathol 1985;16:991-1000.

62. Guyetant S, Rousselett MC, Durigon M, et al. Sex-related C-cell hyperplasia in the normal human thyroid: a quantitative autopsy study. J Clin Endocrinol Metab 1997;87:42-7.

63. Stanta G, Carcangiu ML, Rosai J. The biochemical and immunohistochemical profile of thyroid neoplasia. Pathol Annu 1988;23:129-57.

64. Shin SJ, Treaba D, DeLellis RA. Immunohistochemistry of endocrine tumors. In: Diagnostic immunohistochemistry. Theranostic and genomic applications, 4th ed. Philadelphia: Elsevier Saunders; 2014:322-62.

65. Ali-Rachedi A, Varndell IM, Facer P, et al. Immunocytochemical localisation of katacalcin, a calcium-lowering hormone cleaved from the human calcitonin precursor. J Clin Endocrinol Metab 1983;57:680-2.

66. Zajac JD, Penschow J, Mason T, Tregear G, Colghlan J, Martin TJ. Identification of calcitonin and calcitonin gene-related peptide messenger ribonucleic acid in medullary thyroid carcinoma by hybridization histochemistry. J Clin Endocrinol Metab 1986;62:1037-43.

67. Scopsi L, Ferrari C, Pilotti S, et al. Immunocytochemical localization and identification of prosomatostatin gene products in medullary carcinoma of human thyroid gland. Hum Pathol 1990;21:820-30.

68. Sunday ME, Wolfe HJ, Roos BA, Chin WW, Spindel ER. Gastrin-releasing peptide gene expression in developing, hyperplastic and neoplastic thyroid C-cells. Endocrinology 1988;122:1551-8.

69. Scopsi L, Pilotti S, Rilke F. Immunocytochemical localization in identification of members of the pancreatic polipeptide (PP)-fold family in human thyroid C-cells and medullary carcinomas. Regul Pept 1990;30:89-104.

70. Morpurgo PS, Cappiello V, Verga U, et al. Differential expression of galectin-3 in medullary thyroid carcinoma and C-cell hyperplasia. Clin Endocrinol 2002;57:813-9

71. Ahren B. Regulatory peptides in the thyroid gland —a review on their localization and function. Acta Endocrinol (Copenh) 1991;124:225-32.

72. Nunez EA, Gershon MD. Thyrotropin-induced thyroidal release of 5-hydroxytryptamine and accompanying ultrastructural changes in parafollicular cells. Endocrinology 1983;113:309-17.

73. Gkonos PJ, Tavianini MA, Liu CC, Roos BA. Thyrotropin-releasing hormone gene expression in normal thyroid parafollicular cells. Mol Endocrinol 1989;3:2101-9.

74. Morillo-Bernal J, Fernández-Santos JM, Utrilla JC, et al. Functional expression of the thyrotropin receptor in C-cells: new insights into their involvement in the hypothalamic-pituitary-thyroid axis. J Anat 2009;251:150-8.

75. Papotti M, Kumar U, Volante M, et al. Immunohistochemical detection of somatostatin receptor in types 1-5 in medullary carcinoma of the thyroid. Clin Endocrinol 2001;54:641-9.

76. Blechet C, Lecomte P, deCalan L, et al. Expression of sex steroid hormone receptors in C-cell hyperplasia and medullary thyroid carcinoma. Virchows Arch 2007;450:433-9.

77. Katoh R, Miyagi E, Nakamura N, et al. Expression of thyroid transcription factor-1 in human C-cells and medullary thyroid carcinoma. Hum Pathol 2000;31:386-93.

78. Bejarano PA, Nikiforov YE, Swenson ES, Biddinger PW. Thyroid transcription factor-1, thyroglobulin, cytokeratin 7 and cytokeratin 20 in thyroid neoplasm. Appl Immunohistochem Mol Morphol 2000;8:198-94.

79. DeLellis RA, Rule AH, Spiler I, et al. Calcitonin and carcinoembryonic antigen as tumor markers in medullary thyroid carcinoma. Am J Clin Pathol 1978;70:587-94.

80. Dasovic-Knezevic M, Bormer O, Holm R, et al. Carcinoembryonic antigen in medullary thyroid carcinoma: an immunohistochemical study employing six novel monoclonal antibodies. Mod Pathol 1989:2:610-7.

81. Kommonoth P, Roth J, Saremaslani P, et al. Polysialic acid of the neural cell adhesion molecule in the human thyroid: a marker for medullary thyroid carcinoma and primary C-cell hyperplasia. An immunohistochemical study on 79 thyroid lesions. Am J Surg Pathol 1994;18:399-411.

82. Koporek O, Prinz A, Scheuba C, et al. Tenascin C in medullary thyroid micro carcinoma and C-cell hyperplasia. Virchows Arch 2009;455:43-4.

83. Faggiano A, Talbot M, Lacroix L, et al. Differential expression of galectin-3 in medullary thyroid carcinoma and C-cell hyperplasia. Clin Endocrinol 2002;57:813-9.

84. Mase T, Funahashi H, Kashikawa T, et al. HBME-1 immunostaining in thyroid tumors especially in follicular neoplasm. Endocrinol J 2003;50:173-7.

85. Cavalheiro BG, Junqueira CR, Brandao LG. Expression of matrix metalloproteinase 2 (MMP2) and tissue inhibitor of metalloproteinase 2 (TIMP-2) in medullary thyroid carcinoma. Thyroid 2008;18:865-71.

86. Hinze R, Gimm O, Taubert H, et al. Regulation of proliferation and apoptosis in sporadic and hereditary medullary thyroid carcinoma and putative precursor lesions. Virchows Arch 2000; 437:256-63.

87. Viale G, Roncalli M, Grimelius L, et al. Prognostic value of bcl-2 immunoreactivity in medullary thyroid carcinoma. Hum Pathol 1995;26:945-50.

88. DeLellis RA, May L, Tashjian AH Jr, Wolfe HJ. C-cell granule heterogeneity in man. An ultrastructural immunocytochemical study. Lab Invest 1978;38:263-9.

89. Magno Al, Ward BK, Ratajczak T. The calcium sensing receptor: a molecular perspective. Endocr Rev 2011;32:3-30.

90. Martin TJ, Findlay DM, Sexton MB. Calcitonin. In: Jameson JL, DeGroot LJ, eds. Endocrinology: adult and pediatric, 6th ed. Philadelphia: Saunders/Elsevier; 2010.

91. Beckner KL, Snider RH, Moore CF, et al. Calcitonin in extrathyroidal tissues of man. Acta Endocrinol (Copenh) 1979;92:746-51.

92. Beckner KL, Snider RH, Nylen ES. Procalcitonin in sepsis and systemic inflammation. Br J Pharmacol 2012;159:253-64.

93. Amara SG, Jonas V, Rosenfeld MG, Ong SG, Evans RM. Alternative RNA processing in calcitonin gene expression generates mRNAs encoding different polypeptide products. Nature 1982;298:240-4.

94. Baloch Z, Carayon P, Conte-Devolx B, et al. Laboratory medicine practice guidelines. Laboratory support for the diagnosis and monitoring of thyroid disease. Thyroid 2003;13:3-126.

95. Costante G, Durante C, Francis Z, Schlumberger M, Filetti S. Determination of calcitonin levels in C-cell disease. Nat Clin Prac Endocrinol Metab 2009;5:35-42.

96. Harach HR. Solid cell nests in the thyroid. J Pathol 1988;155:191-200.

97. Williams ED, Toyn CE, Harach HR. The ultimobranchial gland and congenital thyroid abnormalities in man. J Pathol 1989;159:135-41.

98. Fellegara G, Dorji T, Bajimeta MR, Rosai J. "Giant" solid cell nest of the thyroid: a hyperplastic change? Int J Surg Pathol 2009;17:268-9.

99. Cameselle-Teijeiro J, Varela-Duran J, Sambade C, et al. Solid cell nests of the thyroid: the light microscopy and immunohistochemical profile. Hum Pathol 1994;25:684-93.

100. Martin V, Martin L, Viennet G, et al. Ultrastructural features of "solid cell nest" of the human thyroid gland: a study of 8 cases. Ultrastruct Pathol 2000;24:1-5.

101. Nadig J, Weber E, Hedinger C. C-cells in vestiges of the ultimobranchial body in human thyroid glands. Virchows Arch Cell Pathol 1978;27:189-91.

102. Beckner KL, Shultz JJ, Richardson T. Solid and cystic ultimobranchial remnants in the thyroid. Arch Pathol Lab Med 1990;114:1049-52.

103. Rios-Moreno MJ, Galera-Ruiz H, Demiguel M, et al. Immunohistochemical profile of solid cell nest of thyroid gland. Endocr Pathol 2011; 22:35-9.

104. Reis-Filho JS, Preto A, Soares P, et al. p63 expression in solid cell nests of the thyroid: further evidence of a stem cell origin. Mod Pathol 2003; 16:43-8.

105. Preto A, Cameselle-Teijero J, Moldes-Boulossa J, et al. Telomerase expression and proliferative activity suggest a stem cell role for solid cell nests. Mod Pathol 2004;17:819-26.

2 GENES INVOLVED IN THYROID TUMORIGENESIS

Our knowledge of the genetic pathology of thyroid tumors has greatly increased in the past several years. It is now apparent that there is a remarkable correlation between genotype and phenotype, i.e., genetic alterations and histologic appearance. This correlation is more robust than for epithelial tumors in many other organs, indicating that distinct molecular changes are associated with specific stages in a multistep tumorigenic process (fig. 2-1) (1–3).

Alterations of particular genes or gene pathways are linked to specific pathologic features, as in the case of activating mutations of the *TSHR* gene encoding the thyroid-stimulating hormone (TSH)-receptor (TSHR) that are associated with hyperfunctioning thyroid nodules, and mutations of the mitogen-activated protein kinase (MAPK) pathway (e.g., *BRAF*) associated with papillary carcinoma. Conventional karyotyping, DNA content (ploidy) analysis, comparative genomic hybridization, and loss of heterozygosity studies indicate that papillary carcinomas have a stable, normal or near normal complement of chromosomal DNA, while follicular carcinomas (and also follicular adenomas) are often aneuploid, with loss of heterozygosity at various chromosomal sites.

This genotype/phenotype correlation is supported by the now numerous studies on gene expression profiling that have identified molecular signatures for thyroid tumors with specific oncogenic events as well as supposed "markers of malignancy," including some that are used for diagnostic purposes such as galectin 3, CITED1, and keratin 19 (4–7). The analysis of mRNA expression signatures may represent a useful tool for the preoperative diagnosis of thyroid nodules (8). The transfer of knowledge from basic science to potential diagnostic application is also exemplified by recent studies on microRNAs (miRNAs). These are a class of small noncoding RNA molecules with critical functions for cell differentiation that negatively regulate gene expression, including that of

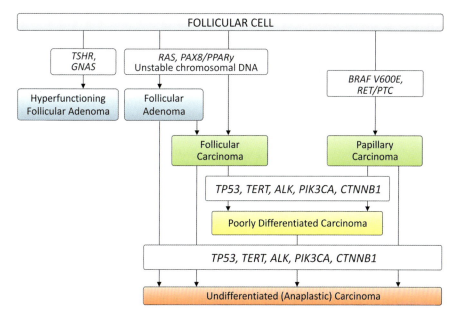

Figure 2-1

MULTISTEP THYROID TUMORIGENESIS

Flow chart showing the main gene mutations and rearrangements.

known oncogene and tumor suppressor proteins (9). Specific miRNA profiles are associated with different types of cancer, including thyroid tumors (10,11). Since miRNA can be analyzed on formalin-fixed routinely processed samples and in fine-needle aspiration biopsy (FNAB) specimens, their use as diagnostic (12–16) and prognostic (16–18) markers appears very promising. In fact, miRNA profiles have been correlated with specific molecular alterations, like *BRAF* and *RAS* mutations, and *RET/PTC* and *PAX8/PPARγ* rearrangements (13). Several studies show that among the targets of dysregulated miRNA are the cell cycle regulator p27 (19), the thyroid hormone receptor (20), and tyrosine kinases like KIT (11) and MET (18), all of which may play a role in the growth of thyroid tumors.

As with other tumor types, the molecular events that shape the biologic and clinical features of thyroid tumors are influenced by environmental factors and the genetics of the patient. The influence of both environment and genetic background explains the remarkable variability in the prevalence of different thyroid carcinoma types and even subtypes throughout the world (2,21).

Environmental factors include iodine availability in the diet and exposure to ionizing radiation, but there are many other factors that still remain to be defined (3,21–23). Iodine deficiency is believed to predispose to follicular and anaplastic carcinomas, while iodine excess has been linked to the *BRAF* V600E mutation in papillary carcinoma (24). Ionizing radiation causes chromosomal alterations and is associated with papillary carcinoma carrying specific gene rearrangements like *RET/PTC*, *ETV6/NTRK3* or *AKAP9/BRAF*, while chemical carcinogenesis probably acts by inducing point mutations in critical genes like *RAS* (3,25). Several studies (26–29) have shown that among radiation-associated tumors (from Hiroshima and Nagasaki survivors of atomic bomb radiation as well as from patients exposed to radiation after the Chernobyl nuclear accident) oncogenic rearrangements predominate over point mutations, and that tumors with rearrangements tend to occur in patients exposed to higher radiation doses, and to develop after a shorter latency period (26–29).

The patient's genetic background is also important: up to approximately one fourth of all medullary carcinomas are familial, either as part of the multiple endocrine neoplasia (MEN) syndromes or without associated extrathyroidal pathology (familial medullary thyroid carcinoma [FNMTC] syndrome). Thyroid tumors originating from follicular cells may also be inherited. They may develop as a component of cancer syndromes dominated by extrathyroidal disease, like familial adenomatous polyposis, where patients develop the cribriform morular variant of papillary carcinoma, or Cowden syndrome, where they develop adenomatous nodules, adenomas, and follicular carcinomas. Tumors also occur in a familial setting where thyroid pathology dominates the clinical picture. It is estimated that approximately 5 percent of all thyroid carcinomas that originate from follicular cells show familial aggregation. These familial carcinomas are almost always of papillary type, and first-degree relatives of patients with tumors have a 5- to 10-fold increased risk of developing papillary carcinoma when compared with the general population (30); relatives of patients with familial thyroid cancer have an increased incidence of multinodular goiter and follicular adenomas (30–32). Although it is not easy to distinguish the influence of the environment from that of the genetic background, many of these familial cases meet the criteria for an hereditary condition that is generically referred to as familial nonmedullary thyroid carcinoma (FNMTC) (31,32). The causative genes are still unknown, but specific susceptibility loci and tumor-associated single-nucleotide polymorphism (SNP) have been identified (33).

Thus, a series of molecular events, influenced by environmental and hereditary factors, underlies the development and the progression of thyroid tumors of follicular cells. While a limited number of early alterations is believed to initiate tumor growth, tumor progression depends on further changes that dysregulate growth factor signaling, adhesion molecules, the cell cycle, cell survival, and other vital cellular functions (2). Both stimulatory and inhibitory factors are likely to be involved in autocrine or paracrine signaling, which may have a critical role in influencing follicular cell proliferation and the rate of progression through a multistage process (34). As such alterations are unraveled, the clearer picture of thyroid tumorigenesis should improve the way thyroid cancer is diagnosed and treated. Preoperative diagnosis would be improved with the application of molecular diagnostics to FNAB specimens while the identification of markers of progression would define targets for therapy in patients with tumors unresponsive to radioactive iodine (2,3). Papillary carcinoma has been selected among the tumors included in the Cancer Genome Atlas (TCGA) (http://cancergenome.nih.gov/), a United States National Institutes of Health effort begun in 2006 to comprehensively evaluate the molecular alterations of human cancers using high throughput molecular analysis. The results of this thorough genomic investigation may contribute important insights and identify markers useful not only for the diagnosis, but also to define the prognosis and to potentially treat thyroid tumors with specific, molecularly targeted therapies.

What follows is an outline of the main genes and molecular pathways involved in thyroid tumorigenesis: the TSH receptor/cAMP pathway, the MAPK pathway that is aberrantly activated because of receptor tyrosine kinase (RET, NTRK1, and other kinases), RAS and BRAF molecular alterations, the PI3K/PTEN/AKT pathway, rearrangement of the *PAX8* and *PPARγ* genes (*PAX8/PPARγ*), the β-catenin/APC/Wnt pathway, *TERT*, and *TP53* (Table 2-1). For molecular genetic alterations that correlate with specific tumor types, the reader is referred to chapter 19, whereas the clinical applications of these tests are briefly discussed in chapter 21.

TSH RECEPTOR/cAMP PATHWAY

The cellular response induced by TSH is largely mediated by cyclic adenosine monophosphate (cAMP) (fig. 2-2). The TSH receptor (TSHR) is a member of the G protein-coupled receptor family and has a complex structure, with a serpentine transmembrane domain with seven loops (35). TSH binding results in conformational changes of the TSHR intracytoplasmic portion that allow the receptor to bind trimeric G proteins. This results in the dissociation of the Gsα subunit from the G protein complex, allowing Gsα to bind and activate membrane-bound adenylate cyclase to produce cAMP.

cAMP exerts its effects in the follicular cell mainly by activating cAMP-dependent protein kinase A, which catalyzes the transfer of phosphate groups from adenosine triphosphate (ATP) to specific serine or threonine residues of selected proteins. Protein kinase A substrates are tissue specific, explaining why the effects of cAMP vary depending on the target cell type (36). In addition, cAMP induces cellular responses independent of protein kinase A. Through EPAC proteins (exchange nucleotide protein directly activated by cAMP), which are cAMP-dependent guanine-nucleotide exchange factors, cAMP activates the small G protein RAP1 (RAS-associated protein 1, a member of the RAS family of small G proteins) which in turn interacts with a variety of downstream targets (37). In the thyroid gland, RAP1 activates BRAF and the MAPK pathway. Thus, in the normal thyroid follicular epithelium, TSH can stimulate all aspects of cell function (iodide uptake and metabolism, thyroid hormone synthesis and release) as well as cell proliferation (36,37).

Activation of the cAMP pathway independent of TSH stimulation occurs in follicular adenomas and hyperplastic thyroid nodules. It is caused by activating mutations in the genes encoding for the TSHR (*TSHR*) or its associated Gsα subunit protein (*GNAS*).

Mutations of *GNAS* (formerly referred to as the *gsp* oncogene), first described in 1990 (38), occur at "hot spots" in codons 201 and 227 (38,39), corresponding to the guanosine triphosphate (GTP) binding domain of the protein. The mutated protein has reduced GTPase activity and, similar to mutated *RAS*, is "locked" in a constitutively active GTP-bound form (36). Activating mutations of *GNAS* characterize growth hormone (GH)-secreting pituitary adenomas and the McCune-Albright syndrome. This syndrome, caused by postzygotic activating mutations of *GNAS*, is defined by the triad of café-au-lait skin pigmentation, polyostotic fibrous dysplasia, and hyperfunctioning endocrinopathies. Patients with the syndrome develop nodular and diffuse goiters (with and without hyperthyroidism), as well as benign thyroid nodules and sometimes even thyroid carcinomas (40). Transgenic mice expressing mutated *GNAS* targeted to the thyroid gland develop hyperthyroidism with foci of hyperplastic thyroid tissue, consistent with the role of *GNAS* mutations in the development of hyperfunctioning nodules in humans (41).

Table 2-1

GENES ALTERED IN THYROID TUMORS

Gene	Chromosomal Site	Protein	Expression	Genetic Alteration
AKT1	14q32.33	AKT1; AKT (a.k.a. Protein Kinase B, PKB) is a family of serine/threonine-specific protein kinases with 3 isoforms: AKT1, AKT2, and AKT3, of which AKT1 is the best studied in human tumors	Ubiquitous; in the thyroid AKT1 and AKT2 are the predominant isoforms	Activating mutations (somatic); oncogenic AKT signaling is the direct result of PTEN/AKT pathway disregulation due to activating *PIK3CA* mutations or *PTEN* inactivation; activating *AKT* mutations also occur in cancer but are less common
ALK	2p23	ALK (Anaplastic Lymphoma Kinase, CD246); belongs to the receptor tyrosine kinase superfamily; binds the growth factors pleiotrophin (PTN) and midkine (MK); a high specificity ligand has not been yet identified and ALK is considered an orphan receptor	ALK is expressed at high level in the developing nervous tissue (central and peripheral); it is expressed at low levels in several mature tissues including the central nervous system	Activating mutations (somatic and germline); rearrangement (somatic); gene amplification (somatic)
BRAF	7q34	Serine-threonine kinase in the MAPK pathway, together with ARAF and CRAF; following activation induced by RAS, RAF proteins phosphorylate and activate MEK, which in turn activates ERK	Ubiquitous; BRAF is the predominant isoform in thyroid follicular cells	Activating mutations (somatic and germline); "hot spot" mutations in exon 15 result in amino acid substitutions that simulate the physiologic activation of the molecule (phosphomimetic mutations); rearrangement (somatic)
CTNNB1	3p22.1	β-catenin, the protein encoded by *CTNNB1*, is both a cell adhesion molecule and a transcription factor for the Wnt signaling pathway	Ubiquitous; in mature cells β-catenin is normally localized to the cell membrane, its nuclear localization indicates activity as transcription factor, the result of Wnt signaling	Activating mutations (somatic); somatic cell *CTNNB1* mutations antagonize β-catenin degradation stabilizing the protein, and thus activate its function as transcription factor
GNAS (*GNAS1*)	20q13.3	GSα: alpha subunit of heterotrimeric G proteins (composed of α, β, and γ subunits, "large" G proteins) activated by G protein-coupled receptors such as TSHr; GSα activates the cAMP-dependent pathway by activating adenylate cyclase	Ubiquitous	Activating mutations (somatic and postzygotic); inactivating mutations (germline)
NTRK1	1q23.1	Neurotrophic tyrosine kinase receptor type 1 protein (TRKA) belongs to the receptor tyrosine kinase superfamily; closely related to TRKB and C; binds with high affinity the nerve growth factor (NGF)	Primarily expressed in the nervous system; normally not expressed in the thyroid; TRKA regulates neuronal differentiation and survival	Rearrangement (somatic); inactivating mutations (germline)
NTRK3	15q25.3	Neurotrophic tyrosine kinase receptor type 3 protein (TRKC) belongs to the receptor tyrosine kinase family; closely related to TRKA and B; binds with high affinity the neurotrophin-3 (NT3) growth factor	Primarily expressed in the nervous system; normally not expressed in the thyroid; TRKC regulates neuronal differentiation and survival	Rearrangement (somatic)
PAX8	2q13	A transcription factor essential for thyroid development and differentiation	Thyroid (follicular cells and to a lesser degree parafollicular C-cells), tubular cells of the kidney, epithelial cells of the fallopian tube; PAX8 is expressed in developing human tissues (thyroid gland, kidney, müllerian structures, nervous system)	Rearrangement (somatic); inactivating mutations (germline)

Table 2-1, continued

GENES ALTERED IN THYROID TUMORS

Gene	Thyroid Disease	Extrathyroid Disease
AKT1	Somatic activating mutations: advanced radio-active iodine refractory thyroid carcinomas	Somatic activating mutations: several human cancers including breast, colonic, and ovarian adenocarcinoma
ALK	Somatic activating mutations: undifferentiated carcinoma; rearrangement (*STRN/ALK, EML4/ALK*): papillary carcinoma, poorly differentiated and undifferentiated carcinomas	*ALK* is activated in several tumor types by rearrangements (anaplastic large cell lymphomas, nonsmall cell lung carcinomas, inflammatory myofibroblastic tumor), somatic activating mutations (neuroblastoma), and sometimes by gene amplification; germline activating mutations: hereditary neuroblastoma
BRAF	Somatic activating mutations (>90% are T1799A transitions in exon 15 that cause a valine to glutamate substitution at residue 600 [Val600Glu or V600E] of the protein activation loop): papillary carcinoma and poorly differentiated or undifferentiated carcinomas originating from papillary carcinoma; rearrangement (*AKAP9/BRAF, AGK/BRAF*): papillary carcinoma	Somatic activating mutations: *BRAF* oncogenic mutations are common in many human cancers including melanoma and adenocarcinomas of the colon; germline gain of function mutations of *BRAF* and of genes encoding other proteins along the RAS-MAPK pathway are associated with Noonan, Costello, and cadiofaciocutaneous syndromes; *BRAF* mutations are typically associated with cardio-faciocutaneous syndromes
CTNNB1	Somatic activating mutations: cribriform morular variant of papillary carcinoma, poorly differentiated and undifferentiated carcinomas	Somatic activating mutations: stabilizing *CTNNB1* mutations occur in several tumors including fibromatosis, colonic and hepatocellular adenocarcinoma, pilomatrichoma, and tumors with a blastematous component (e.g., hepatoblastoma, medulloblastoma, Wilms tumor); germline inactivating mutations of the *APC* gene (in the absence of β-*catenin* mutations) are responsible for tumorigenic Wnt signaling in patients with FAP
GNAS (*GNAS1*)	Somatic activating mutations: hyperfunctioning thyroid nodules/tumors	Somatic activating mutations: GH-secreting pituitary adenomas, fibrous dysplasia of bone; postzygotic activating mutations: McCune-Albright syndrome; germline inactivation: pseudohypoparathyroidism and pseudo-pseudohypoparathyroidism
NTRK1	Rearrangement *(TRK oncogenes-TPM3/NTKR1 [TRK], TPR/NTRK1 [TRK-T1/T2]* and *TFG/NTRK1 [TRK-T3])*: papillary carcinoma	Rearrangement: *NTRK1* can be fused to a variety of gene partners in extrathyroid tumors like lung adenocarcinoma; germline inactivating mutations: congenital insensitivity to pain with anhidrosis (CIPA)
NTRK3	Rearrangement (*ETV6/NTRK3*): papillary carcinoma (radiation associated)	Rearrangement: *ETV6/NTRK3* occurs in congenital fibrosarcoma, congenital mesoblastic nephroma, secretory carcinomas (breast and salivary gland mammary analog tumors), some leukemias
PAX8	Rearrangement (*PAX8/PPARγ*): follicular carcinoma, but also some follicular adenomas and and papillary carcinomas (follicular variant); germline inactivating mutations: congenital hypothyroidism with thyroid dysgenesis	*PAX8* is expressed by several human cancers including renal cell carcinoma, Wilms tumor, ovarian adenocarcinomas, seminoma

Table 2-1, continued

GENES ALTERED IN THYROID TUMORS

Gene	Chromosomal Site	Protein	Expression	Genetic Alteration
PIK3CA	3q26.3	p110α catalytic subunit of of class IA phosphatidylinositol 3-kinase (PI3K); PI3Ks are signal transducer enzymes that through the formation of of PIP3 activate AKT	Ubiquitous	Activating mutation (somatic) clustered to exon 9 and exon 20; *PIK3CA* copy number gains also occur but their tumorigenic role is less defined
PPARγ (*PPARG*)	3p25.2	PPARγ is a nuclear receptor protein of the nuclear hormone receptor superfamily	Highly expressed in adipose tissue and at various levels in many other tissues; PPARγ expression is low in the normal thyroid	Rearrangement (somatic)
PTEN	10q23.31	PTEN, a phosphatase that by converting PIP3 to PIP2 negatively regulates AKT	Ubiquitous	Inactivating mutations (somatic and germline); *PTEN* activity is also lost (in thyroid tumors as well as in many other cancers) by gene deletion and epigenetic modification
H-RAS, K-RAS, N-RAS	11p15.5 (*H-RAS*), 12p12.1 (*K-RAS*), 1p13.2 (*N-RAS*)	Monomeric membrane-bound G proteins ("small" G proteins, homologous to the α subunit of "large" G proteins GSα) of the RAS superfamily of small GTPases; RAS proteins have a critical role in signal transduction and activate the MAPK pathway	Ubiquitous	Activating mutations (somatic and germline); "hot spot" mutations at codons G12 or G13 (GTP binding domain) or at codon Q61 (GTPase domain) result in amino acid subsitutions that "lock" the protein in the active GTP-bound form
RET	10q11.2	RET (REarranged during Transfection); belongs to the receptor tyrosine kinase superfamily; RET ligands belong to the glial cell line-derived neurotrophic factor ligand family (GFLs: GDNF, neurturin, artemin, and persephin) and bind RET in conjunction with one of four coreceptors that are part of the GDNF-family α receptors (GFRα1-4)	Parafollicular calcitonin-producing thyroid C-cells, not expressed at any significant level in follicular thyroid cells; also expressed in brain, thymus, testis, and cells of postulated neural crest origin, including neuroendocrine tissues; RET expression is essential for the early development of the genitourinary system and enteric neurons	Activating mutations (somatic and germline); rearrangement (somatic); inactivating mutations (germline)
TERT	5p15.33	The telomerase enzyme complex is a RNA-dependent reverse transcriptase that maintains telomere ends by addition of the telomere repeat TTAGGG; the enzyme complex includes a protein component with reverse transcriptase activity, encoded by the *TERT* gene, and a RNA component which serves as a template for the telomere repeat encoded by the *TERC* (or *TR*) gene	Germ cells and somatic stem cells; normal somatic cells do not express or have a very low levels of telomerase	Activating mutations of *TERT* promoter (somatic); gene amplification (somatic); epigenetic modifications
TP53	17p13.1	The p53 protein is a transcription factor with tumor suppressive function that controls cell cycle, apoptosis, and genetic stability	Ubiquitous; p53 levels are kept low because the protein is continuously degraded; p53 levels increase as a result of cellular stress or mutations	Inactivating mutations (somatic and germline)
TSHr	14q31	Transmembrane receptor protein for TSH (seven transmembrane domain G protein coupled receptor)	Thyroid follicular cells	Activating mutations (somatic and germline); inactivating mutations (germline)

Table 2-1, continued

GENES ALTERED IN THYROID TUMORS

Gene	Thyroid Disease	Extrathyroid Disease
PIK3CA	Somatic activating mutations: follicular carcinoma, poorly differentiated and undifferentiated carcinomas	Somatic activating mutations: *PIK3CA* oncogenic mutations are common in many human cancers including colonic, breast, and ovarian adenocarcinomas, and glioblastoma
PPARγ (*PPARG*)	Rearrangement (*PAX8/PPARγ, PAX8/PPARG*): follicular carcinoma, but also some follicular adenomas and papillary carcinomas (follicular variant)	*PPARγ* is expressed by several human cancers including breast and prostatic adenocarcinomas; *PPARγ* is involved in the pathogenesis of diabetes, obesity, and atherosclerosis
PTEN	Somatic inactivating mutations: follicular carcinoma and undifferentiated carcinoma; germline inactivating mutations: Cowden syndrome	Loss of *PTEN* activity is common in many human cancers including glioblastoma, endometrial and prostatic adenocarcinoma; germline inactivating mutations: PTEN hamartoma tumor syndromes: Cowden, Bannayan-Riley-Ruvalcaba, Proteus and Proteus-like syndromes; only Cowden syndrome is specifically associated with thyroid disease
H-RAS *K-RAS* *N-RAS*	Somatic activating mutations: hyperplastic nodules, follicular adenoma, follicular carcinoma, papillary carcinoma (follicular variant), poorly differentiated and undifferentiated carcinomas	Somatic activating mutations: *RAS* oncogenic mutations are very common in many human cancers including adenocarcinoma of the colon, pancreas, and lung, melanoma, and acute myeloid leukemia; germline gain of function mutations of *RAS*, and of genes encoding other proteins along the RAS-MAPK pathway are associated with Noonan, Costello, and cardiofaciocutaneous syndromes; *RAS* mutations are typically associated with Noonan syndrome
RET	Somatic activating mutations: medullary carcinoma; rearrangement (*RET/PTC1, -2, -3* and other types): papillary carcinoma; germline activating mutations: multiple endocrine neoplasia type 2 (MEN 2A, MEN 2B), and familial medullary thyroid carcinoma (FMTC)	Rearrangement: *RET* is fused with a variety of gene partners in different extrathyroid tumors, including lung adenocarcinoma and myeloproliferative disorders; germline inactivating mutations: Hirschsprung disease (congenital agangliosis of the colon)
TERT	Somatic activating mutations of *TERT* promoter: papillary carcinoma, follicular carcinoma, poorly differentiated and undifferentiated carcinomas	Telomerase is expressed in approximately 90 percent of human tumors by a variety of mechanisms; somatic mutations of the *TERT* promoter occur in several tumors, more frequently in those of the central nervous system (gliomas, glioblastomas, medulloblastomas), sarcomas (myxoid liposarcoma), and some carcinomas (urothelial and hepatocellular)
TP53	Somatic inactivating mutations: poorly differentiated and undifferentiated carcinomas	Somatic inactivating mutations: *TP53* is the tumor suppressor most commonly mutated in human cancer; germline inactivating mutations: Li-Fraumeni syndrome
TSHr	Somatic activating mutations: hyperfunctioning thyroid nodules/tumors (hyperplastic nodules- "toxic" multinodular goiter, follicular adenoma and follicular carcinoma); activating germline mutations: nonautoimmune autosomal dominant hyperthyroidism; inactivating germline mutations: hereditary TSH resistance (congenital hypothyroidism or euthyroid hyperthyrotropinemia)	

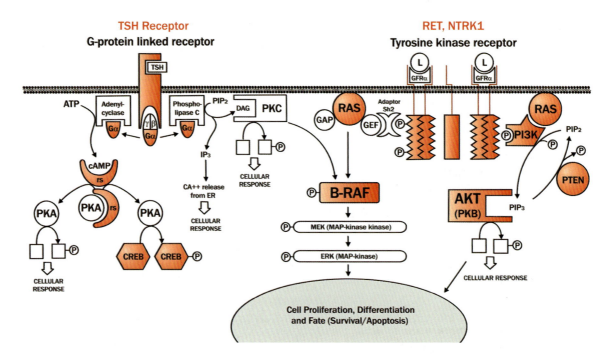

Figure 2-2

PATHWAYS AND MOLECULES ALTERED IN THYROID TUMORS

Many of the molecules altered in thyroid tumors (in red) are involved with classic signaling pathways which mediate communication between epithelial cells and their environment. Membrane receptor proteins, both G-protein linked receptors (e.g. the TSH receptor) and tyrosine kinase receptors (e.g. RET and NTRK1), are often dysregulated by somatic mutations, rearrangements, or other mechanisms. RAS proteins and the MAPK (mitogen-activated protein kinase) protein BRAF are also altered, as a result of point mutations. TSH: thyroid-stimulating hormone; ATP: adenosine-5'-triphosphate; cAMP: cyclic adenosine monophosphate; Gα: Gsα subunit of heterotrimeric G proteins; β: β subunit of heterotrimeric G proteins; γ: γ subunit of heterotrimeric G proteins; rs: regulatory subunit type 1-α of protein kinase A (encoded by *PRKAR1A*); PKA: protein kinase A; CREB: cAMP response element-binding protein (CREB3L2 a CREB3 related protein is rearranged with PPARγ is a few follicular carcinomas); PIPn: phosphatidylinositol n-phosphate; IP3: inositol triphosphate; DAG: diacylglycerol; PKC: protein kinase C; RAS: small GTPase RAS protein; GAP: GTPase activating protein; GEF: guanine nucleotide exchange factor; adaptor SH2: adaptor proteins with Src homology regions; B-RAF: protein kinase BRAF (mitogen-activated protein 3 kinase, MAP3K); MEK: mitogen-activated protein Erk kinase (mitogen-activated protein 2 kinase, MAP2K); ERK: extracellular-signal-regulated kinase (mitogen-activated protein kinase, MAPK); L: ligand; GFRα: GDNF-family α coreceptor; PI3K: phosphoinositide 3-kinase; AKT: AKT kinase (also known as PKB).

Mutations of the *TSHR* gene, first reported in 1993 (42), tend to be concentrated in areas of the gene that correspond to the functionally important domains of the protein, such as the III intracellular loop and VI transmembrane region, both of which are involved in the interaction with G proteins (43), but they may also be spread along the entire length of the molecule. Exon 10, where most alterations occur, is usually analyzed to detect mutations (36). Germline mutations in the *TSHR* gene cause nonautoimmune autosomal dominant hyperthyroidism (44).

The mutated TSHR and Gsα proteins are constitutively active, resulting in increased intracel-

lular cAMP levels and continuous stimulation of thyroid hormone synthesis and secretion. Not surprisingly, hyperplastic thyroid nodules and follicular adenomas with *TSHR* and *GNAS* mutations are "hot" on scintiscan and may be associated with hyperthyroidism (hyperfunctioning or "toxic" thyroid nodules, Plummer adenoma).

Mutations of the *TSHR* and *GNAS* genes have been reported with variable frequency in hyperplastic nodules and follicular adenomas that are hyperfunctioning (36). The variability appears to be mostly due to the techniques used for mutation detection (36,43,45). In general, *TSHR* mutations are more common than those involving *GNAS*. Alterations of other genes participating in cAMP signaling may account for those cases without a *TSHR* or *GNAS* mutation (36). Interestingly, *TSHR* mutations are also present in microscopic, autoradiographically hot foci in approximately 30 percent of euthyroid goiters (46).

In contrast to hyperfunctioning thyroid nodules, *TSHR* or *GNAS* mutations do not generally occur in "cold" thyroid nodules. and have been rarely reported in thyroid carcinoma (36). However, occasional cases of hyperfunctioning thyroid carcinoma with *TSHR* mutations have been described, even among tumors with poorly differentiated histologic features (47,48), and the prevalence of *TSHR* and *GNAS* mutations in thyroid carcinoma may be underestimated (49).

Alterations of other factors related to the cAMP pathway may play a role in the development of cold nodules and thyroid carcinoma. Markedly reduced expression due to allelic loss or promoter methylation of Rap1GAP, a negative regulator of the small G protein RAP1 (see above), has been identified in invasive well-differentiated tumors (both follicular and papillary) as well as in anaplastic carcinoma (50,51). Germline inactivating mutations of the *PRKAR1A* gene, encoding the regulatory subunit type 1α of protein kinase A, a key regulator of cAMP-dependent signaling, cause Carney complex (spotty skin pigmentation, myxomas, schwannomas, and endocrine overactivity), where *PRKAR1A* mutations are found in 45 to 80 percent of cases. Although patients are usually euthyroid, they frequently develop adenomatous thyroid nodules and are at increased risk of developing both follicular and papillary thyroid carcinomas (52–54).

MAPK PATHWAY

The mitogen-activated protein kinase (MAPK) pathway is a cascade of serine/threonine-specific protein kinases (RAF-MEK-ERK) that relays extracellular stimuli to the nucleus to coordinate cellular activities in response to hormones, growth factors, and cytokines that interact with receptor proteins on the cell surface (fig. 2-2). The MAPK pathway regulates important functions such as cell differentiation, proliferation, and fate (survival/apoptosis) and is activated by oncogenic events in many human cancers. Constitutive activation (i.e., activation independent of physiologic stimuli) of the MAPK cascade

represents a crucial event in thyroid tumorigenesis and results from molecular alterations of tyrosine kinase receptor proteins (e.g., RET) or of intracellular downstream effectors like RAS and BRAF (2,3,55). Oncogenic modifications that activate the MAPK pathway are found in approximately 70 percent of well-differentiated thyroid carcinomas of follicular cell derivation. Since specific molecular changes rarely coexist in the same tumor, it follows that alteration of any single component of the pathway may be sufficient to promote tumor growth (2,3,55).

Tyrosine Kinase Receptors (RET, NTRK1, NTRK3, ALK, MET)

Transmembrane receptors with tyrosine kinase activity play a fundamental role in signal transduction, and many are dysregulated in human cancer. More than 20 receptor proteins with tyrosine kinase activity have been identified in the human thyroid gland and several have been implicated with the malignant transformation of thyroid cells (56). The most important of these are RET, NTRK1, NTRK3, ALK, and MET.

The *RET* gene (rearranged during transfection) (57) is located at 10q11.2 and encodes a transmembrane tyrosine-kinase receptor with three isoforms that are generated by alternative splicing of its 3' region (58). The RET protein has an extracellular domain (including ligand binding, cadherin-like and cysteine-rich subdomains) that is involved in the recognition and binding of RET ligands and coreceptors, a transmembrane domain, and an intracellular segment with two tyrosine kinase domains (TK1, TK2) that is required for autophosphorylation of the tyrosine residues within the TK domain of each RET molecule (59). RET ligands are members of the glial cell line–derived neurotrophic factor ligand family (GFLs: GDNF, neurturin, artemin, and persephin) and bind RET in conjunction with coreceptors belonging to the GDNF family α receptors (GFRα 1–4) (fig. 2-2). Thus, ligand-mediated RET activation requires the assembly of a cell surface complex (including RET, its ligand, and a GFRα coreceptor) that causes RET to dimerize in its active configuration and autophosphorylate tyrosine residues. Activation of RET leads to activation of downstream signaling, including the RAS-MAPK kinase and the PI3K/PTEN/AKT pathways (60).

RET is not expressed at any significant level in normal follicular cells, but is instead normally expressed in calcitonin-producing thyroid C-cells. RET is also expressed in brain, thymus, testis, and cells of postulated neural crest origin, including calcitonin-producing thyroid C-cells and a variety of neuroendocrine tissues (adrenal medulla, extra-adrenal paraganglia, sympathetic and enteric ganglia) (61). RET is essential for the development of the genitourinary system and enteric neurons. Mice homozygous for a targeted loss of function *RET* mutation develop to term but demonstrate both renal agenesis or dysgenesis and absence of enteric neurons, but do not have evidence of neoplastic disorders (62). In humans, germline loss of function mutations in *RET* cause Hirschsprung disease (congenital aganglionosis of the colon) (63). On the other hand, *RET* activation is oncogenic and specifically relevant for thyroid tumor development.

Gain of function germline *RET* point mutations cause MEN type 2 (MEN 2A, MEN 2B) and FMTC, representing a paradigm for familial cancer syndromes caused by inherited proto-oncogene activation (64–66). In MEN 2A and FMTC, mutations affect the extracellular cysteine-rich domain of *RET* and are nearly always located either on exon 10 (codons 609, 611, 618, 620) or on exon 11 (codon 634). They almost always involve cysteine residues that are replaced by other amino acids. These cysteine residues are normally engaged in intramolecular disulfide bonds in wild-type RET. The mutation allows the unpaired cysteine residue in a RET monomer to form an aberrant intermolecular disulfide bond with another mutated monomer, causing ligand-independent dimerization and constitutive activation of RET (65).

In MEN 2A, the majority (80 percent or more) of mutations are at codon 634, usually TGC to CGC transitions resulting in the substitution of a cysteine with an arginine residue (Cys634Arg, C634R), not found in FMTC; rare patients with MEN 2A have mutations in the intracellular tyrosine kinase domain. In FMTC, mutations are fairly evenly distributed in the various codons of the extracellular domain and in a few cases are located in the intracellular tyrosine kinase domain (exons 13 and 14) (65). In MEN 2B mutations occur in the intracellular tyrosine kinase domain, virtually all of them (95 percent) in codon 918

(exon 16) resulting in the replacement of a methionine with a threonine residue (Met918Thr, M918T), and the remainder in codon 883 (exon 15). Mutations in the intracellular tyrosine kinase domain induce structural changes of the catalytic core causing constitutive activation of the monomeric form of RET (65).

Given the location of the known clinically relevant mutations, exons 10, 11, 13, 14, 15, and 16 have to be screened in patients with suspected hereditary medullary carcinoma using DNA obtained from peripheral blood samples (65). An important consequence of the diagnosis is the need to perform a total thyroidectomy with central lymph node dissection in asymptomatic kindreds of patients with hereditary medullary carcinomas that carry germline *RET* mutations (see chapter 12) (67).

Since specific *RET* mutations are related not only to the type of syndrome, but also to the aggressiveness of the medullary carcinoma, *RET* mutations have been stratified into risk groups. The highest risk category according to the 2009 Management Guidelines from the American Thyroid Association is exemplified by the codon 918 mutation of MEN 2B, while the codon 634 mutation of MEN 2A belongs to an intermediate risk group (see chapter 12) (65,67).

Both medullary thyroid carcinoma and C-cell hyperplasia occur in transgenic mice with the Cys634Arg or Met918Thr mutation expressed under the control of the calcitonin gene promoter (68,69). Similar tumors have been reported in transgenic mice, with the Cys634Arg mutation fused to the Moloney virus long terminal repeat (70). Transgenic mice constructed with the dopamine β-hydroxylase promoter to direct the expression of Met918Thr develop tumors identical to human ganglioneuromas in the sympathetic nervous system and adrenal medulla (71). Interestingly, mutations of the *GDNF* gene have not been implicated in the development of the MEN 2 syndromes (72).

RET mutations also occur in nonhereditary (sporadic) medullary carcinomas. These mutations have been reported in 30 to 70 percent of cases and in most tumors (approximately 80 percent) are the same codon 918 mutation (M918T) that occurs in most MEN 2B patients. In the remaining cases, mutations have been reported at most of the sites associated with hereditary carcinomas. Somatic *RET* mutations in sporadic medullary carcinomas (and the codon 918 mutation) have been associated with aggressive features and an unfavorable prognosis (see chapter 12) (65,73,74).

RET can also be altered in papillary carcinoma by chromosomal rearrangements that create the *RET/PTC* (papillary thyroid carcinoma) oncogenes (75). Thyroid cancer of follicular cell derivation is among the few epithelial malignancies characterized by specific gene rearrangements, similar to those occurring in hematolymphoid and mesenchymal tumors. Recombination events occur in up to 40 percent of papillary carcinomas (2), and most involve the receptor tyrosine kinase RET. The transforming activity of DNA extracted from papillary carcinoma was initially observed in 1987 (76,77). The oncogene was subsequently sequenced (75), characterized by molecular cytogenetics (78), and shown to be specific for papillary carcinoma (79). *RET/PTC* recombination involves the 3.0 kb intron 11 of *RET* and results from paracentric inversions of the long arm of chromosome 10 where *RET* is located, or from interchromosomal translocations. These recombinations of chromosomal DNA cause in-frame fusion of the distal part of *RET*, including the portion of the gene encoding the entire tyrosine-kinase domain of the protein (from residue E713 to the C-terminus), with heterologous genes (75). The heterologous genes are widely expressed in human tissues, including thyroid follicular cells, where they drive aberrant expression of the RET tyrosine-kinase.

Twelve heterologous genes have been found fused to *RET*, resulting in at least 17 different chimeric sequences because of variable breakpoints (66). These resulting chimeric products are called *RET/PTC*. RET/PTC1 (*RET* fusion with *CCDC6*, coiled-coil domain containing 6 gene, previously known as *H4* or *D10S170*) and *RET/PTC3* (*RET* fusion with *NCOA4*, nuclear coactivator 4 gene, previously known as *RFG*, *ELE1*, or *ARA70*) are both the consequence of paracentric inversions on the long arm of chromosome 10. *RET/PTC1* (*CCDC6/RET*) is detected cytogenetically as an inv10(q11.2q21.2) (78), while the *RET/PTC3* (*NCOA4/RET*) rearrangement at 10q11.2 is cytogenetically undetectable (80). *RET/PTC1* and *RET/PTC3* represent more than 90 percent of all rearrangements in papillary carcinoma, with

RET/PTC1 being found in approximately two thirds and *RET/PTC3* in approximately one third of the *RET/PTC* rearranged cases (81). *RET/PTC2* is caused by the t(10;17)(q11.2;q23) that leads to *RET* fusion with *PRKAR1A* (82), the gene that is inactivated in the germline of patients with the Carney complex (53).

RET/PTC rearrangements are associated with radiation exposure (therapeutic or environmental), the most dramatic evidence of which was the frequent occurrence of *RET* rearrangement in the papillary carcinomas that developed in children after the Chernobyl nuclear reactor accident in 1986 (83,84). The frequency with which *RET*, *CCDC6*, and *NCOA4* (which are several megabases apart along the linear map of chromosome 10) juxtapose in interphase thyrocyte nuclei is believed to predispose the DNA to radiation-induced rearrangement (85). The *RET/PTC* variants different from *RET/PTC1*, *-2*, and *-3*, all of which are very rare, are usually found only in papillary carcinomas from patients with a history of exposure to ionizing radiation, including radiotherapy (65,66).

Several studies using sophisticated high throughput methods of gene analysis are showing that *RET* recombination is not unique to the thyroid gland. For instance, *RET* rearrangement has been demonstrated in 2 percent of lung adenocarcinomas (86,87). It has also been identified in patients with chronic myelomonocytic leukemia (88) and in breast epithelial cells transformed by radiation (89). The rearrangements characterized so far share the same oncogenic properties as *RET/PTC*, but involve different genes from those reported in thyroid tumors (86–88). *RET/PTC1* has been detected in peritoneal carcinomas with papillary features (90) and *RET/PTC3* in a cell line of malignant mesothelioma (91). These important findings indicate that the *RET* gene is "fragile," and that its locus is chromosomally unstable and prone to recombination.

In addition to the fact that they have been isolated from papillary carcinoma, the oncogenic properties of the *RET/PTC* rearrangement are shown in vitro by its ability to cause TSH-independent thyroid cell proliferation and to impair the expression of thyroid differentiation markers (65,66). *RET/PTC* constitutively activates RET tyrosine-kinase signaling and activates downstream RET effectors like the RAS-MAPK kinase and the PI3K/PTEN/AKT pathways (65,66). Transgenic mice with *RET/PTC1* and *RET/PTC3* expression targeted to the thyroid gland develop tumors similar to papillary carcinomas in humans (92,93). Fisher et al. (94) have shown that *RET/PTC* expression in primary cultures of human thyroid follicular cells results in alterations of nuclear morphology typical of papillary carcinoma (irregular nuclear contours, grooves, nuclear clearing, and pseudoinclusions).

The molecular mechanisms of *RET/PTC* oncogenic activation have been clarified: the heterologous genes fused to *RET* have dimerization domains and as the *RET/PTC* chimeric mRNAs are translated into fusion proteins, these domains promote dimerization and thus ligand-independent activation of RET tyrosine kinase (66). Other oncogenic mechanisms include loss of the RET intracellular juxtamembrane domain in the chimeric RET/PTC protein (such domain inhibits RET activation), the delocalization of RET kinase activity from the membrane to the cytoplasm (due to the loss of the transmembrane part of RET in the RET/PTC protein), and dysregulation of the genes fused to *RET* (66).

RET rearrangements are identified in surgical specimens using several methods, but highly sensitive techniques should be avoided for routine molecular diagnosis since they may identify low level recombinations in benign thyroid nodules and even in Hashimoto thyroiditis (95–97). *RET/PTC* usually occurs in thyroid tumors of young patients and children, and in tumors that show a classic papillary histology (98). Several studies have failed to correlate *RET/PTC* with increased morbidity and mortality (98–102).

The *NTRK1* gene, located on chromosome 1 (1q23.1), encodes the neurotropic tyrosine kinase receptor type 1 (NTRK1) protein (also known as TRKA, nerve growth factor receptor tyrosine kinase protein A), which binds the nerve growth factor (NGF) with high affinity. *NTRK1* was originally isolated from human colonic carcinoma as a transforming oncogene activated by a somatic rearrangement involving fusion with the nonmuscular tropomyosin 3 gene (*TPM3*) (103). *NTRK1* is expressed in the peripheral nervous system (sensory spinal and cranial nerve ganglia). Similar to RET, the NTRK1 protein is not present in normal follicular cells, but becomes expressed as a result

of chromosomal rearrangements (referred to as *TRK* rearrangements). These fuse the tyrosine kinase domain of *NTRK1* to the 5'-terminal region of heterologous genes that drive *NRTK1* expression in thyroid follicular cells. The resulting chimeric products exhibit constitutively active tyrosine kinase activity. The rearrangements causing *NTRK1* oncogenic activation include an intrachromosomal recombination of the long arm of chromosome 1 fusing the tyrosine kinase domain of *NTRK1* with the 5'-end region of the *TPM3* gene located at 1q31, resulting in the *TRK* chimeric oncogene, identical to the first *NTRK1* oncogene isolated from colonic carcinoma (104). A second intrachromosomal rearrangement juxtaposes the tyrosine kinase domain of *NTRK1* to the 5'-end of the *TPR* (translocated promoter region) gene localized at 1q25 and results, because of structural variants, in the *TRK-T1* (105) and *TRK-T2* (106) chimeric oncogenes. A third oncogene, *TRK-T3*, is the result of an interchromosomal translocation that fuses the tyrosine kinase domain of *NTRK1* with the 5'-sequence of the *TFG* (*TRK* fused gene) gene on chromosome 3 (3q12.2) (107). In some tumors, *NTRK1* fusion partners are still uncharacterized.

The molecular mechanisms responsible for oncogenic *NTRK1* activation are essentially the same as those described for *RET* (108). Similar to *RET/PTC*, the *TRK*, *TRK-T1/T2*, and *TRK-T3* rearrangements are a feature of papillary carcinoma. Significantly, transgenic mice that express the human *TRK-T1* oncogene in their thyroid glands also develop papillary carcinomas (109). The general clinicopathologic features of tumors with *NTRK1* rearrangement do not seem to be significantly different from those of cases with rearranged *RET*. However, *NTRK1* recombination is believed to be much less common than *RET/PTC*, occurring in approximately 5 percent of papillary carcinomas, with a similar frequency among the three rearrangement types (84).

The *NTRK3* gene, located on chromosome 15 (15q25.3), encodes the neurotrophic tyrosine kinase receptor type 3 (NTRK3) protein (also known as TRKC), which binds the neurotrophin-3 (NT3) growth factor with high affinity. NTRK3 is closely related to NTRK1, is primarily expressed in the central nervous system, and is not normally expressed in the thyroid gland. *NTRK3* fusion to the *ETS variant gene 6* (*ETV6*) results in the *ETV6/NTRK3* oncogene, detected cytogenetically as the t(12;15)(p13;q25). This oncogenic rearrangement has been identified in a variety of tumors (congenital fibrosarcoma, congenital mesoblastic nephroma, and secretory carcinomas of the breast and salivary glands). *ETV6/NTRK3* has also been identified in radiation-associated thyroid carcinomas (28,29). Leeman-Neill et al. (29) detected *ETV6/NTRK3* in approximately 15 percent of radiation-associated papillary carcinomas that developed after the Chernobyl nuclear accident, and in approximately 2 percent of papillary carcinomas not associated with radiation. In thyroid tumors, the fusion points of the chimeric products (usually *ETV6* exon 4-*NTRK3* exon 14) are different from those observed in most extrathyroid neoplasms (*ETV6* exon 5-*NTRK3* exon 13) (29). While no specific link to radiation exposure has been demonstrated for *NTRK1* rearrangements, *ETV6/NTRK3* may be the second most common form of oncogenic rearrangement in radiation-associated papillary carcinoma after *RET/PTC* (28,29). *ETV6/NTRK3* is more common in tumors from patients exposed to higher amounts of radiation (29). The rearrangement is associated with a follicular architecture, as *ETV6/NTRK3*-positive cases are often classified as follicular variant papillary carcinoma or classic papillary carcinoma with a component of follicular growth (28,29). Areas with a solid growth pattern are present in the radiation-associated carcinomas, but not in those unrelated to radiation exposure (29).

The *ALK* proto-oncogene located at 2p23, first identified as the gene rearranged in anaplastic large cell lymphomas, encodes the transmembrane receptor tyrosine kinase ALK (anaplastic lymphoma kinase) (110). ALK and its growth factor ligands pleiotrophin (PTN) and midkine (MK) are involved with the development of the central and peripheral nervous systems, but the physiologic role of ALK is not well understood and a high specificity ligand has not been yet identified. ALK signaling is dysregulated by a variety of changes in several types of cancer in addition to lymphomas, mostly rearrangements (with molecular mechanisms similar to those described for *RET* causing aberrant expression of the tyrosine kinase domain in the intracellular portion of ALK encoded by exons 20-29 of the gene), but also gene amplification, missense mutation, and autocrine/paracrine loops (110). Tumors with *ALK* alterations include carcinomas (nonsmall cell carcinoma of the lung where *ALK* is rearranged with *EML4* or other genes), mesenchymal neoplasms (inflammatory myofibroblastic tumors where *ALK* is rearranged with *TPM4* or other genes), and neuroblastoma (where *ALK* is activated by missense mutations) (110).

In 2012, Hamatani et al. (111) reported *ALK* rearrangement in 10 of 79 (12.6 percent) papillary carcinomas from Hiroshima and Nagasaki survivors of atomic bomb radiation. In 5 cases, *ALK* exon 20 was fused to *EML4* exon 13, in 1 case to *EML4* exon 20, as in the case of *EML4/ALK* rearrangement variants 1 and 2 of nonsmall cell lung carcinoma, respectively. In the remaining 4 cases the gene fused to *ALK* was not characterized (111). An association with solid/trabecular architecture, high radiation dose, and younger age was reported in the cases with rearranged *ALK* (111).

In 2014, the fusion of *ALK* to the *STRN* gene (located at 2p22.2) encoding striatin, a calcium-dependent calmodulin binding protein, was reported in thyroid carcinoma by Kelly et al. (112) and Pérot et al. (113). As in the case of *EML4/ALK*, the genetic change is due to an intrachromosomal rearrangement on the short arm of chromosome 2. The result is a fusion of *ALK* exon 20 with exon 3 of *STRN*, with consequent upregulation of the ALK tyrosine kinase domain (112). Kelly et al. (112) characterized the molecular features of *STRN/ALK* fusion, demonstrating that the ALK kinase inhibitor crizotinib blocks *STRN/ALK* activity. They screened 256 papillary carcinomas, 35 poorly differentiated crcinomas, and 24 undifferentiated (anaplastic) carcinomas for *ALK* rearrangements. The investigators identified *STRN/ALK* in approximately 1 percent of papillary carcinomas, and in approximately 9 percent of poorly differentiated, and 4 percent of undifferentiated thyroid carcinomas. Papillary carcinomas with *STRN/ALK* featured a predominance of follicular growth pattern, as did the papillary carcinoma components associated with poorly and undifferentiated tumors. The investigators identified *EML4/ALK* in only 1 papillary carcinoma, and did not find *EML4/ALK* in the other, more aggressive, types of cancer, nor did they find the rearrangement in papillary carcinomas that developed after radiation exposure following the Chernobyl accident (112).

Pérot et al. (113) identified *STRN/ALK* in an undifferentiated (anaplastic) thyroid carcinoma with a papillary carcinoma component and lung metastases. The *ALK* rearrangement was present in both the papillary and the undifferentiated carcinoma components, and the patient responded to treatment with the ALK kinase inhibitor crizotinib (114). The investigators identified *STRN/ALK* in 2 additional papillary carcinomas out of a series of 75 benign and malignant cases that included 29 papillary carcinomas, 3 poorly differentiated carcinomas with a papillary carcinoma component, and 2 poorly differentiated carcinomas with no identifiable papillary carcinoma, corresponding to an overall prevalence for *STRN/ALK* in papillary carcinoma of approximately 6 percent. Both papillary carcinomas with *STRN/ALK* were reported as conventional (without poorly differentiated features), and the rearrangement was not identified in 11 follicular variant papillary carcinomas (113). No *ALK* rearrangements have been found in follicular carcinomas and adenomas, thyroid oncocytic neoplasms, and medullary carcinoma, or in cases carrying other known thyroid carcinoma driver mutations (*BRAF, RAS, RET/PTC, PAX8/PPARγ*) (112,113). *ALK* rearrangements in thyroid tumors can be identified using the same fluorescence in situ hybridization (FISH) probes and antibodies used to detect the rearrangement in lung carcinomas (112,113).

Activating point mutations in *ALK* exon 23, encoding the tyrosine kinase domain of the protein, were identified in 2 undifferentiated (anaplastic) carcinomas in one series that included a total of 18 undifferentiated cases (115). One tumor harbored the *C3592T* mutation and the other the *G3602A* mutation. Both mutations are novel, different from those found in neurobalastoma, and were not detected in well differentiated papillary or follicular carcinomas (115).

The *MET* proto-oncogene encodes MET (hepatocyte growth factor receptor [HGFR]), a transmembrane receptor tyrosine kinase that binds the hepatocyte growth factor/scatter factor (HGF/SF). HGF/SF is a powerful mitogen for epithelial cells, including thyroid follicular cells. Overexpression of the MET protein has been demonstrated by Western blotting in approximately 60 percent of papillary carcinomas (116), and gene expression studies have shown that *MET* transcripts are consistently over-represented in papillary cancer (4). Since stromal cells of the thyroid gland secrete HGF/SF, it is possible that *MET* is involved in paracrine tumor growth stimulation (117). Other oncogenes may modulate the effect of MET on tumor cell growth. In fact, oncogenic activation of *RET, RAS,* and *BRAF* has been associated with MET overexpression that has been demonstrated in tumors and induced in primary thyroid cell cultures (6,117). Although the clinicopathologic significance of MET overexpression in thyroid carcinoma is unclear, it is likely involved with the growth of papillary carcinoma (116,118). Incidentally, oncogenic activation of *RET, RAS,* and *BRAF* has also been shown to stimulate overexpression of several chemokines (e.g., CXCL1 and CXCL10) that similar to MET may be involved in autocrine/paracrine loops that contribute to commit transformed thyroid cells to a malignant invasive phenotype (34).

Other possible mechanisms of carcinogenesis include signaling through fibroblast growth factor (FGF), vascular endothelial growth factor (VEGF), and other small molecules. Although the genes coding for several tyrosine kinases, including EGFR, VEGFR, PGFR, and KIT, show copy number gains in follicular carcinoma and particularly in anaplastic tumors, activating mutations of these genes are rare (119,120).

RAS

The *H-RAS, K-RAS,* and *N-RAS* genes encode a family of closely related 21-kDa G proteins that play a key role in the intracellular transduction of signals originating at the cell membrane. They were first identified as the transforming oncogenes of the Harvey (*H-RAS*) and Kirsten (*K-RAS*) sarcoma viruses. Human homologues were subsequently identified in tumors and a third human *RAS* gene was designated *N-RAS* for its initial identification in neuroblastoma. *H-RAS, K-RAS,* and *N-RAS* are among the oncogenes most frequently activated in human tumors and play an important role in the malignant transformation and progression of many types of cancer (121,122).

Normal RAS proteins are linked to the inner portion of the cytoplasmic membrane, exhibit guanosine triphosphatase (GTPase) activity, and exist in two forms: an inactive form, linked to guanosine diphosphate (GDP), and an active form, able to bind and hydrolyze guanosine triphosphate (GTP). They convey signals originating from membrane receptor proteins to the MAPK cascade and other pathways, including the PI3K/PTEN/AKT pathway, which activate the transcription of target genes in the nucleus, leading to cell growth and proliferation (fig. 2-2). Oncogenic *RAS* activation is typically due to point mutations of the gene affecting the GTP-binding domain (exon 2, codons G12 or G13) or the GTPase domain (exon 3, codon Q61) which "lock" the protein in the active GTP-bound form. Transgenic mice with thyroid-specific expression of mutated *RAS* develop tumors with features of follicular adenomas, follicular carcinomas, papillary carcinomas, and poorly differentiated carcinomas (123,124).

Constitutive activation of all three *RAS* oncogenes (*K-RAS*, *N-RAS*, and *H-RAS*) has been identified in tumors originating from the follicular epithelium of the thyroid gland covering the entire spectrum, from follicular adenomas to anaplastic carcinomas. It has been reported in 5 to 10 percent of hyperplastic thyroid nodules (25). Oncogenic *RAS* activation also occurs in medullary carcinoma (125–127).

A meta-analysis of the *RAS*-mutated thyroid tumors of follicular cell derivation, including only cases with mutations confirmed by direct sequencing, has shown that *RAS* mutations are, overall, more common in malignant tumors than in benign ones ($p<10^{-8}$) (25). This meta-analysis also showed that codon 61 *N-RAS* mutations are more frequent in follicular carcinomas than in adenomas ($p<0.03$), that codon 61 *H-RAS* mutations are more frequent in follicular carcinomas than in benign nodules ($p<0.02$), and that codon 12 and 13 *K-RAS* mutations are more frequent in malignant tumors (follicular and papillary) than in benign nodules ($p<10^{-4}$). There is, however, marked variability in the prevalence and specific types of *RAS* mutations reported in different series. This is likely due to a variety of causes, including specific methodologies for mutation detection, case selection, and the impact of environmental factors. In fact, the prevalence of oncogenic *RAS* may be higher in areas of iodine deficiency (128) and may be influenced by other environmental factors such as food-borne carcinogens (3,25). In thyroid tumors derived from follicular cells, mutations at codon 61 of *N-RAS* and, to a lesser degree, of *H-RAS*, are those more frequently detected (25).

RAS mutations are reported with similar frequencies (ranging from 20 to 50 percent) in follicular carcinoma, follicular adenoma, and the follicular variant of papillary carcinoma. Mutated *RAS* represents, therefore, a marker for follicular-patterned thyroid lesions (3).

RAS mutations are uncommon in conventional papillary carcinomas but are frequently detected in both poorly differentiated and undifferentiated thyroid carcinomas, indicating that they have a role in tumor progression. In fact, *RAS* may be implicated with aneuploidy in follicular tumors (129) and *RAS* mutations have been associated with thyroid carcinomas with aggressive clinicopathologic features and unfavorable prognosis (130–132).

In medullary carcinoma, oncogenic activation of *RAS* appears mutually exclusive with that of *RET*. *RAS* mutations have been found in up to approximately 80 percent of medullary carcinomas that do not have *RET* mutations, germline (MEN 2 or FMTC syndromes) or somatic (sporadic cases), and in less than 5 percent of *RET* mutated cases. The mutations more frequently identified are in *H-RAS* and *K-RAS,* while *N-RAS* mutations are uncommon (125–127).

BRAF

Oncogenic activation of *BRAF* is the most common molecular alteration of papillary thyroid carcinoma. BRAF, together with ARAF and CRAF, is a serine-threonine kinase in the MAPK pathway encoded by a gene located at 7q34. Following activation induced by RAS binding and recruitment to the cell membrane, RAF proteins phosphorylate and activate MEK, which in turn activates ERK. Activated ERK phosphorylates cytoplasmic proteins and translocates to the nucleus to regulate the transcription of genes involved with cell differentiation, proliferation, and survival (fig. 2-2) (133).

Among the three RAF proteins, BRAF, the most important isoform in thyroid follicular cells, has the highest basal kinase activity and is the strongest activator of MEK (133,134). Like other kinases, it has a bilobed catalytic core structure with an ATP binding site in a deep cleft located between the lobes. In its inactive conformation, BRAF is stabilized by hydrophobic interactions between the activation segment in the C lobe and the glycine-rich phosphate binding loop (P loop, the ATP binding site) in the N lobe. While *ARAF* and *CRAF* gene mutations are rare, *BRAF* activating mutations occur in many human cancers, notably melanoma and colorectal adenocarcinoma, but also ovarian and lung adenocarcinomas (135). Most mutations are clustered at the activation segment or at the P loop. These mutations disrupt the inactive BRAF conformation by allowing new interactions that fold the kinase into a catalytically active form (136,137).

In *BRAF* exon 15, a thymine to adenine transversion at the nucleotide 1799 (T1799A) results in the replacement of a hydrophobic valine with glutamic acid at residue (codon) 600, in the activation segment of the protein (Val600Glu, V600E). This mutation accounts for about 90 percent of all of the 65 or more known *BRAF* mutations. The amino acid replacement mimics the phosphorylation that physiologically activates the *BRAF* (phosphomimetic mutation), and as result of the *BRAF* V600E mutation the protein becomes constitutively active, independent of RAS. *BRAF* V600E represents more than 95 percent of all *BRAF* mutations in thyroid tumors (3). Other forms of mutant *BRAF* are rare and include the replacement of a lysine with glutamic acid at residue 601 of the protein (Lys601Glu, K601E) and small insertions or deletions close to codon 600 (138–142). Mutated BRAF proteins have been divided into a high activity group (exemplified by the *V600E* and the *K601E* mutations), an intermediate activity group, and an impaired activity group, according to the extent and mechanisms of MEK activation (136). Unlike the case of the V600E mutation, the modalities through which some uncommon BRAF mutated proteins activate downstream targets are complex (143) and not fully understood (141).

BRAF mutational analysis is easy to perform using a variety of methods. The first reports of *BRAF* oncogenic activation in thyroid carcinoma in 2003 (144,145) have been followed by many others that have demonstrated an impressive association of *BRAF* V600E with the papillary histotype. In fact, *BRAF* V600E is virtually restricted to the papillary carcinomas and the poorly differentiated and anaplastic carcinomas derived from them (138,146,147). *BRAF* V600E specificity is confirmed by its detection in the peripheral blood of patients with papillary carcinoma (148) and, interestingly, in papillary carcinomas arising within struma ovarii (149,150). Among papillary carcinomas, the association is strongest with the tall cell variant and very weak with the follicular variant. *BRAF* K601E and other uncommon mutations different from *BRAF* V600E are usually reported only in the follicular variant of papillary carcinoma (141,151), although *BRAF* K601E has also been identified in rare follicular adenomas (55) and carcinomas (152). Examples of "false positive" cytology specimens with a *BRAF* V600E mutation are extremely rare (153).

The oncogenic role of *BRAF* has been proven by numerous in vitro models (34,154,155) and by the development of papillary carcinomas in transgenic mice with *BRAF* V600E expression targeted to the thyroid (156,157). *BRAF* V600E is believed to be important not only for thyroid tumor initiation, but also to have a relevant role in promoting invasion and progression (158,159). Invasion in papillary carcinoma is associated with the induction of epithelial-mesenchymal transition (160), and the *BRAF* V600E mutation is linked to remodeling of extracellular matrix, deregulation of cell adhesion, and changes consistent with epithelial-mesenchymal transition during progression of *BRAF* V600E mutated papillary carcinoma to poorly differentiated thyroid cancer (159).

Papillary carcinomas with *BRAF* V600E are associated with reduced expression of genes required for thyroid hormone biosynthesis (e.g., thyroid peroxidase and thyroglobulin) and with decreased expression of the sodium iodide symporter (NIS) that is responsible for iodide uptake in the follicular cell (157,161–163). This suggests that tumors with *BRAF* V600E may be more likely to loose their differentiation and become refractory to radioactive iodine treatment, as apparently confirmed by the high prevalence of *BRAF* V600E in radioactive iodine-refractory thyroid carcinomas (164). In fact, many studies have associated the mutation with aggressive clinical features and poor outcome (142,146,163,165–168). However, not all the reports have shown this association (151,169–172). According to a retrospective study conducted at 13 medical centers in the United States, Europe, Australia, and Japan, *BRAF* V600E is significantly associated with increased cancer-related mortality among patients with papillary carcinoma, but the association is not independent of conventional clinicopathologic parameters (173). The possibility that *BRAF* V600E may not be present in all neoplastic cells within a given tumor, but only in neoplastic cell subclones, can confound a clear definition of the prognostic impact of *BRAF* V600E in thyroid cancer (174–177).

An increase over time in the proportion of carcinomas of conventional (classic) papillary histotype carrying *BRAF* V600E has been reported (178,179). The mutation has been associated with high iodine content in natural drinking water (24).

BRAF point mutations are not typical of papillary carcinomas related to radiation exposure (180,181). However, a rare oncogenic form of *BRAF* resulting from a paracentric inversion of chromosome 7 that juxtaposes *BRAF* (located at 7q34) with the gene *AKAP9* (located at 7q21-22) has been identified in approximately 10 percent of papillary carcinomas that developed with a 5- to 6-year latency period in children after exposure to the Chernobyl radioactive fallout (181). The AKAP9/BRAF fusion protein has elevated kinase activity since it contains the BRAF kinase domain but lacks its autoinhibitory amino-terminal portion. In vitro, the transforming activity of *AKAP9/BRAF* is comparable with that of the *BRAF* V600E mutation (181). Fusion of *BRAF* to *AGK* (encoding the mitochondrial protein acylglycerol kinase) has been identified in 1 of 26 pediatric radiation-associated thyroid carcinomas that developed after the Chernobyl nuclear accident. *AGK/BRAF* is the consequence of an intrachromosomal rearrangement at 7q34 (where both genes are located), and as in the case of AKAP9/BRAF, the AGK/BRAF fusion protein lacks the BRAF autoinhibitory amino-terminal domain. The tumor with *AGK/BRAF* had the features of a conventional papillary carcinoma, and the rearrangement was not found in tumor controls not related to radiation (28).

PI3K/PTEN/AKT PATHWAY

Phosphatidylinositol 3-kinase (PI3K)/AKT signaling regulates many important cellular functions, including proliferation, survival, and me-tabolism. Activation of this important pathway is common to many human tumors, including those originating in the thyroid gland (182–184).

PI3Ks are a family of signal transducer enzymes that phosphorylate the 3 position hydroxyl group of the inositol ring of phosphatidylinositol (fig. 2-2). The PI3K family is divided in three classes. Class I PI3Ks are heterodimeric molecules activated by G-protein coupled receptors and tyrosine kinase receptors. They consist of a regulatory and a catalytic subunit and are further subdivided into IA and IB subsets. Class IA PI3Ks are composed of one of five regulatory subunits attached to one of three catalytic subunits (p110α, β, or δ). Among the isoforms of the p110 catalytic subunits, the best studied is the class IA-type α, encoded by the *PIK3CA* gene that is mutated or amplified in human cancers, including colonic and gastric adenocarcinomas and glioblastomas (185–187).

AKT (protein kinase B [PKB]) is a family of serine/threonine-specific protein kinases with three isoforms, AKT1, AKT2, AKT3. The name AKT does not refer to the protein function but to its viral oncogene homologue (v-AKT), the designation of which is due to the viral oncogene isolation from the AKR mouse strain ("T" for transforming replaced the "R"). Of the three isoforms, AKT1, the one originally isolated, is ubiquitously expressed and best studied in human tumors; AKT2 is preferentially expressed in insulin-responsive tissues; AKT3 has restricted expression (brain, heart, and kidneys). The three AKT isoforms are expressed in the normal thyroid gland, but AKT1 and AKT2 predominate (182,188).

Activation of PI3K results in the formation of phosphatidylinositol 3,4,5, triphosphate (PIP3), which recruits to the cytosolic aspect of the cell membrane proteins with pleckstrin homology (PH) domains such as AKT (fig. 2-2) (187). The PH domain binds phosphoinositides with high affinity, and once correctly localized to the membrane via PIP3 binding, AKT can be phosphorylated at two sites critical for activation of the protein, threonine 308 by PDK1 (phosphoinositide-dependent kinase-1) and serine 473 by several kinases including mTORC2 (mammalian target of rapamycin complex 2) (189), and AKT itself (by autophosphorylation) (186,187,190). Activated AKT phosphorylates and interacts with numerous targets in the cytoplasm and in the nucleus, and subcellular localization of AKT appears to be an important factor in determining its biologic effects.

AKT signaling is activated by tyrosine kinases and RAS (although apparently not by downstream effectors along the MAPK cascade such as BRAF) (187,190). If we consider that oncogenic activation of RAS proteins and of tyrosine kinases (e.g., RET) is a frequent molecular alteration in thyroid cancer, it is possible that AKT acts as a common central regulator of thyroid oncogene function, thus playing a crucial role in thyroid tumorigenesis. Negative regulation of AKT is important for tumor suppression. It is achieved by PTEN (see below), a phosphatase that opposes PI3K activity by converting PIP3 back to PIP2, as well as by protein phosphatases that directly dephosphorylate AKT, or by disruption of AKT protein stabilization in the cytoplasm (187,190).

Activation of the PI3K/PTEN/AKT pathway occurs in thyroid carcinoma, particularly in follicular as opposed to papillary histotypes, and may have an important role in their progression to anaplastic cancer. Dysregulated AKT signaling has been linked to both loss of PTEN function (see below) as well as to activating mutations or to copy number gains of the *PIK3CA* gene (190). Moreover, mutations of the *AKT1* gene that constitutively activate AKT signaling have been identified in approximately 15 percent of high-grade, aggressive, radioactive iodine-refractory forms of thyroid cancer (164). Although these mutations may be focal within the tumor, they have been associated with tumor progression (164). *PIK3CA* gene mutations are clustered on exons 9 and 20, encoding the helical domain and the kinase domain of the protein, respectively. These mutations have been reported up to approximately 10 percent of follicular carcinomas and in up to approximately 25 percent of anaplastic thyroid cancers, though rarely in papillary carcinomas (less than 5 percent). Copy number gains of *PIK3CA* appear more common than mutations (having been identified in approximately 25 percent of follicular carcinomas and in up to 40 percent of anaplastic carcinomas), but their tumorigenic role is less defined (119,190–193).

PTEN (phosphatase and tensin homolog deleted on chromosome 10) is a dual function lipid and protein phosphatase that preferentially dephosphorylates phosphoinositide substrates, and by converting PIP3 to PIP2 negatively regulates AKT (fig. 2-2) (183,194). The *PTEN* gene mapped at 10q23.31 is a tumor suppressor often inactivated through different mechanisms that vary according to the tumor type. PTEN activity is lost by somatic *PTEN* gene mutations in several cancers (notably endometrial and prostatic adenocarcinoma, glioblastoma and other gliomas), although gene deletion and epigenetic modification (e.g., gene silencing by promoter methylation) appear more common than inactivating mutations (183,195).

Loss of function germline *PTEN* mutations are responsible for Cowden syndrome, an autosomal dominant condition characterized by multiple benign tumors and hamartomatous proliferations at various sites (196). Thyroid carcinoma, almost always of follicular type, develops in approximately 10 percent of the patients and is one of the major criteria required for the clinical diagnosis of the syndrome. Multicentric adenomatous thyroid nodules and thyroiditis are present in approximately two thirds of patients with Cowden syndrome (197–199).

While transgenic mice with a *PTEN* homozygous deletion are not viable, heterozygous *PTEN* +/- mice develop tumors at multiple sites, resembling Cowden syndrome in humans, including thyroid tumors (200). *PTEN* mutations have been reported in sporadic thyroid tumors with an overall frequency and distribution among tumor types similar to that of *PIK3CA* activating mutations. *PTEN* is mutated in up to approximately 10 percent of follicular carcinomas, in 5 to 15 percent of anaplastic carcinomas, and rarely in papillary carcinoma. Decreased PTEN mRNA and protein levels (201–203), however, appear to be more frequent than *PTEN* mutations, indicating that loss of heterozygosity or epigenetic mechanisms, different from gene inactivation by mutation, are a more common cause for reduced PTEN function (190). *PTEN* promoter methylation appears to have an important role (203,204) and the prevalence of methylation has been correlated with genetic alterations of *PIK3CA* (204). *PTEN* and *PIK3CA* gene mutations and *PIK3CA* copy number gain rarely coexist in well-differentiated tumors, suggesting the independent role of each alteration for the activation of the PI3K/ PTEN/AKT pathway. The fact that in poorly differentiated and anaplastic carcinomas these alterations may overlap with each other, as well as with other genetic changes like *BRAF* mutation, is consistent with the proposed role of the PI3K/ PTEN/AKT pathway in thyroid tumor progression (119,164,190–193).

PPARγ REARRANGEMENT

The *PAX8/PPARγ* (*PAX8/PPRG*) rearrangement, originally described by Kroll et al. (205), is the result of the t(2;3)(q13;p25) translocation that involves the short arm of chromosome 3, a recombination hotspot detected by cytogenetic analysis in follicular carcinomas (206). The rearrangement fuses a full length transcript (exons 1-6) of the *PPARγ* gene (*PPSRG*, mapped at 3p25) in frame with the proximal 7-9 exons of *PAX8* (mapped at 2q13), including its promoter region. The rearrangement variably splices out exons 8 and 9 of *PAX8*, resulting in some variation of the amino acid sequence predicted for the fusion protein (PAX8 PPARγ fusion protein [PPFP]) that has at its N terminus PAX8, including its DNA binding domain, and PPARγ at the C terminus with all its functional domains (205).

PPARγ (peroxisomal proliferator-activated receptor is a member of the nuclear hormone receptor superfamily that includes thyroid hormone, retinoic acid, and androgen and estrogen receptors. These receptors share several features, including a central DNA binding domain and a carboxyl-terminal domain responsible for ligand binding. PPARγ protein forms heterodimers with retinoid X receptors (RXRs) and these heterodimers, together with coactivators, activate the transcription of target genes.

PPARγ expression is very high in adipose tissue, and genes regulated by PPARγ control adipocyte function and differentiation. The action of thiazolidinediones, a class of drugs used to treat type 2 diabetes, is mediated by their binding to PPARγ, and PPARγ has been implicated in the pathogenesis of diabetes, obesity, and atherosclerosis. In addition to adipose tissue, PPARγ is expressed at various levels in many human tissues (liver, kidney, small and large intestine) but its level is very low in the thyroid gland in the absence of the *PAX8/PPARγ* rearrangement (207,208).

PAX8 (paired box gene 8) encodes a transcription factor essential for the genesis of thyroid follicular cell lineages and for the maintenance of a differentiated thyroid follicular cell phenotype.

In fact, the PAX8 protein controls and activates the transcription of the main proteins responsible for thyroid follicular cell function (such as thyroglobulin, thyroperoxidase, and sodium/iodide symporter) and *PAX8* mutations have been identified in cases of congenital hypothyroidism with thyroid dysgenesis (209,210).

PAX8 is expressed in embryonal human tissues, in particular, in the developing thyroid gland, kidney, müllerian structures, nervous system, and human placenta. In the adult, PAX8 is expressed by thyroid follicular cells (and to a lesser degree also by C-cells), tubular cells of the kidney, and epithelial cells of the fallopian tube. Since PAX8 is expressed by follicular cells, its promoter drives the expression of the rearranged PAX8/PPARγ protein, which can be detected by immunohistochemistry using antibodies against PPARγ. Strong nuclear immunoreactivity for PPARγ is considered a surrogate marker for the chromosomal rearrangement, but the correlation with immunohistochemistry is not perfect and confirmation by molecular methods (such as reverse transcriptase-polymerase chain reaction [RT-PCR]) may be necessary (211). The oncogenic properties of the PAX8/PPARγ protein are being elucidated and have been related to interference with wild-type PPARγ or PAX8 function, the novel intrinsic properties of the rearranged protein, or a combination of these (207,208).

In the original report from Kroll et al. (205), the *PAX8/PPARγ* rearrangement was present in 5 of 8 follicular carcinomas but not in the papillary carcinomas or in the benign thyroid nodules analyzed. It was subsequently found not only in follicular carcinomas but also in follicular adenomas (211–213), and in the follicular variant of papillary carcinoma (214), although not in aggressive tumors such as anaplastic thyroid cancer (164,212).

Although not specifically associated with radiation exposure, *PAX8/PPARγ* has been reported in follicular variant papillary carcinomas that developed after the Chernobyl nuclear accident (27,28).

A second rearranged form of the *PPARγ* gene was identified by Kroll et al. (215) in a follicular carcinoma with a t(3;7)(p25;q34). In this case, a full length transcript of *PPARγ* was fused in frame with exons 1 and 2 of the *CREB3L2* gene (mapped at 7q34). cAMP response element binding proteins (CREB) are a group of transcription factors that bind short DNA sequences called cAMP response elements (CRE) with a basic leucine zipper (bZIP) domain. CREB3L2 (acronym for "cAMP responsive element binding protein 3-like 2," also known as BBF2H7) is a CREB3- related protein with a transmembrane domain that is believed to be cleaved by proteolysis in response to endoplasmic reticulum stress (216). The cleaved fragments of CREB3L2 translocate into the nucleus where they bind to cAMP-responsive element DNA sequences to activate the transcription of target genes (216). *CREB3L2/PPARγ* has been shown to stimulate thyroid cell proliferation and to reduce the expression of thyroglobulin in vitro. The observation that *PPARγ* is involved in more than one rearrangement points to its role in thyroid tumorigenesis and suggests that 3p25, also a common site of loss of heterozygosity, is a breakpoint hot spot (208). Interestingly, the *CREB3L2* gene is fused to *FUS* as a result of the t(7;16)(q33;p11) that is a feature of low-grade fibromyxoid sarcoma (217). *CREB3L2/PPARγ* is much less common than *PAX8/PPARγ*, with an estimated prevalence lower than 3 percent among follicular carcinomas. It has been reported in one radiation-associated follicular variant papillary carcinoma that developed in a child exposed to the Chernobyl radioactive fallout (28). *CREB3L2/PPARγ* has not been identified in benign or non-neoplastic thyroid tissue (215).

ß-CATENIN/APC/Wnt SIGNALING

β-catenin, encoded by the *CTNNB1* gene, is a multifunctional protein with a critical role in both cell adhesion and transcription. It is also a key effector of Wnt signaling, a pathway that regulates cell fate and differentiation during embryonal life (218–220). In normal mature cells, in the absence of Wnt signaling, β-catenin is mostly bound to cadherins at the cell membrane adherens junctions, where it functions as an intracellular anchor protein that helps connect cadherins to the actin cytoskeleton of the cell (218–220). Free β-catenin levels are low because β-catenin is rapidly destroyed by ubiquitin-proteasome degradation. Such degradation requires the phosphorylation of β-catenin at critical Ser and Thr residues and a multiprotein destruction complex that includes the adenomatous polyposis coli protein (APC) and axin. Both are necessary for β-catenin phosphorylation by the glycogen synthase kinase-3b (GSK3b) and other kinases that target β-catenin for degradation by the proteasome.

During embryogenesis, physiologic Wnt signaling antagonizes β-catenin degradation and β-catenin is diverted to the nucleus, binds transcription factors, and stimulates the expression of various target genes (including *CCND1* encoding cyclinD1 and *MYC*) that promote cell proliferation and regulate differentiation (218). Thus, localization of β-catenin to the nucleus is a marker of its activity as a transcription factor, while its localization to the cell membrane marks its activity in cell adhesion.

β-catenin transcriptional activity resulting in cellular proliferation occurs when its binding to the cadherins is lost (e.g., due to decreased cadherin expression), when β-catenin degradation is ineffective (e.g., due to inactivating mutations in *APC* as in the case of familial adenomatous polyposis, or to *CTNNB1* mutations that disrupt phosphorylation sites and thus stabilize β-catenin), or when Wnt signaling is activated (218–221).

The function of β-catenin is dysregulated by stabilizing *CTNNB1* mutations in a variety of tumors that include colonic cancer, hepatocellular carcinoma, pilomatricoma, and tumors with a blastematous component (hepatoblastoma, medulloblastoma, Wilms tumor) (220).

In the thyroid gland, oncogenic signaling through β-catenin occurs in the cribriform morular variant of papillary carcinoma, in the setting of familial adenomatous polyposis with germline *APC* mutations, and in sporadic cases. Both inactivating *APC* mutations and *CTNNB1* exon 3 mutations that stabilize β-catenin have been found in the sporadic cribriform morular variant of papillary carcinoma (222,223).

Loss of membrane expression of E-cadherin and β-catenin is generally associated with tumor progression and unfavorable outcome in patients with thyroid carcinoma (224–227). β-catenin nuclear localization and *CTNNB1* mutation, are found in anaplastic thyroid carcinomas. They are also present in some poorly differentiated tumors, but absent in well-differentiated papillary or follicular carcinoma, indicating that activation of this pathway has a role in thyroid tumor progression (225,226,228).

TERT

Telomeres are the terminal portion of chromosomes. They are approximately 10 to 15 kilobases long and are characterized by short repetitive DNA sequences (TTAGGG in vertebrates). Telomeres protect chromosome integrity by preventing their degradation and uncontrolled fusion/breaking cycles with other chromosomes, and are the cell "mitotic clock" (229).

The special role of telomeres in cellular replication has been known and investigated for a long time. In the 1930s, it was observed that telomeres have distinctive features and do not get involved in aberrant chromosome fusion (230). Since DNA polymerase uses an RNA primer and synthesizes DNA exclusively in the 5' to 3' direction, the replication of the end of linear DNA is problematic (the "end replication problem" of Watson) (231). It was realized that telomeres get shorter with each replication cycle (by approximately 50 to 200 base pairs) (232), explaining why mature human diploid cells divide only a limited number of times (the "Hayflick limit") (233), before entering cellular senescence. In fact, critically short telomeric DNA elicits a DNA damage response (DDR) mediated by the p53 pathway, resulting in cell cycle arrest and eventually death by apoptosis (229).

Telomerase (telomere terminal transferase), a RNA-dependent reverse transcriptase complex, adds new DNA repeats to the chromosome ends, thus maintaining telomere length and extending the life span of the cell. Telomerase includes two main units: TERT (telomerase reverse transcriptase), the enzyme core protein with the reverse transcriptase domain encoded by the *TERT* gene, and TERC (telomerase RNA component, also known as TR, telomerase RNA), the RNA component that provides the template for telomeric DNA elongation encoded by *TERC* (or *TR*) (234). Additional components of telomerase are the dyskerin protein and the telomerase Cajal body protein 1 (TCAB1). In vivo, the telomerase complex is localized to the Cajal body, a subnuclear organelle 0.3 to 1.0 μm in diameter, visible in the nucleus of proliferating cells (e.g. embryonic cells) or metabolically active cells (e.g., neurons). The telomerase complex synthetizes DNA during the S phase and into the M phase of the cell cycle. It preferentially elongates the shortest telomeres; the extent of telomere elongation is very sensitive to the level of telomerase in the nucleus (234).

Telomerase activation can render a cell immortal and therefore is tightly regulated. Telomerase is active in embryonic cells, but in adult cells it is silenced and telomere shortening is the general default state of human proliferating cells (229). Telomerase activity is retained in the undifferentiated germ cells of adult males (spermatogonia) and in the stem cell compartment of a self-renewing tissue, so that telomere length is stable in the undifferentiated germ cell population, while it decreases only slightly with time in somatic stem cells (234).

Telomere shortening in adult stem cells impairs regeneration, resulting in the disruption of tissue homeostasis. Short telomeres have been linked to a variety of diseases, including inflammatory, neurological, cardiovascular, and degenerative disorders (e.g., ulcerative colitis, chronic liver disease and cirrhosis, dementia, Parkinson disease, heart failure). Telomere syndromes (234), due to inherited mutations of the telomerase complex genes or of other genes encoding components of the Shelterin and CST complexes that are also necessary for telomere maintenance, include dyskeratosis congenita (due to *TERT*, *TERC*, or other telomere maintenance gene mutations), as well as idiopathic pulmonary fibrosis (due to *TERT* and *TERC* mutations in approximately 10 and 1 to 3 percent of cases, respectively), and aplastic anemia (due to *TERT* or *TERC* mutations, with each gene mutated in approximately 4 percent of cases) (234).

Short telomeres have also been linked to tumor development. In the presence of mutations that disable the DNA damage response (e.g., inactivating *TP53* mutations), a cell with critically short telomeres continues to replicate and the unprotected chromosomes undergo aberrant recombination with cycles of breakage/fusion ("telomeric crisis") resulting in aneuploidy, genomic instability, and oncogenic mutations. If telomere length can be maintained above a critically short level, these cells can escape telomeric crisis-induced death, continue to grow, and form a tumor (229). Since unlimited cellular proliferation is one of the defining features of cancer, neoplastic cells must have in place telomere-maintaining mechanisms, regardless of whether telomere alterations play a role in tumor development. In fact, telomerase is expressed in approximately 90 percent of human tumors. The molecular mechanisms that activate telomerase in human tumors are not entirely clear and include *TERT* gene amplification, induction of *TERT* transcription by oncogenes (e.g., *c-MYC*), and epigenetic changes (229).

In 2013, two seminal articles showed that a high proportion of malignant melanomas had C>T transition mutations at two hot spots in the promoter of *TERT* at positions -124 (*C228T*) and -146 (*C250T*) (-1 being the base just upstream of the A of the ATG start codon for DNA transcription) (235,236). These mutations are mutually exclusive and create a novel binding site for transcription factors of the ETS family, thus promoting *TERT* transcription (235,236), with a 2- to 4-fold increase in *TERT* transcriptional activity measured in cell lines carrying the mutations (236). The MAPK kinase pathway (activated by *RAS* or *BRAF*) induces the expression of ETS family transcription factors. *TERT* promoter mutations were found to be associated with the *BRAF* V600E mutation in melanoma samples, with a potential to further increase the transcription of *TERT* in *BRAF*-mutated tumors (235). *C228T* or *C250T* mutations were found in approximately one third of primary melanomas and in 85 percent of metastatic tumors, but appear uncommon in melanocytic nevi (235).

The same mutations in the *TERT* promoter were subsequently identified in a variety of tumors, with the highest prevalence in those of the central nervous system (gliomas, glioblastomas, medulloblastomas), sarcomas (myxoid liposarcoma), and some carcinomas (urothelial and hepatocellular carcinomas) (237). Tumors have been classified as *TERT*-low, when the prevalence of *TERT* promoter mutations is 0 to 15 percent and *TERT*-high when the prevalence is higher than 15 percent (237). Since telomerase is physiologically active in the stem cell compartment of self-renewing tissues (e.g., hematopoietic parenchyma, gastrointestinal epithelium), most tumors with a high prevalence of *TERT* promoter mutations originate from organs with a stable population of cells that does not undergo constant turnover, where telomerase is not normally expressed (237).

In human tumors where telomerase is not active (approximately 10 percent), telomere length is maintained by the alternative lengthening of telomeres (ALT) pathway (238) in which telomeres are lengthened by mechanisms that involve homologous recombination of telomeric DNA. What causes the ALT pathway to become active is currently unknown, but inactivation of the ATRX/DAXX chromatin remodeling complex is considered the hallmark of ALT. *TERT* promoter and *ATRX* mutations are mutually exclusive, suggesting that they endow neoplastic cells with equivalent growth advantages (237).

Thyroid tissue does not normally express *TERT*, but *TERT* expression and telomerase activity is seen in tumors originating from follicular cells and in medullary carcinoma (239,240). As in the case of malignancies originating at other sites, *TERT* expression or telomerase activity are often found in tumors of advanced stage and are usually associated with poor survival (240). In addition to full-length *TERT* transcripts, three shorter splice variants have been identified in thyroid tumors. Carcinomas usually have short telomeres, high telomerase enzymatic activity, and express a high fraction of full-length *TERT* transcripts. The opposite is generally true for benign thyroid nodules that have long telomeres, low telomerase activity, and low full-length *TERT* transcript levels (241).

In 2013, following the identification of *TERT* promoter mutations in melanoma, the same *C228T* and *C250T* mutations were reported in tumors derived from follicular cells, revealing that they represent a common mechanism for *TERT* activation and telomere maintenance (242–245). Thyroid tumors of follicular derivation originate from cells that are stable, with a low proliferative rate. The finding of *TERT* promoter mutations is thus consistent with the hypothesis that these mutations occur in tissues that do not normally undergo continuous self-renewal (237).

The reported ranges for *TERT* promoter mutations are 5 to 25 percent for papillary carcinoma, 10 to 35 percent for follicular carcinoma, 20 to 50 percent for poorly differentiated carcinoma, and 30 to 50 percent for undifferentiated (anaplastic) carcinoma, with an evident relative increase of the mutation rate among less differentiated, aggressive histiotypes (242–247). As in the case of melanomas and other tumors with *TERT* promoter mutations *C228T* and *C250T* are mutually exclusive. The *C228T* is more common than the *C250T* mutation (by at least 5 fold in most series), across all tumor histiotypes (242–244, 247). *TERT* promoter mutations have not been identified in normal thyroid parenchyma, lymphocytic thyroiditis, hyperplastic thyroid nodules, or follicular adenomas (244,246,247), with the exception of one series that reported *C228T* mutations in 1 of 58 conventional follicular adenomas and in 3 of 18 adenomas with atypical features (248).

Several series have shown an association between *BRAF* V600E (or *BRAF* V600E and *RAS* mutations) and *TERT* promoter mutations, supporting the concept that MAPK-induced expression of transcription factors of the ETS family may further enhance the expression of *TERT*, as in the case of melanoma (242,244,246,247). *TERT* promoter mutations are emerging as a very powerful prognostic marker. In differentiated thyroid carcinomas, follicular or papillary, they are associated with older age, large tumor size, extrathyroidal extension, stage III or IV disease at presentation, distant metastases, and persistent disease (243,246,247), and may be an independent predictor of disease-specific mortality, particularly relevant for papillary carcinoma (243,246). No link between *TERT* promoter mutation and exposure to ionizing radiation (243,246) or dietary iodine intake (247) has been demonstrated.

Activation of the ALT pathway has been shown in a subset of medullary carcinomas (240), but no *TERT* promoter mutations were identified (243,244,246).

TUMOR PROTEIN p53

The tumor protein p53 (p53), with reference to its apparent electrophoretic mass, is a transcription factor that regulates the cell cycle encoded by the *TP53* gene mapped to chromosome 17p13.1 (249). In normal cells, p53 is continually produced but levels are kept low through proteasome-dependent degradation. Protein levels increase as result of cellular stress or mutations that prevent efficient p53 degradation and result in the accumulation of ineffective

p53. Proper expression of the gene is essential to prevent cancer development and germline loss of function. *TP53* mutations cause the Li-Fraumeni syndrome, characterized by a wide range of malignant tumors (breast carcinoma, gliomas, leukemia, and sarcoma) occurring at a young age (249).

TP53 is the prototype of a tumor suppressor gene through its effects on cell cycle control, apoptosis, and maintenance of genetic stability (249). Although p53 has many functions (249), tumor suppressing p53 activities are related to its ability to prevent cells with damaged DNA to proliferate. The p53 protein mediates cell cycle arrest (at the G1 or G2/M phases) in response to DNA damage. This arrest allows DNA repair mechanisms, some of which are directly stimulated by p53, to correct the damage. In the presence of severe, nonrecoverable DNA alterations, p53 promotes programmed cell death by apoptosis, thus avoiding replication of abnormal cell clones. Cancer cells with impaired p53 function are at selective advantage and permit the accumulation of genetic damage with chromosomal instability (249).

Alterations of p53 function occur in most human cancers and *TP53* is mutated in about 50 percent of them, often as a late event in tumor progression. Over 75 percent of *TP53* mutations are small nucleotide changes that lead to the expression of a mutant protein or, less commonly, to its complete absence. Over 90 percent occur in the DNA-binding domain (residues 92-292) (249), and *TP53* exons 5 to 8 or 9 are those usually screened for mutation detection.

Mutations in thyroid carcinomas are no different from those of cancers at other sites. They appear restricted to poorly differentiated and undifferentiated histotypes (250–253), and are uncommon in differentiated thyroid tumors, including cases related to radiation exposure (254). Recovery of p53 function in cultured cells derived from human thyroid carcinoma is accompanied by reacquisition of cell differentiation with induced reexpression of thyroglobulin, thyroperoxidase, and TSHR, as well as by a marked reduction in cell proliferation (255,256).

REFERENCES

1. Wynford-Thomas D. Origin and progression of thyroid epithelial tumours: cellular and molecular mechanisms. Horm Res 1997;47:145-57.
2. Kondo T, Ezzat S, Asa SL. Pathogenetic mechanisms in thyroid follicular-cell neoplasia. Nat Rev Cancer 2006;6:292-306.
3. Nikiforov YE, Nikiforova MN. Molecular genetics and diagnosis of thyroid cancer. Nat Rev Endocrinol 2011;7:569-80.
4. Huang Y, Prasad M, Lemon WJ, et al. Gene expression in papillary thyroid carcinoma reveals highly consistent profiles. Proc Natl Acad Sci U S A 2001;98:15044-9.
5. Aldred MA, Huang Y, Liyanarachchi S, et al. Papillary and follicular thyroid carcinomas show distinctly different microarray expression profiles and can be distinguished by a minimum of five genes. J Clin Oncol 2004;22:3531-9.
6. Giordano TJ, Kuick R, Thomas DG, et al. Molecular classification of papillary thyroid carcinoma: distinct BRAF, RAS, and RET/PTC mutation-specific gene expression profiles discovered by DNA microarray analysis. Oncogene 2005;24:6646-56.
7. Griffith OL, Melck A, Jones SJ, Wiseman SM. Meta-analysis and meta-review of thyroid cancer gene expression profiling studies identifies important diagnostic biomarkers. J Clin Oncol 2006;24:5043-51.
8. Alexander EK, Kennedy GC, Baloch ZW, et al. Preoperative diagnosis of benign thyroid nodules with indeterminate cytology. N Engl J Med 2012;367:705-15.
9. Croce CM. Causes and consequences of microRNA dysregulation in cancer. Nat Rev Genet 2009;10:704-14.
10. Lu J, Getz G, Miska EA, et al. MicroRNA expression profiles classify human cancers. Nature 2005;435:834-8.
11. He H, Jazdzewski K, Li W, et al. The role of microRNA genes in papillary thyroid carcinoma. Proc Natl Acad Sci U S A 2005;102:19075-80.
12. Pallante P, Visone R, Croce CM, Fusco A. Deregulation of microRNA expression in follicular-cell-derived human thyroid carcinomas. Endocr Relat Cancer 2010;17:F91-104.
13. Nikiforova MN, Tseng GC, Steward D, Diorio D, Nikiforov YE. MicroRNA expression profiling of thyroid tumors: biological significance and diagnostic utility. J Clin Endocrinol Metab 2008;93:1600-8.
14. Chen YT, Kitabayashi N, Zhou XK, Fahey TJ 3rd, Scognamiglio T. MicroRNA analysis as a potential diagnostic tool for papillary thyroid carcinoma. Mod Pathol 2008;21:1139-46.
15. Kitano M, Rahbari R, Patterson EE, et al. Expression profiling of difficult-to-diagnose thyroid histologic subtypes shows distinct expression profiles and identify candidate diagnostic microRNAs. Ann Surg Oncol 2011;18:3443-52.
16. Dettmer MS, Perren A, Moch H, Komminoth P, Nikiforov YE, Nikiforova MN. MicroRNA profile of poorly differentiated thyroid carcinomas: new diagnostic and prognostic insights. J Mol Endocrinol 2014;52:181-9.
17. Chou CK, Chen RF, Chou FF, et al. miR-146b is highly expressed in adult papillary thyroid carcinomas with high risk features including extrathyroidal invasion and the BRAF(V600E) mutation. Thyroid 2010;20:489-94.
18. Yip L, Kelly L, Shuai Y, et al. MicroRNA signature distinguishes the degree of aggressiveness of papillary thyroid carcinoma. Ann Surg Oncol 2011;18:2035-41.
19. Visone R, Russo L, Pallante P, et al. MicroRNAs (miR)-221 and miR-222, both overexpressed in human thyroid papillary carcinomas, regulate p27Kip1 protein levels and cell cycle. Endocr Relat Cancer 2007;14:791-8.
20. Jazdzewski K, Boguslawska J, Jendrzejewski J, et al. Thyroid hormone receptor beta (THRB) is a major target gene for microRNAs deregulated in papillary thyroid carcinoma (PTC). J Clin Endocrinol Metab 2011;96:E546-53.
21. Williams ED, Abrosimov A, Bogdanova T, et al. Morphologic characteristics of Chernobyl-related childhood papillary thyroid carcinomas are independent of radiation exposure but vary with iodine intake. Thyroid 2008;18:847-52.
22. Pellegriti G, De Vathaire F, Scollo C, et al. Papillary thyroid cancer incidence in the volcanic area of Sicily. J Natl Cancer Inst 2009;101:1575-83.
23. Ward MH, Kilfoy BA, Weyer PJ, Anderson KE, Folsom AR, Cerhan JR. Nitrate intake and the risk of thyroid cancer and thyroid disease. Epidemiology 2010;21:389-95.
24. Guan H, Ji M, Bao R, et al. Association of high iodine intake with the T1799A BRAF mutation in papillary thyroid cancer. J Clin Endocrinol Metab 2009;94:1612-7.
25. Vasko V, Ferrand M, Di Cristofaro J, Carayon P, Henry JF, de Micco C. Specific pattern of RAS oncogene mutations in follicular thyroid tumors. J Clin Endocrinol Metab 2003;88:2745-52.
26. Hamatani K, Eguchi H, Ito R, et al. RET/PTC rearrangements preferentially occurred in papillary thyroid cancer among atomic bomb survivors exposed to high radiation dose. Cancer Res 2008;68:7176-82.

27. Leeman-Neill RJ, Brenner AV, Little MP, et al. RET/PTC and PAX8/PPARγ chromosomal rearrangements in post-Chernobyl thyroid cancer and their association with iodine-131 radiation dose and other characteristics. Cancer 2013;119:1792-9.

28. Ricarte-Filho JC, Li S, Garcia-Rendueles ME, et al. Identification of kinase fusion oncogenes in post-Chernobyl radiation-induced thyroid cancers. J Clin Invest 2013;123:4935-44.

29. Leeman-Neill RJ, Kelly LM, Liu P, et al. ETV6-NTRK3 is a common chromosomal rearrangement in radiation-associated thyroid cancer. Cancer 2014;120:799-807.

30. Hemminki K, Eng C, Chen B. Familial risks for nonmedullary thyroid cancer. J Clin Endocrinol Metab 2005;90:5747-53.

31. Kebebew E. Hereditary non-medullary thyroid cancer. World J Surg 2008;32:678-82.

32. Bonora E, Tallini G, Romeo G. Genetic predisposition to familial nonmedullary thyroid cancer: an update of molecular findings and state-of-the-art studies. J Oncol 2010;2010:385206.

33. de la Chapelle A. Unraveling the genetic predisposition to differentiated thyroid carcinoma. J Clin Endocrinol Metab 2013;98:3974-6.

34. Melillo RM, Castellone MD, Guarino V, et al. The RET/PTC-RAS-BRAF linear signaling cascade mediates the motile and mitogenic phenotype of thyroid cancer cells. J Clin Invest 2005;115:1068-81.

35. Farid NR, Szkudlinski MW. Minireview: structural and functional evolution of the thyrotropin receptor. Endocrinology 2004;145:4048-57.

36. Krohn K, Führer D, Bayer Y, et al. Molecular pathogenesis of euthyroid and toxic multinodular goiter. Endocr Rev 2005;26:504-24.

37. Borland G, Smith BO, Yarwood SJ. EPAC proteins transduce diverse cellular actions of cAMP. Br J Pharmacol 2009;158:70-86.

38. Lyons J, Landis CA, Harsh G, et al. Two G protein oncogenes in human endocrine tumors. Science 1990;249:655-9.

39. O'Sullivan C, Barton CM, Staddon SL, Brown CL, Lemoine NR. Activating point mutations of the gsp oncogene in human thyroid adenomas. Mol Carcinog 1991;4:345-9.

40. Collins MT, Sarlis NJ, Merino MJ, et al. Thyroid carcinoma in the McCune-Albright syndrome: contributory role of activating Gs alpha mutations. J Clin Endocrinol Metab 2003;88:4413-7.

41. Michiels FM, Caillou B, Talbot M, et al. Oncogenic potential of guanine nucleotide stimulatory factor alpha subunit in thyroid glands of transgenic mice. Proc Natl Acad Sci U S A 1994;91:10488-92.

42. Parma J, Duprez L, Van Sande J, et al. Somatic mutations in the thyrotropin receptor gene cause hyperfunctioning thyroid adenomas. Nature 1993;365:649-51.

43. Parma J, Duprez L, Van Sande J, et al. Diversity and prevalence of somatic mutations in the thyrotropin receptor and Gs alpha genes as a cause of toxic thyroid adenomas. J Clin Endocrinol Metab 1997;82:2695-701.

44. Duprez L, Parma J, Van Sande J, et al. Germline mutations in the thyrotropin receptor gene cause non-autoimmune autosomal dominant hyperthyroidism. Nat Genet 1994;7:396-401.

45. Trulzsch B, Krohn K, Wonerow P, et al. Detection of thyroid-stimulating hormone receptor and Gsalpha mutations in 75 toxic thyroid nodules by denaturing gradient gel electrophoresis. J Mol Med (Berl) 2001;78:684-91.

46. Krohn K, Wohlgemuth S, Gerber H, Paschke R. Hot microscopic areas of iodine-deficient euthyroid goitres contain constitutively activating TSH receptor mutations. J Pathol 2000;192:37-42.

47. Spambalg D, Sharifi N, Elisei R, Gross JL, Medeiros-Neto G, Fagin JA. Structural studies of the thyrotropin receptor and Gs alpha in human thyroid cancers: low prevalence of mutations predicts infrequent involvement in malignant transformation. J Clin Endocrinol Metab 1996;81:3898-901.

48. Russo D, Tumino S, Arturi F, et al. Detection of an activating mutation of the thyrotropin receptor in a case of an autonomously hyperfunctioning thyroid insular carcinoma. J Clin Endocrinol Metab 1997;82:735-8.

49. Nikiforova MN, Wald AI, Roy S, Durso MB, Nikiforov YE. Targeted next-generation sequencing panel (ThyroSeq) for detection of mutations in thyroid cancer. J Clin Endocrinol Metab 2013;98:E1852-60.

50. Nellore A, Paziana K, Ma C, et al. Loss of Rap-1GAP in papillary thyroid cancer. J Clin Endocrinol Metab 2009;94:1026-32.

51. Zuo H, Gandhi M, Edreira MM, et al. Downregulation of Rap1GAP through epigenetic silencing and loss of heterozygosity promotes invasion and progression of thyroid tumors. Cancer Res 2010;70:1389-97.

52. Stratakis CA, Courcoutsakis NA, Abati A, et al. Thyroid gland abnormalities in patients with the syndrome of spotty skin pigmentation, myxomas, endocrine overactivity, and schwannomas (Carney complex). J Clin Endocrinol Metab 1997;82:2037-43.

53. Kirschner LS, Carney JA, Pack SD, et al. Mutations of the gene encoding the protein kinase A type I-alpha regulatory subunit in patients with the Carney complex. Nat Genet 2000;26:89-92.

54. Lodish MB, Stratakis CA. Rare and unusual endocrine cancer syndromes with mutated genes. Semin Oncol 2010;37:680-90.

55. Soares P, Trovisco V, Rocha AS, et al. BRAF mutations and RET/PTC rearrangements are alternative events in the etiopathogenesis of PTC. Oncogene 2003;22:4578-80.

56. Tanaka K, Nagayama Y, Nakano T, et al. Expression profile of receptor-type protein tyrosine kinase genes in the human thyroid. Endocrinology 1998;139:852-8.

57. Takahashi M, Ritz J, Cooper GM. Activation of a novel human transforming gene, ret, by DNA rearrangement. Cell 1985;42:581-8.

58. Takahashi M, Buma Y, Iwamoto T, Inaguma Y, Ikeda H, Hiai H. Cloning and expression of the ret proto-oncogene encoding a tyrosine kinase with two potential transmembrane domains. Oncogene 1988;3:571-8.

59. Ichihara M, Murakumo Y, Takahashi M. RET and neuroendocrine tumors. Cancer Lett 2004; 204:197-211.

60. Lai AZ, Gujral TS, Mulligan LM. RET signaling in endocrine tumors: delving deeper into molecular mechanisms. Endocr Pathol 2007;18:57-67.

61. Pachnis V, Mankoo B, Costantini F. Expression of the c-ret proto-oncogene during mouse embryogenesis. Development 1993;119:1005-17.

62. Schuchardt A, D'Agati V, Larsson-Blomberg L, Costantini F, Pachnis V. Defects in the kidney and enteric nervous system of mice lacking the tyrosine kinase receptor Ret. Nature 1994;367:380-3.

63. Lyonnet S, Bolino A, Pelet A, et al. A gene for Hirschsprung disease maps to the proximal long arm of chromosome 10. Nat Genet 1993;4:346-50.

64. Mulligan LM, Kwok JB, Healey CS, et al. Germline mutations of the RET proto-oncogene in multiple endocrine neoplasia type 2A. Nature 1993;363:458-60.

65. de Groot JW, Links TP, Plukker JT, Lips CJ, Hofstra RM. RET as a diagnostic and therapeutic target in sporadic and hereditary endocrine tumors. Endocr Rev 2006;27:535-60.

66. Castellone MD, Santoro M. Dysregulated RET signaling in thyroid cancer. Endocrinol Metab Clin North Am 2008;37:363-74, viii.

67. American Thyroid Association Guidelines Task Force, Kloos RT, Eng C, et al. Medullary thyroid cancer: management guidelines of the American Thyroid Association. Thyroid 2009;19:565-612.

68. Acton DS, Velthuyzen D, Lips CJ, Hoppener JW. Multiple endocrine neoplasia type 2B mutation in human RET oncogene induces medullary thyroid carcinoma in transgenic mice. Oncogene 2000;19:3121-5.

69. Reynolds L, Jones K, Winton DJ, et al. C-cell and thyroid epithelial tumours and altered follicular development in transgenic mice expressing the long isoform of MEN 2A RET. Oncogene 2001;20:3986-94.

70. Kawai K, Iwashita T, Murakami H, et al. Tissue-specific carcinogenesis in transgenic mice expressing the RET proto-oncogene with a multiple endocrine neoplasia type 2A mutation. Cancer Res 2000;60:5254-60.

71. Sweetser DA, Froelick GJ, Matsumoto AM, et al. Ganglioneuromas and renal anomalies are induced by activated RET(MEN2B) in transgenic mice. Oncogene 1999;18:877-86.

72. Marsh DJ, Zheng Z, Arnold A, et al. Mutation analysis of glial cell line-derived neurotrophic factor, a ligand for an RET/coreceptor complex, in multiple endocrine neoplasia type 2 and sporadic neuroendocrine tumors. J Clin Endocrinol Metab 1997;82:3025-8.

73. Schilling T, Burck J, Sinn HP, et al. Prognostic value of codon 918 (ATG-->ACG) RET proto-oncogene mutations in sporadic medullary thyroid carcinoma. Int J Cancer 2001;95:62-6.

74. Elisei R, Cosci B, Romei C, et al. Prognostic significance of somatic RET oncogene mutations in sporadic medullary thyroid cancer: a 10-year follow-up study. J Clin Endocrinol Metab 2008;93:682-7.

75. Grieco M, Santoro M, Berlingieri MT, et al. PTC is a novel rearranged form of the ret proto-oncogene and is frequently detected in vivo in human thyroid papillary carcinomas. Cell 1990;60:557-63.

76. Fusco A, Grieco M, Santoro M, et al. A new oncogene in human thyroid papillary carcinomas and their lymph-nodal metastases. Nature 1987;328:170-2.

77. Bongarzone I, Pierotti MA, Monzini N, et al. High frequency of activation of tyrosine kinase oncogenes in human papillary thyroid carcinoma. Oncogene 1989;4:1457-62.

78. Pierotti MA, Santoro M, Jenkins RB, et al. Characterization of an inversion on the long arm of chromosome 10 juxtaposing D10S170 and RET and creating the oncogenic sequence RET/PTC. Proc Natl Acad Sci U S A 1992;89:1616-20.

79. Santoro M, Carlomagno F, Hay ID, et al. Ret oncogene activation in human thyroid neoplasms is restricted to the papillary cancer subtype. J Clin Invest 1992;89:1517-22.

80. Minoletti F, Butti MG, Coronelli S, et al. The two genes generating RET/PTC3 are localized in chromosomal band 10q11.2. Genes Chromosomes Cancer 1994;11:51-7.

81. Tallini G, Asa SL. RET oncogene activation in papillary thyroid carcinoma. Adv Anat Pathol 2001;8:345-54.

82. Sozzi G, Bongarzone I, Miozzo M, et al. A t(10;17) translocation creates the RET/PTC2 chimeric transforming sequence in papillary thyroid carcinoma. Genes Chromosomes Cancer 1994;9:244-50.

83. Nikiforov YE, Rowland JM, Bove KE, Monforte-Munoz H, Fagin JA. Distinct pattern of ret oncogene rearrangements in morphological variants of radiation-induced and sporadic thyroid papillary carcinomas in children. Cancer Res 1997;57:1690-4.

84. Rabes HM, Demidchik EP, Sidorow JD, et al. Pattern of radiation-induced RET and NTRK1 rearrangements in 191 post-Chernobyl papillary thyroid carcinomas: biological, phenotypic, and clinical implications. Clin Cancer Res 2000;6:1093-103.

85. Nikiforova MN, Stringer JR, Blough R, Medvedovic M, Fagin JA, Nikiforov YE. Proximity of chromosomal loci that participate in radiation-induced rearrangements in human cells. Science 2000;290:138-41.

86. Lipson D, Capelletti M, Yelensky R, et al. Identification of new ALK and RET gene fusions from colorectal and lung cancer biopsies. Nat Med 2012;18:382-4.

87. Kohno T, Ichikawa H, Totoki Y, et al. KIF5B-RET fusions in lung adenocarcinoma. Nat Med 2012;18:375-7.

88. Ballerini P, Struski S, Cresson C, et al. RET fusion genes are associated with chronic myelomonocytic leukemia and enhance monocytic differentiation. Leukemia 2012;26:2384-9.

89. Unger K, Wienberg J, Riches A, et al. Novel gene rearrangements in transformed breast cells identified by high-resolution breakpoint analysis of chromosomal aberrations. Endocr Relat Cancer 2010;17:87-98.

90. Flavin R, Jackl G, Finn S, et al. RET/PTC rearrangement occurring in primary peritoneal carcinoma. Int J Surg Pathol 2009;17:187-97.

91. Ogino H, Yano S, Kakiuchi S, et al. Novel dual targeting strategy with vandetanib induces tumor cell apoptosis and inhibits angiogenesis in malignant pleural mesothelioma cells expressing RET oncogenic rearrangement. Cancer Lett 2008;265:55-66.

92. Santoro M, Chiappetta G, Cerrato A, et al. Development of thyroid papillary carcinomas secondary to tissue-specific expression of the RET/PTC1 oncogene in transgenic mice. Oncogene 1996;12:1821-6.

93. Powell DJ Jr, Russell J, Nibu K, et al. The RET/PTC3 oncogene: metastatic solid-type papillary carcinomas in murine thyroids. Cancer Res 1998;58:5523-8.

94. Fischer AH, Taysavang P, Jhiang SM. Nuclear envelope irregularity is induced by RET/PTC during interphase. Am J Pathol 2003;163:1091-100.

95. Ishizaka Y, Kobayashi S, Ushijima T, Hirohashi S, Sugimura T, Nagao M. Detection of retTPC/PTC transcripts in thyroid adenomas and adenomatous goiter by an RT-PCR method. Oncogene 1991;6:1667-72.

96. Fusco A, Chiappetta G, Hui P, et al. Assessment of RET/PTC oncogene activation and clonality in thyroid nodules with incomplete morphological evidence of papillary carcinoma: a search for the early precursors of papillary cancer. Am J Pathol 2002;160:2157-67.

97. Rhoden KJ, Unger K, Salvatore G, et al. RET/papillary thyroid cancer rearrangement in nonneoplastic thyrocytes: follicular cells of Hashimoto's thyroiditis share low-level recombination events with a subset of papillary carcinoma. J Clin Endocrinol Metab 2006;91:2414-23.

98. Adeniran AJ, Zhu Z, Gandhi M, et al. Correlation between genetic alterations and microscopic features, clinical manifestations, and prognostic characteristics of thyroid papillary carcinomas. Am J Surg Pathol 2006;30:216-22.

99. Bongarzone I, Vigneri P, Mariani L, Collini P, Pilotti S, Pierotti MA. RET/NTRK1 rearrangements in thyroid gland tumors of the papillary carcinoma family: correlation with clinicopathological features. Clin Cancer Res 1998;4:223-8.

100. Soares P, Fonseca E, Wynford-Thomas D, Sobrinho-Simões M. Sporadic ret-rearranged papillary carcinoma of the thyroid: a subset of slow growing, less aggressive thyroid neoplasms? J Pathol 1998;185:71-8.

101. Tallini G, Santoro M, Helie M, et al. RET/PTC oncogene activation defines a subset of papillary thyroid carcinomas lacking evidence of progression to poorly differentiated or undifferentiated tumor phenotypes. Clin Cancer Res 1998;4:287-94.

102. Santoro M, Papotti M, Chiappetta G, et al. RET activation and clinicopathologic features in poorly differentiated thyroid tumors. J Clin Endocrinol Metab 2002;87:370-9.

103. Martin-Zanca D, Hughes SH, Barbacid M. A human oncogene formed by the fusion of truncated tropomyosin and protein tyrosine kinase sequences. Nature 1986;319:743-8.

104. Radice P, Sozzi G, Miozzo M, et al. The human tropomyosin gene involved in the generation of the TRK oncogene maps to chromosome 1q31. Oncogene 1991;6:2145-8.

105. Greco A, Pierotti MA, Bongarzone I, et al. TRK-T1 is a novel oncogene formed by the fusion of TPR and TRK genes in human papillary thyroid carcinomas. Oncogene 1992;7:237-42.

106. Greco A, Miranda C, Pagliardini S, Fusetti L, Bongarzone I, Pierotti MA. Chromosome 1 rearrangements involving the genes TPR and NTRK1 produce structurally different thyroid-specific TRK oncogenes. Genes Chromosomes Cancer 1997;19:112-23.

107. Greco A, Mariani C, Miranda C, et al. The DNA rearrangement that generates the TRK-T3 oncogene involves a novel gene on chromosome 3 whose product has a potential coiled-coil domain. Mol Cell Biol 1995;15:6118-27.

108. Pierotti MA. Chromosomal rearrangements in thyroid carcinomas: a recombination or death dilemma. Cancer Lett 2001;166:1-7.

109. Russell JP, Powell DJ, Cunnane M, et al. The TRK-T1 fusion protein induces neoplastic transformation of thyroid epithelium. Oncogene 2000;19:5729-35.

110. Mariño-Enríquez A, Dal Cin P. ALK as a paradigm of oncogenic promiscuity: different mechanisms of activation and different fusion partners drive tumors of different lineages. Cancer Genet 2013;206:357-73.

111. Hamatani K, Mukai M, Takahashi K, Hayashi Y, Nakachi K, Kusunoki Y. Rearranged anaplastic lymphoma kinase (ALK) gene in adult-onset papillary thyroid cancer amongst atomic bomb survivors. Thyroid 2012;22:1153-9.

112. Kelly LM, Barila G, Liu P, et al. Identification of the transforming STRN-ALK fusion as a potential therapeutic target in the aggressive forms of thyroid cancer. Proc Natl Acad Sci U S A 2014;111:4233-8.

113. Pérot G, Soubeyran I, Ribeiro A, et al. Identification of a recurrent STRN/ALK fusion in thyroid carcinomas. PLoS One 2014;9:e87170.

114. Godbert Y, Henriques de Figueiredo B, Bonichon F, et al. Remarkable response to crizotinib in woman with anaplastic lymphoma kinase-rearranged anaplastic thyroid carcinoma. J Clin Oncol 2014. [Epub ahead of print]

115. Murugan AK, Xing M. Anaplastic thyroid cancers harbor novel oncogenic mutations of the ALK gene. Cancer Res 2011;71:4403-11.

116. Di Renzo MF, Olivero M, Serini G, et al. Overexpression of the c-MET/HGF receptor in human thyroid carcinomas derived from the follicular epithelium. J Endocrinol Invest 1995;18:134-9.

117. Ivan M, Bond JA, Prat M, Comoglio PM, Wynford-Thomas D. Activated ras and ret oncogenes induce over-expression of c-met (hepatocyte growth factor receptor) in human thyroid epithelial cells. Oncogene 1997;14:2417-23.

118. Belfiore A, Gangemi P, Costantino A, et al. Negative/low expression of the Met/hepatocyte growth factor receptor identifies papillary thyroid carcinomas with high risk of distant metastases. J Clin Endocrinol Metab 1997;82:2322-8.

119. Liu Z, Hou P, Ji M, Guan H, et al. Highly prevalent genetic alterations in receptor tyrosine kinases and phosphatidylinositol 3-kinase/akt and mitogen-activated protein kinase pathways in anaplastic and follicular thyroid cancers. J Clin Endocrinol Metab 2008;93:3106-16.

120. Ricarte-Filho JC, Matsuse M, Lau C, et al. Absence of common activating mutations of the epidermal growth factor receptor gene in thyroid cancers from American and Japanese patients. Int J Cancer 2012;130:2215-7; author reply 2217-8.

121. Bos JL. Ras oncogenes in human cancer: a review. Cancer Res 1989;49:4682-9.

122. Malumbres M, Barbacid M. RAS oncogenes: the first 30 years. Nat Rev Cancer 2003;3:459-65.

123. Rochefort P, Caillou B, Michiels FM, et al. Thyroid pathologies in transgenic mice expressing a human activated Ras gene driven by a thyroglobulin promoter. Oncogene 1996;12:111-8.

124. Vitagliano D, Portella G, Troncone G, et al. Thyroid targeting of the N-ras(Gln61Lys) oncogene in transgenic mice results in follicular tumors that progress to poorly differentiated carcinomas. Oncogene 2006;25:5467-74.

125. Moura MM, Cavaco BM, Pinto AE, Leite V. High prevalence of RAS mutations in RET-negative sporadic medullary thyroid carcinomas. J Clin Endocrinol Metab 2011;96:E863-8.

126. Boichard A, Croux L, Al Ghuzlan A, et al. Somatic RAS mutations occur in a large proportion of sporadic RET-negative medullary thyroid carcinomas and extend to a previously unidentified exon. J Clin Endocrinol Metab 2012;97:E2031-5.

127. Ciampi R, Mian C, Fugazzola L, et al. Evidence of a low prevalence of RAS mutations in a large medullary thyroid cancer series. Thyroid 2013;23:50-7.

128. Shi YF, Zou MJ, Schmidt H, et al. High rates of ras codon 61 mutation in thyroid tumors in an iodide-deficient area. Cancer Res 1991;51:2690-3.

129. Castro P, Soares P, Gusmao L, Seruca R, Sobrinho-Simoes M. H-RAS 81 polymorphism is significantly associated with aneuploidy in follicular tumors of the thyroid. Oncogene 2006;25:4620-7.

130. Basolo F, Pisaturo F, Pollina LE, et al. N-ras mutation in poorly differentiated thyroid carcinomas: correlation with bone metastases and inverse correlation to thyroglobulin expression. Thyroid 2000;10:19-23.

131. Garcia-Rostan G, Zhao H, Camp RL, et al. Ras mutations are associated with aggressive tumor phenotypes and poor prognosis in thyroid cancer. J Clin Oncol 2003;21:3226-35.

132. Volante M, Rapa I, Gandhi M, et al. RAS mutations are the predominant molecular alteration in poorly differentiated thyroid carcinomas and bear prognostic impact. J Clin Endocrinol Metab 2009;94:4735-41.

133. Marais R, Light Y, Paterson HF, Mason CS, Marshall CJ. Differential regulation of Raf-1, A-Raf, and B-Raf by oncogenic ras and tyrosine kinases. J Biol Chem 1997;272:4378-83.

134. Peyssonnaux C, Eychene A. The Raf/MEK/ERK pathway: new concepts of activation. Biol Cell 2001;93:53-62.
135. Davies H, Bignell GR, Cox C, et al. Mutations of the BRAF gene in human cancer. Nature 2002;417:949-54.
136. Wan PT, Garnett MJ, Roe SM, et al. Mechanism of activation of the RAF-ERK signaling pathway by oncogenic mutations of BRAF. Cell 2004;116:855-67.
137. Roskoski R Jr. RAF protein-serine/threonine kinases: structure and regulation. Biochem Biophys Res Commun 2010;399:313-7.
138. Trovisco V, Vieira de Castro I, Soares P, et al. BRAF mutations are associated with some histological types of papillary thyroid carcinoma. J Pathol 2004;202:247-51.
139. Trovisco V, Soares P, Soares R, Magalhaes J, Sa-Couto P, Sobrinho-Simões M. A new BRAF gene mutation detected in a case of a solid variant of papillary thyroid carcinoma. Hum Pathol 2005;36:694-7.
140. Carta C, Moretti S, Passeri L, et al. Genotyping of an Italian papillary thyroid carcinoma cohort revealed high prevalence of BRAF mutations, absence of RAS mutations and allowed the detection of a new mutation of BRAF oncoprotein (BRAF(V599Ins)). Clin Endocrinol (Oxf) 2006;64:105-9.
141. De Falco V, Giannini R, Tamburrino A, et al. Functional characterization of the novel T599I-VKSRdel BRAF mutation in a follicular variant papillary thyroid carcinoma. J Clin Endocrinol Metab 2008;93:4398-402.
142. Lupi C, Giannini R, Ugolini C, et al. Association of BRAF V600E mutation with poor clinicopathological outcomes in 500 consecutive cases of papillary thyroid carcinoma. J Clin Endocrinol Metab 2007;92:4085-90.
143. Garnett MJ, Rana S, Paterson H, Barford D, Marais R. Wild-type and mutant B-RAF activate C-RAF through distinct mechanisms involving heterodimerization. Mol Cell 2005;20:963-9.
144. Kimura ET, Nikiforova MN, Zhu Z, Knauf JA, Nikiforov YE, Fagin JA. High prevalence of BRAF mutations in thyroid cancer: genetic evidence for constitutive activation of the RET/PTC-RAS-BRAF signaling pathway in papillary thyroid carcinoma. Cancer Res 2003;63:1454-7.
145. Cohen Y, Xing M, Mambo E, et al. BRAF mutation in papillary thyroid carcinoma. J Natl Cancer Inst 2003;95:625-7.
146. Nikiforova MN, Kimura ET, Gandhi M, et al. BRAF mutations in thyroid tumors are restricted to papillary carcinomas and anaplastic or poorly differentiated carcinomas arising from papillary carcinomas. J Clin Endocrinol Metab 2003;88:5399-404.
147. Xing M. BRAF mutation in thyroid cancer. Endocr Relat Cancer 2005;12:245-62.
148. Cradic KW, Milosevic D, Rosenberg AM, Erickson LA, McIver B, Grebe SK. Mutant BRAF(T1799A) can be detected in the blood of papillary thyroid carcinoma patients and correlates with disease status. J Clin Endocrinol Metab 2009;94:5001-9.
149. Flavin R, Smyth P, Crotty P, et al. BRAF T1799A mutation occurring in a case of malignant struma ovarii. Int J Surg Pathol 2007;15:116-20.
150. Schmidt J, Derr V, Heinrich MC, et al. BRAF in papillary thyroid carcinoma of ovary (struma ovarii). Am J Surg Pathol 2007;31:1337-43.
151. Trovisco V, Soares P, Preto A, et al. Type and prevalence of BRAF mutations are closely associated with papillary thyroid carcinoma histotype and patients' age but not with tumour aggressiveness. Virchows Arch 2005;446:589-95.
152. Pennelli G, Vianello F, Barollo S, et al. BRAF(K601E) mutation in a patient with a follicular thyroid carcinoma. Thyroid 2011; 21:1393-6.
153. Kim SW, Lee JI, Kim JW, et al. BRAFV600E mutation analysis in fine-needle aspiration cytology specimens for evaluation of thyroid nodule: a large series in a BRAFV600E-prevalent population. J Clin Endocrinol Metab 2010;95:3693-700.
154. Mitsutake N, Miyagishi M, Mitsutake S, et al. BRAF mediates RET/PTC-induced mitogen-activated protein kinase activation in thyroid cells: functional support for requirement of the RET/PTC-RAS-BRAF pathway in papillary thyroid carcinogenesis. Endocrinology 2006;147:1014-9.
155. Liu D, Liu Z, Condouris S, Xing M. BRAF V600E maintains proliferation, transformation, and tumorigenicity of BRAF-mutant papillary thyroid cancer cells. J Clin Endocrinol Metab 2007;92:2264-71.
156. Knauf JA, Ma X, Smith EP, et al. Targeted expression of BRAFV600E in thyroid cells of transgenic mice results in papillary thyroid cancers that undergo dedifferentiation. Cancer Res 2005;65:4238-45.
157. Chakravarty D, Santos E, Ryder M, et al. Small-molecule MAPK inhibitors restore radioiodine incorporation in mouse thyroid cancers with conditional BRAF activation. J Clin Invest 2011;121:4700-11.
158. Nucera C, Porrello A, Antonello ZA, et al. B-Raf(V600E) and thrombospondin-1 promote thyroid cancer progression. Proc Natl Acad Sci U S A 2010;107:10649-54.
159. Knauf JA, Sartor MA, Medvedovic M, et al. Progression of BRAF-induced thyroid cancer is associated with epithelial-mesenchymal transition requiring concomitant MAP kinase and TGFβ signaling. Oncogene 2011;30:3153-62.

160. Vasko V, Espinosa AV, Scouten W, et al. Gene expression and functional evidence of epithelial-to-mesenchymal transition in papillary thyroid carcinoma invasion. Proc Natl Acad Sci U S A 2007;104:2803-8.

161. Durante C, Puxeddu E, Ferretti E, et al. BRAF mutations in papillary thyroid carcinomas inhibit genes involved in iodine metabolism. J Clin Endocrinol Metab 2007;92:2840-3.

162. Riesco-Eizaguirre G, Gutierrez-Martinez P, Garcia-Cabezas MA, Nistal M, Santisteban P. The oncogene BRAF V600E is associated with a high risk of recurrence and less differentiated papillary thyroid carcinoma due to the impairment of Na+/I- targeting to the membrane. Endocr Relat Cancer 2006;13:257-69.

163. Xing M. BRAF mutation in papillary thyroid cancer: pathogenic role, molecular bases, and clinical implications. Endocr Rev 2007;28:742-62.

164. Ricarte-Filho JC, Ryder M, Chitale DA, et al. Mutational profile of advanced primary and metastatic radioactive iodine-refractory thyroid cancers reveals distinct pathogenetic roles for BRAF, PIK3CA, and AKT1. Cancer Res 2009;69:4885-93.

165. Xing M, Westra WH, Tufano RP, et al. BRAF mutation predicts a poorer clinical prognosis for papillary thyroid cancer. J Clin Endocrinol Metab 2005;90:6373-9.

166. Kim TY, Kim WB, Rhee YS, et al. The BRAF mutation is useful for prediction of clinical recurrence in low-risk patients with conventional papillary thyroid carcinoma. Clin Endocrinol (Oxf) 2006;65:364-8.

167. Elisei R, Ugolini C, Viola D, et al. BRAF(V600E) mutation and outcome of patients with papillary thyroid carcinoma: a 15-year median follow-up study. J Clin Endocrinol Metab 2008;93:3943-9.

168. Basolo F, Torregrossa L, Giannini R, et al. Correlation between the BRAF V600E mutation and tumor invasiveness in papillary thyroid carcinomas smaller than 20 millimeters: analysis of 1060 cases. J Clin Endocrinol Metab 2010;95:4197-205.

169. Fugazzola L, Puxeddu E, Avenia N, et al. Correlation between B-RAFV600E mutation and clinico-pathologic parameters in papillary thyroid carcinoma: data from a multicentric Italian study and review of the literature. Endocr Relat Cancer 2006;13:455-64.

170. Ito Y, Yoshida H, Maruo R, et al. BRAF mutation in papillary thyroid carcinoma in a Japanese population: its lack of correlation with high-risk clinicopathological features and disease-free survival of patients. Endocr J 2009;56:89-97.

171. Pelttari H, Schalin-Jäntti C, Arola J, Löyttyniemi E, Knuutila S, Välimäki MJ. BRAF V600E mutation does not predict recurrence after long-term follow-up in TNM stage I or II papillary thyroid carcinoma patients. APMIS 2012;120:380-6.

172. Sancisi V, Nicoli D, Ragazzi M, Piana S, Ciarrocchi A. BRAFV600E mutation does not mean distant metastasis in thyroid papillary carcinomas. J Clin Endocrinol Metab 2012;97:E1745-9.

173. Xing M, Alzahrani AS, Carson KA, et al. Association between BRAF V600E mutation and mortality in patients with papillary thyroid cancer. JAMA 2013;309:1493-501.

174. Guerra A, Fugazzola L, Marotta V, et al. A High Percentage of BRAFV600E alleles in papillary thyroid carcinoma predicts a poorer outcome. J Clin Endocrinol Metab 2012;97:2333-40.

175. Guerra A, Sapio MR, Marotta V, et al. The primary occurrence of BRAF(V600E) is a rare clonal event in papillary thyroid carcinoma. J Clin Endocrinol Metab 2012;97:517-24.

176. Ghossein RA, Katabi N, Fagin JA. Immunohistochemical detection of mutated BRAF V600E supports the clonal origin of BRAF-induced thyroid cancers along the spectrum of disease progression. J Clin Endocrinol Metab 2013;98:E1414-21.

177. de Biase D, Cesari V, Visani M, et al. High sensitivity brafmutation analysis: BRAF V600E is acquired early during tumor development but is heterogeneously distributed in a subset of papillary thyroid carcinomas. J Clin Endocrinol Metab 2014;99:E1530-8.

178. Mathur A, Moses W, Rahbari R, et al. Higher rate of BRAF mutation in papillary thyroid cancer over time: a single-institution study. Cancer 2011;117:4390-5.

179. Jung CK, Little MP, Lubin JH, et al. The increase in thyroid cancer incidence during the last four decades is accompanied by a high frequency of BRAF mutations and a sharp increase in RAS mutations. J Clin Endocrinol Metab 2014;99:276-85.

180. Lima J, Trovisco V, Soares P, et al. BRAF mutations are not a major event in post-Chernobyl childhood thyroid carcinomas. J Clin Endocrinol Metab 2004;89:4267-71.

181. Ciampi R, Knauf JA, Kerler R, et al. Oncogenic AKAP9-BRAF fusion is a novel mechanism of MAPK pathway activation in thyroid cancer. J Clin Invest 2005;115:94-101.

182. Ringel MD, Hayre N, Saito J, et al. Overexpression and overactivation of Akt in thyroid carcinoma. Cancer Res 2001;61:6105-11.

183. Sansal I, Sellers WR. The biology and clinical relevance of the PTEN tumor suppressor pathway. J Clin Oncol 2004;22:2954-63.

184. Engelman JA, Luo J, Cantley LC. The evolution of phosphatidylinositol 3-kinases as regulators of growth and metabolism. Nat Rev Genet 2006;7:606-19.

185. Leevers SJ, Vanhaesebroeck B, Waterfield MD. Signalling through phosphoinositide 3-kinases: the lipids take centre stage. Curr Opin Cell Biol 1999;11:219-25.

186. Vogt PK, Kang S, Elsliger MA, Gymnopoulos M. Cancer-specific mutations in phosphatidylinositol 3-kinase. Trends Biochem Sci 2007;32:342-9.

187. Cully M, You H, Levine AJ, Mak TW. Beyond PTEN mutations: the PI3K pathway as an integrator of multiple inputs during tumorigenesis. Nat Rev Cancer 2006;6:184-92.

188. Staal SP. Molecular cloning of the akt oncogene and its human homologues AKT1 and AKT2: amplification of AKT1 in a primary human gastric adenocarcinoma. Proc Natl Acad Sci U S A 1987;84:5034-7.

189. Sarbassov DD, Guertin DA, Ali SM, Sabatini DM. Phosphorylation and regulation of Akt/PKB by the rictor-mTOR complex. Science 2005;307:1098-101.

190. Paes JE, Ringel MD. Dysregulation of the phosphatidylinositol 3-kinase pathway in thyroid neoplasia. Endocrinol Metab Clin North Am 2008;37:375-87, viii-ix.

191. Santarpia L, El-Naggar AK, Cote GJ, Myers JN, Sherman SI. Phosphatidylinositol 3-kinase/akt and ras/raf-mitogen-activated protein kinase pathway mutations in anaplastic thyroid cancer. J Clin Endocrinol Metab 2008;93:278-84.

192. Garcia-Rostan G, Costa AM, Pereira-Castro I, et al. Mutation of the PIK3CA gene in anaplastic thyroid cancer. Cancer Res 2005;65:10199-207.

193. Hou P, Liu D, Shan Y, et al. Genetic alterations and their relationship in the phosphatidylinositol 3-kinase/Akt pathway in thyroid cancer. Clin Cancer Res 2007;13:1161-70.

194. Maehama T, Dixon JE. PTEN: a tumour suppressor that functions as a phospholipid phosphatase. Trends Cell Biol 1999;9:125-8.

195. Eng C. PTEN: one gene, many syndromes. Hum Mutat 2003;22:183-98.

196. Liaw D, Marsh DJ, Li J, et al. Germline mutations of the PTEN gene in Cowden disease, an inherited breast and thyroid cancer syndrome. Nat Genet 1997;16:64-7.

197. Longy M, Lacombe D. Cowden disease. Report of a family and review. Ann Genet 1996;39:35-42.

198. Pilarski R, Eng C. Will the real Cowden syndrome please stand up (again)? Expanding mutational and clinical spectra of the PTEN hamartoma tumour syndrome. J Med Genet 2004;41:323-6.

199. Hobert JA, Eng C. PTEN hamartoma tumor syndrome: an overview. Genet Med 2009;11:687-94.

200. Di Cristofano A, Pesce B, Cordon-Cardo C, Pandolfi PP. PTEN is essential for embryonic development and tumour suppression. Nat Genet 1998;19:348-55.

201. Bruni P, Boccia A, Baldassarre G, et al. PTEN expression is reduced in a subset of sporadic thyroid carcinomas: evidence that PTEN-growth suppressing activity in thyroid cancer cells mediated by p27kip1. Oncogene 2000;19:3146-55.

202. Gimm O, Perren A, Weng LP, et al. Differential nuclear and cytoplasmic expression of PTEN in normal thyroid tissue, and benign and malignant epithelial thyroid tumors. Am J Pathol 2000;156:1693-700.

203. Alvarez-Nunez F, Bussaglia E, Mauricio D, et al. PTEN promoter methylation in sporadic thyroid carcinomas. Thyroid 2006;16:17-23.

204. Hou P, Ji M, Xing M. Association of PTEN gene methylation with genetic alterations in the phosphatidylinositol 3-kinase/AKT signaling pathway in thyroid tumors. Cancer 2008;113:2440-7.

205. Kroll TG, Sarraf P, Pecciarini L, et al. PAX8-PPAR-gamma1 fusion oncogene in human thyroid carcinoma. Science 2000;289:1357-60.

206. Jenkins RB, Hay ID, Herath JF, et al. Frequent occurrence of cytogenetic abnormalities in sporadic nonmedullary thyroid carcinoma. Cancer 1990;66:1213-20.

207. McIver B, Grebe SK, Eberhardt NL. The PAX8/PPAR gamma fusion oncogene as a potential therapeutic target in follicular thyroid carcinoma. Curr Drug Targets Immune Endocr Metabol Disord 2004;4:221-34.

208. Eberhardt NL, Grebe SK, McIver B, Reddi HV. The role of the PAX8/PPARgamma fusion oncogene in the pathogenesis of follicular thyroid cancer. Mol Cell Endocrinol 2010;321:50-6.

209. Macchia PE, Lapi P, Krude H, et al. PAX8 mutations associated with congenital hypothyroidism caused by thyroid dysgenesis. Nat Genet 1998;19:83-6.

210. De Felice M, Di Lauro R. Thyroid development and its disorders: genetics and molecular mechanisms. Endocr Rev 2004;25:722-46.

211. Nikiforova MN, Biddinger PW, Caudill CM, Kroll TG, Nikiforov YE. PAX8-PPARgamma rearrangement in thyroid tumors: RT-PCR and immunohistochemical analyses. Am J Surg Pathol 2002;26:1016-23.

212. Marques AR, Espadinha C, Catarino AL, et al. Expression of PAX8-PPAR gamma 1 rearrangements in both follicular thyroid carcinomas and adenomas. J Clin Endocrinol Metab 2002;87:3947-52.

213. Cheung L, Messina M, Gill A, et al. Detection of the PAX8-PPAR gamma fusion oncogene in both follicular thyroid carcinomas and adenomas. J Clin Endocrinol Metab 2003;88:354-7.

214. Castro P, Rebocho AP, Soares RJ, et al. PAX8-PPARgamma rearrangement is frequently detected in the follicular variant of papillary thyroid carcinoma. J Clin Endocrinol Metab 2006;91:213-20.

215. Lui WO, Zeng L, Rehrmann V, et al. CREB3L2-PPARgamma fusion mutation identifies a thyroid signaling pathway regulated by intramembrane proteolysis. Cancer Res 2008;68:7156-64.

216. Kondo S, Saito A, Hino S, et al. BBF2H7, a novel transmembrane bZIP transcription factor, is a new type of endoplasmic reticulum stress transducer. Mol Cell Biol 2007;27:1716-29.

217. Mertens F, Fletcher CD, Antonescu CR, et al. Clinicopathologic and molecular genetic characterization of low-grade fibromyxoid sarcoma, and cloning of a novel FUS/CREB3L1 fusion gene. Lab Invest 2005;85:408-15.

218. Peifer M, Polakis P. Wnt signaling in oncogenesis and embryogenesis—a look outside the nucleus. Science 2000;287:1606-9.

219. Saadeddin A, Babaei-Jadidi R, Spencer-Dene B, Nateri AS. The links between transcription, beta-catenin/JNK signaling, and carcinogenesis. Mol Cancer Res 2009;7:1189-96.

220. Polakis P. Wnt signaling in cancer. Cold Spring Harb Perspect Biol 2012;4(5). pii: a008052.

221. Morin PJ, Sparks AB, Korinek V, et al. Activation of beta-catenin-Tcf signaling in colon cancer by mutations in beta-catenin or APC. Science 1997;275:1787-90.

222. Cameselle-Teijeiro J, Ruiz-Ponte C, Loidi L, Suarez-Penaranda J, Baltar J, Sobrinho-Simões M. Somatic but not germline mutation of the APC gene in a case of cribriform-morular variant of papillary thyroid carcinoma. Am J Clin Pathol 2001;115:486-93.

223. Xu B, Yoshimoto K, Miyauchi A, et al. Cribriform-morular variant of papillary thyroid carcinoma: a pathological and molecular genetic study with evidence of frequent somatic mutations in exon 3 of the beta-catenin gene. J Pathol 2003;199:58-67.

224. von Wasielewski R, Rhein A, Werner M, et al. Immunohistochemical detection of E-cadherin in differentiated thyroid carcinomas correlates with clinical outcome. Cancer Res 1997;57:2501-7.

225. Garcia-Rostan G, Camp RL, Herrero A, Carcangiu ML, Rimm DL, Tallini G. Beta-catenin dysregulation in thyroid neoplasms: downregulation, aberrant nuclear expression, and CTNNB1 exon 3 mutations are markers for aggressive tumor phenotypes and poor prognosis. Am J Pathol 2001;158:987-96.

226. Kurihara T, Ikeda S, Ishizaki Y, et al. Immunohistochemical and sequencing analyses of the Wnt signaling components in Japanese anaplastic thyroid cancers. Thyroid 2004;14:1020-9.

227. Wiseman SM, Masoudi H, Niblock P, et al. Derangement of the E-cadherin/catenin complex is involved in transformation of differentiated to anaplastic thyroid carcinoma. Am J Surg 2006;191:581-7.

228. Garcia-Rostán G, Tallini G, Herrero A, D'Aquila TG, Carcangiu ML, Rimm DL. Frequent mutation and nuclear localization of beta-catenin in anaplastic thyroid carcinoma. Cancer Res 1999;59:1811-5.

229. Bernardes de Jesus B, Blasco MA. Telomerase at the intersection of cancer and aging. Trends Genet 2013;29:513-20.

230. Muller HJ. The remaking of chromosomes. The Collecting Net-Woods Hole. 1938;13:181-98.

231. Watson JD. Origin of concatemeric T7DNA. Nat New Biol 1972;239:197–201.

232. Olovnikov AM. A theory of marginotomy. The incomplete copying of template margin in enzymic synthesis of polynucleotides and biological significance of the phenomenon. J Theor Biol 1973;41:181-90.

233. Hayflick L, Moorhead PS. The serial cultivation of human diploid cell strains. Exp Cell Res 1961;25:585–621.

234. Armanios M, Blackburn EH. The telomere syndromes. Nat Rev Genet 2012;13:693-704.

235. Horn S, Figl A, Rachakonda PS, et al. TERT promoter mutations in familial and sporadic melanoma. Science 2013;339:959-61.

236. Huang FW, Hodis E, Xu MJ, Kryukov GV, Chin L, Garraway LA. Highly recurrent TERT promoter mutations in human melanoma. Science 2013;339:957-9.

237. Killela PJ, Reitman ZJ, Jiao Y, et al. TERT promoter mutations occur frequently in gliomas and a subset of tumors derived from cells with low rates of self-renewal. Proc Natl Acad Sci U S A 2013;110:6021-6.

238. Bryan TM, Englezou A, Dalla-Pozza L, Dunham MA, Reddel RR. Evidence for an alternative mechanism for maintaining telomere length in human tumors and tumor-derived cell lines. Nat Med 1997;3:1271-4.

239. Saji M, Xydas S, Westra WH, et al. Human telomerase reverse transcriptase (hTERT) gene expression in thyroid neoplasms. Clin Cancer Res 1999;5:1483-9.

240. Wang N, Xu D, Sofiadis A, et al. Telomerase-dependent and independent telomere maintenance and its clinical implications in medullary thyroid carcinoma. J Clin Endocrinol Metab 2014;99:E1571-9.

241. Wang Y, Meeker AK, Kowalski J, et al. Telomere length is related to alternative splice patterns of telomerase in thyroid tumors. Am J Pathol 2011;179:1415-24.

242. Landa I, Ganly I, Chan TA, et al. Frequent somatic TERT promoter mutations in thyroid cancer: higher prevalence in advanced forms of the disease. J Clin Endocrinol Metab 2013;98:1562-6.

243. Liu T, Wang N, Cao J, et al. The age- and shorter telomere-dependent TERT promoter mutation in follicular thyroid cell-derived carcinomas. Oncogene 2014;33:4978-84.

244. Liu X, Bishop J, Shan Y, et al. Highly prevalent TERT promoter mutations in aggressive thyroid cancers. Endocr Relat Cancer 2013;20:603-10.

245. Vinagre J, Almeida A, Pópulo H, et al. Frequency of TERT promoter mutations in human cancers. Nat Commun 2013;4:2185.

246. Melo M, da Rocha AG, Vinagre J, et al. TERT promoter mutations are a major indicator of poor outcome in differentiated thyroid carcinomas. J Clin Endocrinol Metab 2014;99:E754-65.

247. Liu X, Qu S, Liu R, et al. TERT promoter mutations and their association with BRAF V600E mutation and aggressive clinicopathological characteristics of thyroid cancer. J Clin Endocrinol Metab 2014;99:E1130-6.

248. Wang N, Liu T, Sofiadis A, et al. TERT promoter mutation as an early genetic event activating telomerase in follicular thyroid adenoma (FTA) and atypical FTA. Cancer 2014;120:2965-79.

249. Levine AJ, Oren M. The first 30 years of p53: growing ever more complex. Nat Rev Cancer 2009;9:749-58.

250. Ito T, Seyama T, Mizuno T, et al. Unique association of p53 mutations with undifferentiated but not with differentiated carcinomas of the thyroid gland. Cancer Res 1992;52:1369-71.

251. Donghi R, Longoni A, Pilotti S, Michieli P, Della Porta G, Pierotti MA. Gene p53 mutations are restricted to poorly differentiated and undifferentiated carcinomas of the thyroid gland. J Clin Invest 1993;91:1753-60.

252. Dobashi Y, Sugimura H, Sakamoto A, et al. Stepwise participation of p53 gene mutation during dedifferentiation of human thyroid carcinomas. Diagn Mol Pathol 1994;3:9-14.

253. Quiros RM, Ding HG, Gattuso P, Prinz RA, Xu X. Evidence that one subset of anaplastic thyroid carcinomas are derived from papillary carcinomas due to BRAF and p53 mutations. Cancer 2005;103:2261-8.

254. Nikiforov YE, Nikiforova MN, Gnepp DR, Fagin JA. Prevalence of mutations of ras and p53 in benign and malignant thyroid tumors from children exposed to radiation after the Chernobyl nuclear accident. Oncogene 1996;13:687-93.

255. Fagin JA, Tang SH, Zeki K, Di Lauro R, Fusco A, Gonsky R. Reexpression of thyroid peroxidase in a derivative of an undifferentiated thyroid carcinoma cell line by introduction of wild-type p53. Cancer Res 1996;56:765-71.

256. Moretti F, Farsetti A, Soddu S, et al. p53 reexpression inhibits proliferation and restores differentiation of human thyroid anaplastic carcinoma cells. Oncogene 1997;14:729-40.

3 GENERAL FEATURES OF THYROID TUMORS

INCIDENCE OF THYROID CARCINOMA

Thyroid carcinoma is by far the most common type of endocrine gland malignancy, even though it represents only about 1 percent of all clinically detectable human cancers. The number of estimated new thyroid cancer cases in the United States in 2013 is 60,220, and the number of estimated deaths for the same period is 1,850 (1). The incidence rate of thyroid cancer has been increasing sharply since the mid-1990s, and it is the fastest increasing cancer in both men and women. Some studies suggest that the rise is due to the increased detection of small tumors through ultrasound and confirmation via fine-needle aspiration, while others argue that it is in part real, and involves both small and large tumors (1).

THYROID TUMORS AND IODINE DEFICIENCY

Dietary iodine deficiency, historically known to be the major cause of endemic goiter, is also linked to the development of thyroid carcinoma, particularly of the follicular type (2). Conversely, papillary carcinoma is more frequent in regions of adequate or high dietary iodine intake. In areas of iodine deficiency, the relative frequency of papillary carcinoma increases after iodine supplementation, but it is not clear whether this is due to an absolute increase in the incidence of papillary carcinoma or a drop in the incidence of follicular carcinoma (3).

A significant decrease in the number of undifferentiated (anaplastic) carcinomas has been noted following dietary iodine administration, both in Europe and South America (4). A higher dietary intake of iodine has also been found to be associated with a high frequency of thyroiditis (5).

THYROID TUMORS AND RADIATION EXPOSURE

During the first half of this century, low-dose radiation to the head and neck region of children and adolescents was a common form of therapy for disorders such as "thymic enlargement," tonsillar hypertrophy, tuberculous adenitis, hemangiomas, nevi, eczema, and acne. The average dose was about 600 rads. In the United States, approximately 1,000,000 people were subjected to this treatment, which resulted in a variety of thyroid diseases later in life, particularly in women. Approximately one fourth of the population at risk developed thyroid nodules, with the risk being substantially greater if the radiation was given before the age of 7 years (6,7). Most of these nodules (about 75 percent) were benign and showed the features of nodular hyperplasia, follicular adenoma (rare), lymphocytic thyroiditis, oncocytic change, focal fibrosis, and atrophy (8–12). The treatment for these benign follicular nodules was the same as for those seen in the general population, i.e., lobectomy or subtotal thyroidectomy, depending on their size and number. The incidence of recurrence after surgery, which was similar to that seen in nonirradiated patients, was substantially decreased if thyroid hormone was given postoperatively to suppress thyroid-stimulating hormone (TSH) secretion (13).

There was also an increased occurrence of carcinoma in this population, supporting the belief that irradiation is the most clearly documented etiologic factor for thyroid malignancy. Most of the tumors were papillary carcinomas (7,14–16). The incidence of this tumor type among irradiated patients having a thyroid operation ranged from 20 to over 50 percent in the various series, and it partially depended on the extent of the operation and the thoroughness of the pathologic examination (17,18). The median latency period for the development of malignancy was approximately 20 years. Many of these papillary carcinomas showed evidence of multicentricity and/or intraglandular spread and cervical lymph node involvement, perhaps more than in those occurring in the general population, but the long-term prognosis of patients was the same (6).

Other structures in the region are also subject to radiation-induced neoplasia. Benign and (less commonly) malignant tumors of salivary glands, parathyroid glands, bone, and soft tissues have been reported in this population, emphasizing the need for continued surveillance (19,20). Isolated examples of postradiation thyroid lymphoma also have been reported (21).

Thyroid carcinoma and other thyroid abnormalities also result from high-dose radiation to the region, such as that administered for Hodgkin lymphoma, breast carcinoma, and other malignant neoplasms (10,22–27). In contrast, the risk of thyroid cancer due to the use of medical diagnostic X rays is small, if present at all (28).

The dramatic increase in the incidence of thyroid carcinoma in individuals exposed to the accident at the nuclear power plant at Chernobyl in 1986 (29,30) provided definitive evidence that exposure to ^{131}I in childhood is associated with an increased risk of thyroid cancer (31). The Chernobyl cohort was overwhelmingly composed of papillary carcinomas (32), and is further discussed in chapter 7. Suffice to say here that the morphologic features of Chernobyl-related childhood papillary thyroid carcinomas seem to be independent of radiation exposure. Specifically, and in contrast with others (33), we found no significant differences between papillary thyroid carcinomas from radiation-exposed children from Belarus/Ukraine/Russian Federation and those from children from the same countries who had not been exposed to radiation (33a). Rather, the differences observed seemed to be related to dietary iodine levels, suggesting that iodine deficiency could increase the incidence and reduce the latency, thus influencing tumor morphology and aggressiveness (34).

THYROID TUMORS IN CHILDHOOD

The morphologic appearance of the thyroid tumors and tumor-like conditions developing in infants and children does not differ significantly from that of the corresponding lesions in adults; however, their relative frequency does. The most important difference is the higher frequency of carcinoma in the former, to the point that, in some recent series, the malignant tumors surpass the benign processes (35,36). It has been estimated that the risk of malignancy in a solitary thyroid nodule is about 50 percent in patients under 25 years of age and 75 percent in patients under 15 years of age.

Among the malignancies, papillary carcinoma comprises by far most of the cases, and its relative frequency is even higher than in adults (37–39). This is followed by the familial form of medullary carcinoma and by oncocytic neoplasms (40). In some older series, there is also a fair number of follicular carcinomas, but we suspect that many of them would be regarded as follicular variants of papillary carcinoma by current criteria (41,42). In the pediatric series of Sierk et al. (38), not a single case of nononcocytic follicular carcinoma was found on a review of 32 patients. Undifferentiated carcinomas are almost nonexistent in this age group, and poorly differentiated carcinomas are very rare.

The papillary carcinomas occurring in children tend to have extensive solid and/or squamous areas. They are associated with a higher frequency of cervical lymph node and lung metastases than their adult counterparts, but the overall prognosis is still excellent (43–48). A few cases of congenital papillary carcinoma have been reported (49). In recent series, the history of previous irradiation to the neck was present in about 25 percent of the patients. This figure is substantially lower than in series published before 1970, in some of which it was as high as 80 percent (38). Some of the reported cases have been seen in children who had undergone successful multimodal management of malignant tumors such as acute leukemia or nephroblastoma (50). As with adult cases, the presence of aneuploidy in pediatric thyroid malignancies does not seem to correlate with either the extent of the disease at diagnosis or patient outcome (50).

REFERENCES

1. Siegel R, Naishadham D, Jemal A. Cancer statistics, 2013. CA Cancer J Clin 2013;63:11-30.
2. Schlumberger MJ. Papillary and follicular thyroid carcinoma. N Engl J Med 1998;338:297-306.
3. Ezaki H, Ebihara S, Fujimoto Y, et al. Analysis of thyroid carcinoma based on material registered in Japan during 1977-1986 with special reference to predominance of papillary type. Cancer 1992;70:808-14.
4. Harach HR, Ceballos GA. Thyroid cancer, thyroiditis and dietary iodine: a review based on the Salta, Argentina model. Endocr Pathol 2008;19:209-20.
5. Harach HR, Williams ED. Thyroid cancer and thyroiditis in the goitrous region of Salta, Argentina, before and after iodine prophylaxis. Clin Endocrinol (Oxf) 1995;43:701-6.
6. Pottern LM, Kaplan MM, Larsen PR, et al. Thyroid nodularity after childhood irradiation for lymphoid hyperplasia: a comparison of questionnaire and clinical findings. J Clin Epidemiol 1990;43:449-60.
7. Schneider AB. Radiation-induced thyroid tumors. Endocrinol Metab Clin North Am 1990;19:495-508.
8. Fjälling M, Tisell LE, Carlsson S, Hansson G, Lundberg LM, Odën A. Benign and malignant thyroid nodules after neck irradiation. Cancer 1986;58:1219-24.
9. Hanson GA, Komorowski RA, Cerletty JM, Wilson SD. Thyroid gland morphology in young adults: normal subjects versus those with prior low-dose neck irradiation in childhood. Surgery 1983;96:984-8.
10. Kaplan MM, Garnick MB, Gelber R, et al. Risk factors for thyroid abnormalities after neck irradiation for childhood cancer. Am J Med 1983;74:272-80.
11. Komorowski RA, Hanson GA. Morphologic changes in the thyroid following low-dose childhood radiation. Arch Pathol Lab Med 1977;101:36-9.
12. Spitalnik PF, Straus FH II. Patterns of human thyroid parenchymal reaction following low-dose childhood irradiation. Cancer 1978;41:1098-105.
13. Fogelfeld L, Wiviott MB, Shore-Freedman E, et al. Recurrence of thyroid nodules after surgical removal in patients irradiated in childhood for benign conditions. N Engl J Med 1989;320:835-40.
14. Hempelmann LH, Hall WJ, Phillips M, Cooper RA, Ames WR. Neoplasms in persons treated with x-rays in infancy: fourth survey in 20 years. J Natl Cancer Inst 1975;55:519-30.
15. Schneider AB, Pinsky S, Bekerman C, Ryo UY. Characteristics of 108 thyroid cancers detected by screening in a population with a history of head and neck irradiation. Cancer 1980;46:1218-27.
16. Schneider AB, Recant W, Pinsky SM, Ryo UY, Bekerman C, Shore-Freedman E. Radiation-induced thyroid carcinoma. Clinical course and results of therapy in 296 patients. Ann Intern Med 1986;105:405-12.
17. Calandra DB, Shah KH, Lawrence AM, Paloyan E. Total thyroidectomy in irradiated patients. A twenty-year experience in 206 patients. Ann Surg 1985;202:356-60.
18. Wilson SD, Komorowski R, Cerletty J, Majewski JT, Hooper M. Radiation-associated thyroid tumors: extent of operation and pathology technique influence the apparent incidence of carcinoma. Surgery 1983;94:663-9.
19. Schneider AB, Shore-Freedman E, Ryo UY, Bekerman C, Favus M, Pinsky S. Radiation-induced tumors of the head and neck following childhood irradiation. Prospective studies. Medicine (Baltimore) 1985;64:1-15.
20. Schneider AB, Shore-Freedman E, Weinstein RA. Radiation-induced thyroid and other head and neck tumors: occurrence of multiple tumors and analysis of risk factors. J Clin Endocrinol Metab 1986;63:107-12.
21. Bisbee AC, Thoeny RH. Malignant lymphoma of the thyroid following irradiation. Cancer 1975;35:1296-9.
22. Carr RF, LiVolsi VA. Morphologic changes in the thyroid after irradiation for Hodgkin's and non-Hodgkin's lymphoma. Cancer 1989;64:825-9.
23. Satran L, Sklar C, Dehner L, Kim T, Nesbit M. Thyroid neoplasm after high-dose radiotherapy. Am J Pediatr Hematol Oncol 1983;5:307-9.
24. Tang TT, Holcenberg JS, Duck SC, Hodach AE, Oechler HW, Camitta BM. Thyroid carcinoma following treatment for acute lymphoblastic leukemia. Cancer 1980;46:1572-6.
25. Acharya S, Sarafoglou K, LaQuaglia M, et al. Thyroid neoplasms after therapeutic radiation for malignancies during childhood or adolescence. Cancer 2003;97:2397-403.
26. Huang J, Walker R, Groome PG, Shelley W, Mackillop WJ. Risk of thyroid carcinoma in a female population after radiotherapy for breast carcinoma. Cancer 2001;92:1411-8.
27. Hancock SL, Cox RS, McDougall IR. Thyroid diseases after treatment of Hodgkin's disease. N Engl J Med. 1991;325:599-605.

28. Inskip PD, Ekbom A, Galanti MR, Grimelius L, Boice JD Jr. Medical diagnostic x rays and thyroid cancer. J Natl Cancer Inst 1995;87:1613-21.
29. Williams ED. Chernobyl and thyroid cancer. J Surg Oncol 2006;94:670-7.
30. Tronko MD, Howe GR, Bogdanova TI, et al. A cohort study of thyroid cancer and other thyroid diseases after the Chernobyl accident: thyroid cancer in Ukraine detected during first screening. J Natl Cancer Inst 2006;98:897-903.
31. Cardis E, Kesminiene A, Ivanov V, et al. Risk of thyroid cancer after exposure to 131I in childhood. J Natl Cancer Inst 2005;97:724-32.
32. LiVolsi VA, Abrosimov AA, Bogdanova T, et al. The Chernobyl thyroid cancer experience: pathology. Clin Oncol (R Coll Radiol) 2011;23:261-7.
33. Nikiforov Y, Gnepp DR. Pediatric thyroid cancer after the Chernobyl disaster. Pathomorphologic study of 84 cases (1991-1992) from the Republic of Belarus. Cancer 1994;74:748-66.
33a. LiVolsi VA, Abrosimov AA, Bogdanova T, et al. The Chernobyl thyroid cancer experience: pathology. Clin Oncol (R Coll Radiol) 2011;23:261-7.
34. Williams ED, Abrosimov A, Bogdanova T, et al. Morphologic characteristics of Chernobyl-related childhood papillary thyroid carcinomas are independent of radiation exposure but vary with iodine intake. Thyroid 2008;18:847-52.
35. Gorlin JB, Sallan SE. Thyroid cancer in childhood. Endocrinol Metab Clin North Am 1990:19;649-62.
36. Gupta A, Ly S, Castroneves LA, et al. A standardized assessment of thyroid nodules in children confirms higher cancer prevalence than in adults. J Clin Endocrinol Metab 2013;98:3238-45.
37. Goepfert H, Dichtel WJ, Samaan NA. Thyroid cancer in children and teenagers. Arch Otolaryngol 1984;110:72-5.
38. Sierk A, Askin FB, Reddick RL, Thomas CG Jr. Pediatric thyroid cancer. Pediatr Pathol 1990; 10:877-93.
39. Mizukami Y, Michigishi T, Nonomura A, et al. Carcinoma of the thyroid at a young age—a review of 23 patients. Histopathology 1992;20:63-6.
40. Hayles AB, Kennedy RL, Beahrs OH, Woolner LB. Carcinoma of the thyroid gland in children. AMA Am J Dis Child 1955;90:705-15.
41. Bongiovanni AM, DiGeorge AM. Cancer of the thyroid in childhood and adolescence. Am J Med Sci 1963;246:734-49.
42. Winship T, Rosvoll RV. Childhood thyroid carcinoma. Cancer 1961;14:734-43.
43. Lamberg BA, Karkinen-Jaaskelainen M, Franssila KO. Differentiated follicle-derived thyroid carcinoma in children. Acta Paediatr Scand 1989; 78:419-25.
44. Samuel AM, Sharma SM. Differentiated thyroid carcinomas in children and adolescents. Cancer 1991;67:2186-90.
45. Schlumberger M, De Vathaire F, Travagli JP, et al. Differentiated thyroid carcinoma in childhood: long term follow-up of 72 patients. J Clin Endocrinol Metab 1987;65:1088-94.
46. Grigsby PW, Gal-or A, Michalski JM, Doherty GM. Childhood and adolescent thyroid carcinoma. Cancer 2002;95:724-9.
47. Farahati J, Bucsky P, Parlowsky T, Mäder U, Reiners C. Characteristics of differentiated thyroid carcinoma in children and adolescents with respect to age, gender, and histology. Cancer 1997;80:2156-62.
48. Collini P, Massimino M, Leite SF, et al. Papillary thyroid carcinoma of childhood and adolescence: a 30-year experience at the Istituto Nazionale Tumori in Milan. Pediatr Blood Cancer 2006;46:300-6.
49. Mills SE, Allen MS Jr. Congenital occult papillary carcinoma of the thyroid gland. Hum Pathol 1986;17:1179-81.
50. Vane D, King DR, Boles ET Jr. Secondary thyroid neoplasms in pediatric cancer patients: increased risk with improved survival. J Pediatr Surg 1984; 19:855-60.

4 CLASSIFICATION OF THYROID TUMORS

Several classification systems for thyroid tumors have been proposed, but none is entirely satisfactory. Pierre Masson (1), after struggling with the task for years, stated in frustration, "No classification is more difficult to establish than that of thyroid epitheliomas. Their pleomorphism is almost the rule; very few are adapted to a precise classification." As to the pathologist's ability to distinguish benign from malignant thyroid tumors, he commented, "Of all cancers, thyroid epitheliomas teach, perhaps, the greatest lesson of humility to histopathologists … Many pathologists agree with me in never giving a prognosis on an epithelial thyroid tumor without reservation."

As with many other tumor classification systems in other sites, those that have been applied to thyroid neoplasms are based on a haphazard combination of architectural, cytologic, histogenetic, grading, and (lately) molecular genetic features (1–5). The most important group, by far, is that of the primary epithelial neoplasms. Since in the thyroid gland there are only two major types of epithelial cells, i.e., the follicular cell and the C-cell, the first major division of the corresponding tumors is into those exhibiting follicular cell differentiation and those featuring C-cell differentiation, with an exceedingly small third group showing differentiation along both cell lines. This classification scheme, which we have adopted for this Fascicle, is essentially the same as that proposed by the World Health Organization in 2005 (2).

There is only one major type of thyroid neoplasm exhibiting predominant evidence of C-cell differentiation: the malignant tumor that carries the time-honored designation of medullary carcinoma (including its variants). For the tumors featuring follicular cell differentiation, the situation is considerably more complex.

Neoplasms of follicular cells have been customarily classified into benign and malignant. The benign tumors are generically designated as follicular adenomas. It follows that their malignant counterpart should be designated as follicular adenocarcinomas. This is rarely done, however. Instead, the better-differentiated members of the group have been traditionally divided into two major categories, follicular and papillary (initially on the basis of their architectural features), while the lesser-differentiated types, whether still recognizable as epithelial or having a sarcoma-like appearance, have been designated as undifferentiated or anaplastic. The criteria for the recognition of follicular and papillary carcinomas have changed in recent years (thus, the presence of papillae is no longer necessary for the diagnosis of papillary carcinoma), but the two names have been retained.

This superficially simple scheme is considerably modified and complicated by two factors. The first is the occurrence in some tumors of follicular cell derivation, whether follicular or papillary, of a variety of cytoplasmic changes, either singly or in combination: oncocytic, clear, squamous, and mucinous. Some of these changes are inconsequential, but others have definite behavioral connotations and are therefore of importance.

The other important consideration is that not all follicular or papillary carcinomas are well-differentiated tumors. Instead, some exhibit poorly differentiated morphologic features; this is just as important (or perhaps more so) from a prognostic and therapeutic standpoint as whether they belong to the follicular or papillary group (3). The higher the grade of the tumor, the less significant it becomes to assign it to either a follicular or papillary category: it is important for the better differentiated tumors, less so for the poorly differentiated ones, and unwarranted (and generally not feasible) for the undifferentiated categories. This approach is similar to that being adopted in many other sites (e.g., soft tissue tumors), in the sense that considerations based on tumor grading are being progressively incorporated into the traditional cytoarchitecturally-based schemes.

Since some of the morphologic features present in these tumors (i.e., clear cell changes) cross classification lines, we thought it useful to list and discuss them separately from the major classification scheme, mainly for differential diagnosis purposes.

As a final comment, it should be pointed out that the terms *goiter* and *struma* simply refer to enlargement of the thyroid gland, whatever its cause. In fact, the terms have been applied in popular language to any type of swelling in the anterolateral region of the neck, Virchow being allegedly the first to suggest that they should be restricted to thyroid swellings. Currently, they are more frequently used for non-neoplastic thyroid conditions (i.e., nodular hyperplasia, Hashimoto thyroiditis). To avoid confusion, these terms should never be used without a qualifier, if at all.

The classification of thyroid neoplasms adopted for this Fascicle is the following:

PRIMARY TUMORS

Epithelial Tumors
  Tumors of Follicular Cells
    Benign: Follicular adenoma
      Conventional
      Variants
    Malignant: Carcinoma
      Well differentiated
        Follicular carcinoma
        Papillary carcinoma
          Classic
          Variants
      Poorly differentiated
        Insular carcinoma
        Others
      Undifferentiated (anaplastic)
  Tumors of C- (and related neuroendocrine) cells
    Medullary carcinoma
    Others

Tumors of Follicular and C-cells
Sarcomas
Malignant Lymphoma and related Hematopoietic Neoplasms
Miscellaneous Tumors

Tumor types and subtypes that cross lines in the above classification due to the presence of particular cytologic features include the following:

Tumors with oncocytic (Hürthle cell) features
  Oncocytic adenoma (Hürthle cell adenoma)
  Oncocytic carcinoma (Hürthle cell carcinoma)
  Papillary oncocytic (Hürthle cell) tumors
Tumors with clear cell features
Tumors with squamous features
Tumors with mucinous features

SECONDARY TUMORS AND TUMOR-LIKE LESIONS

Furthermore, the well-differentiated carcinomas of follicular cells listed in the "official" classification may be subdivided into eight types by the sequential application of three criteria: 1) *nuclear features* (presence or absence of papillary thyroid carcinoma (PTC)-type nuclei); 2) *cytoplasmic features* (presence or absence of oncocytic change); and 3) *architectural features* (papillary versus follicular pattern of growth). Although this may not qualify as a bonafide classification, we have found it useful for didactic purposes and as a template on which to test the clinical, immunohistochemical, and molecular genetic findings of these tumors. In this regard, it is of interest that every box of the scheme (Table 4-1) contains a documented tumor type (with the possible exception of the papillary variant of follicular carcinoma).

Table 4-1

SCHEMATIC VIEW OF WELL-DIFFERENTIATED THYROID CARCINOMAS COMPOSED OF FOLLICULAR CELLS

Nucleus	Cytoplasm	Pattern of Growth	Tumor Type
PTC[a]-Type	Nononcocytic	Papillary	Papillary carcinoma, classic
		Follicular	Papillary carcinoma, follicular variant
	Oncocytic	Papillary	Papillary carcinoma, oncocytic variant
		Follicular	Papillary carcinoma, oncocytic follicular variant
Not PTC-Type	Nononcocytic	Follicular	Follicular carcinoma, classic
		Papillary	Follicular carcinoma, papillary variant
	Oncocytic	Follicular	Follicular carcinoma, oncocytic variant
		Papillary	Follicular carcinoma, oncocytic papillary variant

[a] PTC = papillary thyroid carcinoma.

REFERENCES

1. Masson P. Human tumors. Histology, diagnosis, and technique (English translation), 2nd ed. Detroit: Wayne State Univ, 1970:588-9.
2. DeLellis RA, Lloyd RV, Heitz PU, Eng C, eds. Pathology and genetics of tumours of endocrine organs. World Health Organization Classification of Tumours, Lyon: IARC Press; 2004.
3. Zampi G, Carcangiu ML, Rosai J, guest eds. Thyroid tumor pathology. Proceedings of an International Workshop held in San Miniato, Italy, October 1984. Sem Diagn Pathol 1985;2:1-146.
4. LiVolsi V. Surgical pathology of the thyroid. Major problems in pathology, vol. 22, 2nd ed. Philadelphia: WB Saunders; 1990.
5. Nikiforov Y, Biddinger PW, Thompson LD, eds. Diagnostic pathology and molecular genetics of the thyroid. A comprehensive guide for practicing thyroid pathology, 2nd ed. Philadelphia: Lippincott Williams & Wilkins; 2009.

5

FOLLICULAR THYROID ADENOMA AND VARIANTS

FOLLICULAR ADENOMA

Definition. *Follicular adenoma* is a benign encapsulated tumor showing evidence of follicular cell differentiation. Sometimes the tumor is simply designated as *adenoma* without a qualifier, since all of the currently recognized types of thyroid adenoma are of follicular cell nature. All other adjectives applied to thyroid adenomas refer to subtypes or variants of follicular adenoma.

General Features. Follicular adenoma is a common neoplasm. In a review of 300 consecutive autopsies performed at Yale University on patients aged 20 years or older, 9 adenomas were found, for an incidence of 3 percent (1). In an analogous study of 300 cases examined in Sao Paulo, Brazil, the frequency of adenoma was similar: 12 adenomas were found, for an incidence of 4.3 percent (2). There seems to be no relationship between the overall frequency of adenoma and the level of iodine in the diet; however, it has been claimed that solitary autonomously functioning thyroid nodules ("toxic adenomas") are more common in areas of iodine deficiency (3). Patients with Cowden (multiple hamartoma) syndrome develop thyroid adenomas with great frequency, and also have an increased incidence of nodular hyperplasia (4).

Adenomas are usually solitary, but instances in which two or more adenomas are seen in the same gland occur, even when strict criteria for their distinction from hyperplastic nodules are applied (basically, the presence or absence of a continuous fibrous capsule). Most adenomas occur in otherwise normal glands, but they are also seen in glands affected by lymphocytic/ Hashimoto or granulomatous thyroiditis, nodular hyperplasia, or other lesions (5).

Most adenomas are located in one or another of the two thyroid lobes, but a few affect primarily the isthmus. No predilection for one lobe or a portion of a lobe has been noted.

The assumption that follicular adenoma, being a neoplastic process, has a clonal origin

(whereas the reverse should be true for nodular hyperplasia) has been explored by analyzing the X chromosomes in mice (6) and humans (7,8), with widely discrepant results. In one study from Korea, all of five totally encapsulated nodules were clonal, whereas all but one of five unencapsulated nodules were polyclonal. Also, the capsule tended to be thicker in clonal than in polyclonal nodules (9). Unfortunately, these satisfying results have not been duplicated by others. Thus, Apel et al. (10) found that only seven of their hyperplastic nodules were polyclonal whereas as many as 18 morphologically similar hyperplastic nodules were clonal.

Clinical Features. Most patients with follicular adenomas of the thyroid gland are middle aged, and women are most often affected. Although indisputable cases of adenoma in children and in the elderly also occur, the chance of an alternative diagnosis, particularly carcinoma, is higher in these two age groups.

Most patients with follicular adenomas are euthyroid and present with a painless lump in the neck. Pressure-related symptoms, mainly resulting from tracheal compression, may occur with larger lesions. Sudden growth, sometimes associated with pain, may be present; this is usually the result of intratumoral hemorrhage. On isotopic scan, the adenoma is usually "cold" (hypofunctional), sometimes "cool" or "warm" (functional), and only exceptionally "hot" (hyperfunctional) (see chapter 21). Many patients with follicular adenomas have elevated circulating levels of thyroglobulin (11), but few of the tumors are associated with clinical hyperthyroidism ("toxic" adenomas, discussed later).

Gross Findings. Adenomas are usually round or oval. They are characteristically surrounded by a complete fibrous capsule that varies in thickness but is usually thin (figs. 5-1, 5-2). The presence of an unduly thick and irregularly shaped capsule should raise suspicion for follicular carcinoma.

The size of follicular adenomas is highly variable. They are rarely described as microscopic

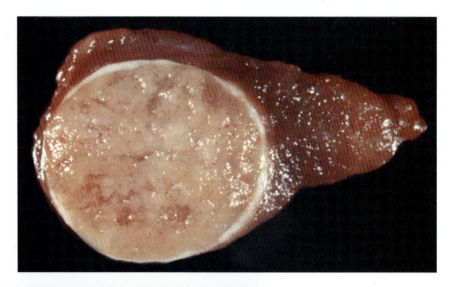

Figure 5-1

FOLLICULAR ADENOMA

Typically, the lesion is single and surrounded by a thin fibrous capsule. The cut surface is tan, homogeneous, and solid. The thyroid gland surrounding the adenoma has a normal appearance.

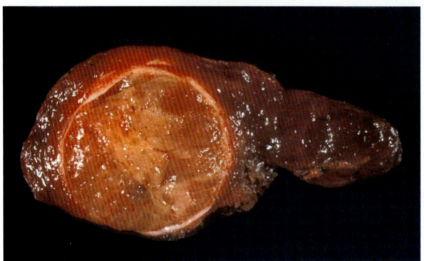

Figure 5-2

FOLLICULAR ADENOMA

Another example of the gross appearance of a follicular adenoma.

findings, however, perhaps because at this stage their distinction from a hyperplastic nodule is nearly impossible. Most adenomas have a diameter between 1 and 3 cm at the time of excision, but occasional lesions are considerably larger and weigh several hundred grams. Their consistency is rubbery or firm. In uncomplicated cases, the cut surface is usually homogeneous, bulging, and without internal lobulations.

The color of the adenoma largely depends on the cell composition and amount of colloid present. It is usually grayish white in the trabecular/solid and hyalinizing trabecular variants and tan in adenomas showing follicle formation with colloid deposition, in which case the hue is dependent on the relative proportion of cells and colloid and on the degree of vascularity (fig. 5-3).

Secondary changes that are seen at the gross level in adenomas, although not as frequently as in hyperplastic nodules, include hemorrhage, fibrosis, calcification, ossification, and cystic degeneration (figs. 5-4, 5-5). Fresh tumor necrosis is unusual as a spontaneous event in adenoma but is now being observed with greater frequency (especially in the oncocytic type) as a complication of fine-needle aspiration (fig. 5-6).

Microscopic Findings. Follicular adenomas exhibit a bewildering variety of architectural patterns, but the architecture is usually uniform in an individual lesion. Less commonly, an admixture of two or more patterns is seen. Except for the special variants listed separately, the variations in architecture mostly depend on the degree of cellularity, presence and size of

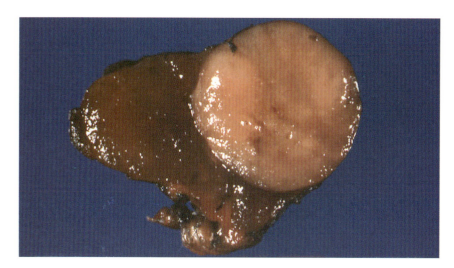

Figure 5-3

FOLLICULAR ADENOMA

The bulging on the cut surface is typical of highly cellular follicular adenomas.

Figure 5-4

FOLLICULAR ADENOMA

This adenoma has undergone extensive secondary changes in the form of massive hemorrhage and peritumoral fibrosis. The fresh hemorrhage may be spontaneous or secondary to a fine-needle aspiration.

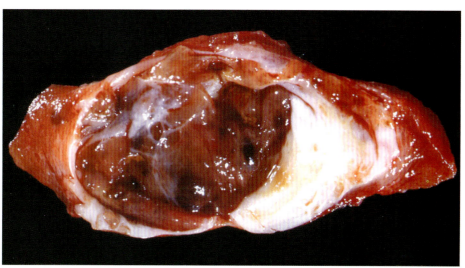

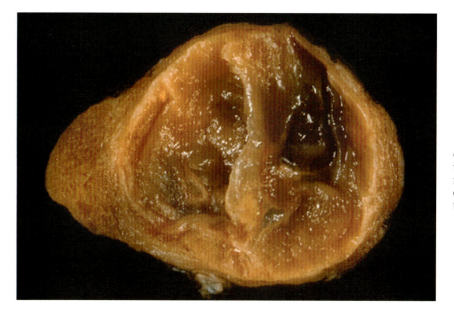

Figure 5-5

FOLLICULAR ADENOMA

Marked cystic degeneration is evident in this tumor. It is likely that most "primary thyroid cysts" represent follicular adenomas exhibiting an extreme form of this phenomenon.

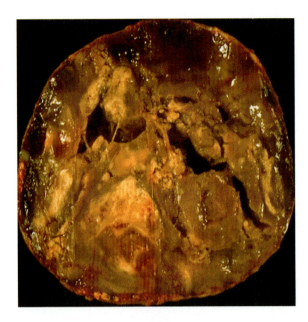

Figure 5-6

FOLLICULAR ADENOMA

This follicular adenoma shows marked necrosis, hemorrhage, and cystic changes.

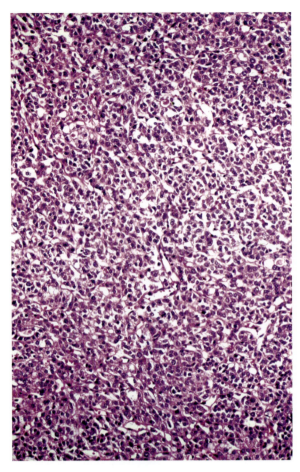

Figure 5-7

FOLLICULAR ADENOMA

Low-power view of a highly cellular follicular adenoma.

follicles, and pattern of growth of the nonfollicular component, if any.

Follicular adenomas of conventional types are traditionally divided among the following categories (figs. 5-7–5-9):

Trabecular/Solid. This tumor subtype is very cellular and grows in either a trabecular or diffuse (solid) fashion, with the formation of few or no follicles (12). It is sometimes also referred to as *embryonal* because of its morphologic resemblance to a developing thyroid gland in a very early (prefollicular) stage.

Microfollicular. In this tumor, neoplastic follicles are formed but are smaller than those of the neighboring gland. The ratio of cells to lumen is greatly altered in favor of the former, and the amount of colloid present is minimal. This subtype is sometimes designated as *fetal*, following embryologic analogies similar to those mentioned with the previous type.

Normofollicular (Simple). The pattern of growth of this tumor is follicular throughout, and the size of the follicles approaches that of the non-neoplastic gland.

Macrofollicular (Colloid). The neoplastic follicles in this tumor are larger and full of colloid, thus resembling those seen in hyperplastic nodules.

Most follicular adenomas belong to one of the first two categories, either entirely or partially. The larger and more colloid-like the follicles in a benign follicular nodule, the less likely that the lesion is a true neoplasm. Sometimes one or more sharply outlined but unencapsulated trabecular/solid nodules are seen within an adenoma with an otherwise normofollicular or macrofollicular appearance. These have been referred to as *foci of secondary proliferation* or *secondary growth centers* (13).

Although the histologic differences between these subtypes are striking, they are of no clinical relevance. Perhaps their only practical value is that the more cellular a follicular nodule is, the more one should search for evidence of malignancy.

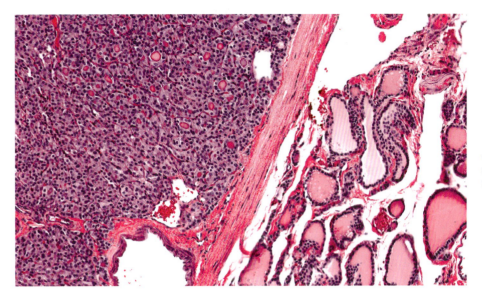

Figure 5-8

FOLLICULAR ADENOMA
A hypercellular follicular adenoma is surrounded by a smooth, sharply outlined capsule.

The cells of follicular adenoma tend to be polygonal, with normochromatic nuclei that are round to oval with smooth contours; the latter is an important point in the differential diagnosis with the follicular variant of papillary carcinoma. Variations in nuclear size and shape are minimal, except for the special variants (see below). Mitoses are usually absent or scanty. The presence of more than an occasional mitosis should raise the index of suspicion for carcinoma. The cytoplasm is acidophilic to amphophilic and moderately abundant. Cell borders are usually well defined.

The lumens of the neoplastic follicles contain variable amounts of colloid that may exhibit an amphophilic or pale eosinophilic staining quality. If the appearance of the colloid is strongly and homogeneously eosinophilic throughout, the alternative possibility that the lesion is a follicular variant of papillary carcinoma should be considered. In rare instances, the lumens of adenomatous follicles contain calcium oxalate crystals. It is much more common, however, for these crystals to be found in the thyroid tissue outside "hot" nodules, where they are interpreted as a sign of suppression.

The capsule of an adenoma is continuous and made of fibrous tissue within which vessels of various sizes are found (figs. 5-8, 5-10–5-12). It is common for the capsule to contain almond-shaped or ovoid masses of smooth muscle, representing areas of localized thickening ("cushions") of the wall of blood vessels (14).

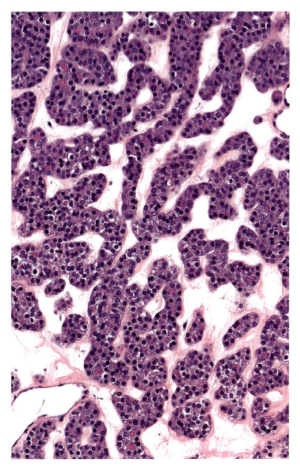

Figure 5-9

FOLLICULAR ADENOMA
A striking trabecular pattern of growth and an edematous stroma are seen.

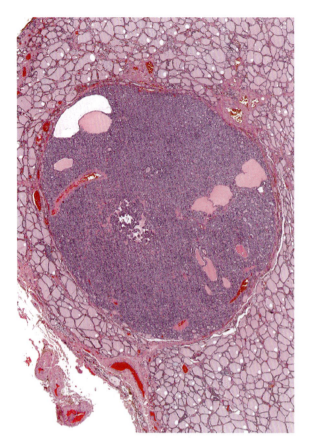

Figure 5-10

FOLLICULAR ADENOMA OR HYPERPLASTIC NODULE?

This highly cellular nodule is partially surrounded by an incomplete, extremely thin capsule. It is debatable whether this should be regarded as a follicular adenoma or a solitary (dominant) expression of nodular hyperplasia. The noncommittal term "benign follicular nodule" can be used in such instances.

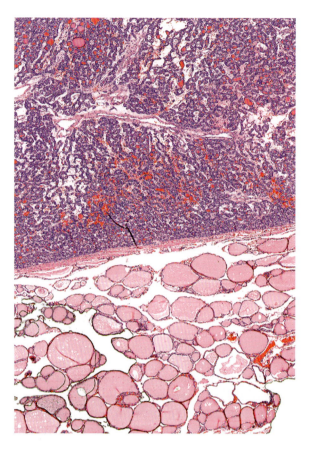

Figure 5-11

FOLLICULAR ADENOMA

This is the minimal thickness that the fibrous shell around the tumor should have in order to qualify as a capsule, thus identifying the lesion as an adenoma.

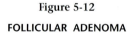

Figure 5-12

FOLLICULAR ADENOMA

The capsule of this adenoma is well formed and of smooth contours. The surrounding thyroid gland shows some fibrosis and atrophic follicles, probably due to compression by the tumor.

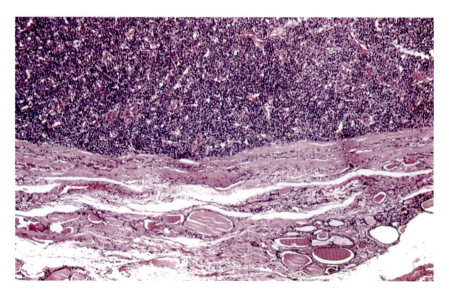

Parenthetically, these peculiar structures are more common in hyperplastic nodules and rare in carcinomas (15). Evans (16) made the interesting and unexpected observation that the capsule is generally thinner in follicular adenomas than in follicular carcinomas. The interface between the tumor and the inner side of the capsule is usually sharp but can also be irregular due to herniation or entrapment of tumor cells. The adjacent gland is often compressed and atrophic, particularly with larger adenomas.

The stromal component of the adenoma is usually more abundant in the central portion, where it tends to exhibit a loose, edematous quality. Degenerative alterations such as recent or old hemorrhage, thrombosis, edema, myxoid change, fibrosis and hyalinization, calcification, metaplastic ossification, and cyst formation occur. The fibrosis, if present, tends to be centrally located, with a stellate, scar-like configuration.

Squamous metaplasia is exceptionally rare, but it can occur as a focal event, sometimes secondarily to necrosis, whether spontaneous or induced by a fine-needle aspiration (17). Whenever squamous metaplasia is present, the alternative possibility that the tumor is a carcinoma, particularly of papillary type, should be considered.

Similarly, the presence of sharply outlined fibrohyaline septa running across the tumor (most often at the periphery, beneath the capsule, and having an appearance reminiscent of colloid) is not a common feature of follicular adenoma. Their presence should raise the possibility of an alternative diagnosis, particularly the follicular variant of papillary carcinoma.

Follicular adenomas are well-vascularized tumors. The intermingling of tumor cells and vessels within the lesion is intimate, and it is not unusual to find isolated follicular cells (or sometimes small cell clusters) within the vascular lumens. This finding, probably of artifactual nature, is of no diagnostic significance if limited to vessels within the tumor (as opposed to capsular vessels). In some adenomas, the number and prominence of vessels is such as to simulate a vascular neoplasm.

Immunohistochemical Findings. The immunohistochemical (and enzyme histochemical) profile of follicular adenomas mirrors that of the normal follicle (18). Reactivity for thyroglobulin is the rule. This is more intense in the cytoplasm of the tumor cells but is also evident in the intraluminal colloid, both at a light and electron microscopic level (18–20). In general, the degree of the thyroglobulin staining in the adenoma is less intense than in the adjacent gland. Positivity is also consistently present for thyroxine and triiodothyronine. Staining for thyroglobulin is particularly useful diagnostically in the more solid and cellular types of adenomas (as well as in follicular carcinomas) by showing droplet-like foci of positivity in tiny follicles not easily discernible in routinely stained sections.

Keratin reactivity is uniformly present. The keratins expressed in follicular adenomas, like those found in the normal follicle, are of low molecular weight, as befits simple epithelial structures. Schelfhout et al. (21) found consistently high expression of cytokeratins (CK) 8 and 18 in both follicular adenomas and normal follicles. The reactivity for CK19 in both situations was only focal and weak. Keratins of high molecular weight are absent. Vimentin is often coexpressed with keratin, with a pattern and frequency similar to those observed in the normal gland and in follicular carcinomas (22,23).

The neoplastic follicles are surrounded by a well-developed basement membrane, which can be demonstrated with the periodic acid–Schiff (PAS) stain, silver reactions, or through the immunohistochemical detection of its main components, i.e., laminin and type IV collagen (24,25). This may be useful in delineating small follicles in cellular lesions that appear solid on routinely stained sections.

The enzyme histochemical pattern of follicular adenomas also recapitulates that of the normal follicle. There is positivity for 5 α-nucleotidase, α-naphthyl acetate esterase, and acid phosphatase, and negativity for adenosine triphosphatase and alkaline phosphatase (26).

The lectin receptors expressed by the cells of follicular adenomas are the same as those of normal follicular cells, but the binding in the neoplastic lesion is said to be significantly stronger (27,28). Metallothionein, a low molecular weight protein thought to be involved in the intracellular storage of essential metals, is commonly expressed in both benign and malignant tumors of follicular cells but substantially less so by the normal gland (29).

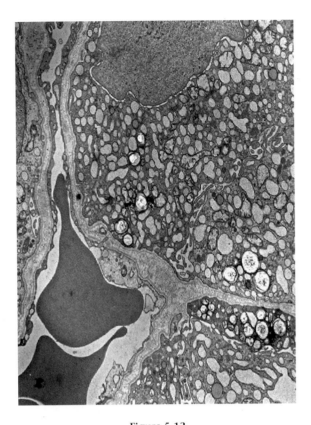

Figure 5-13

FOLLICULAR ADENOMA

Ultrastructurally, the tumor cells have a small number of mitochondria, abundant and somewhat dilated granular endoplasmic reticulum, scattered lysosomes, and intertwining microvilli. Parallel basal lamina belonging to the follicular epithelial cells and the adjacent endothelial cells from a blood vessel are shown. (Courtesy of Dr. R. Erlandson, New York, NY.)

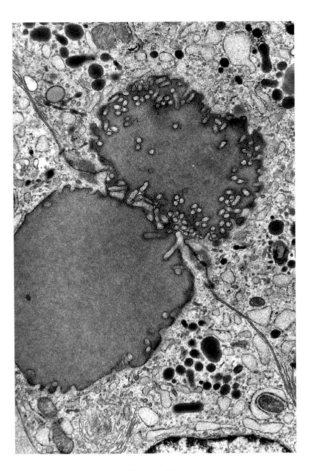

Figure 5-14

FOLLICULAR ADENOMA

This electron micrograph shows well-developed lamina into which microvilli project. Clusters of lysosomes are visible in the cytoplasm of the tumor cells, together with mitochondria, granular endoplasmic reticulum, and a well-developed Golgi apparatus. (Courtesy of Dr. R. Erlandson, New York, NY.)

Claims have been made that the following markers are absent or rare in follicular adenoma but consistently expressed by follicular carcinoma: ceruloplasmin; iron-binding proteins (lactoferrin, transferrin, ferritin); tissue polypeptide antigen (30–32); tumor-associated carbohydrate antigens CA50 and CA19-9 (particularly the former) (33); and leu-7 antigen (HNK-1) (34). Obviously, independent confirmation of these rather surprising results is needed before employing them for diagnostic purposes.

Ultrastructural Findings. The cells of follicular adenomas have no distinctive features at the ultrastructural level. Their appearance is similar to that of nodular hyperplasia and the normal thyroid gland. The granular endoplasmic reticulum and the Golgi apparatus are well developed, and there are abundant ribosomes and polyribosomes (fig. 5-13). Accumulations of phagolysosomal bodies are seen in the apical portion of the cytoplasm, and the cell surface is covered with microvilli (fig. 5-14). Cilia are present in most instances. The follicular cells rest on a continuous basal lamina (35).

Molecular Genetic Findings. See chapter 19.

Cytologic Findings. See chapter 20.

Differential Diagnosis. The differential diagnosis of follicular adenoma of conventional type includes a "dominant" hyperplastic nodule, a minimally invasive follicular carcinoma, and the encapsulated follicular variant of papillary carcinoma (36–38). On gross examination, a typical uncomplicated adenoma has a more homogeneous cut surface than nodular hyperplasia and lacks the internal lobulation of the latter. Microscopically, a diagnosis of adenoma should be favored over that of a dominant hyperplastic nodule if the lesion is single, completely encapsulated, leads to compression of the surrounding thyroid gland, and has a uniform microscopic appearance that is substantially different from that of the rest of the gland. By using these criteria, most nodules with a trabecular, solid, or microfollicular pattern of growth are diagnosed as adenomas, whereas most of those with a normofollicular or macrofollicular pattern of growth are called hyperplastic nodules, acknowledging the fact that exceptions occur in both directions. Features that favor a hyperplastic nodule are the presence of inflammation, so-called Sanderson polsters, and papillary projections within dilated follicles. In most thyroid glands with hyperplastic nodules, smaller nodules of similar appearance are detected in the remainder of the gland. However, if the nodule in question fulfills all the criteria of an adenoma (including total encapsulation), it should be so designated, even if there is more than one or if the rest of the organ shows nodular hyperplastic changes.

Sometimes the distinction between nodular hyperplasia and neoplasia is impossible, as is also the case in most other endocrine organs. We prefer to use the noncommittal term *benign follicular nodule* for these lesions, followed by an explanatory note (fig. 5-10).

Treatment. The standard therapy for follicular adenoma limited to one lobe (whether conventional or one of the variants) is surgical removal in the form of lobectomy. Enucleation of the adenoma (nodulectomy) should not be attempted, because if the final diagnosis is that of a minimally invasive follicular or papillary carcinoma, the operation will have been inadequate. The lobectomy is often accompanied by an isthmusectomy for aesthetic reasons, and sometimes a subtotal thyroidectomy is carried out. A total or near-total thyroidectomy is unnecessary for this lesion.

Suppression of the adenoma with L-thyroxine and treatment of the toxic adenoma with ^{131}I have been employed, but in general, the results have been disappointing (39,40).

ADENOMA VARIANTS

Several more or less distinct variants of follicular adenoma have been described, mainly on the basis of the microscopic features (41,42). Although most have no special clinical significance, their recognition is important to avoid confusion with lesions that have more ominous connotations. These variants are described below, except for oncocytic adenoma (Hürthle cell adenoma) and adenoma with clear cell change (including signet ring adenoma), which are discussed in chapters 10 and 11, respectively.

Adenoma with Bizarre Nuclei

In some adenomas, *scattered bizarre nuclei* are found that are characterized by a huge size (10 times or more than those of the adjacent cells), irregular shape, and striking hyperchromasia (fig. 5-15) (42). These nuclei tend to occur in clusters. They are analogous to the nuclei seen in many other endocrine tumors (such as parathyroid adenoma and paraganglioma) and should not be taken, by themselves, as a sign of malignancy. Actually, they occur more often in follicular adenomas than in carcinomas, as is also the case in the parathyroid glands.

Hyalinizing Trabecular Adenoma

Hyalinizing trabecular adenoma is the name proposed by Carney et al. (43) for a distinctive type of thyroid neoplasm previously described by Ward et al. (44) as "hyaline cell tumor of the thyroid with massive accumulation of cytoplasmic filaments," and even before by Pierre Masson and by Rahel Ziphin (who credited her chief, Theodor Langhans, for its original identification) (45).

Grossly, these tumors are yellow-tan and well circumscribed or encapsulated, not significantly different from conventional adenomas. Microscopically, the main distinguishing features are the prominent hyaline appearance (both extracellular due to the perivascular deposition of collagen, and intracellular due to the accumulation of intermediate filaments) and the trabecular arrangement of the tumor cells (fig. 5-16). The trabecula can be straight or curved in the form of ribbons and festoons (fig. 5-17). Some of the tumor cells are inserted perpendicularly into the walls of small blood vessels. In other areas, the cells are arranged in

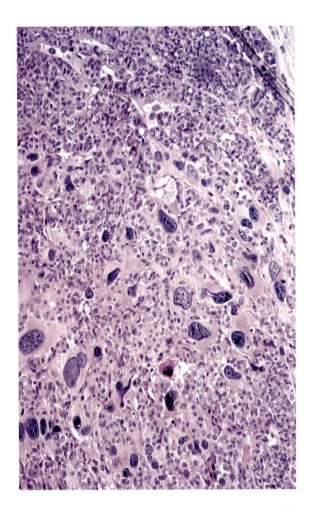 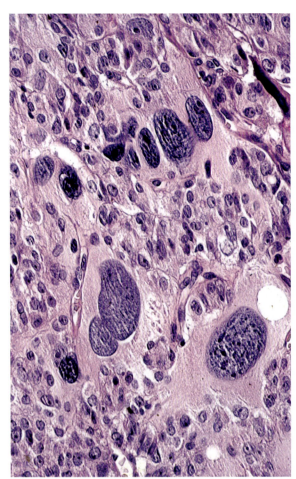

Figure 5-15

FOLLICULAR ADENOMA WITH BIZARRE NUCLEI

Left: Tumor cells with giant nuclei tend to appear as clusters, surrounded by unremarkable follicular cells. They are not a sign of malignancy, but probably an expression of degenerative change.

Right: High-power view.

compact clusters reminiscent of the "Zellballen" of paraganglioma, hence the alternative (but rarely used) designation of this adenoma variant as *paraganglioma-like* (46,47).

Follicular formation is minimal or absent; the few follicles present tend to be irregularly shaped and may feature papillary infoldings. The nuclei are round, oval, or elongated, sometimes markedly so. Some nuclei exhibit grooves, pseudoinclusions, and perinuclear vacuoles (figs. 5-18, 5-19) (48). Chan et al. (49) suggested that the latter feature is due to the presence of "nuclear rods," which represent aggregates of intranuclear filaments. Mitoses are usually absent. The cytoplasm has acidophilic, amphophilic, or

clear-staining qualities, and the cell borders are sharply outlined (fig. 5-20).

A subtle morphologic feature present in almost all cases is the so-called *cytoplasmic yellow bodies*, which appear as roughly spherical, slightly refractile, pale yellow structures measuring 2 to 5 μm in diameter, often surrounded by a clear halo of retracted cytoplasm and sometimes causing indentation and molding of the nucleus. Alas, these formations are also detected in some cases of Hürthle cell carcinoma, papillary carcinoma, and follicular carcinoma (50,51).

Immunohistochemically, the profile of hyalinizing trabecular adenoma is heterogeneous (52). Most tumor cells are reactive for

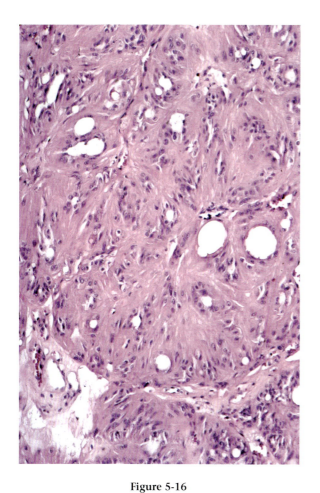

Figure 5-16

HYALINIZING TRABECULAR ADENOMA

At low-power, extensive hyaline changes throughout the tumor are seen.

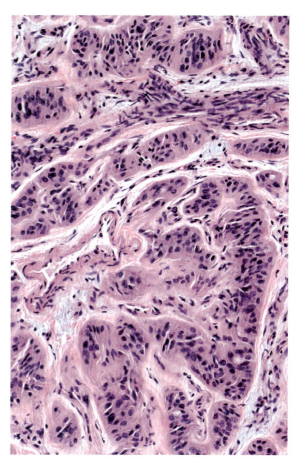

Figure 5-17

HYALINIZING TRABECULAR ADENOMA

In this tumor the trabecular pattern of growth is particularly evident.

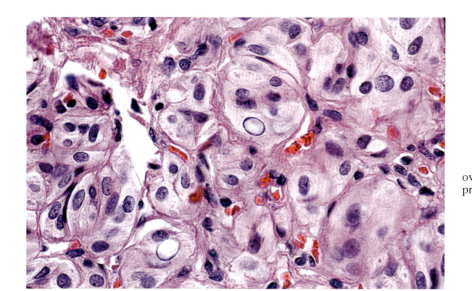

Figure 5-18

HYALINIZING TRABECULAR ADENOMA

Most of the nuclei have an ovoid shape, and some show prominent pseudoinclusions.

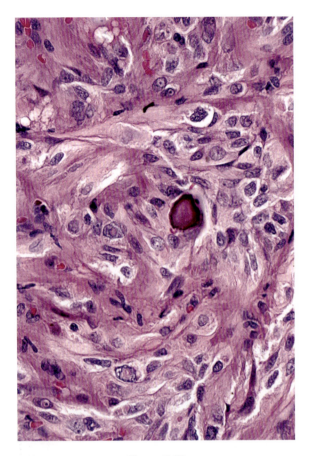

Figure 5-19

HYALINIZING TRABECULAR ADENOMA

Most of the tumor cells have oval to spindle-shaped nuclei. A well-developed psammoma body is present.

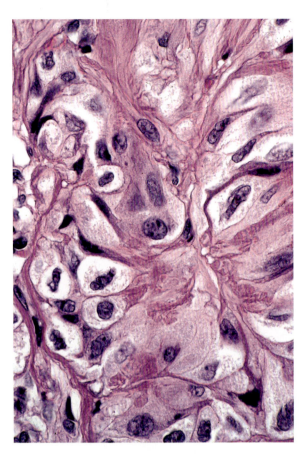

Figure 5-20

HYALINIZING TRABECULAR ADENOMA

Many of the tumor cells are elongated, and some of the nuclei are grooved.

thyroglobulin, thyroid transcription factor (TTF)-1, and keratin, and negative for calcitonin, in keeping with their presumed follicular origin (fig. 5-21). Some of these tumors, however, exhibit argyrophilia and immunohistochemical reactivity for neuron-specific enolase (NSE), chromogranin A, neurotensin, and α-endorphin. These findings raise the possibility of dual follicular and neuroendocrine differentiation (53–55). Staining for galectin-3 is highly variable, but rarely as intense as in papillary carcinoma (48). The homogeneous eosinophilic material seen in the stroma in hematoxylin and eosin (H&E)-stained sections reacts immunohistochemically for laminin and type IV collagen, indicating basement membrane accumulation (fig. 5-22) (54).

A peculiar immunohistochemical finding is the strong membrane positivity that is seen with the proliferation marker MIB-1 (Ki-67) (fig. 5-23) (56). The unexpected location (in the cell membrane rather than in the nucleus) and the fact that only some antibody clones give this result suggest that we are dealing with an artifact (although, as artifacts go, it is pretty spectacular) (57).

Ultrastructurally, the main features of this neoplasm are packing by intermediate filaments of the cytoplasm of the tumor cells and an abundance of intracellular and extracellular basal lamina material, suggesting a deregulation of secretory pathways (55,58,59).

By definition, hyalinizing trabecular adenoma is regarded as a benign neoplasm. However, it shares several morphologic features with papillary carcinoma, such as the above-described nuclear features, the occasional occurrence of psammoma body-like formations (fig. 5-19), a

76

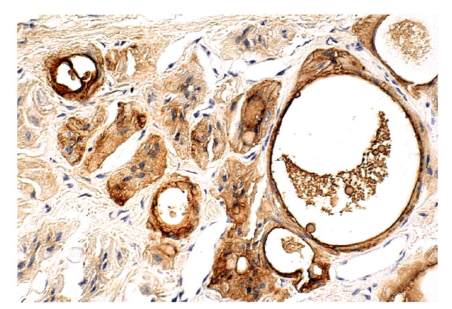

Figure 5-21

HYALINIZING TRABECULAR ADENOMA

Intraluminal and cytoplasmic thyroglobulin immunoreactivity is evident.

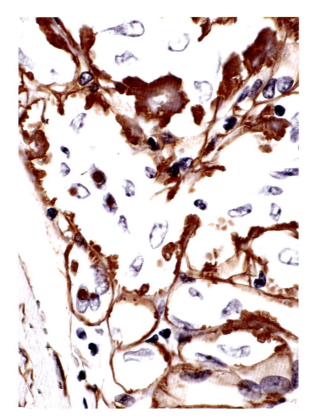

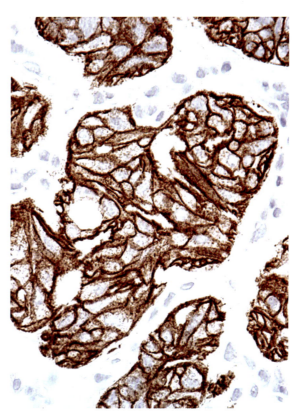

Figure 5-22

HYALINIZING TRABECULAR ADENOMA

The tumor cells are surrounded by abundant basal lamina material, here shown with an immunohistochemical stain for type IV collagen. The deposition of this material is partially responsible for the hyaline appearance of the tumor at the light microscopic level.

Figure 5-23

HYALINIZING TRABECULAR ADENOMA

Strong immunostaining of the cell membrane of the tumor cells with the proliferating marker MIB-1 (Ki-67). This peculiar phenomenon, which is probably of artifactual nature, is seen with some antibody clones but not with others.

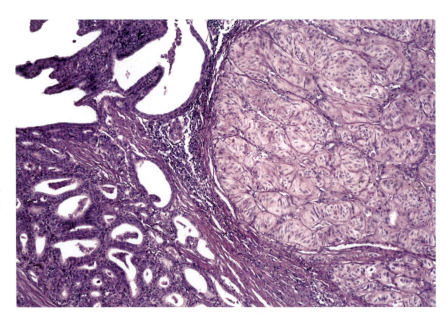

Figure 5-24

HYALINIZING TRABECULAR ADENOMA AND PAPILLARY CARCINOMA

A typical hyalinizing trabecular adenoma pattern (right), and a lesion with the features of a papillary carcinoma (left) are seen side by side, in a cervical lymph node metastasis.

similar expression of high molecular weight keratins (42a,58), and similarities at the molecular genetic level (although the latter two claims have been disputed [see chapter 19]) (61–64). We have also seen several examples of papillary carcinoma merging with hyalinizing trabecular adenoma; one of these tumors had metastasized to the cervical lymph nodes, and the metastases focally had a hyalinizing trabecular adenoma-like pattern (fig. 5-24). Several of the reported cases of hyalinizing trabecular adenoma have occurred against a background of Hashimoto thyroiditis or in patients with a history of radiation to the neck, two common antecedents of papillary carcinoma (65). This combination of findings suggests that hyalinizing trabecular adenoma and papillary carcinoma are probably related.

A somewhat related issue is the occasional occurrence of neoplasms having the cytoarchitectural features of hyalinizing trabecular adenoma but exhibiting capsular and/or vascular invasion. These extremely unusual tumors have been designated *hyalinizing trabecular carcinomas*, which seems logical enough, but their place in the scheme of thyroid neoplasia remains uncertain (65–67). Other authors have proposed using a noncommittal term, such as *hyalinizing trabecular tumor* or *hyalinizing trabecular neoplasm*, to cover the group (68,69). The fact still remains that nearly all of the reported tumors having a hyalinizing trabecular morphology behave in a benign fashion and should therefore be treated conservatively. Specifically, lobectomy is the therapy of choice for them (43,53,70).

Adenolipoma and Adenochondroma

Adenolipoma (also known as *thyrolipoma, adenolipomatosis*, and *hamartomatous adiposity of thyroid gland*) is an exceptionally rare type of follicular adenoma in which the neoplastic follicles are separated by islands of mature adipose tissue (71–73). The lesion is probably not a true mixed tumor with epithelial and mesenchymal components, as the name implies, but rather a follicular adenoma in which the stroma has undergone adipose metaplasia, in a way similar to that also seen in the normal gland, nodular hyperplasia, papillary carcinoma, and, with a much greater frequency, amyloid goiter (74). In one reported case, the adipose tissue within the adenoma had foci of extramedullary hematopoiesis (75).

Adenochondroma has a mixed tumor-like appearance similar to that of adenolipoma, but one in which the stromal component is made up of lobules of mature cartilaginous tissue (fig. 5-25) (76,77). The epithelial and cartilaginous components were sharply demarcated in both of the reported cases.

Atypical Adenoma (Including Spindle Cell Adenoma)

Hazard and Kenyon (42) proposed the term *atypical adenoma* for follicular adenomas having a gross or microscopic appearance which

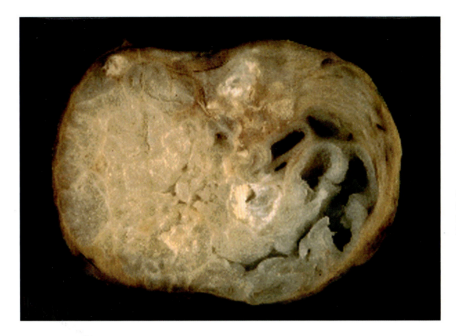

Figure 5-25

FOLLICULAR ADENOMA WITH EXTENSIVE CARTILAGINOUS METAPLASIA (ADENOCHONDROMA)

The lobular configuration and shiny white appearance of the cartilaginous component in this tumor is evident. (Courtesy of Dr. M. Pea, Vicenza, Italy.)

departed from the norm. Specifically, they included in this category (which comprised 2.3 percent of their cases) those adenomas characterized by: 1) closely packed follicles, often lacking lumens; 2) solid columns, often with little intervening stroma; and/or 3) sheet-like or diffusely cellular masses. In their article, they also illustrated cases in which the tumor cells had spindle-shaped nuclei. Grossly, atypical adenomas are said to be more fleshy and more solid than the usual adenoma. The concept of atypical adenoma thus defined is too broad and imprecise; it merges with the trabecular/solid and microfollicular subtypes of follicular adenoma and perhaps even with the hyalinizing trabecular variety. It is possible that some "atypical adenomas" represent the preinvasive phase of a follicular carcinoma (78), but theoretically this may also be true of some conventional adenomas.

The World Health Organization describes as "atypical" those adenomas in which "cellular proliferation is more pronounced and the architectural and cytological patterns are less regular," thus perpetuating the vague and imprecise connotations of the term (79). As a result, atypical adenoma has become, for too many pathologists, a wastebasket term in which any adenoma that looks peculiar or worrisome, even for reasons such as spontaneous necrosis or undue mitotic activity, is included. Since hypercellularity seems the most important cri-

terion that authors have used to place a thyroid adenoma into an atypical category (55,80), it would seem better to designate these lesions *cellular* or *hypercellular adenomas* and to delete the term atypical adenoma altogether (75). In any event, the more "atypical" or cellular an adenoma (regardless of the terminology used), the more important it is to examine it carefully to rule out capsular or vascular invasion.

As above mentioned, some follicular adenomas formerly included in the "atypical" category have a component of spindle cells. When this component predominates, the tumor can be called *spindle cell adenoma*. The metaplastic follicular nature of the spindle cell is demonstrated by their immunohistochemical profile (81). The differential diagnosis includes all other types of thyroid tumors made up of spindle cells , i.e., schwannoma, solitary fibrous tumor, so-called SETTLE, and the spindle cell form of anaplastic carcinoma.

Adenoma with Papillary Features

On occasion, otherwise typical follicular adenomas have papillary or pseudopapillary structures that may be confused with those of papillary carcinoma (figs. 5-26, 5-27). Most of these adenomas are composed of normal-sized (normofollicular) or large (macrofollicular) follicles. It is characteristic for the papillary formations to be short, blunt, and nonbranching, and

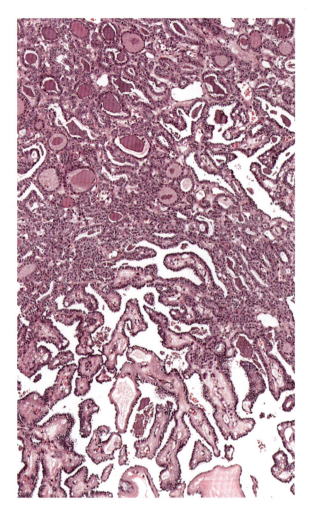

Figure 5-26

FOLLICULAR ADENOMA WITH PAPILLARY FEATURES

The partially papillary pattern of growth of this tumor is evident, but the nuclear and other features of papillary carcinoma were absent.

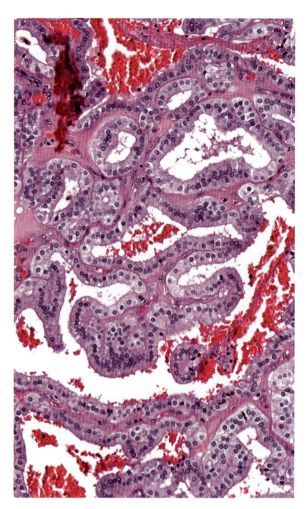

Figure 5-27

FOLLICULAR ADENOMA WITH PAPILLARY FEATURES

The partially papillary appearance of this follicular adenoma may induce to a misdiagnosis of papillary carcinoma, but on higher-power examination the nuclei were basally located, smoothly contoured, and not optically clear, leading to the right diagnosis.

to face the lumens of cystically dilated follicles. A central fibrovascular core is poorly developed or absent. Instead, the stroma is likely to be edematous and to enclose numerous follicles. More important, the follicular cells lining these structures are tall cuboidal or columnar, with basally located nuclei that tend to be perfectly round and normochromatic or hyperchromatic, i.e., substantially different from those typically seen in papillary carcinoma (82). Immunohistochemically, staining for keratin in formalin-fixed, paraffin-embedded material is usually patchy and limited to the low molecular weight

forms of this marker, in contrast to the diffuse and intense staining usually seen in papillary carcinoma.

These papillary structures in adenoma are equivalent in all regards to those seen with higher frequency in hyperplastic nodules and, as in the latter, are probably an expression of localized hyperactivity. Indeed, some of the adenomas featuring these structures are hyperfunctioning ("toxic") (83). The use of the term papillary adenoma for these lesions is objectionable on several grounds (83). Many of the formations in question do not qualify morphologically

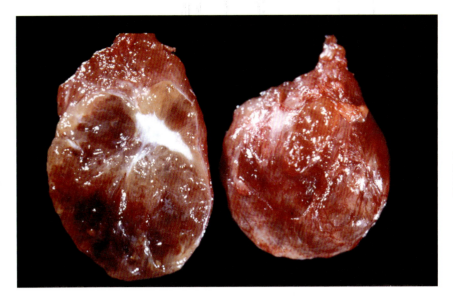

Figure 5-28

"HOT" ADENOMA

A hyperfunctioning ("hot") follicular adenoma. The tumor is soft, bulges on the surface, and has a dark red color due to the high degree of vascularization.

as true papillae. More important, the term papillary adenoma has also been used in the past for encapsulated papillary lesions having all of the features of papillary carcinoma, including characteristic nuclear changes and psammoma bodies. We regard such lesions as encapsulated papillary carcinomas and therefore exclude them from any category of follicular adenoma. It is therefore preferable to designate the type of adenoma described in this section as *adenoma with papillary features*. Other terms that have been employed are *adenoma with papillary architecture*, *adenoma with papillary hyperplasia*, and *hyperplastic papillary adenoma* (83,84). Yet another option that has been suggested, presumably tongue-in-cheek, is that of *papillary variant of follicular adenoma*. The term is actually accurate, but its use is only likely to increase the semantic confusion that already exists.

"Toxic" Adenoma

Toxic adenoma, also known as *hyperfunctioning adenoma* or *Plummer adenoma*, is a follicular adenoma accompanied by clinical evidence of thyroid hyperfunction, usually of a mild degree (fig. 5-28). Such a lesion appears "hot" on a scintigram. The term "toxic" should not be applied to all hot adenomas, however, but only to those in which clinical manifestations occur. Thus defined, toxic adenoma is a rarity (only about 1 percent of all adenomas) and a clinical rather than pathologic entity.

In many clinical papers on toxic adenoma, no attempt was made to distinguish the true adenomas from the substantially more frequent hyperplastic nodules on pathologic grounds (85). Nevertheless, several microscopic correlates of clinically hyperfunctioning thyroid adenomas exist. Such an adenoma is likely to be microfollicular or normofollicular and to contain pseudopapillary formations of the type described earlier. The lining cells tend to be tall cuboidal rather than flattened, and the nuclear to cytoplasmic ratio is likely to be decreased due to cytoplasmic prominence (86,87). At the ultrastructural level, the features are those of very actively secreting follicular cells, comparable to those seen in diffuse hyperplasia (Graves disease) (88). This includes a prominent rough endoplasmic reticulum, well-developed Golgi apparatus, numerous lysosomes, and innumerable slender apical microvilli and pseudopods (35).

REFERENCES

1. Silverberg SG, Vidone RA. Adenoma and carcinoma of the thyroid. Cancer 1966;19:1053-62.

2. Bisi H, Fernandes VS, Asato de Camargo RY, Koch L, Abdo AH, de Brito T. The prevalence of unsuspected thyroid pathology in 300 sequential autopsies, with special reference to the incidental carcinoma. Cancer 1989;64:1888-93.

3. Belfiore A, Sava L, Runello F, Tomaselli L, Vigneri R. Solitary autonomously functioning thyroid nodules and iodine deficiency. J Clin Endocrinol Metab 1983;56:283-7.

4. Brownstein MH, Wolf M, Bikowski JB. Cowden's disease: a cutaneous marker of breast cancer. Cancer 1978;41:2393-8.

5. Feinmesser M, Murray D, Colapinto N, Asa SL. Granulomatous and lymphocytic thyroiditis associated wih a follicular adenoma. Endocr Pathol 1992;3:105-9.

6. Thomas GA, Williams D, Williams ED. The clonal origin of thyroid nodules and adenomas. Am J Pathol 1989;134:141-7.

7. Hicks DG, LiVolsi VA, Neidich JA, Puck JM, Kant JA. Clonal analysis of solitary follicular nodules in the thyroid. Am J Pathol 1990;137:553-62.

8. Namba H, Matsuo K, Fagin JA. Clonal composition of benign and malignant human thyroid tumors. J Clin Invest 1990;86:120-5

9. Chung DH, Kang GH, Kim WH, Ro JY. Clonal analysis of a solitary follicular nodule of the thyroid with the polymerase chain reaction method. Mod Pathol 1999;12:265-71.

10. Apel RL, Ezzat S, Bapat BV, Pan N, LiVolsi VA, Asa SL. Clonality of thyroid nodules in sporadic goiter. Diagn Mol Pathol 1995;4:113-21.

11. Shlossberg AH, Jacobson JC, Ibbertson HK. Serum thyroglobulin in the diagnosis and management of thyroid carcinoma. Clin Endocrinol (Oxf) 1979;10:17-27.

12. Volante M, Papotti M. A practical diagnostic approach to solid/trabecular nodules in the thyroid. Endocr Pathol 2008;19:75-81.

13. Harach HR, Sánchez SS, Williams ED. Pathology of the autonomously functioning (hot) thyroid nodule. Ann Diagn Pathol 2002;6:10-9.

14. Hazard JB. Nomenclature of thyroid tumours. In: Young S, Inman DR, eds. Thyroid neoplasia; Proceedings of the 2nd Imperial Cancer Research Fund symposium held in London in April, 1967. London: Academic Press; 1968:3-38.

15. Sapino A, Cassoni P, Papotti M, Bussolati G. Muscular cushions of the vessel wall at the periphery of thyroid nodules. Mod Pathol 1999;12:879-84.

16. Evans HL. Follicular neoplasms of the thyroid. A study of 44 cases followed for a minimum of 10 years, with emphasis on differential diagnosis. Cancer 1984;54:535-40.

17. LiVolsi VA, Merino MJ. Squamous cells in the human thyroid gland. Am J Surg Pathol 1978;2:133-40.

18. Davila RM, Bedrossian CW, Silverberg AB. Immunocytochemistry of the thyroid in surgical and cytologic specimens. Arch Pathol Lab Med 1988;112:51-6.

19. Kawaoi A, Okano T, Nemoto N, Shikata T. Production of thyroxine (T4) and triiodothyronine (T3) in nontoxic thyroid tumors. An immunohistochemical study. Virchows Arch A Pathol Anat Histol 1981;390:249-57.

20. Nakayama I, Noguchi S, Yamashita H, et al. Immunoelectron microscopic localization of thyroglobulin in human follicular adenoma. Acta Pathol Jpn 1983;33:1139-50.

21. Schelfhout LJ, Van Muijen GN, Fleuren GJ. Expression of keratin 19 distinguishes papillary thyroid carcinoma from follicular carcinomas and follicular thyroid adenoma. Am J Clin Pathol 1989;92:654-8.

22. Buley ID, Gatter KC, Heryet A, Mason DY. Expression of intermediate filament proteins in normal and diseased thyroid glands. J Clin Pathol 1987;40:136-42.

23. Viale G, Dell'Orto P, Coggi G, Gambacorta M. Coexpression of cytokeratins and vimentin in normal and diseased thyroid glands. Lack of diagnostic utility of vimentin immunostaining. Am J Surg Pathol 1989;13:1034-40.

24. Kendall CH, Sanderson PR, Cope J, Talbot IC. Follicular thyroid tumours: a study of laminin and type IV collagen in basement membrane and endothelium. J Clin Pathol 1985;38:1100-5.

25. Miettinen M, Virtanen I. Expression of laminin in thyroid gland and thyroid tumors: an immunohistologic study. Int J Cancer 1984;34:27-30.

26. Cohen MB, Miller TR, Beckstead JH. Enzyme histochemistry and thyroid neoplasia. Am J Clin Pathol 1986;85:668-73.

27. González-Cámpora R, Sanchez Gallego F, Martin Lacave I, Mora Marin J, Montero Linares C, Galera-Davidson H. Lectin histochemistry of the thyroid gland. Cancer 1988;62:2354-62.

28. Sasano H, Rojas M, Silverberg SG. Analysis of lectin binding in benign and malignant thyroid nodules. Arch Pathol Lab Med 1989;113:186-9

29. Nartey N, Cherian MG, Banerjee D. Immunohistochemical localization of metallothionein in human thyroid tumors. Am J Pathol 1987;129:177-82.

30. Barresi G, Tuccari G. Iron-binding proteins in thyroid tumours. An immunocytochemical study. Pathol Res Pract 1987;182:344-51.

31. Tuccari G, Barresi G. Immunohistochemical demonstration of ceruloplasmin in follicular adenomas and thyroid carcinomas. Histopathology 1987;11:723-31.

32. Tuccari G, Barresi G. Tissue polypeptide antigen in thyroid tumours of follicular cell origin: an immunohistochemical re-evaluation for diagnostic purposes. Histopathology 1990;16:377-81.

33. Vierbuchen M, Schröder S, Uhlenbruck G, Ortmann M, Fischer R. CA 50 and CA 19-9 antigen expression in normal, hyperplastic, and neoplastic thyroid tissue. Lab Invest 1989;60:726-32.

34. Ghali VS, Jimenez EJS, Garcia RL. Distribution of Leu-7 antigen (HNK-1) in thyroid tumors: its usefulness as a diagnostic marker for follicular and papillary carcinomas. Hum Pathol 1992;23:21-5.

35. Sobrinho-Simões M, Nesland JM, Johannessen JV. Ultrastructural features of neoplastic lesions of the thyroid gland. In: Russo J, Sommers SC, eds. Tumor diagnosis by electron microscopy. New York: Field, Rich, & Associates; 1989:53-92.

36. Baloch ZW, Livolsi VA. Follicular-patterned lesions of the thyroid: the bane of the pathologist. Am J Clin Pathol 2002;117:143-50.

37. Serra S, Asa SL. Controversies in thyroid pathology: the diagnosis of follicular neoplasms. Endocr Pathol 2008;19:156-65.

38. Chetty R. Follicular patterned lesions of the thyroid gland: a practical algorithmic approach. J Clin Pathol 2011;64:737-41.

39. Gharib H, James EM, Charboneau JW, Naessens JM, Offord KP, Gorman CA. Suppressive therapy with levothyroxine for solitary thyroid nodules. A double-blind controlled clinical study. N Engl J Med 1987;317:70-5.

40. Goldstein R, Hart IR. Follow-up of solitary autonomous thyroid nodules treated with 131I. N Engl J Med 1983;309:1473-6.

41. Faquin WC. The thyroid gland: recurring problems in histologic and cytologic evaluation. Arch Pathol Lab Med 2008;132:622-32.

42. Hazard JB, Kenyon R. Atypical adenoma of the thyroid. Arch Pathol 1954;58:554-63.

43. Carney JA, Ryan J, Goellner JR. Hyalinizing trabecular adenoma of the thyroid gland. Am J Surg Pathol 1987;11:583-91.

44. Ward JV, Murray D, Horvath E, Kovacs K, Baumal R. Hyaline cell tumor of the thyroid with massive accumulation of cytoplasmic microfilaments [Abstract]. Lab Invest 1982;46:88A.

45. Carney JA. Hyalinizing trabecular tumors of the thyroid gland: quadruply described but not by the discoverer. Am J Surg Pathol 2008;32:622-34.

46. Bronner MP, LiVolsi VA, Jennings TA. PLAT: paraganglioma-like adenomas of the thyroid. Surg Pathol 1988;1:383-9.

47. Libbey NP, Hemstreet MK, Butmarc JR, Tibbetts LM, Tucci JR. Paraganglioma-like adenomas of the thyroid (PLAT): incidental lesions with unusual features in a patient with nodular goiter. Endocr Pathol 1997;8:143-51.

48. Gaffney RL, Carney JA, Sebo TJ, et al. Galectin-3 expression in hyalinizing trabecular tumors of the thyroid gland. Am J Surg Pathol 2003;27:494-8.

49. Chan JK, Tse CC, Chiu HS. Hyalinizing trabecular adenoma-like lesion in multinodular goitre. Histopathology 1990;16:611-14.

50. Rothenberg HJ, Goellner JR, Carney JA. Hyalinizing trabecular adenoma of the thyroid gland: recognition and characterization of its cytoplasmic yellow body. Am J Surg Pathol 1999;23:118-25.

51. Rothenberg HJ, Goellner JR, Carney JA. Prevalence and incidence of cytoplasmic yellow bodies in thyroid neoplasms. Arch Pathol Lab Med 2003;127:715-7.

52. Papotti M, Riella P, Montemurro F, Pietribiasi F, Bussolati G. Immunophenotypic heterogeneity of hyalinizing trabecular tumours of the thyroid. Histopathology 1997;31:525-33.

53. Katoh R, Jasani B, Williams ED. Hyalinizing trabecular adenoma of the thyroid. A report of three cases with immunohistochemical and ultrastructural studies. Histopathology 1989;15:211-24.

54. Sambade C, Franssila K, Cameselle-Teijeiro J, Nesland J, Sobrinho-Simões M. Hyalinizing trabecular adenoma: a misnomer for a peculiar tumor of the thyroid gland. Endocr Pathol 1991;2:83-91.

55. Sambade C, Sarabando F, Nesland JM, Sobrinho-Simões M. Hyalinizing trabecular adenoma of the thyroid. Hyalinizing spindle cell tumor of the thyroid with dual differentiation (variant of the so-called hyalinizing trabecular adenoma). Ultrastruct Pathol 1989;13:275-80.

56. Hirokawa M, Carney JA. Cell membrane and cytoplasmic staining for MIB-1 in hyalinizing trabecular adenoma of the thyroid gland. Am J Surg Pathol 2000;24:575-8.

57. Del Sordo R, Sidoni A. MIB-1 cell membrane reactivity: a finding that should be interpreted carefully. Appl Immunohistochem Mol Morphol 2008;16:568.

58. Li M, Carcangiu ML, Rosai J. Abnormal intracellular and extracellular distribution of basement membrane material in papillary carcinoma and hyalinizing trabecular tumors of the thyroid: implication for deregulation of secretory pathways. Hum Pathol 1997;28:1366-72.

59. Katoh R, Kakudo K, Kawaoi A. Accumulated basement membrane material in hyalinizing trabecular tumors of the thyroid. Mod Pathol 1999;12:1057-61.

60. Fonseca E, Nesland JM, Sobrinho-Simões M. Expression of stratified epithelial-type cytokeratins in hyalinizing trabecular adenomas supports their relationship with papillary carcinomas of the thyroid. Histopathology 1997;31:330-5.

61. Cheung CC, Boerner SL, MacMillan CM, Ramyar L, Asa SL. Hyalinizing trabecular tumor of the thyroid: a variant of papillary carcinoma proved by molecular genetics. Am J Surg Pathol 2000;24:1622-6.

62. Papotti M, Volante M, Giuliano A, et al. RET/PTC activation in hyalinizing trabecular tumors of the thyroid. Am J Surg Pathol 2000;24:1615-21.

63. Hirokawa M, Carney JA, Ohtsuki Y. Hyalinizing trabecular adenoma and papillary carcinoma of the thyroid gland express different cytokeratin patterns. Am J Surg Pathol 2000;24:877-81.

64. Salvatore G, Chiappetta G, Nikiforov YE, et al. Molecular profile of hyalinizing trabecular tumours of the thyroid: high prevalence of RET/PTC rearrangements and absence of B-raf and N-ras point mutations. Eur J Cancer 2005;41:816-21.

65. Molberg K, Albores-Saavedra J. Hyalinizing trabecular carcinoma of the thyroid gland. Hum Pathol 1994;25:192-7.

66. McCluggage WG, Sloan JM. Hyalinizing trabecular carcinoma of thyroid gland. Histopathology 1996;28:357-62.

67. González-Cámpora R, Fuentes-Vaamonde E, Hevia-Vázquez A, Otal-Salaverri C, Villar-Rodriguez JL, Galera-Davidson H. Hyalinizing trabecular carcinoma of the thyroid gland: report of two cases of follicular cell thyroid carcinoma with hyalinizing trabecular pattern. Ultrastruct Pathol 1998;22:39-46.

68. Nosé V, Volante M, Papotti M. Hyalinizing trabecular tumor of the thyroid: an update. Endocr Pathol 2008;19:1-8.

69. LiVolsi VA. Hyalinizing trabecular tumor of the thyroid: adenoma, carcinoma, or neoplasm of uncertain malignant potential? Am J Surg Pathol 2000;24:1683-4.

70. Carney JA, Hirokawa M, Lloyd RV, Papotti M, Sebo TJ. Hyalinizing trabecular tumors of the thyroid gland are almost all benign. Am J Surg Pathol 2008;32:1877-89.

71. DeRienzo D, Truong L. Thyroid neoplasms containing mature fat: a report of two cases and review of the literature. Mod Pathol 1989;2:506-10.

72. Schröder S, Böcker W, Hüsselmann H, Dralle H. Adenolipoma (thyrolipoma) of the thyroid gland: report of two cases and review of the literature. Virchows Arch A Pathol Anat Histopathol 1984;404:99-103.

73. Gnepp DR, Ogorzalek JM, Heffess CS. Fat-containing lesions of the thyroid gland. Am J Surg Pathol 1989;13:605-12.

74. Hamed G, Heffess CS, Shmookler BM, Wenig BM. Amyloid goiter. A clinicopathologic study of 14 cases and review of the literature. Am J Clin Pathol 1995;104:306-12.

75. Schmid C, Beham A, Seewann HL. Extramedullary haematopoiesis in the thyroid gland. Histopathology 1989;15:423-5.

76. Visonà A, Pea M, Bozzola L, Stracca-Pansa V, Meli S. Follicular adenoma of the thyroid gland with extensive chondroid metaplasia. Histopathology 1991;18:278-9.

77. Wolvos TA, Chong FK, Razvi SA, Tully GL 3rd. An unusual thyroid tumor: a comparison to a literature review of thyroid teratomas. Surgery 1985;97:613-7.

78. Tzen CY, Huang YW, Fu YS. Is atypical follicular adenoma of the thyroid a preinvasive malignancy? Hum Pathol 2003;34:666-9.

79. Hedinger CE, Williams ED, Sobin LH. Histological typing of thyroid tumours. In: Hediger CE, ed. International histological classification of tumours, Vol 11, 2nd ed. Berlin: Springer-Verlag; 1988.

80. Lang W, Georgii A, Stauch G, Kienzle E. The differentiation of atypical adenomas and encapsulated follicular carcinomas in the thyroid gland. Virchows Arch A Pathol Anat Histol 1980;385:125-41.

81. Matoso A, Easley SE, Mangray S, Jacob R, DeLellis RA. Spindle cell foci in the thyroid gland: an immunohistochemical analysis. Appl Immunohistochem Mol Morphol 2011;19:400-7.

82. LiVolsi VA. Surgical pathology of the thyroid. In: Major problems in pathology; Vol 22 [series] Philadelphia: WB Saunders; 1990.

83. Vickery AL Jr. Thyroid papillary carcinoma. Pathological and philosophical controversies. Am J Surg Pathol 1983;7:797-807.

84. Mai KT, Landry DC, Thomas J, et al. Follicular adenoma with papillary architecture: a lesion mimicking papillary thyroid carcinoma. Histopathology 2001;39:25-32.

85. Horst W, Rösler H, Schneider C, Labhart A. 306 cases of toxic adenoma: clinical aspects, findings in radioiodine diagnostics, radiochromatography and histology; results of 131-I and surgical treatment. J Nucl Med 1967;8:515-28.

86. Campbell WL, Santiago HE, Perzin KH, Johnson PM. The autonomous thyroid nodule: correlation of scanappearance and histopathology. Radiology 1973;107:133-8.

87. Hamburger JI. Solitary autonomously functioning thyroid lesions. Diagnosis, clinical features and pathogenetic considerations. Am J Med 1975;58:740-8.

88. Panke TW, Croxson MS, Parker JW, Carriere DP, Rosoff L Sr, Warner NE. Triiodothyronine-secreting (toxic) adenoma of the thyroid gland: light and electron microscopic characteristics. Cancer 1978;41:528-37.

6 FOLLICULAR THYROID CARCINOMA

Follicular thyroid carcinoma is a malignant epithelial tumor showing evidence of follicular cell differentiation and not belonging to any of the distinctive types of thyroid carcinoma. Generically, any malignant thyroid tumor with phenotypic and/or architectural features indicative of follicular cell differentiation could be regarded as a follicular carcinoma. The difficulty with this approach is that it results in lumping into one category tumor types that vary considerably in their morphologic appearance and, more importantly, natural history (1). The substantial differences that exist among these tumors would be obscured and the result would be inappropriate therapeutic and prognostic conclusions (2). Tumors that have enough distinctive features to be excluded from the category of follicular carcinoma "not otherwise specified" are therefore discussed in other sections of this Fascicle, and include the following:

Follicular Variant of Papillary Carcinoma. This tumor is thought to belong to the papillary family of neoplasms despite its predominantly or exclusively follicular pattern of growth (see chapter 7).

Follicular Carcinoma, Oncocytic Variant (Hürthle Cell Carcinoma). Most oncocytic thyroid tumors have a follicular pattern of growth, although they are often admixed with trabecular or solid areas. We believe that these lesions differ enough from other follicular tumors to justify considering them separately (see chapter 10).

Poorly Differentiated (Including "Insular") Carcinoma. Most of these tumors probably represent poorly differentiated types of follicular carcinoma; however, others with a similar appearance have been found to have a close link with papillary carcinoma. Because of these histogenetic considerations and the unfavorable prognostic connotations associated with this pattern, we prefer to place these tumors in a category of their own (see chapter 8).

In series originating from noniodine-deficient regions, the frequency of follicular carcinoma among thyroid malignancies ranges from 5 to 15 percent of all thyroid cancers (3–5). Unfortunately, not much weight can be given to these figures considering the lack of consistency with which the term follicular carcinoma is used. Nevertheless, it seems established that, in iodine-deficient areas, the incidence of this tumor type is 30 to 40 percent (3–6). Interestingly, iodide addition to the diet results in an increase in papillary carcinoma and a corresponding decrease in follicular carcinoma (4,7,8).

Whether thyroid nodular hyperplasia not related to iodine deficiency ("sporadic") is associated with a higher incidence of follicular carcinoma remains a controversial issue. If there is indeed an increased incidence, it seems to be of such a minimal nature that it becomes insignificant from a clinical standpoint.

Even more controversial is the alleged relationship between follicular carcinoma and dyshormonogenetic goiter. Here the difficulty is compounded by the fact that dyshormonogenetic glands may acquire multinodular, hypercellular, atypical, and pseudoinvasive features (9). Therefore, some pathologists do not accept a diagnosis of follicular carcinoma arising in a dyshormonogenetic gland unless the tumor has metastasized. We think this is an unreasonably restrictive approach. We believe that the criteria for malignancy should be the same regardless of whether the gland is the site of this genetically determined abnormality or not. In any event, enough metastasizing thyroid carcinomas arising in such glands are now on record to indicate that their frequency may indeed be increased (9,10).

Follicular carcinoma is more prevalent in women; the average age of occurrence is 10 years older than for those with papillary carcinoma (11). It typically presents as a solitary thyroid nodule that is nearly always "cold" on scintigraphic examination and unaccompanied by cervical adenopathy. It is rare for follicular carcinoma to be "hot" and even rarer to result in clinically evident signs of hyperthyroidism,

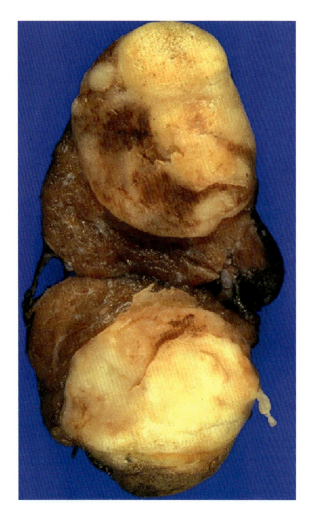

Figure 6-1

MINIMALLY INVASIVE FOLLICULAR CARCINOMA

The tumor is encapsulated, has a homogeneous light tan appearance, and contains small foci of hemorrhage. The features are indistinguishable from those of a cellular follicular adenoma.

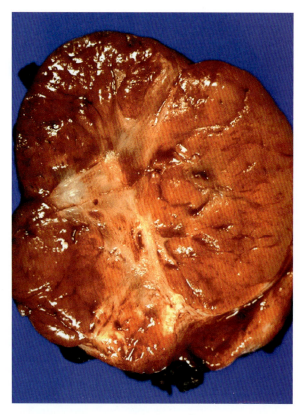

Figure 6-2

MINIMALLY INVASIVE FOLLICULAR CARCINOMA

The tumor has a fleshy appearance and an irregularly shaped central scar.

but several well-documented cases are on record (12,13). Occasionally, distant metastases (particularly to the bone) are the first manifestations of the disease. In contrast to papillary carcinoma, it is unusual for follicular carcinoma to be clinically occult (14).

Once the special types of carcinoma listed above have been eliminated, there remains a relatively homogeneous form of thyroid malignancy to which the term follicular carcinoma is well suited. Still, from a morphologic and prognostic standpoint, this tumor is traditionally divided into two major categories on the basis of the degree of invasiveness: 1) minimally invasive or encapsulated and 2) widely invasive. There is little overlap between these two types, of which the former is by far the most common.

MINIMALLY INVASIVE (ENCAPSULATED) TYPE

Gross Findings. The gross appearance of this tumor does not differ appreciably from that of a follicular adenoma. It is generally round and of variable size (although almost always larger than 1 cm in diameter) and is light tan to brown, with a solid, bulging cut surface (figs. 6-1, 6-2). Secondary hemorrhagic, cystic, and fibrotic changes occur as frequently as in adenomas. The capsule that surrounds the tumor tends to be thicker and more irregular than in adenomas (figs. 6-3, 6-4) (15). It is unusual for capsular or blood vessel invasion to be identifiable on gross examination.

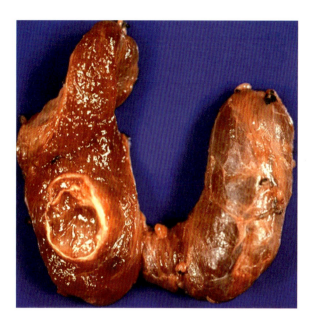

Figure 6-3

MINIMALLY INVASIVE FOLLICULAR CARCINOMA

It is common for this type of tumor to have a capsule that is thicker and more irregular than that of an adenoma, as shown in this case. This tumor, which also had prominent cystic changes, metastasized to the iliac bone.

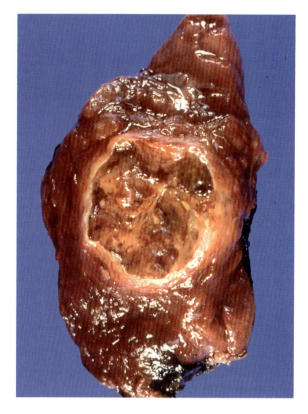

Figure 6-4

MINIMALLY INVASIVE FOLLICULAR CARCINOMA

The tumor is surrounded by a thick capsule and shows extensive cystic degenerative changes.

Microscopic Findings. The cytoarchitectural features of minimally invasive follicular carcinoma resemble those of its benign counterpart. The carcinomas, however, have more hypercellular forms (corresponding to the embryonal, fetal, and atypical forms of the adenoma), and few exhibit a normofollicular or macrofollicular (colloid) appearance. The index of suspicion should be raised whenever encountering a follicular neoplasm with a solid, trabecular, microfollicular, or atypical pattern of growth (16,17). Mitotic figures are easily seen and nuclei are large and have conspicuous nucleoli (18,19). Despite this, the diagnosis of malignancy depends primarily on the demonstration of unequivocal capsular or vascular invasion (20). Because of the crucial significance of invasion, a detailed description is in order.

Capsular Invasion. It has been traditionally accepted that a tumor must penetrate the entire thickness of the capsule to be regarded as having unequivocal capsular invasion (fig. 6-5). Irregularities of contour along the capsular inner border or clusters of follicular cells embedded within the capsule are not sufficient. A serious interpretive problem is created by the presence of a small nodule of tumor cells lying immediately outside an intact capsule. The two possible explanations for this phenomenon are invasion of the capsule not apparent at that particular level (which would imply the diagnosis of carcinoma) and occurrence of an independent follicular nodule adjacent to the larger one (which would not). Irregular outlines and similarity of cytoarchitectural features favor the former interpretation, which could be explained as a narrow focus of capsular invasion with a more expansile (mushroom-like) extracapsular component. The opposite features, together with the presence of additional similar nodules in the remaining thyroid gland, would be more in keeping with the latter interpretation. In any event, demonstration of a capsular break through serial sectioning or submission of additional material is necessary before labeling the tumor as malignant.

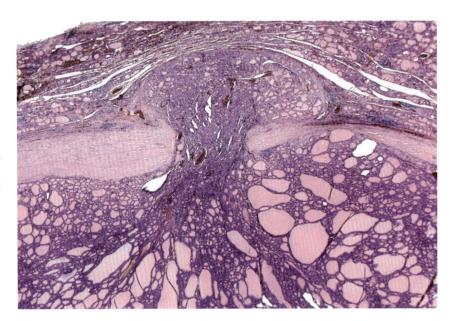

Figure 6-5

MINIMALLY INVASIVE FOLLICULAR CARCINOMA

There is total interruption of the capsule by the tumor, which then grows into the adjacent thyroid tissue in a typical mushroom-like fashion.

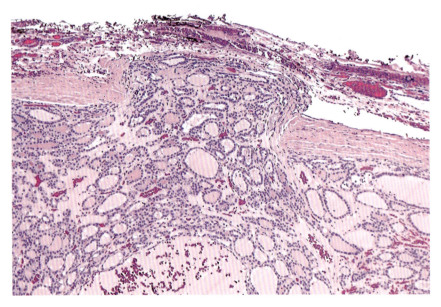

Figure 6-6

MINIMALLY INVASIVE FOLLICULAR CARCINOMA

Total capsular interruption by the tumor growth, which also shows an area highly suggestive of vascular invasion.

It follows that the initial sampling of a grossly encapsulated follicular-patterned tumor should provide a thorough representation of the capsule (ideally of its total circumference unless the tumor is excessively large) (see chapter 21) (21). When a follicular carcinoma invades into and through the capsule, it usually does not permeate the surrounding parenchyma; instead, a new fibrous capsule is often formed at the leading edge. When the expansile extracapsular component becomes very large but is covered by this newly formed capsule, the tumor may resemble a dumb-

bell or may appear as an irregular nodule partially divided in two by an apparent septum.

As already mentioned, the fibrous capsule tends to be thicker in carcinomas than in adenomas and the interface with the tumor more irregular (figs. 6-6–6-8) (15,21,22). A possible explanation of these seemingly paradoxical findings is that the capsule of an adenoma is merely the result of the condensation of preexistent stromal fibers by the expanding mass, whereas that of the carcinoma probably possesses, in addition, a component of newly

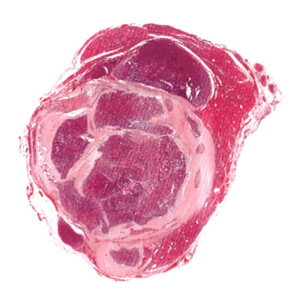

Figure 6-7

MINIMALLY INVASIVE FOLLICULAR CARCINOMA

Note the marked thickening of the capsule and the numerous areas of capsular invasion.

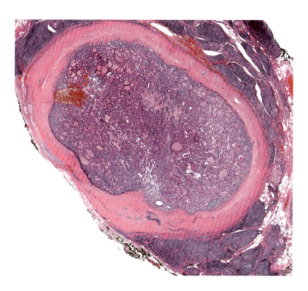

Figure 6-8

FOLLICULAR NEOPLASM WITH THICK NONINVADED CAPSULE

Tumors in which the capsule is unduly thick should be regarded as suspicious for follicular carcinoma or the follicular variant of papillary carcinoma. Evidence of capsular of vascular invasion should be sought after thorough sampling.

laid down collagen fibers as an expression of host response to the malignancy.

Foci of capsular invasion should be distinguished from capsular rupture resulting from a fine-needle aspiration biopsy (FNAB) procedure. The latter should be suspected when the area in question has a fissure-like quality, contains foci of recent or old hemorrhage, and exhibits florid stromal reparative changes (23).

Another mimic of capsular invasion is the pseudoinvasion resulting from herniation of tumor tissue when the section for histology has been taken perpendicularly to a previous capsule cut made by the surgeon or pathologist on the fresh specimen. To avoid this trap, it is advisable to disregard the areas at the very edge of the section in which the tumor appears to be enwrapping an abrupt cross section of the capsule (figs. 6-9, 6-10) (24).

Vascular Invasion. Invasion of blood vessels by tumor cells is a much more reliable predictor of clinical aggressiveness than capsular invasion (25–27). The criteria for its recognition, therefore, need to be just as stringent if not more so (16,17,28–32). The vessel in question should be located within the capsule or immediately

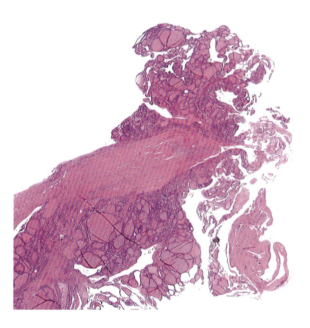

Figure 6-9

FOLLICULAR NEOPLASM WITH RUPTURED CAPSULE

If the capsule of a follicular tumor is torn during surgery or gross dissection, the herniated tumor tissue may simulate capsular invasion. A diagnosis of capsular invasion should not be made if only one edge of the capsule is identified and the tumor tissue appears ragged and disrupted.

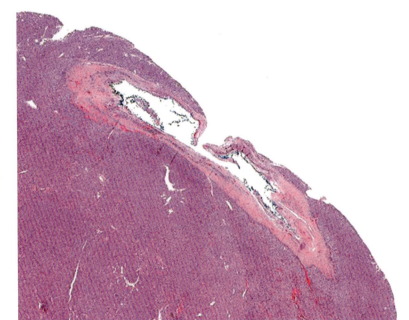

Figure 6-10

FOLLICULAR NEOPLASM

The capsule of this tumor is turned into iteself after being artifactually torn, creating a false impression of capsular invasion.

outside it (rather than within the tumor itself) (figs. 6-11, 6-12). It should be of large (i.e., venous rather than capillary) caliber and should have an identifiable endothelial lining. The intravascular cells should have a clear-cut epithelial appearance (fig. 6-13). They should project into the vessel lumen in a thrombus-like fashion, in such a way that they partly or completely obliterate it. Most importantly, they should be attached at some point to the vessel wall (figs. 6-11–6-13) (32). A cluster of follicular cells found floating in the vascular lumen may be the result of artifactual detachment at surgery or gross examination and should therefore be discounted. Another feature to be regarded as insufficient evidence of vascular invasion is the close intermingling of follicular cells and vessels within the capsule. This may be the result of the labyrinthine configuration of those vessels coupled with the sometimes marked irregularity of the interface between tumor cells and capsule.

There is some controversy regarding the significance of the endothelial layer often seen over the tumor nests protruding into the vascular lumen. Some observers consider this evidence that vascular invasion has not yet occurred, arguing that one component of the vessel wall is still present between the tumor cells and the vascular lumen. Others, ourselves included, not only regard its presence as com-

patible with a diagnosis of vascular invasion, but view it as corroborating evidence for this occurrence (16). According to this interpretation, the reason for its presence would be analogous to that operating in ordinary thrombi, i.e., an attempt at organization and recanalization.

Because it is sometimes difficult to decide whether an intracapsular nest of tumor cells is located within a vessel or not, attempts have been made to facilitate this determination with the use of special stains. In general, the results have been disappointing, mostly because of the peculiar nature of the capsular vessels. Despite their large caliber, the walls are partially or sometimes completely devoid of a continuous smooth muscle layer or an elastic lamina (fig. 6-14) (16). As a result, elastic tissue stains, trichrome stains, or immunocytochemical reactions for smooth muscle actin are often useless. Immunostains for endothelial cells, such as CD31, CD34 (not very specific), factor VIII-related antigen (which tends to diffuse out), Ulex europaeus agglutinin I (very labile), FLI-1 (which, being a nuclear marker, does not delineate continuously the vessel in question), and ERG (V-ETS avian erythroblastosis virus E26 oncogene homologue) are more useful (fig. 6-15) (32–36). The results with any of these markers are sometimes negative in structures indubitably representing vessels, whether for

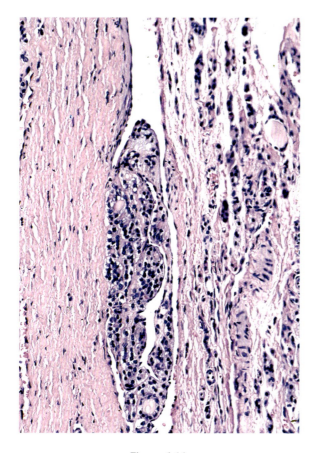

Figure 6-11

VASCULAR INVASION IN FOLLICULAR CARCINOMA

A tumor thrombus fills and distends the lumen of a capsular vessel and is attached to the vessel wall. The vessel has a characteristically thin quality.

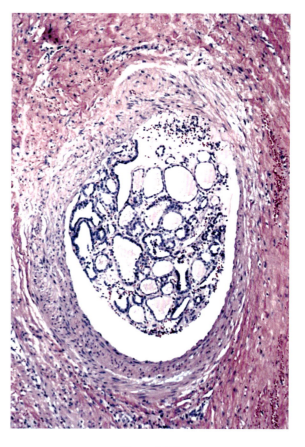

Figure 6-12

VASCULAR INVASION IN FOLLICULAR CARCINOMA

It is unusual for invaded capsular vessels to have a wall as thick as that exhibited in this case. The attachment of tumor to the vessel wall is evident.

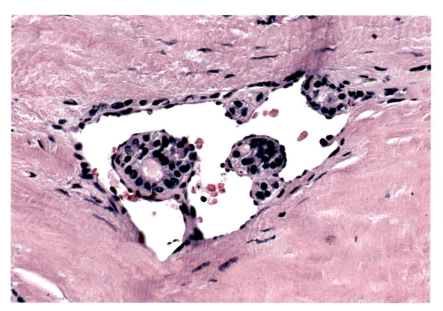

Figure 6-13

VASCULAR INVASION IN FOLLICULAR CARCINOMA

Tumor thrombi protrude into the vascular lumen in a polyp-like fashion. Most are covered by an attenuated layer of endothelial cells, in a fashion similar to that seen in ordinary thrombi.

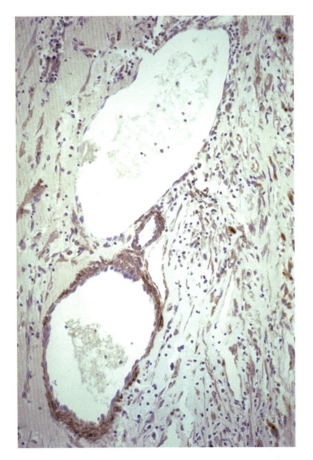

Figure 6-14

CAPSULAR VESSEL

An immunostain for smooth muscle actin shows that some capsular vessels have a thin layer of smooth muscle whereas others (probably of lymphatic nature) lack it almost completely. A tumor growing in this area could easily reach the vascular lumen.

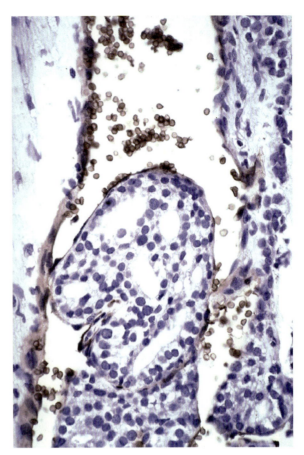

Figure 6-15

VASCULAR INVASION IN FOLLICULAR CARCINOMA

The blood vessel invasion of this follicular carcinoma is confirmed with staining for Ulex europaeus agglutinin I. The endothelial cells are positive, including those covering the tumor thrombus. The intravascular red blood cells are also reactive.

technical reasons, delayed fixation, or true lack of marker expression.

Invasion of capsular blood vessels by tumor can be simulated by reactive proliferations of the vascular structures themselves, which acquire a variety of patterns, including papillary endothelial hyperplasia (so-called Masson lesion) and Kaposi sarcoma-like features (figs. 6-16, 6-17) (37–40). Some of these are probably the expression of organization and recanalization of thrombi (whether spontaneous or following FNAB), others are induced by angiogenic factors secreted by the tumor cells, and still others are secondary to blood vessel invasion by tumor that is not apparent in the section examined, as suggested

by the fact that they are more commonly seen in follicular carcinomas than in follicular adenomas (40). The performance of serial sections and immunostains for vessel-related cells and tumor cells are useful in this situation (fig. 6-18).

Another type of change that can be seen in the capsular vessels of follicular carcinoma is the "muscular cushion" already described in chapter 5 in connection with follicular adenoma. This change has no diagnostic or prognostic significance (41).

Rare examples of follicular carcinomas have been described that have a prominent spindle cell component (42,43), a rhabdoid phenotype (44), or a peculiar glomeruloid pattern of growth (45).

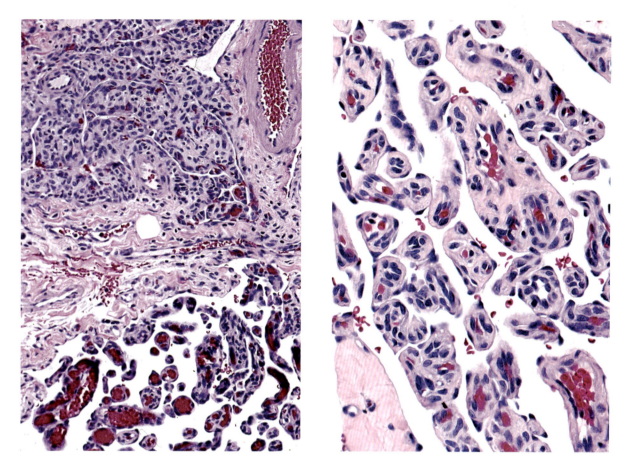

Figure 6-16

VASCULAR PROLIFERATION IN FOLLICULAR NEOPLASM

Left: The extremely cellular proliferation in the capsular vessels can simulate capsular and vascular invasion by tumor. The upper half has a more solid appearance, whereas the lower half has the features of intravascular papillary endothelial hyperplasia (so-called Masson hemangioma).

Right: High-power view of the component with the features of intravascular papillary endothelial hyperplasia.

Immunohistochemical and Ultrastructural Findings. The main phenotypical and ultrastructural features of follicular carcinoma do not differ from those of follicular adenoma, but some immunohistochemical differences have been described. These include increased expression of COX-2, loss of expression of BCL-2, loss of the RAP1GAP protein, increased expression of human telomerase reverse transcriptase, higher titers of the cell proliferation markers MCM2 and cyclin D1, increased expression of matrix metalloproteinases (especially MMP2), expression of p27, and abnormalities of retinoid acid receptor in the carcinomas. None of these differences is of proven diagnostic use (46–60). Ultrastructurally, the solid/trabecular areas of

follicular carcinoma show a lesser degree of differentiation than those with a follicular pattern of growth, and are more similar to poorly differentiated carcinoma (fig. 6-19) (61,62).

Molecular Genetic Findings. See chapter 19.

Cytologic Findings. See chapter 20.

Differential Diagnosis. The differential diagnosis of minimally invasive follicular carcinoma includes follicular adenoma, a dominant nodule of nodular hyperplasia, the follicular variant of papillary carcinoma, and the tubular (follicular) variant of medullary carcinoma (63,64). Of these, the most common and most difficult is the distinction with follicular adenoma. This is not surprising since many features are shared by the two neoplasms. As already mentioned, the

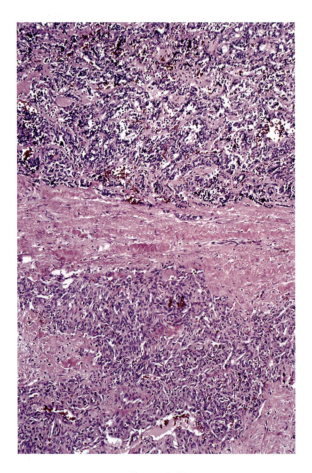

Figure 6-17

**VASCULAR PROLIFERATION
IN FOLLICULAR NEOPLASM**

The florid vascular proliferation on both sides of the capsule of a follicular tumor simulates massive capsular invasion.

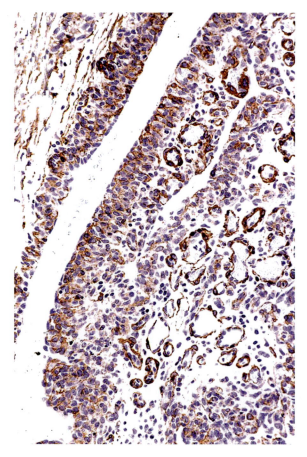

Figure 6-18

**VASCULAR PROLIFERATION
IN FOLLICULAR NEOPLASM**

The endothelial nature of many of the cells is evident with an immunostain for CD31.

distinction is largely based on the detection of capsular or blood vessel invasion in the carcinoma.

There are two matters of practical importance that need to be addressed. The first issue is whether there is such a thing as a *noninvasive follicular carcinoma*, i.e., a follicular carcinoma lacking capsular or vascular invasion. From a theoretical standpoint, the answer must of necessity be "yes," because it is inconceivable that all follicular carcinomas are "born" with capsular or vascular invasion in them. At a practical or "managerial" level, the answer is generally "no." Only when a noninvasive encapsulated follicular tumor shows clear-cut signs of malignancy in the form of high mitotic activity (including atypical forms), widespread nuclear

atypia with undue nucleolar prominence (rather than the occasional bizarre hyperchromatic nucleus), and necrosis, or when it is associated with documented distant metastases, should this diagnostic term be considered. When thus defined, noninvasive carcinoma is exceptional indeed. The few cases we have seen have shared many of the nuclear/cytoplasmic features of poorly differentiated (insular) carcinoma, and we suspect that a more thorough sampling would have revealed the presence of invasion.

The second issue concerns how to handle well-differentiated follicular neoplasms in which the capsular interruption is "incomplete," in the sense of involving only the inner half or being represented by tumor islands embedded

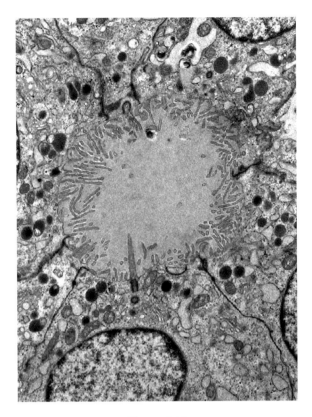

Figure 6-19

FOLLICULAR CARCINOMA

The follicular tumor cells shown in this electron micrograph converge toward a central lumen that contains moderately electron-dense granular material consistent with colloid. Numerous long microvilli are seen on the luminal side of the tumor cells, as well as single cilium. Other features include junctional complexes, lysosomes, and a moderately well-developed endoplasmic reticulum. The appearance is indistinguishable from that of a follicular adenoma. (Courtesy of Dr. R. Erlandson, New York, NY.)

within the capsule, a situation in which there is considerable interobserver variability. The Chernobyl group of thyroid pathologists (65) recommended the adoption of the following terminology when facing this situation: for tumors showing definite (complete) capsular invasion and no papillary carcinoma-type nuclear changes: *follicular carcinoma*; for tumors showing questionable capsular invasion: *follicular tumor of uncertain malignant potential (FT-UMP)* if papillary carcinoma-type nuclear changes are absent, and well-differentiated tumor of uncertain malignant potential (WDT-UMP) if papillary carcinoma-type nuclear changes are questionable (incomplete).

Most of the authors of this Fascicle look favorably at this proposal, with the understanding that "UMP" tumors do not represent a distinct category on either morphologic or immunohistochemical grounds (66,67). One of us (JR) is inclined to avoid the term carcinoma even for tumors in which capsular invasion is complete as long as: 1) the capsule is thin, inconspicuous, regular, and with an inner smooth surface; 2) there is no blood vessel invasion; 3) papillary carcinoma-type nuclear features are absent; and 4) the tumor is well differentiated throughout, both at an architectural and cytologic level.

The above proposal has generated a lot of controversy and a good deal of criticism. One concern is the potential for a low level of interobserver and intraobserver reproducibility, although the few studies that have been carried out so far looking into this aspect have shown that such a level is not significantly different whether a UMP category is included or not (68,69). The legitimate concern has been expressed that UMP might become a "wastebasket" for many follicular lesions that do not fit comfortably into the minimally invasive category. A second issue relates to the acceptance (or lack thereof) of this terminology by surgeons and endocrinologists. Pathologists who use this nomenclature more often than not will receive a call from one of the clinicians asking if the lesion is "benign" or "malignant" (we all have difficulty in dealing with uncertainty!). Patients may also call asking the same question. The approach that some of us (RAD) have taken is to classify lesions of this type as *follicular adenomas with focal atypical features* (rather than atypical adenomas), accompanied by a note indicating that the findings are insufficiently well-developed to warrant an unequivocal diagnosis of malignancy, that in all likelihood the lesion will behave in a favorable fashion, and that lobectomy is likely to be adequate therapy.

Spread and Metastases. Because a sine qua non for the diagnosis of minimally invasive follicular carcinoma is for the capsular invasion to be *minimal*, it follows that direct extension into the perithyroid tissue is never a feature at the time of presentation. Recurrence in the residual gland after lobectomy is also rare. Lymph node metastases to the neck are the exception. Whenever they are observed in a tumor presumed to be

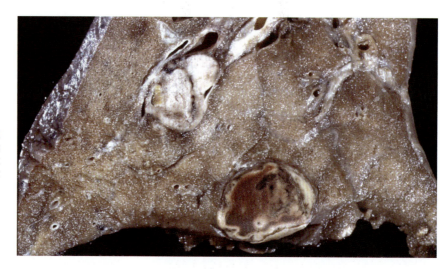

Figure 6-20

LUNG METASTASIS OF FOLLICULAR CARCINOMA

This well-circumscribed intrapulmonary nodule was the largest of several metastatic lung foci of a thyroid follicular carcinoma.

a follicular carcinoma, the alternative possibilities of follicular variant of papillary carcinoma, oncocytic carcinoma, and poorly differentiated carcinoma should be considered.

The most common sites for metastases in follicular carcinoma are lung and bone, particularly the latter (figs. 6-20, 6-21) (70). Sometimes bone metastases (which are usually osteolytic) are the first manifestation of the disease. A pathologic fracture of a long bone due to a metastasis of a previously silent follicular thyroid carcinoma is a well-known form of presentation. Bones most often involved are long bones (such as the femur) and flat bones (particularly the pelvis and sternum but also skull) (71). Another unusual but documented site of metastases of thyroid follicular carcinoma is the skin (72).

Bone metastases can feature follicular structures so well differentiated as to closely simulate those of non-neoplastic thyroid gland (73). This is the source for the picturesque but oxymoronic and deservedly obsolete term, *benign metastasizing goiter*. The high degree of differentiation is also demonstrated by the ability of the follicular structures to incorporate radioactive iodine, a feature that is exploited for diagnostic and therapeutic purposes.

Metastatic follicular thyroid carcinoma may be simulated microscopically by endolymphatic sac tumor (74), thyroid-like follicular carcinoma of kidney (75), and intrahepatic cholangiocarcinoma (76,77), all of which are exceptional occurrences. In turn, ovarian metastases of follicular thyroid carcinoma may be mistakenly interpreted as struma ovarii (78).

Treatment and Prognosis. The optimal therapy for minimally invasive follicular carcinoma remains just as controversial as that for papillary carcinoma. Some authors advocate total thyroidectomy followed by the administration of radioactive iodine (79,80). Others, ourselves included, believe that a more conservative approach, i.e., a lobectomy or subtotal thyroidectomy without radioactive iodine administration, will result in similar if not identical survival curves (81–83). In the absence of prospective randomized studies, the issue remains open.

Metastatic disease is generally treated with radioactive iodine. Excision or external radiation therapy can also be used, depending on the site and number of metastases. Bone metastases are rarely cured, but excellent long-term palliation can be achieved (80).

The overall prognosis of patients with minimally invasive follicular carcinoma is excellent, perhaps as good as that of papillary carcinoma. This is not immediately apparent when evaluating the extant literature on the subject. The main problem is that, in most of these papers (particularly those published in surgical or clinical journals), the term follicular carcinoma is used in a generic sense, thereby including neoplasms with a distinctly less favorable outcome, such as widely invasive and poorly differentiated carcinomas (84). An additional source of difficulty is that, in some series, no distinction is made between the patients who developed metastases after thyroidectomy and those who already had them at the time of the initial diagnosis, i.e., those who presented with stage III disease (15).

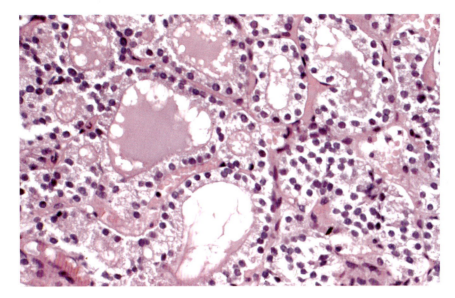

Figure 6-21

BONE METASTASIS OF FOLLICULAR CARCINOMA

The tumor is extremely well differentiated and indistinguishable from a follicular adenoma.

The few studies that have dealt exclusively with the minimally invasive type of follicular carcinoma that was limited to the thyroid gland at the time of surgery have shown a cure rate of over 95 percent (18). This figure has reached 100 percent in some series in which capsular invasion was the sole criterion for malignancy, leading some authors to question the diagnostic significance of the latter finding (82,85–87). The indolent nature and excellent prognosis of these tumors was made apparent by the lack of encapsulated, well-differentiated, follicular patterned carcinomas in a large series of fatal thyroid carcinomas (84). It is because of these figures that, as indicated above, we have taken an increasingly conservative approach to this tumor type, and are following the recommendations of the Chernobyl group of thyroid pathologists group by avoiding the word carcinoma for those neoplasms in which the evidence of capsular or blood vessel invasion is questionable (65,89).

It seems to us that there is room for a clinically significant subdivision of minimally invasive (encapsulated) follicular carcinomas, which would take into account the fact that there are marked prognostic differences among those tumors that show invasion of only the capsule, and those that show vascular invasion (14), with or without capsular invasion and the fact that among those with vascular invasion, there seems to be a prognostic difference depending on the number of vessels involved. The subdivision in question, which represents a departure from the classic scheme and which will therefore need to be validated by clinico-pathologic studies, is shown in Table 6-1.

A somewhat similar proposal has been made by D'Avanzo et al. (90), although using a terminology that we find confusing and potentially misleading, i.e., calling minimally invasive the tumors with capsular invasion only, and moderately invasive those with vascular invasion (with or without capsular invasion).

In cases of follicular carcinoma with metastatic involvement of lung or bone, adverse prognostic factors include multiplicity of sites, older patient age at the time of discovery of the metastases, and absence of radioactive iodine uptake by the metastases. In one series (which also included some "moderately differentiated" types and probably some widely invasive tumors), the overall survival rates were 53 percent at 5 years, 38 percent at 10 years, and 30 percent at 15 years (91).

WIDELY INVASIVE TYPE

As the name indicates, this tumor shows extensive areas of invasion at the gross and microscopic level, and therefore, the differentiation from adenoma is obvious (fig. 6-22). Often, the mass lacks evidence of preexisting encapsulation altogether. Lang et al. (92) suggested including in this category those encapsulated follicular neoplasms in which four or more capsular vessels are invaded, a criterion that we have adopted for the proposal seen in Table 6-1.

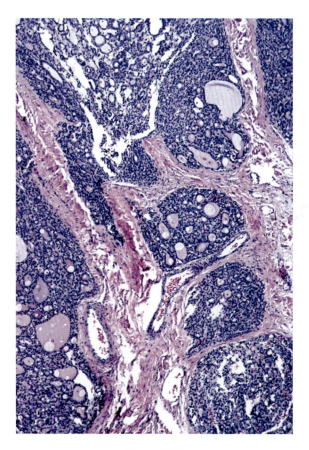

Figure 6-22

WIDELY INVASIVE FOLLICULAR CARCINOMA

This follicular carcinoma invades the thyroid gland in a multinodular fashion, with no evidence of capsule formation.

Table 6-1

PROPOSED SUBDIVISION OF MINIMALLY INVASIVE (ENCAPSULATED) FOLLICULAR CARCINOMAS

With capsular (but no vascular) invasion

With limited vascular invasion (<4 vessels, with or without capsular invasion)

With extensive vascular invasion (≥4 vessels, with or without capsular invasion)

Microscopically, some of these tumors look similar to their minimally invasive counterpart. Most, however, exhibit features suggestive of malignancy at the cytoarchitectural level, such as a solid, nesting, or trabecular pattern of growth; high mitotic activity; marked nuclear hyperchromasia; and necrosis. These features overlap considerably with those of poorly differentiated carcinoma (see chapter 8). This similarity is also maintained at the behavioral level, since widely invasive follicular carcinoma is associated with a distant metastatic rate (mainly to lung and bone but also brain and liver) and mortality rate roughly comparable to those for poorly differentiated carcinoma (93). Lang et al. (92) found that 80 percent of their patients with widely invasive carcinomas had metastases and about 20 percent died of tumor. Woolner et al. (94,95) found a 50 percent death rate for patients with widely invasive tumors, as opposed to only 3 percent for those with minimally invasive tumors.

The incidence of widely invasive follicular carcinoma compared to that of the minimally invasive type greatly depends on the liberality of the pathologist in making the former diagnosis. In our experience, widely invasive follicular carcinoma is an uncommon neoplasm.

REFERENCES

1. LiVolsi VA, Asa SL. The demise of follicular carcinoma of the thyroid gland. Thyroid 1994;4:233-6.
2. Sobrinho-Simões M, Eloy C, Magalhães J, Lobo C, Amaro T. Follicular thyroid carcinoma. Mod Pathol 2011;24:S10-8.
3. Cuello C, Correa P, Eisenberg H. Geographic pathology of thyroid carcinoma. Cancer 1969; 23:230-9
4. Williams ED. Pathology and natural history. In: Duncan W, ed. Thyroid cancer. Berlin: Springer-Verlag; 1980:47-55. (Duncan W, ed. Recent results in cancer research; Vol 73.)
5. Williams ED, Doniach I, Bjarnason O, Michie W. Thyroid cancer in an iodide rich area: histopathologic study. Cancer 1977;39:215-22.
6. Grebe SK, Hay ID. Follicular thyroid cancer. Endocrinol Metab Clin North Am 1995;24:761-801.
7. Harach HR, Escalante DA, Oñativia A, Lederer Outes J, Saravia Day E, Williams ED. Thyroid carcinoma and thyroiditis in an endemic goitre region before and after iodine prophylaxis. Acta Endocrinol (Copenh) 1985;108:55-60.
8. Hofstadter F. Frequency and morphology of malignant tumours of the thyroid before and after the introduction of iodine prophylaxis. Virchows Arch A Pathol Anat Histol 1980;385:263-70.
9. Vickery AL Jr. The diagnosis of malignancy in dyshormonogenetic goitre. Clin Endocrinol Metab 1981;10:317-35.
10. Cooper DS, Axelrod L, DeGroot LJ, Vickery AL Jr, Maloof F. Congenital goiter and the development of metastatic follicular carcinoma with evidence for a leak of nonhormonal iodide: clinical, pathological, kinetic, and biochemical studies and a review of the literature. J Clin Endocrinol Metab 1981;52:294-306.
11. Lang W, Choritz H, Hundeshagen H. Risk factors in follicular thyroid carcinomas. A retrospective follow-up study covering a 14-year period with emphasis on morphological findings. Am J Surg Pathol 1986;10:246-55.
12. Paul SJ, Sisson JC. Thyrotoxicosis caused by thyroid cancer. Endocrinol Metab Clin North Am 1990;19:593-612.
13. Harach HR, Sánchez SS, Williams ED. Pathology of the autonomously functioning (hot) thyroid nodule. Ann Diagn Pathol 2002;6:10-9.
14. Boehm T, Rothouse L, Wartofsky L. Metastatic occult follicular thyroid carcinoma. JAMA 1976;235:2420-1.
15. Evans HL. Follicular neoplasms of the thyroid. A study of 44 cases followed for a minimum of 10 years, with emphasis on differential diagnosis. Cancer 1984;54:535-40.
16. Franssila KO, Ackerman LV, Brown CL, Hedinger CE. Follicular carcinoma. Semin Diagn Pathol 1985;2:101-22.
17. Hazard JB, Kenyon R. Atypical adenoma of the thyroid. Arch Pathol 1954;58:554-63.
18. Mazzaferri EL, Oertel JE. The pathology and prognosis of thyroid cancer. In: Kaplan EL, ed. Surgery of the thyroid and parathyroid glands. Clinical Surgery International, Vol 6. Edinburgh: Churchill Livingstone; 1983:23-5.
19. Arif S, Patel J, Blanes A, Diaz-Cano SJ. Cytoarchitectural and kinetic features in the histological evaluation of follicular thyroid neoplasms. Histopathology 2007;50:750-63.
20. Goldstein NS, Czako P, Neill JS. Metastatic minimally invasive (encapsulated) follicular and Hurthle cell thyroid carcinoma: a study of 34 patients. Mod Pathol 2000;13:123-30.
21. Yamashina M. Follicular neoplasms of the thyroid. Total circumferential evaluation of the fibrous capsule. Am J Surg Pathol 1992;16:392-400.
22. Westra WH, Phelps TH, Hruban RH, Isacson C. Surgical pathology dissection: an illustrated guide, 2nd ed, New York: Springer-Verlag; 2006.
23. LiVolsi VA, Merino MJ. Worrisome histologic alterations following fine-needle aspiration of the thyroid (WHAFFT). Pathol Annu 1994;29:99-120.
24. Rosai J, Kuhn E, Carcangiu ML. Pitfalls in thyroid tumour pathology. Histopathology 2006;49:107-20.
25. Brennan MD, Bergstralh EJ, van Heerden JA, McConahey WM. Follicular thyroid cancer treated at the Mayo Clinic, 1946 through 1970: initial manifestations, pathologic findings, therapy, and outcome. Mayo Clin Proc 1991;66:11-22.
26. Ghossein R. Encapsulated malignant follicular cell-derived thyroid tumors. Endocr Pathol 2010;21:212-8.
27. Collini P, Sampietro G, Pilotti S. Extensive vascular invasion is a marker of risk of relapse in encapsulated non-Hürthle cell follicular carcinoma of the thyroid gland: a clinicopathological study of 18 consecutive cases from a single institution with a 11-year median follow-up. Histopathology 2004;44:35-9.
28. Hazard JB, Kenyon R. Encapsulated angioinvasive carcinoma (angioinvasive adenoma) of the thyroid gland. Am J Clin Pathol 1954;24:755-66.
29. Kahn NF, Perzin KH. Follicular carcinoma of the thyroid: an evaluation of the histology criteria used for diagnosis. Pathol Annu 1983;18:221-53.

30. Warren S. Invasion of blood vessels in thyroid cancer. Am J Clin Pathol 1956;26:64-5.

31. Warren S. Significance of invasion of blood vessels of the thyroid gland. Arch Pathol 1931;11:255-7.

32. Mete O, Asa SL. Pathological definition and clinical significance of vascular invasion in thyroid carcinomas of follicular epithelial derivation. Mod Pathol 2011;24:1545-52.

33. González-Cámpora R, Montero C, Martin-Lacave I, Galera-Davidson H. Demonstration of vascular endothelium in thyroid carcinomas using Ulex europaeus I agglutinin. Histopathology 1986;10:261-6.

34. Harach HR, Jasani B, Williams ED. Factor VIII as a marker of endothelial cells in follicular carcinoma of the thyroid. J Clin Pathol 1983;36:1050-4.

35. Stephenson TJ, Griffiths DW, Mills PM. Comparison of Ulex europaeus I lectin binding and factor VIII-related antigen as markers of vascular endothelium in follicular carcinoma of the thyroid. Histopathology 1986;10:251-60.

36. Chan K. Newly available antibodies with practical applications in surgical pathology. Int J Surg Pathol 2013;21:553-72.

37. Baloch ZW, LiVolsi VA. Intravascular Kaposi's-like spindle cell proliferation of the capsular vessels of follicular-derived thyroid carcinomas. Mod Pathol 1998;11:995-8.

38. Chebib I, Opher E, Richardson ME. Vascular and capsular pseudoinvasion in thyroid neoplasms. Int J Surg Pathol 2009;17:449-51.

39. Papotti M, Arrondini M, Tavaglione V, Veltri A, Volante M. Diagnostic controversies in vascular proliferations of the thyroid gland. Endocr Pathol 2008;19:175-83.

40. Tse LL, Chan I, Chan JK. Capsular intravascular endothelial hyperplasia: a peculiar form of vasoproliferative lesion associated with thyroid carcinoma. Histopathology 2001;39:463-8.

41. Sapino A, Cassoni P, Papotti M, Bussolati G. Muscular cushions of the vessel wall at the periphery of thyroid nodules. Mod Pathol 1999;12:879-84.

42. Mizukami Y, Nonomura A, Michigishi T, Noguchi M, Ishizaki T. Encapsulated follicular thyroid carcinoma exhibiting glandular and spindle cell components. A case report. Pathol Res Pract 1996;192:67-71.

43. Giusiano-Courcambeck S, Denizot A, Secq V, De Micco C, Garcia S. Pure spindle cell follicular carcinoma of the thyroid. Thyroid 2008;18:1023-5.

44. Chetty R, Govender D. Follicular thyroid carcinoma with rhabdoid phenotype. Virchows Arch 1999;435:133-6.

45. Cameselle-Teijeiro J, Pardal F, Eloy C, et al. Follicular thyroid carcinoma with an unusual glomeruloid pattern of growth. Hum Pathol 2008;39:1540-7.

46. Barresi G, Tuccari G. Iron-binding proteins in thyroid tumours. An immunocytochemical study. Pathol Res Pract 1987;182:344-51.

47. Tuccari G, Barresi G. Immunohistochemical demonstration of ceruloplasmin in follicular adenomas and thyroid carcinomas. Histopathology 1987;11:723-31.

48. Tuccari G, Barresi G. Tissue polypeptide antigen in thyroid tumours of follicular cell origin: an immunohistochemical re-evaluation for diagnostic purposes. Histopathology 1990;16:377-81.

49. Vierbuchen M, Schröder S, Uhlenbruck G, Ortmann M, Fischer R. CA 50 and CA 19-9 antigen expression in normal, hyperplastic, and neoplastic thyroid tissue. Lab Invest 1989;60:726-32.

50. Haynik DM, Prayson RA. Immunohistochemical expression of cyclooxygenase 2 in follicular carcinomas of the thyroid. Arch Pathol Lab Med 2005;129:736-41.

51. Haynik DM, Prayson RA. Immunohistochemical expression of Bcl-2, Bcl-x, and Bax in follicular carcinomas of the thyroid. Appl Immunohistochem Mol Morphol 2006;14:417-21.

52. Schmid KW, Farid NR. How to define follicular thyroid carcinoma? Virchows Arch 2006;448:385-93.

53. Wang SL, Chen WT, Wu MT, Chan HM, Yang SF, Chai CY. Expression of human telomerase reverse transcriptase in thyroid follicular neoplasm: an immunohistochemical study. Endocrine Pathol 2005;16:211-8.

54. Cho Mar K, Eimoto T, Nagaya S, Tateyama H. Cell proliferation marker MCM2, but not Ki67, is helpful for distinguishing between minimally invasive follicular carcinoma and follicular adenoma of the thyroid. Histopathology 2006;48:801-7.

55. Asa SL. The role of immunohistochemical markers in the diagnosis of follicular-patterned lesions of the thyroid. Endocr Pathol 2005;16:295-309.

56. Abulkheir IL, Mohammad DB. Value of immunohistochemical expression of p27 and galectin-3 in differentiation between follicular adenoma and follicular carcinoma. Appl Immunohistochem Mol Morphol 2012;20:131-40.

57. Seybt TP, Ramalingam P, Huang J, Looney SW, Reid MD. Cyclin D1 expression in benign and differentiated malignant tumors of the thyroid gland: diagnostic and biologic implications. Appl Immunohistochem Mol Morphol 2012;20:124-30.

58. Arif S, Patel J, Blanes A, Diaz-Cano SJ. Cytoarchitectural and kinetic features in the histological evaluation of follicular thyroid neoplasms. Histopathology 2007;50:750-63.

59. Cho Mar K, Eimoto T, Tateyama H, Arai Y, Fujiyoshi Y, Hamaguchi M. Expression of matrix metalloproteinases in benign and malignant follicular thyroid lesions. Histopathology 2006;48: 286-94.

60. Gauchotte G1, Lacomme S, Brochin L, et al. Retinoid acid receptor expression is helpful to distinguish between adenoma and well-differentiated carcinoma in the thyroid. Virchows Arch 2013;462:619-32.

61. Massi D, Santucci M, Bianchi S, Vezzosi V, Zampi G. Ultrastructural features of solid/trabecular areas in differentiated thyroid carcinoma. Ultrastruct Pathol 2001;25:13-20.

62. Cavallari V, Albiero F, Cicciarello R, et al. Morphological changes of follicular cell basal borders and basement membranes in benign and malignant nodular lesions of the thyroid gland: an ultrastructural study. Ultrastruct Pathol 2004;28:199-207.

63. Fonseca E, Soares P, Cardoso-Oliveira M, Sobrinho-Simões M. Diagnostic criteria in well-differentiated thyroid carcinomas. Endocr Pathol 2006;17:109-17.

64. Baloch ZW, LiVolsi VA. Follicular-patterned afflictions of the thyroid gland: reappraisal of the most discussed entity in endocrine pathology. Endocr Pathol 2014;25:12-20.

65. Williams ED. Two proposals regarding the terminology of thyroid tumors. Int J Surg Pathol 2000;8:181-183 (Guest Editorial).

66. Rosai J. Handling of thyroid follicular patterned lesions. Endocr Pathol 2005;16:279-83.

67. Papotti M, Rodriguez J, De Pompa R, Bartolazzi A, Rosai J. Galectin-3 and HBME-1 expression in well-differentiated thyroid tumors with follicular architecture of uncertain malignant potential. Mod Pathol 2005;18:541-6.

68. Franc B, de la Salmonière P, Lange F, et al. Interobserver and intraobserver reproducibility in the histopathology of follicular thyroid carcinoma. Hum Pathol 2003;34:1092-100.

69. Hofman V, Lassalle S, Bonnetaud C, et al. Thyroid tumours of uncertain malignant potential: frequency and diagnostic reproducibility. Virchows Arch 2009;455:21-33.

70. Massin JP, Savoie JC, Garnier H, Guiraudon G, Leger FA, Bacourt F. Pulmonary metastases in differentiated thyroid carcinoma. Study of 58 cases with applications for the primary tumor treatment. Cancer 1984;53:982-92.

71. Nagamine Y, Suzuki J, Katakura R, Yoshimoto T, Matoba N, Takaya K. Skull metastasis of thyroid carcinoma. Study of 12 cases. J Neurosurg 1985;63:526-31.

72. Quinn TR, Duncan LM, Zembowicz A, Faquin WC. Cutaneous metastases of follicular thyroid carcinoma: a report of four cases and a review of the literature. Am J Dermatopathol 2005;27:306-12.

73. Tickoo SK, Pittas AG, Adler M, et al. Bone metastases from thyroid carcinoma: a histopathologic study with clinical correlates. Arch Pathol Lab Med 2000;124:1440-7.

74. Bisceglia M, D'Angelo VA, Wenig BM. Endolymphatic sac papillary tumor (Heffner tumor). Adv Anat Pathol 2006;13:131-8.

75. Dhillon J, Tannir NM, Matin SF, Tamboli P, Czerniak BA, Guo CC. Thyroid-like follicular carcinoma of the kidney with metastases to the lungs and retroperitoneal lymph nodes. Hum Pathol 2011;42:146-50.

76. Fornelli A, Bondi A, Jovine E, Eusebi V. Intrahepatic cholangiocarcinoma resembling a thyroid follicular neoplasm. Virchows Arch 2010;456:339-42.

77. Chablé-Montero F, Shah BS, Montante-Montes de Oca D, Angeles-Angeles A, Henson DE, Albores-Saavedra J. Thyroid-like cholangiocarcinoma of the liver: an unusual morphologic variant with follicular, trabecular and insular patterns. Ann Hepatol 2012;11:961-5.

78. Young RH, Jackson A, Wells M. Ovarian metastasis from thyroid carcinoma 12 years after partial thyroidectomy mimicking struma ovarii: report of a case. Int J Gynecol Pathol 1994;13:181-5.

79. Clark OH. Total thyroidectomy: the treatment of choice for patients with differentiated thyroid cancer. Ann Surg 1982;196:361-70.

80. Harness JK, Thompson NW, McLeod MK, Eckhauser FE, Lloyd RV. Follicular carcinoma of the thyroid gland: trends and treatment. Surgery 1984;96:972-80.

81. Schroder DM, Chambors A, France CJ. Operative strategy for thyroid cancer. Is total thyroidectomy worth the price? Cancer 1986;58:2320-8.

82. Thompson LD, Wieneke JA, Paal E, Frommelt RA, Adair CF, Heffess CS. A clinicopathologic study of minimally invasive follicular carcinoma of the thyroid gland with a review of the English literature. Cancer 2001;91:505-24.

83. Heffess CS, Thompson LD. Minimally invasive follicular thyroid carcinoma. Endocr Pathol 2001;12:417-22.

84. Brennan MD, Bergstralh EJ, van Heerden JA, McConahey WM. Follicular thyroid cancer treated at the Mayo Clinic, 1946 through 1970: initial manifestations, pathologic findings, therapy, and outcome. Mayo Clin Proc 1991;66:11-22.

85. Cady B, Rossi R, Silverman M, Wool M. Further evidence of the validity of risk group definition in differentiated thyroid carcinoma. Surgery 1985;98:1171-8.

86. Iida F. Surgical significance of capsule invasion of adenoma of the thyroid. Surg Gynecol Obstet 1977;144:710-2.

87. van Heerden JA, Hay ID, Goellner JR, et al. Follicular thyroid carcinoma with capsular invasion alone: a nonthreatening malignancy. Surgery 1992;112:1130-6.

88. Piana S, Frasoldati A, Di Felice E, Gardini G, Tallini G, Rosai J. Encapsulated well-differentiated follicular-patterned thyroid carcinomas do not play a significant role in the fatality rates from thyroid carcinoma. Am J Surg Pathol 2010;34:868-72.

89. Carcangiu ML. Minimally invasive follicular carcinoma. Endocr Pathol 1997;8:231-4.

90. D'Avanzo A, Treseler P, Ituarte PH, et al. Follicular thyroid carcinoma: histology and prognosis. Cancer 2004;100:1123-9.

91. Schlumberger M, Tubiana M, De Vathaire F, et al. Long-term results of treatment of 283 patients with lung and bone metastases from differentiated thyroid carcinoma. J Clin Endocrinol Metab 1986;63:960-7.

92. Lang W, Choritz H, Hundeshagen H. Risk factors in follicular thyroid carcinomas. A retrospective follow-up study covering a 14-year period with emphasis on morphological findings. Am J Surg Pathol 1986;10:246-55.

93. Carcangiu ML, Zampi G, Rosai J. Poorly differentiated ("insular") thyroid carcinoma. A reinterpretation of Langhans' "wuchernde Struma." Am J Surg Pathol 1984;8:655-68.

94. Woolner LB. Thyroid carcinoma: pathologic classification with data on prognosis. Semin Nucl Med 1971;1:481-502.

95. Woolner LB, Beahrs OH, Black BM, McConahey WM, Keating FR Jr. Classification and prognosis of thyroid carcinoma. A study of 885 cases observed in a thirty year period. Am J Surg 1961;102:354-87.

7 PAPILLARY THYROID CARCINOMA AND VARIANTS

PAPILLARY CARCINOMA

Definition. *Papillary thyroid carcinoma* (PTC) is a malignant epithelial tumor showing evidence of follicular cell differentiation and characterized by a set of distinctive nuclear features. Papillae may or may not be present.

General Features. PTC is the most common type of thyroid cancer (65 to 80 percent of thyroid cancers in the United States) (1). Its relative incidence compared with that of follicular carcinoma seems to be greater in areas of high iodine intake (2,3).

There is a well-documented association between radiation exposure to the neck and the subsequent development of PTC (4–7). In most of the cases, the radiation was given during childhood, and the average interval until the development of the malignancy was about 20 years (8). PTC also developed shortly after the administration of high-dose radiation to the neck for malignant disease (9–14). In two large series, the number of patients with PTC who gave a history of previous irradiation to the neck were 6.0 (8) and 6.6 (15) percent, respectively. The relationship between radiation exposure of the thyroid and the development of PTC got its most dramatic confirmation from the explosion and fire at the nuclear power plant in Chernobyl in the former USSR in April 1986, which was followed by an "epidemic" of thyroid carcinomas, mostly in children who were under the age of 15 at the time of the accident (some in utero), and overwhelmingly of the papillary type (16–20).

It has been suggested that there may be an increased incidence of PTC in patients with Graves disease, but this has not been conclusively proven (21–26). The incidence of Graves disease in PTC patients is 4 percent. In those patients with Graves disease who develop thyroid carcinoma, the thyroid-stimulating antibodies that are responsible for this autoimmune disorder may play a role in the genesis of the tumor (27).

PTC is also said to be more common in thyroid glands affected by lymphocytic/ Hashimoto thyroiditis (28–30). We find the reported evidence for this claim to be much more convincing than that for Graves disease but feel that a definite statistical relationship remains to be proven. Hyperplastic nodules or adenomas are present in about 40 percent of the thyroid glands harboring PTC, but the two events are probably unrelated (8).

Cases of PTC have been reported in a familial setting (31), in patients with ataxia-telangiectasia (32), as a component of a type of multiple endocrine neoplasia (MEN) syndrome (33), and in association with parathyroid tumors (34), carotid body tumors (35), and a variety of colorectal abnormalities. The latter include sporadic adenocarcinoma, polyposis coli, Gardner syndrome, and Cowden syndrome (36). Whether the coexistence of these neoplasms is significant or coincidental is not always clear (37). Some of the cases of synchronous PTC and parathyroid adenoma have occurred in patients with a history of previous irradiation to the neck (34).

Clinical Features. PTC is more common in women. The ratio of women to men in most series ranges between 2:1 and 4:1 (8,38–42) but is substantially higher in Japan (9–13:1). The mean age at the time of diagnosis ranges from 31 to 49 years in the various series. Several authors have noted a shift to a younger age range in recent years, perhaps due to earlier diagnosis (43,44). PTC constitutes 90 percent or more of all cases of thyroid carcinoma in childhood (41). Congenital cases have been described, especially in the population exposed to the Chernobyl nuclear accident (18).

Nearly all patients present with clinically evident disease in the neck (40,45,46). In one series, this was located in the thyroid gland alone in 67 percent, in the thyroid gland plus

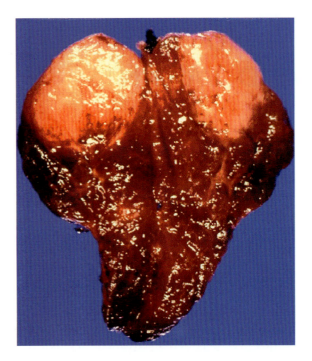

Figure 7-1

PAPILLARY CARCINOMA

This bisected thyroid gland shows a papillary carcinoma at one pole. The tumor is well circumscribed but not encapsulated, bulges on the surface, and has a granular solid appearance.

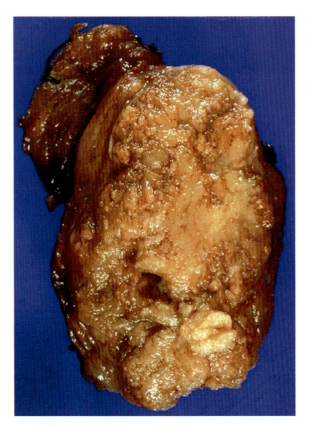

Figure 7-2

PAPILLARY CARCINOMA

This large papillary carcinoma shows invasive features and a predominantly solid appearance, with marked granularity suggestive of papillary formations. Uninvolved thyroid gland is seen in the upper left corner.

cervical nodes in 13 percent, and in cervical nodes alone in 20 percent of the cases (8).

Most PTCs are "cold" lesions on thyroid scan, but well-documented cases have presented as autonomously functioning (hot) nodules (47).

Gross Findings. Grossly, the typical PTC presents as an invasive neoplasm with ill-defined margins, a firm consistency, and a granular cut surface (figs. 7-1, 7-2). The color is usually whitish, and calcifications may be apparent. The size is extremely variable, with a mean diameter of 2 to 3 cm (48). The percentage of tumors measuring 1.5 cm or less in diameter ranges in various series from 13.7 percent (49) to 64.0 percent (50). This wide variation in size probably reflects either the type of material examined or the tendency of some patient populations to consult late in the course of the disease. Most of the variations in the gross appearance of the tumor are related to its variants and are discussed with them later in this chapter. This applies to the well-circumscribed and fleshy appearance

resembling adenoma that can be exhibited by the follicular variant, and the partial or complete cystic change that can be seen in some of the encapsulated types (formerly designated papillary cystadenocarcinomas).

Fresh tumor necrosis is exceptional in PTC. Its detection in the absence of a previous fine-needle aspiration biopsy should suggest an alternative diagnosis or the emergence of a more aggressive (i.e., poorly differentiated or undifferentiated) component within the tumor.

An interesting curiosity that has been documented in several instances is the fact that if a PTC develops in a "black thyroid" (chapter 1), the tumor itself is usually nonpigmented, suggesting a diminished function of thyroid peroxidase in the tumor cells (51).

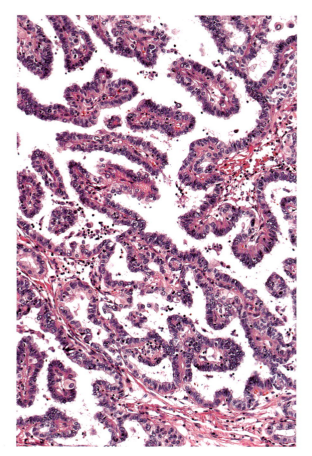

Figure 7-3

PAPILLARY CARCINOMA

The tumor is composed of an intricate network of randomly oriented, branching papillae.

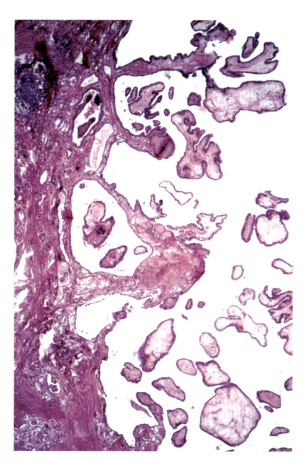

Figure 7-4

PAPILLARY CARCINOMA

The papillae are separated from each other by abundant watery material.

Microscopic Findings. The two morphologic features that best characterize typical PTCs are the papillae and the nuclear changes, although not necessarily in that order of importance.

Papillae. As in papillary tumors in other locations, the papillae of PTC are formed by a central fibrovascular stalk covered by a neoplastic epithelial lining (figs. 7-3–7-5). The better-developed papillae are long, with a complex arborizing pattern. Others are straight and slender, arranged in a parallel, regimented fashion; still others are short and stubby, standing in a "picket-fence" configuration from a straight base. In some instances, the papillae are tightly packed, resulting in pseudosolid or pseudotrabecular configurations. When these areas are cut perpendicularly to the long axis of the papillae, the resulting images may resemble rosettes.

The thickness and composition of the papillary stalk is variable. In most instances, it is made up of loose connective tissue and variously sized thin-walled vessels. In some cases, it is swollen by edema fluid or occupied by abundant acellular hyaline material (figs. 7-6, 7-7). Sometimes it is infiltrated by lymphocytes or clusters of macrophages, some of which may be foamy or hemosiderin-laden. Psammoma bodies (discussed below) and other calcific concretions may be present. In exceptionally rare instances, PTC contains mature adipose tissue (52). It is not unusual to find round structures with the appearance of follicles containing colloid in their lumens within the papillary stalks.

For papillae to qualify as such, they need to contain a central fibrovascular stalk, in contrast to the infolding epithelium of benign lesions.

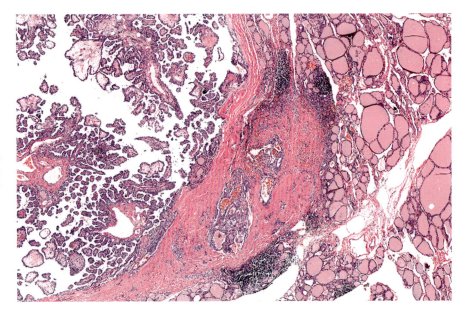

Figure 7-5

PAPILLARY CARCINOMA

A highly papilliferous pattern at growth is seen in a partially encapsulated tumor.

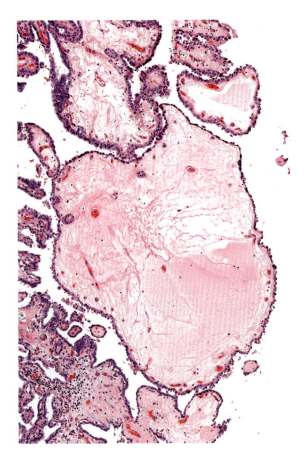

Figure 7-6

PAPILLARY CARCINOMA

Markedly edematous papillae vaguely resemble the villi of a hydatidiform mole.

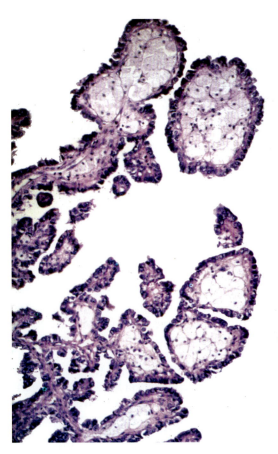

Figure 7-7

PAPILLARY CARCINOMA

The stroma of the papillae contains scattered foamy macrophages in an edematous background.

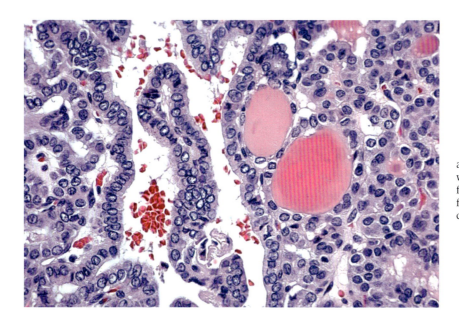

Figure 7-8

PAPILLARY CARCINOMA

The left side of this tumor has a typical papillary configuration, whereas the right side displays follicular structures. The nuclear features are similar in the two components.

This requirement is sound, but exceptions exist. The "abortive" papillae of some variants of PTC are devoid of a stalk, but their presence may represent the first clue to the diagnosis. Conversely, in some benign conditions such as diffuse hyperplasia, nodular hyperplasia, or adenoma with papillary hyperplasia, the papillary structures within them may contain fibrovascular stalks.

In its most characteristic form, PTC has a great predominance of papillary structures throughout the tumor; however, it is rare for it to be composed exclusively of papillae (53). In most cases, the papillae are interspersed with neoplastic follicles that have similar nuclear features (fig. 7-8). The ratio of papillae to follicles varies from case to case, and can be described by the expressions "with papillary predominance" or "with follicular predominance," depending on the case, although this is probably unnecessary. The term *mixed carcinoma* should not be used for these tumors. As long as the cells in the follicles have the nuclear features seen in the papillae (see below), the tumor is a PTC. When the follicular predominance over the papillae is complete, the tumor should be termed the follicular variant of PTC.

Nuclear Features. The nuclei of the cells of PTC, most of which are round or slightly oval, display a set of abnormalities that have greater diagnostic significance than the papillae themselves. These abnormalities are divided into two major categories. The first and most important is the morphologic variation of a common theme, i.e., a remodeling of the nuclear envelope, which is manifested in the form of circumferential membrane irregularities (garlands); subtle indentations, crenelations, and folds; and crescent (semilunar) shapes in the form of pseudoinclusions or as prominent longitudinal grooves (54). The pseudoinclusions, which represent deep cytoplasmic invaginations into the nucleus, appear as acidophilic, inclusion-like round structures, sharply outlined and slightly eccentric, with a crescent-shaped rim of compressed chromatin on one side (figs. 7-9, 7-10) (55,56). They are similar in appearance (and probably in their mechanism of formation) to those seen in other neoplasms of a variety of organs, such as glioblastoma multiforme, pheochromocytoma, and malignant melanoma. The nuclear grooves are more common in oval nuclei and are usually parallel to the long axis (fig. 7-11). Sometimes two or more grooves are seen in the same nucleus, running side by side; they are similar to those seen in granulosa cell tumors of the ovary and in the cells of Langerhans cell histiocytosis, among others (57,58).

It has recently been shown in a very elegant fashion that these various morphologic features are seen at better advantage following immunostaining for nuclear membrane-associated proteins, such as lamin A and emerin (59,60). They are also clearly demonstrated in tridimensional reconstructions by confocal microscope analysis (61).

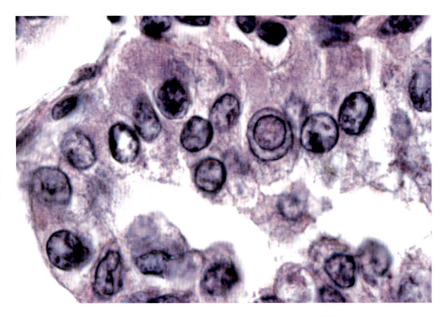

Figure 7-9

PAPILLARY CARCINOMA

A prominent nuclear pseudo-inclusion is seen near the center of the field, typically bound by a thick cell membrane. The inside of the pseudoinclusion is made up of acidophilic cytoplasm.

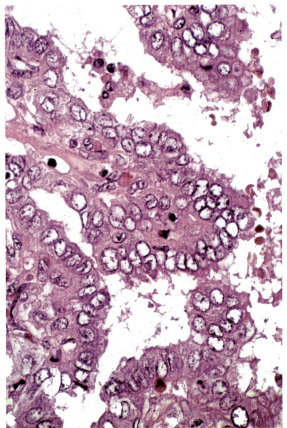

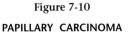

Figure 7-10

PAPILLARY CARCINOMA

Markedly overlapping, optically clear nuclei have irregular cell membranes and occasional nuclear grooves.

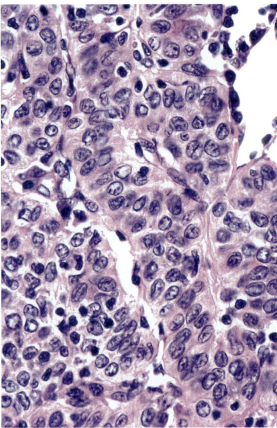

Figure 7-11

PAPILLARY CARCINOMA

The tumor has a solid/trabecular rather than a papillary or follicular architecture, but is recognized as PTC because of the oval nuclei with numerous grooves.

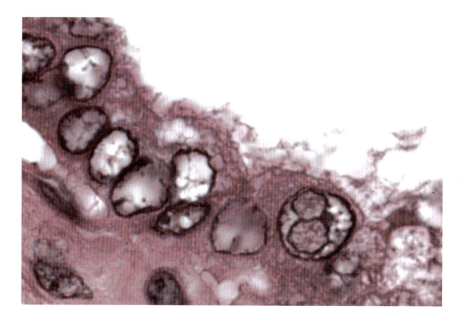

Figure 7-12

PAPILLARY CARCINOMA

High-power view of the nuclei, one of which contains two huge pseudoinclusions.

The second consistent feature of the nucleus of PTC cells is represented by an empty appearance of the nucleoplasm, which seems almost totally devoid of chromatin strands (figs. 7-10, 7-12) (62). The inner aspect of the nuclear membrane is irregularly thickened by the apposition of chromatin material. The nucleolus, which may be prominent, is often pushed aside against the nuclear membrane. These nuclei have been variously described as pale, clear, optically clear, watery, empty, ground glass, and "Orphan Annie's eyes" (63). Nuclei with these alterations are enlarged and often have an overlapping quality, even in very thin sections. Their appearance has been likened to tiles on a roof or an egg basket (fig. 7-10) (64).

The ground-glass appearance is well shown in fixed, paraffin-embedded material (regardless of the fixative used) but is inconspicuous or absent in frozen sections or smears from the same cases (fig. 7-13) (65,66). In formalin-fixed tissue, it is said to vary depending on the concentration of the formalin (67). These observations led to the conclusion that it represents an artifact of fixation or embedding. Even if this were the case, we strongly suspect that it reflects some intrinsic physicochemical alteration of the chromatin structure or associated nuclear proteins, which should be distinguished from the nuclear "bubbles" (pseudopseudoinclusions) of the type seen in many other sites and conditions, and which surely represent an

artifact of some sort. When these bubbles are present, they tend to be evident in most of the follicular cells of the field being examined, to be multiple in the individual nuclei, to have a uniform size and shape, and to be colorless (instead of having the pale acidophilic staining quality similar to that of the adjacent cytoplasm that is typical of PTC-related pseudoinclusions) (fig. 7-14) (68).

Clear nuclei are present in the morules sometimes focally seen in otherwise typical PTC and in a greater number in the cribriform-morular variant of PTC. In this instance, the clearing is due to the accumulation of microfilaments containing biotin (69,70).

Exceptionally, some or most of the cells of PTC exhibit spindle-shaped nuclei (71–73). The presence of these nuclei, which are bland appearing, with fine chromatin and inconspicuous nucleoli, should raise the differential diagnosis with spindle cell follicular adenoma, the spindle cell variant of medullary carcinoma, a variety of mesenchymal tumors, and, most importantly, the spindle cell form of anaplastic carcinoma (74).

Mitotic figures are exceptional or absent in PTC, a feature that correlates with their low proliferative activity as measured by bromodeoxyuridine labeling or MIB-1 (Ki-67) staining (75). Presence of more than an occasional number should suggest the emergence of a poorly differentiated neoplasm (76).

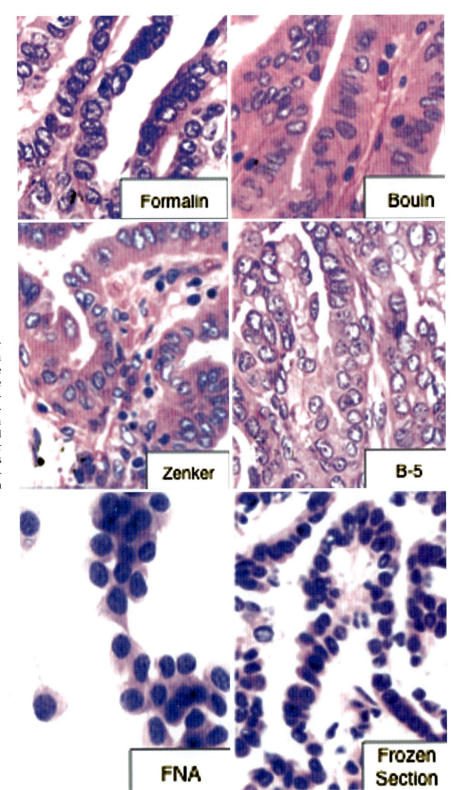

Figure 7-13

PAPILLARY CARCINOMA

Nuclear features of the tumor cells of a papillary carcinoma after various procedures. The ground-glass appearance of the nuclei is evident in the paraffin-embedded material, regardless of whether the fixation was carried out in buffered formalin, Bouin fluid, Zenker fluid, or B5; conversely, it is not appreciable in a touch preparation (FNA) or in a frozen section.

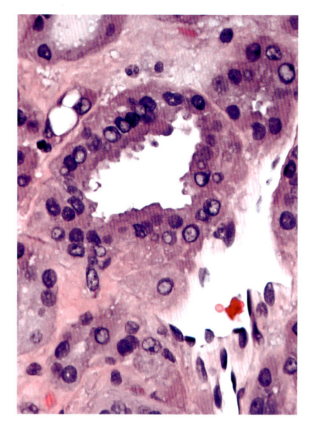

Figure 7-14

PAPILLARY CARCINOMA

Nuclear "bubbles" simulate pseudoinclusions. This artifact is present in most of the tumor cells.

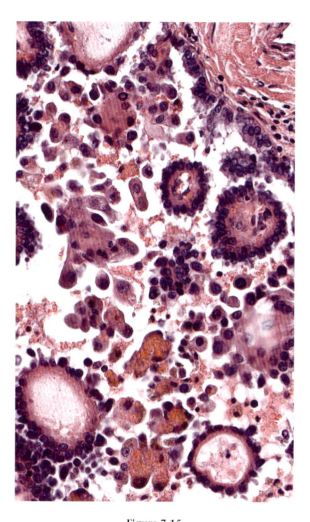

Figure 7-15

PAPILLARY CARCINOMA

The hobnail appearance of the tumor cells lining the papillae is said to be associated with a more aggressive clinical course.

Other Morphologic Features. In contrast to the highly distinctive nuclear qualities, the cytoplasm of PTC cells is nondescript in most instances. It is modest in amount, and slightly to moderately eosinophilic to amphophilic. Variations include pale cells, cells with a finely granular cytoplasm (due to the richness of mitochondria), and cells with a diffusely acidophilic cytoplasm (due to cytoplasmic filaments and resulting in a squamoid appearance).

Recently, another morphologic variation of PTC has been described, allegedly associated with aggressive behavior and characterized by the presence of prominent hobnail features of the tumor cells often associated with micropapillary features (fig. 7-15) (77–80). Additional studies are needed to see whether this pattern qualifies as a bonafide variant like those described below.

In addition to the papillary and follicular patterns, PTC can grow in solid or trabecular formations. Solid areas are detected in about 25 percent of the cases (38). Usually this is a focal change, but it may involve most or all of the neoplasm (fig. 7-16). This should not be taken as evidence that the tumor has become undifferentiated or even poorly differentiated, as long as the typical nuclear features of PTC persist. Squamous metaplasia is also common PTC, having been recorded in 20 to 40 percent of the cases (figs. 7-17, 7-18) (8,38). It can be focal or extensive. In its most characteristic form, squamous metaplasia presents as concentric whorls of keratinized

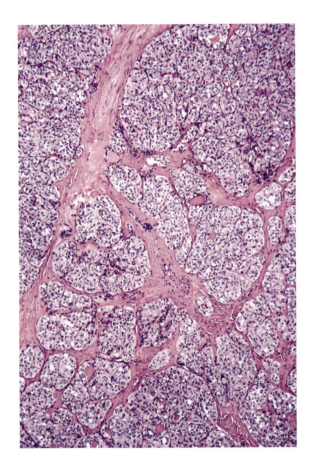 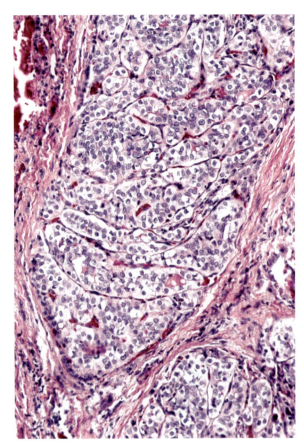

Figure 7-16

PAPILLARY CARCINOMA

Left: The pattern of growth is predominantly solid, and the individual tumor nests are separated from each other by wide fibrous bands.

Right: A predominantly trabecular pattern of growth within a sharply outlined tumor nest is seen.

Figure 7-17

PAPILLARY CARCINOMA

Focus of squamous metaplasia. This is a common finding in PTC.

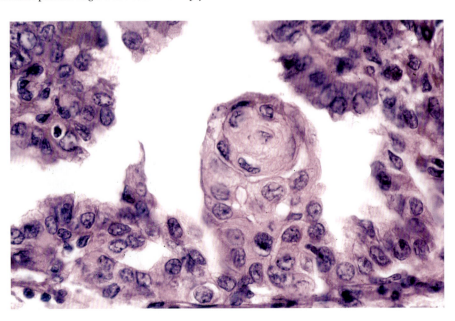

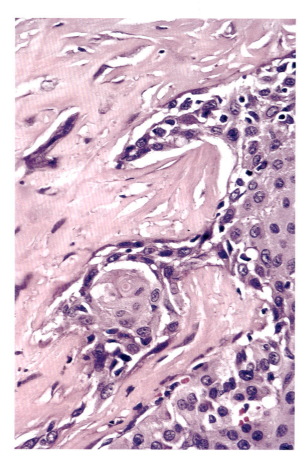

Figure 7-18

PAPILLARY CARCINOMA

The tumor shows extensive squamous metaplasia.

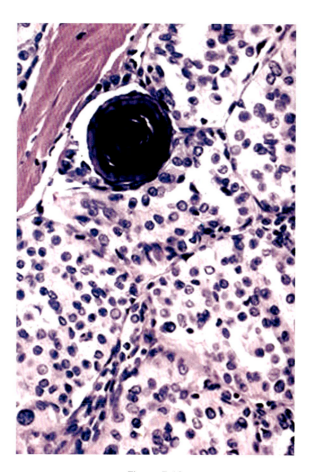

Figure 7-19

PAPILLARY CARCINOMA

This predominantly solid tumor is identified as PTC because of the nuclear features, the sharply outlined fibrohyaline band in the upper left corner, and the presence of a well-formed psammoma body.

cells surrounded by papillary foci. Squamous metaplasia is most common in tumor foci surrounded by abundant stromal tissue.

Another structure classically associated with PTC is the psammoma body, which is a round calcific concretion that exhibits concentric lamination (figs. 7-19, 7-20). Psammoma bodies are found in about 50 percent of the cases and are particularly common in tumors that feature a predominantly papillary growth pattern. Their mechanism of formation is controversial. Osteopontin produced by macrophages has been implicated in their development (81). We find appealing the hypothesis that the nidus for their genesis is a single necrotic tumor cell, upon which successive layers of calcium salt have been deposited (fig. 7-21) (82).

Psammoma bodies are not specific for PTC; however, they are so exceptionally rare in benign

thyroid diseases that their detection should immediately suggest the presence of PTC (83,84). If found in an area of inflammation and dense fibrosis, they likely represent the residua ("fossils" or "tombstones") of a PTC that has regressed at that site (fig. 7-22). If found in an otherwise normal thyroid, chances are high that a PTC is present a few microns away, and thus they represent an indication for the submission of the entire specimen (85). If present in an otherwise normal cervical lymph node, there is a high probability that the node is involved by a metastatic PTC that is not apparent at that particular level.

Although the most characteristic location of psammoma bodies is near the tip of the papillary stalk, they are also numerous in intrathyroid

113

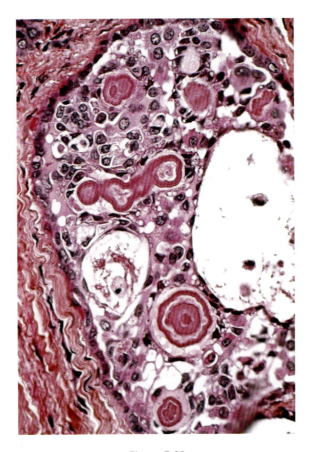

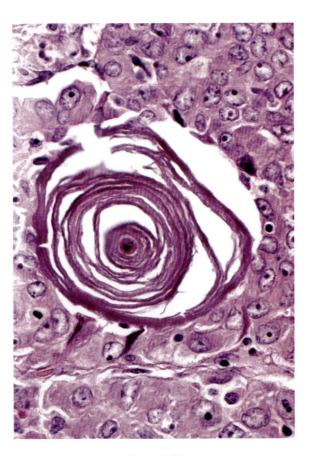

Figure 7-20

PAPILLARY CARCINOMA

Numerous psammoma bodies are seen in an early stage of formation.

Figure 7-21

PAPILLARY CARCINOMA

A large psammoma body shows typical concentric laminations. The single necrotic cell in the center probably represents the initial nidus for the formation of this structure.

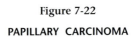

Figure 7-22

PAPILLARY CARCINOMA

Numerous psammoma bodies are scattered in a fibrous background. This appearance is highly suggestive of a regressed PTC.

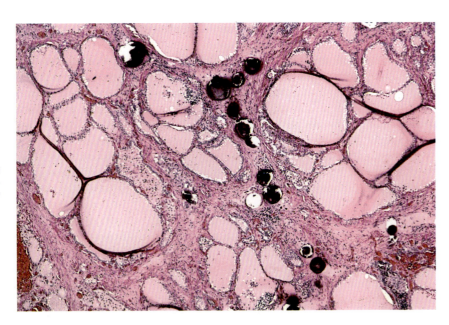

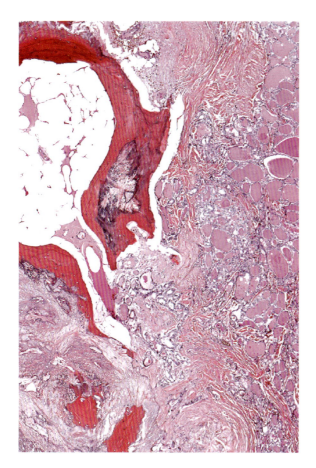

Figure 7-23

PAPILLARY CARCINOMA

Osseous metaplasia of the tumor stroma.

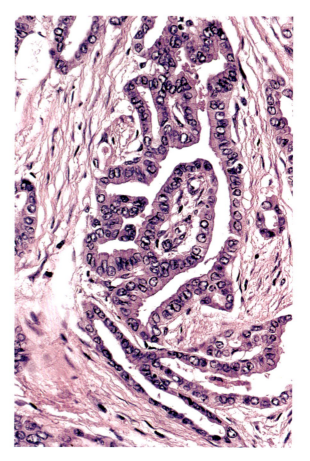

Figure 7-24

PAPILLARY CARCINOMA

Highly invasive tumor, intermixed with an abundant cellular stroma.

tumor emboli within lymph vessels. They can also be found in the stroma between neoplastic follicles or in the midst of a solid epithelial component (fig. 7-19). Psammoma body-like formations located within the lumens of follicles should be disregarded. In most instances, they are the result of inspissated secretion and are more commonly seen in connection with oncocytic neoplasms (see chapter 10).

Psammoma bodies have also been described in follicular carcinomas, but we suspect that most of these cases would presently be classified as the follicular variant of PTC. They also occur in medullary carcinoma and have even been described in carcinoma metastatic to the thyroid gland (86). Other types of calcification are associated with PTC such as metaplastic ossification (fig. 7-23), but this feature does not have the diagnostic significance of the psammoma body.

An abundant fibrous stroma is a common feature of PTC (fig. 7-24) (53). In most instances, it presents in the form of wide hyaline bands that traverse the tumor and divide it incompletely into irregularly shaped and often angulated lobules. The fibrosing tendencies of this tumor are particularly evident at the advancing edge. Some of this stromal reaction has a very cellular ("desmoplastic") appearance (87). Occasionally, it acquires a quality resembling nodular fasciitis, fibromatosis, or inflammatory myofibroblastic tumor, to the point of obscuring the neoplastic component (figs. 7-25, 7-26) (88–94). In other cases, it exhibits prominent myxoid foci, elastosis, and deposits of amyloid, the latter potentially leading to a mistaken diagnosis of medullary carcinoma (95–97).

Figure 7-25

PAPILLARY CARCINOMA

The outer aspect and cut surface of this PTC is accompanied by abundant nodular fasciitis-like stroma. The bulk of the mass was formed by this exuberant myofibroblastic proliferation.

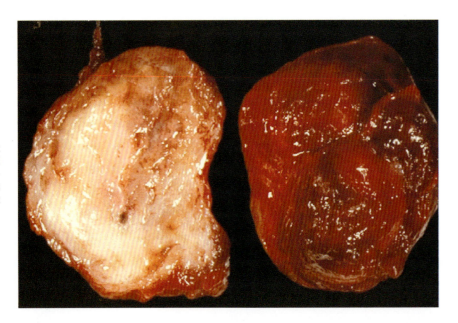

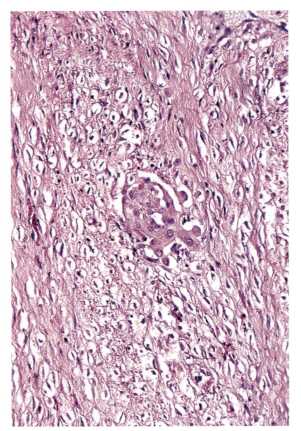
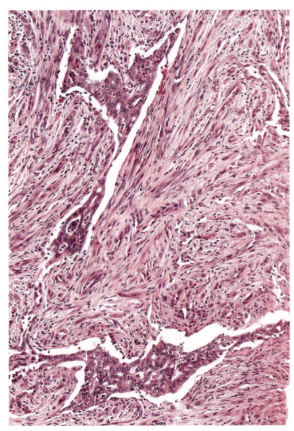

Figure 7-26

PAPILLARY CARCINOMA

Left: The exuberant stromal reaction present in this case has a nodular fasciitis-like appearance which hides the tumor.
Right: In other areas of the specimen, the true nature of the process is revealed by the presence of tumor islands surrounded by the florid reactive stromal proliferation.

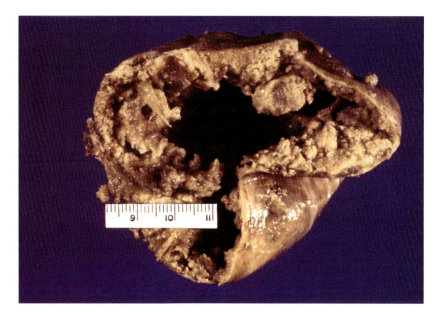

Figure 7-27

PAPILLARY CARCINOMA

Extensive cystic degeneration, a secondary change, can be seen in the primary tumor as well as in the nodal metastases. Its presence may result in an underdiagnosis of benign cyst. Thorough sampling of the specimen is essential in cases of this type.

The vascularity of PTC is greater than that of follicular neoplasms (98). Approximately one third of PTCs show a lymphocytic infiltration that is moderate to marked. This change tends to be more pronounced at the tumor periphery and within the fibrovascular papillary stalks. In most instances, it probably represents a host reaction to the tumor (99); in others, it may be the expression of preexisting autoimmune thyroiditis (100,101).

The stroma of PTC may contain aggregates of cells immunoreactive for S-100 protein, which have been interpreted as Langerhans or dendritic cells (102,103). Scattered multinucleated giant cells of a non-neoplastic histiocytic nature are often present, and are particularly conspicuous in cytologic preparations (104). They probably represent a response to leakage of colloid into the interstitium, and should be distinguished from the scattered pleomorphic tumor cells occasionally seen in PTC, analogous to those seen in other endocrine neoplasms and devoid of clinical significance, and the anaplastic giant cells of undifferentiated carcinoma, which has ominous implications (105).

Secondary cystic changes are common (figs. 7-27, 7-28). The more papillary the tumor, the more likely that these changes are present. Most of these cysts are lined by papillary formations diagnostic of the entity, but others are covered by a very attenuated, single-layered, flat epithelium with a deceptively benign appearance.

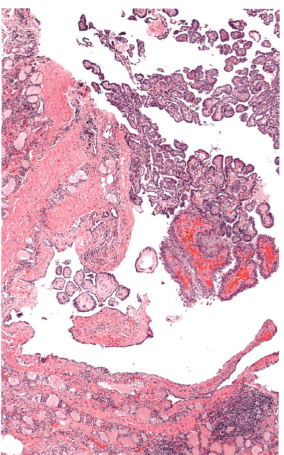

Figure 7-28

PAPILLARY CARCINOMA

There are prominent cystic changes.

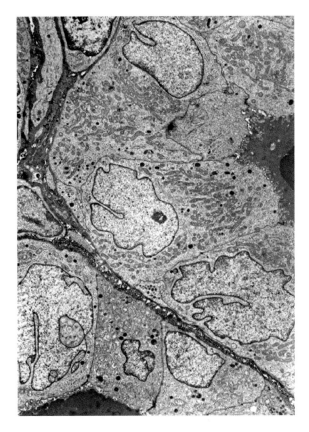

Figure 7-29

PAPILLARY CARCINOMA

The cells lining the papillae in the electron micrograph are tall cuboidal. The cytoplasm contains a large number of mitochondria and scattered lysosomes. The nucleus is characteristically indented, corresponding to the grooves seen in light microscopic preparations. (Courtesy of Dr. R. Erlandson, New York, NY.)

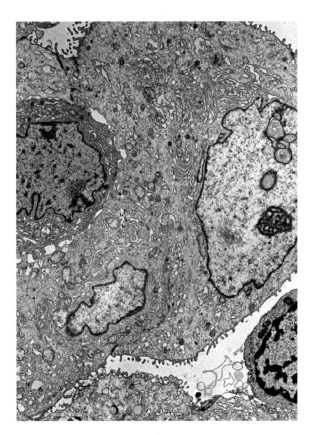

Figure 7-30

PAPILLARY CARCINOMA

This tumor was metastatic to a supraclavicular lymph node. Ultrastructurally, the nucleus of a tumor cell shows cytoplasmic invaginations. Microvillous differentiation is seen at the surface. (Courtesy of Dr. R. Erlandson, New York, NY.)

Blood vessel invasion is not as common or as diagnostically important as in follicular carcinoma, but it does occur. In one series, it was found in 7 percent of the cases (8). Invasion of lymph vessels is a much more common phenomenon, but it is not always easy to detect. When lymphatic invasion is extensive, the possibility of the tumor belonging to the diffuse sclerosing variant should be considered. The issue of multicentricity is discussed in the section Spread and Metastases.

Microscopic Grading. The overwhelming majority of PTCs have the nuclear and architectural features already described. A few exhibit nuclear pleomorphism, hyperchromasia, mitotic activity, foci of necrosis, and other features traditionally regarded as unfavorable

(98,106,107). Such tumors have been designated "high-grade" or "poorly differentiated" PTC and are described further in the next chapter. In the Mayo Clinic experience, PTCs thought to have a microscopic grade higher than 1 comprised only 6.2 percent of the cases (108).

Ultrastructural Findings. The characteristic nuclei of PTC cells exhibit finely dispersed chromatin, a highly folded nuclear membrane, and an apparent paucity of nuclear pores (figs. 7-29, 7-30) (55,56,109–111). The nuclear folds may result in large invaginations within the nucleus that correspond to the inclusion-like formations seen with the light microscope, both in histologic and cytologic preparations. The cytoplasm is rich in mitochondria, lysosomes, and filaments. The latter are particularly numerous

118

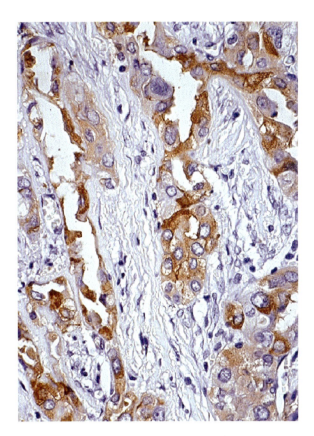

Figure 7-31

PAPILLARY CARCINOMA

Immunohistochemical positivity for thyroglobulin is evident in this PTC. Most of the tumor cells show cytoplasmic reactivity that ranges from moderate to strong.

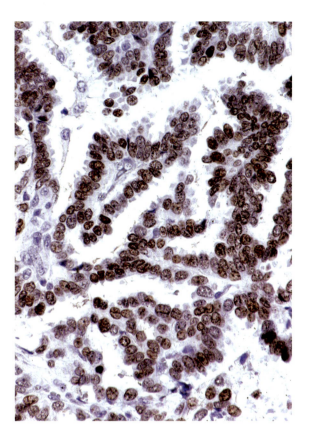

Figure 7-32

PAPILLARY CARCINOMA

Strong thyroid transcription factor (TTF)-1 immunostaining of the nuclei of PTC is seen.

in foci of squamous metaplasia, where they may be accompanied by keratohyaline granules. The apical surface exhibits microvillous differentiation (fig. 7-30).

Immunohistochemical Findings. PTC cells are consistently positive for thyroglobulin, although the intensity of the reaction is less pronounced than in follicular neoplasms (fig. 7-31) (112–114). The tumor cells are also immunoreactive for TTF-1, keratin, and vimentin, with frequent coexpression of these markers in the same cell (figs. 7-32, 7-33) (115–119).

The keratins expressed are not only of the low molecular weight type present in the normal thyroid gland but also those of high molecular weight, in keeping with the tendency of the tumor to undergo squamous metaplasia (fig. 7-34) (120–122). Keratin 19 is the keratin that has been

most thoroughly investigated as a corroborating tool for the diagnosis of PTC, together with galectin-3 and HBME-1 (123). Because these three markers are not usually encountered in the normal thyroid gland or in benign or malignant follicular neoplasms, it has been claimed by several authors that their presence strongly supports the diagnosis of PTC (124–126), particularly if used as part of a battery of markers (127,128). Our own experience indicates that these three markers (particularly HBME-1) usually stain the cells of PTC (often in a very intense fashion) while being negative in the benign conditions above mentioned (116,128,129). Unfortunately, the abnormal follicular epithelium of Hashimoto thyroiditis also tends to express them in a focal, but often intense fashion, thus considerably diminishing their diagnostic utility. In other

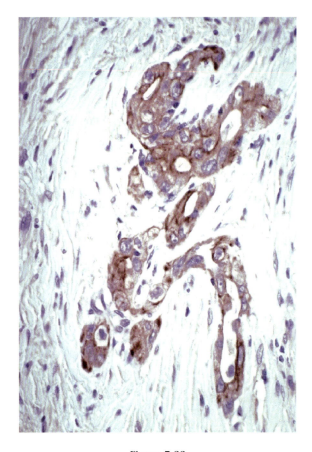

Figure 7-33

PAPILLARY CARCINOMA

Immunohistochemical positivity for pankeratin is seen in the invasive component of the tumor, which is surrounded by a prominent desmoplastic reaction. Keratin reactivity is particularly prominent in these invasive foci.

words, the sensitivity of these markers is high, but the specificity is not, at least in our experience. As a result, we and others do not rely on them for the diagnosis of PTC (123,130,131). Another interesting parallel between the cells of PTC and those of Hashimoto thyroiditis is their frequent strong immunoreactivity for S-100 protein (132) and p63 (133).

Other markers that have been detected in the cells of PTC (unfortunately of not much diagnostic use, despite the sometimes extravagant claims made) are epithelial membrane antigen (EMA) (134); CA125 (135); CD15 (136); involucrin (137); alpha-1-antitrypsin (138); alpha-1-antichymotrypsin (139); p75 neurotrophin receptor (140); estrogen receptors (141); fibronectin-1, calretinin, p16, SFTPB, and CITED1 (128); ICAM-1 (142); procollagen III peptide (143); and insulin-like growth factor 1 (144). p27kip1 is significantly decreased in PTC when compared with the normal or hyperplastic thyroid gland (145,146). Strangely, CD56 is said to be positive in all thyroid lesions except papillary carcinoma (147,148).

Contrary to general belief, traditional mucin stains are positive in a considerable number of PTCs, whether in the colloid, luminal border, or cytoplasm (149). This correlates with the immunohistochemical demonstration of mucins, simple mucin antigens, and histo-blood group antigens in the cells of these tumors (but also in follicular carcinomas) (150). EMA and Alcian blue stain the apical membrane of the PTC cells lining

Figure 7-34

PAPILLARY CARCINOMA

The pankeratin stain is intensely positive in all the cells of this PTC.

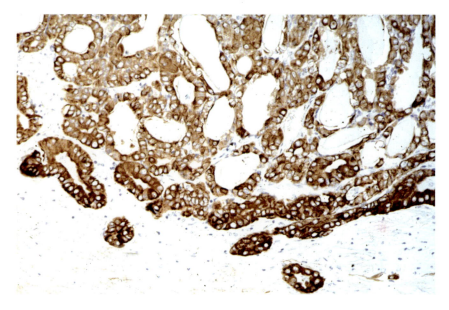

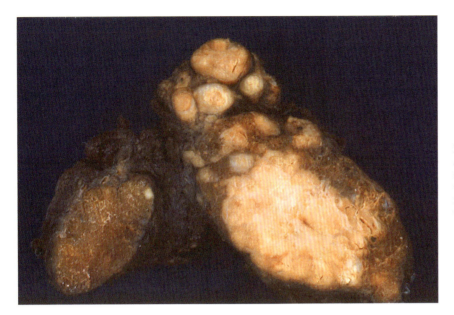

Figure 7-35

PAPILLARY CARCINOMA

A large tumor mass in the lower half of the specimen is accompanied by numerous smaller nodules in the rest of the gland, as an example of either multicentricity or intrathyroidal tumor spread.

the papillae, but not those of the benign papillae of diffuse or nodular hyperplasia (151).

Molecular Genetic Findings. See chapter 19.

Cytologic Findings. See chapter 20.

Spread and Metastases. One of the most notable features of PTC is its tendency for multiple involvement of the gland (fig. 7-35). Controversy exists as to whether this phenomenon is the result of intrathyroidal lymph vessel spread or of "true" multicentric transformation of the follicular epithelium. It is our impression, supported by clonality studies, that both mechanisms operate (152,153). The incidental finding of two or more microscopic foci of PTC widely separate from each other, and having an identical microscopic appearance, favors multiple independent tumors ("true" multicentricity), as does the finding of two separate PTCs having a different histology. The finding of multiple ipsilateral foci of PTC (especially if within vascular spaces) obviously suggests intrathyroid spread.

In most reported series, the incidence of multicentricity ranges from 18 to 22 percent (8). Outstanding exceptions are the 87.5 percent reported by Russell et al. (154) in a whole-mount study of 80 well-differentiated thyroid carcinomas (most of which were of the papillary type), and the 78.1 percent recorded by Katoh et al. (155). It is obvious that the frequency of this phenomenon is directly dependent on the thoroughness of the sampling, although the lib-

erality of the pathologist in interpreting minimal microscopic changes probably also plays a role.

Extrathyroid extension into the soft tissues of the neck occurs in 10 to 34 percent of cases, according to various series (8,38,42,49,101,156,157). The growth takes place along fascial planes and perineural spaces and within skeletal muscle (fig. 7-36). It can also involve, by direct extension, the parathyroid glands, especially when the latter are located within the thyroid, a common occurrence (158). In advanced stages, PTC extends directly into larynx, trachea, esophagus, or skin (fig. 7-37) (159,160). The anatomic manner of invasion of the trachea has been proposed as a criterion for the pathologic staging of PTC (161).

PTC has a great propensity to metastasize to cervical lymph nodes (fig. 7-38) (162). In one series, 35 percent of the patients had clinically evident lymphadenopathy at the time of presentation (8). Even in cases thought to be negative on palpation, microscopic examination reveals metastatic tumor in approximately 50 percent (163). The incidence of nodal metastases is said to be higher in the PTCs with an invasive pattern of growth, hobnail features, loss of cohesiveness/polarity, or micropapillary structures (164,165). A similar claim has been made for PTCs featuring so-called tumor sprouts (165). The deposits are usually on the same side as the tumor, but bilateral involvement occurs in about 10 percent of the cases (166).

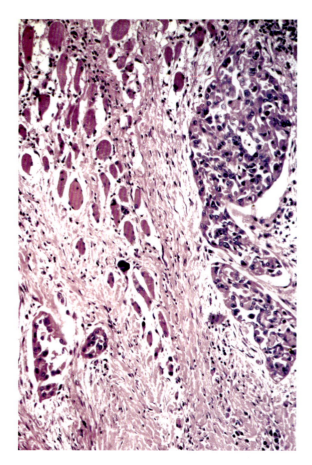

Figure 7-36

PAPILLARY CARCINOMA

Extrathyroid extension of the tumor, with entrapment and atrophy of surrounding skeletal muscle fibers.

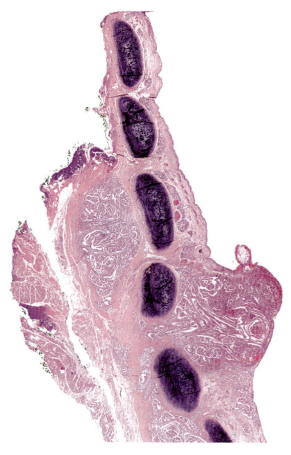

Figure 7-37

PAPILLARY CARCINOMA

Tracheal invasion by tumor, with preservation of tracheal cartilaginous rings.

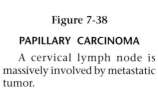

Figure 7-38

PAPILLARY CARCINOMA

A cervical lymph node is massively involved by metastatic tumor.

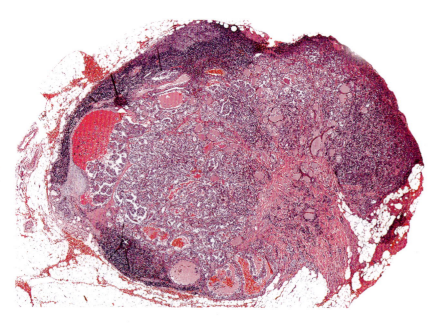

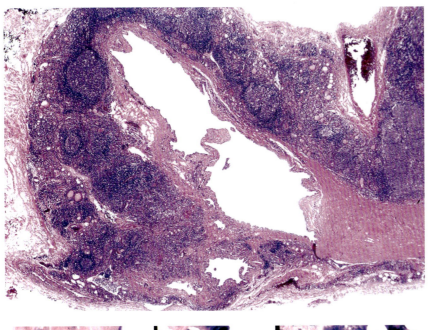

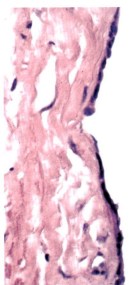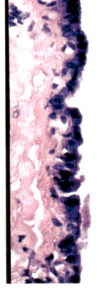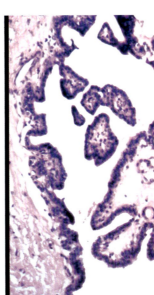

Figure 7-39

PAPILLARY CARCINOMA

Top: Nodal metastasis of papillary carcinoma with marked secondary cystic degeneration. This lesion can be easily mistaken for a benign branchial cleft cyst.

Bottom: High-power view of three areas of the lining of the cystic nodal metastasis. The panel on the left shows a covering of flattened endothelial-like cells, almost impossible to identify as thyroid follicular cells in hematoxylin and eosin (H&E)-stained sections; the cells in the central panel are suspicious of cancer because of their cuboidal shape and overlapping; the papillary structures in the right panel establish the diagnosis and emphasize the importance of thorough sampling.

Spread to mediastinal nodes is usually secondary to extensive cervical disease. A Japanese group has suggested the performance of sentinel node biopsy to estimate the amount of metastatic nodal burden, but the technique has not gained popularity (167).

Nodal metastases of PTC tend to undergo cystic degeneration or to grow in an obvious papillary pattern, even when these features are not well developed in the primary tumor. The cystic change may be so pronounced as to result in a misdiagnosis of branchial cleft cyst on microscopic examination (fig. 7-39) (168,169). The presence of papillae, nuclear abnormalities, or psammoma bodies provides the clue for the diagnosis, which can be easily confirmed with a thyroglobulin stain. Another pitfall in this situation is the presence of dilated high endothelial venules simulating PTC (170).

Blood-borne metastases also occur, although less commonly than with most other thyroid malignant tumors. The incidence ranges from 4 to 14 percent in the various series (8,10,38,42,171–173). The lung is by far the

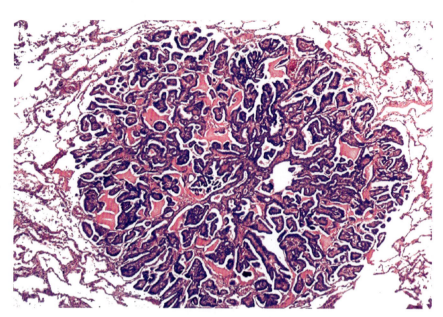

Figure 7-40

PAPILLARY CARCINOMA METASTATIC TO LUNG

The nodule grows freely inside the pulmonary parenchyma and displays an exuberance of papillary formations.

most common site for these deposits, which can occur in the absence of cervical nodal involvement (fig. 7-40) (174). The lung metastases may have a "miliary" (micronodular) appearance, be large and rounded (macronodular), or result in diffuse pulmonary infiltration ("snowflake" pattern) (172). Other documented sites of involvement are the skeletal system, liver, central nervous system, kidney, pancreas, breast, soft tissues, and skin, the latter showing a predilection for the scalp (fig. 7-41) (175–178).

Treatment. The treatment of PTC is controversial and probably will remain so until a proper prospective study is carried out. In the past, the standard approach in many institutions was the performance of a total thyroidectomy, together with radical lymph node dissection on the side of the tumor. The rationale for this aggressive approach was the high frequency of intraglandular spread or multicentricity and of regional lymph node metastases. The performance of a formal cervical lymphadenectomy has been largely abandoned, partly because it fails to remove many of the first-station lymph nodes but mainly because no detectable improvements in prognosis have been documented as a result of this formidable operation (179–181). Currently, the most common surgical approach toward these nodes is to leave them undisturbed if they appear grossly normal, and to perform a modified lymph node dissection (with preservation of the sternomastoid muscle) if they appear involved.

As for the thyroid gland itself, some groups strongly advocate total thyroidectomy followed by the administration of radioactive iodine for the purpose of ablating any possible metastatic sites (15,40,182–184). Other groups regard this approach as unnecessarily radical and maintain that similarly good results can be obtained with a lesser operation followed by suppression of thyroid-stimulating hormone secretion, without the addition of radioactive iodine postoperatively (185–190).

Our own experience (8) and the evaluation of two large series on the subject (189,191) suggest that the latter, more conservative approach is just as effective, and perhaps preferable, for most of the cases, i.e., those PTCs clinically and scintigraphically localized to one lobe, not belonging to one of the microscopically unfavorable variants (such as diffuse sclerosing, tall cell, or columnar cell), and occurring in low-risk patients (women under the age of 50 years or men under the age of 40 years). The specific type of operation, whether lobectomy, lobectomy with isthmusectomy, or subtotal thyroidectomy, seems to be of no great significance. We question the advisability of performing a nodulectomy, with the definite risk of leaving gross tumor behind, and of carrying out a total thyroidectomy, with the small but ever-present risk of inducing hypoparathyroidism or recurrent laryngeal nerve injury, two potentially serious complications.

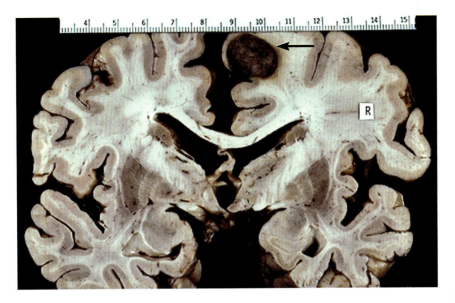

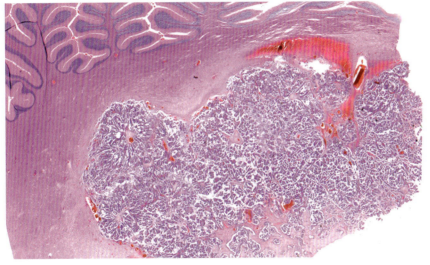

Figure 7-41

PAPILLARY CARCINOMA

Top: Brain metastasis of a papillary thyroid carcinoma, an unusual event. (Courtesy of Dr. N. Kostich, Minneapolis, MN.)

Bottom: Microscopic view of a cerebellar metastasis.

Blood-borne metastases are treated with ^{131}I. Those in the lungs respond in a high percentage of cases, whereas those located in the skeletal system are more resistant (192).

Prognosis. The overall probability of long-term survival for patients with PTC is excellent, to the point that in some series, the figures are not significantly different from those of the normal population of similar age (44,108). The incidence of tumor deaths in most large series is about 5 percent (8,193). The factors listed below are associated with prognosis. Some have been grouped to construct prognostic scoring systems (such as AMES and MACIS, the former developed at the Lahey Clinic and the latter proposed by the Mayo Clinic (see Table 21-5) (194).

Age. This is of paramount importance. In most series, no tumor deaths from papillary carcinoma are seen below the age of 40 years, and the probability of a fatal outcome increases exponentially with each decade (8, 156,195–198).

Gender. In most series, women fare better than men, but the difference is not as striking as for age (46,197,199). Cady et al. (156) proposed dividing patients with well-differentiated (including papillary) carcinomas into two groups on the basis of the two factors listed above: a *low-risk group* (composed of men 40 years old or younger and women 50 years old or younger) and a *high-risk group* (older patients). Almost all deaths from PTC occur in the latter.

Lack of Concomitant Hashimoto Thyroiditis. Cases of PTC not associated with Hashimoto thyroiditis seem to present with a more aggressive clinical stage and to have a high recurrence rate (200). A possibly related claim is that lymphocytic infiltration surrounding or inside the tumor is a predictor of a favorable prognosis (201).

Tumor Size. The probability of tumor recurrence increases when the tumor size exceeds 5 cm. The best prognosis is associated with PTCs measuring 1.5 cm in diameter or less (108).

Multiplicity. Tumors in which this feature is easily detectable are associated with an increased chance of nodal and pulmonary metastases and a corresponding decrease in disease-free survival rate (8). This feature is further discussed in this chapter in connection with the microcarcinoma variant of PTC.

Blood Vessel Invasion. According to most authors, this feature is of only modest prognostic impact, barely significant at the statistical level (8,39,43,202).

Invasiveness. Infiltrative tumors do much worse than those that are partially or completely surrounded by a capsule, a feature that is further discussed in connection with the encapsulated variant of PTC (203).

Extrathyroid Extension. This feature, which is a direct consequence of the degree of invasiveness and the location of the tumor, constitutes one of the worst morphologic prognostic signs in PTC, being associated with an over sixfold increase in the number of tumor deaths (8). As a matter of fact, of all the pathologic features of PTC not exhibiting poor differentiation or dedifferentiation, the presence of extrathyroid disease has the most significant bearing on prognosis (42,49,197).

Lymph Node Metastases. Whereas the mere presence of metastatic PTC in cervical lymph nodes does not have much clinical significance, the finding of extracapsular invasion in those metastatic nodes is a significant indicator of disease recurrence and poorer prognosis (204).

Distant Metastases. The occurrence of lung metastasis is associated with a moderate but obvious deleterious effect on prognosis (particularly if its radiographic appearance is macronodular rather than "miliary" or "snowflake"). The development of bone metastases carries an ominous prognostic significance, even when the tumors concentrate ^{131}I (8,172,205).

Aneuploidy. See chapter 19.

High Microscopic Grade. This rare event, which is related to the following item, is associated with a more aggressive clinical course (108).

Tumor Prognostic Scores. EORTC, AGES (206), MACIS (207,208).

Progression to a Poorly Differentiated (Including Insular) or Undifferentiated (Anaplastic) Pattern. These two types of dedifferentiation, which have an adverse prognostic significance (particularly the latter) are discussed in chapter 19.

BRAF. In several recent studies, *BRAF* V600E-mutated PTCs have been found to be associated with markers of poor prognosis, including old patient age, male gender, extrathyroid invasion, lymph node metastases, and high tumor stage at presentation. They have also been associated with recurrent or persistent disease and even reduced survival (see chapter 19)

The features associated with a good prognosis, other than those indirectly mentioned in the above paragraphs, include total encapsulation, pushing margins of growth, and cystic changes (8). These three features often coexist. It has also been suggested that patients with PTC featuring aggregates of S-100 protein–positive cells in the stroma fare better than those without this finding (102). However, this claim has not been confirmed in other studies (103).

Features that are not statistically significant prognostic indicators include a history of head and neck irradiation in childhood (193), relative numbers of papillae and follicles, presence and type of fibrosis, presence and amount of squamous metaplasia, presence and number of psammoma bodies (but see Bai et al. [208]), and presence or absence of cervical lymph node metastases (8).

In our experience, the presence of trabecular or solid areas does not have an adverse impact on prognosis as long as the typical nuclear features of PTC are retained (14), but others claim otherwise (89,98). Another parameter that does not carry prognostic significance in most series is the type of therapy employed, as already commented upon (8,44,185,186,209).

Immunohistochemical Profile. Of the numerous markers that have been investigated in PTC at the immunohistochemical level, hardly any are independent indicators of prognosis (210).

PAPILLARY CARCINOMA VARIANTS

Papillary Microcarcinoma

In its latest edition (published in 2004), the World Health Organization (WHO) Committee for the Classification of Thyroid Tumors (211) defines this variant as a PTC that is found incidentally and measures 1 cm or less in diameter. The term *papillary microcarcinoma*, originally proposed by Hazard (212), roughly corresponds to the entity formerly known as *occult sclerosing carcinoma* (213), *nonencapsulated sclerosing tumor* (212), and *occult papillary carcinoma* (214).

Papillary microcarcinoma is a very common finding in population-based autopsy studies and in carefully examined specimens of partial or total thyroidectomies performed for other reasons (215–222). The reported incidence in autopsy material in the various series ranges from 5.6 to 35.6 percent. The latter figure is from Finland and is based on a detailed study of 101 cases (223). The authors of that paper estimated that, if serial sections of the glands had been taken, the total number of detected tumors would have reached the astonishing figure of 308.

These studies have also shown that the prevalence of this tumor increases steeply from birth to adulthood and remains constant afterwards. Due to their small size, papillary microcarcinomas are easily missed at the gross level unless a careful and systematic search for them is carried out (fig. 7-42).

Some tumors are so small that they are totally undetectable grossly. The extreme manifestation of this phenomenon is the instance in which the tumor involvement is limited to a single follicle (fig. 7-43) (224).

Microscopically, the prototypical example of this entity has an irregular, scar-like configuration (fig. 7-44). The neoplastic elements predominate at the periphery of the fibrotic area, but others are seen entrapped in the center. The general attributes of PTC are present, including typical nuclear changes, psammoma bodies, and occasionally well-formed papillae. In most areas, however, the tumor cells display a follicular or solid architecture, a feature expected of a PTC growing in such a sclerotic milieu.

Some papillary microcarcinomas are accompanied by little or no fibrosis (fig. 7-43A). Others are totally surrounded by an extremely thick fibrous

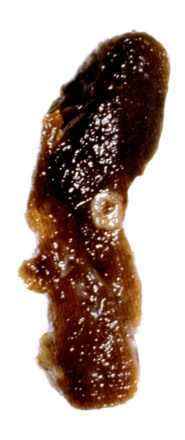

Figure 7-42

PAPILLARY MICROCARCINOMA

This tumor, which is unusually well circumscribed and focally cystic, measures less than 1 cm in diameter.

capsule that may be focally calcified (fig. 7-45). A variation is represented by the presence of tumor both inside and outside the capsule, sometimes in roughly equivalent amounts, and sometimes with the extracapsular component predominating (fig. 7-46). In such cases, the component located within the capsule tends to have a predominantly follicular configuration, whereas that on the outside is likely to feature a more conventional papillary pattern of growth.

It is difficult to analyze genetic alterations in papillary microcarcinomas due to their small size, but several studies have shown that they carry the same changes found in larger tumors (see chapter 19).

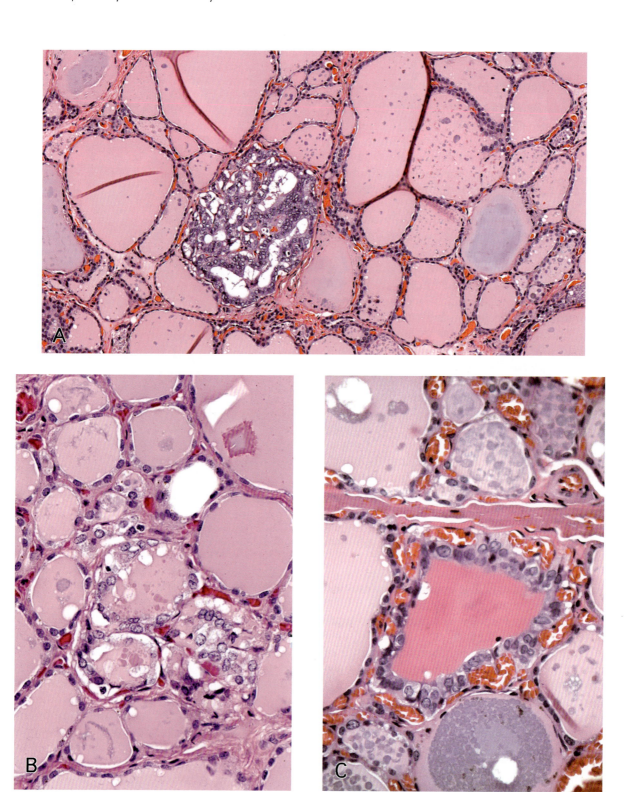

Figure 7-43

PAPILLARY MICROCARCINOMA

Three examples of papillary carcinoma measuring less than 1 cm and therefore qualifying as papillary microcarcinomas. The tumor in C seems to be composed of a single follicle.

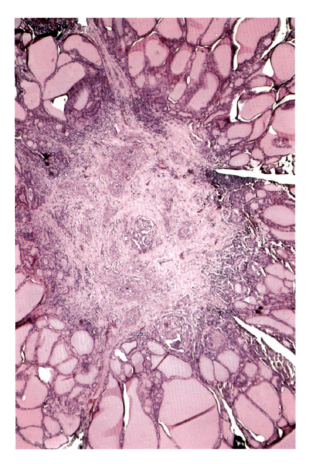

Figure 7-44

PAPILLARY MICROCARCINOMA

Typical low-power view of papillary microcarcinoma. The tumor edges have an infiltrative pattern and there is a pronounced stromal proliferation.

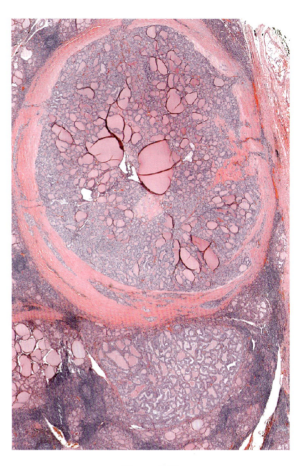

Figure 7-45

PAPILLARY MICROCARCINOMA

This papillary microcarcinoma (follicular variant) is surrounded by a thick capsule which is minimally invaded at several points. There is also a large tumor nest outside the capsule at the bottom.

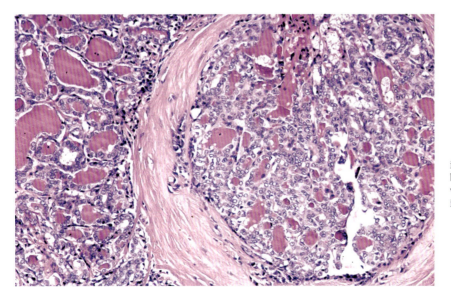

Figure 7-46

PAPILLARY MICROCARCINOMA

This papillary microcarcinoma is encapsulated but accompanied by an extracapsular component which is actually larger than the intracapsular original neoplasm.

The fact that these lesions exhibit malignant behavior has been proven by the repeated demonstration that they can metastasize to regional nodes (225–227). Furthermore, exceptional examples metastasizing through the bloodstream and resulting in fatalities are on record (228–232). In such instances, however, the metastases were generally present at the time of the initial examination. For tumors discovered incidentally in thyroid glands excised for other reasons, the chances of metastases developing later are extremely low. Overall, the prognosis of patients with papillary microcarcinoma is excellent: in one series, 93 percent of the patients were free of disease on follow-up, and there was no instance of distant metastases (8).

Features that may modify negatively this remarkably favorable outlook include the following: 1) absence of peritumoral fibrosis or inflammatory infiltrate. It has been hypothesized that such tumors, although fulfilling the current WHO definition of papillary microcarcinoma, are actually early stages of conventional PTC; 2) tall cells are more frequently associated with multicentricity, extrathyroid extension, and nodal metastases than conventional papillary microcarcinomas; 3) several studies have suggested that *BRAF* V600E may be a marker of poor prognosis; and 4) tumors that express S100A4 protein have more lymph node metastases (233,234).

Although some dissenting voices remain (235), most authors, ourselves included, favor a conservative therapeutic approach to papillary microcarcinoma lacking unfavorable features and found incidentally in a lobectomy done for other reasons (236). Specifically, we do not advocate completion of the thyroidectomy or radioiodine remnant ablation under those circumstances.

In order to reinforce this position, and knowing that the repercussions of a "cancer" diagnosis are much greater than those justified by the biologic potential of this tumor subtype, a group of thyroid pathologists meeting in Porto (Portugal) in 2003 proposed to rename this entity in a way that would avoid those potential untoward effects while still accurately reflecting its nature (237,238). In what became known as "the Porto proposal," they chose the term *papillary microtumor,* making it clear that it specifically applied to the most common situation, i.e., a single focus of PTC measuring 1 cm in diameter or less, contained within the thyroid gland of an adult patient, and found incidentally at thyroidectomy done for another reason. Excluded from this proposal (and therefore still to be called papillary microcarcinomas) are 1) tumors occurring in children or adolescents under the age of 19 years; 2) multiple tumors greater than 1 cm once their respective diameters are added; 3) tumors invading the thyroid (pseudo) capsule; 4) tumors accompanied by blood vessel invasion; and 5) tumors with tall cell features.

Encapsulated Variant

One of the most distinctive features of PTC is its tendency to invade the surrounding gland. In most cases, the interface between the tumor periphery and the normal tissue is irregular and devoid of a capsule. In others, there is focal evidence of capsular formation, but this is associated with areas of obvious invasion. A type of PTC exists that is totally surrounded by a fibrous capsule that may be intact or only focally infiltrated by tumor growth (fig. 7-47). This type, designated the *encapsulated variant of papillary carcinoma,* comprises about 10 percent of all PTCs (8,225,239,240). In the past, tumors with these features were sometimes designated *papillary adenomas* (241). The fact that they can be associated with cervical lymph node metastases is enough evidence that these lesions should be regarded as potentially malignant, although to a much lesser degree than the usual invasive PTC (8,225,240,242,243). The main differential diagnosis is with follicular adenoma with papillary hyperplasia, which lacks PTC-type nuclear changes (see chapter 5) (244).

When thus defined, encapsulated PTC confers an excellent prognosis. Regional nodal metastases may be present, but blood-borne metastases are rare, and the survival rate is nearly 100 percent (240,242,245).

The term encapsulated PTC (without further qualifiers) should be restricted to encapsulated tumors having, in addition to the required nuclear changes, a typical papillary architecture. Those encapsulated tumors having the same nuclear features but exhibiting a follicular pattern of growth should be regarded instead as encapsulated follicular variants of PTC. They are discussed in the next section.

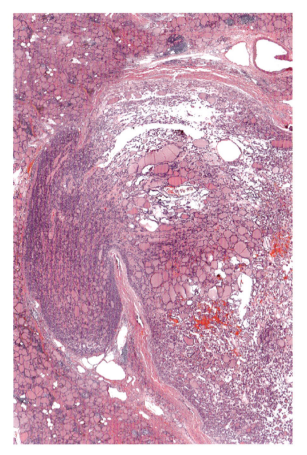

Figure 7-47

ENCAPSULATED VARIANT

Extensive capsular invasion is seen, resulting in a mushroom-like configuration.

Follicular Variant

The designation of *follicular variant of PTC* (FVPTC) is given to a PTC with an exclusively or almost exclusively follicular (rather than papillary) pattern of growth (196,227,246,247). This lesion represents the extreme expression of the fact that nearly all PTCs are composed of an admixture of papillae and follicles, and that the latter may predominate over the former (248,249).

In its most typical ("infiltrative") form, this variant shares many features with conventional PTC: capsule formation is absent, stromal invasion is obvious (often accompanied by a desmoplastic or hyaline reaction, fibrous and fibrohyaline septa separating the neoplastic follicles are common and sometimes extensive, and scattered psammoma bodies may be found in the interfollicular stroma (fig. 7-48).

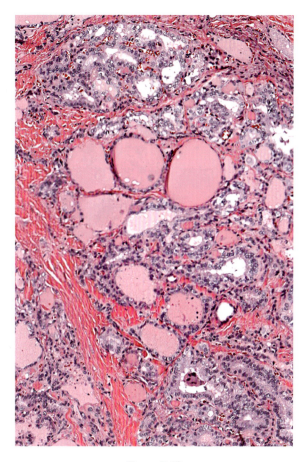

Figure 7-48

FOLLICULAR VARIANT

Admixture of microfollicles with typical nuclear changes and normal-sized follicles lined by unremarkable follicular cells. It is not always possible to decide whether the latter are entrapped normal follicles or neoplastic follicles that have undergone so-called terminal differentiation.

The follicles themselves offer several clues of their nature resulting from disruption of their architecture (250). Some are markedly elongated, resembling tubular glands, whereas others exhibit irregularities of their lining epithelium, with formations of folds, ridges, buds, and other intraluminal protrusions that probably represent rudimentary attempts to form papillae. Most importantly, the nuclei of the cells lining the follicles have features analogous to those of conventional PTC (figs. 7-49–7-51). In rare instances, the cytoplasm may exhibit focal or extensive oncocytic features (fig. 7-52). The colloid within the lumens of the neoplastic follicles often has a strong and homogeneous eosinophilic quality and a scalloped

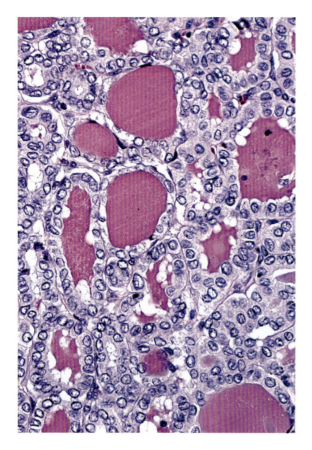

Figure 7-49

FOLLICULAR VARIANT

Typical appearance of the follicular variant of papillary carcinoma. The clear nuclei overlap and the colloid stains a homogeneous deep red.

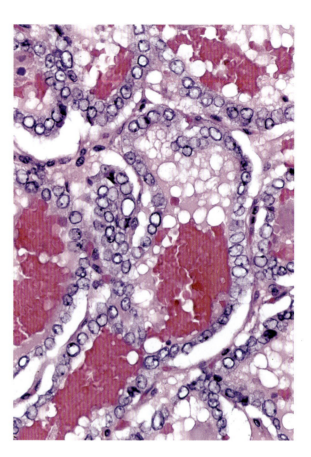

Figure 7-50

FOLLICULAR VARIANT

The contour of the follicles is irregular in this example.

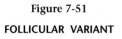

Figure 7-51

FOLLICULAR VARIANT

It is not unusual for the neoplastic follicles of this variant to have an elongated tubular shape.

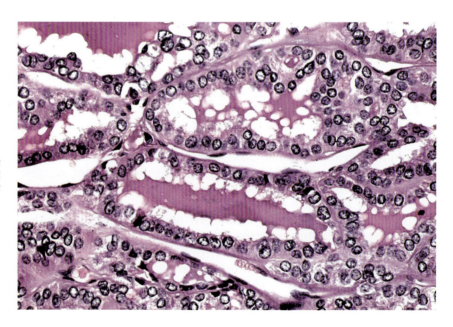

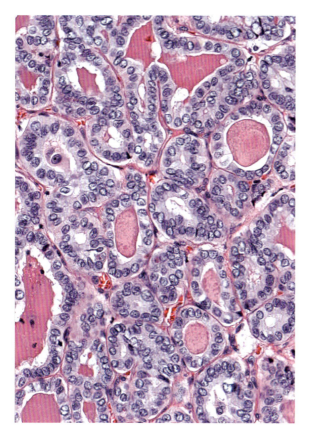

Figure 7-52

FOLLICULAR VARIANT

The pattern of growth is follicular throughout.

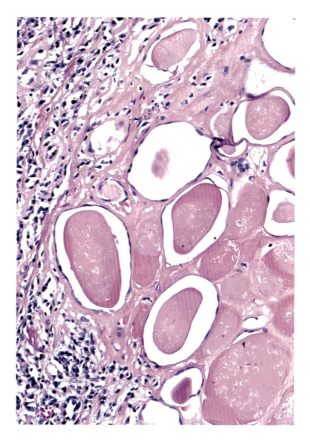

Figure 7-53

FOLLICULAR VARIANT

A subcapsular focus of "dried-up" follicles results from the hyaline appearance of the intraluminal colloid and the abundant stroma. The nature and significance of this peculiar change are not known.

configuration, the latter similar to that seen in markedly hyperplastic glands (figs. 7-49–7-51). On occasion, there is a subcapsular rim composed of neoplastic follicles and stroma having a peculiar homogeneous pink appearance ("dried-up" follicles) (fig. 7-53). Exceptionally, calcium oxalate crystals are found in the lumen. The intratumoral lymph vessel density is higher in FVPTC than in either follicular adenoma or follicular carcinoma (251).

Unusual variations of FVPTC are the rare cases in which the neoplastic follicles are cystically dilated, thus simulating nodular hyperplasia ("macrofollicular variant") (figs. 7-54, 7-55) (252–254); the cases in which minute neoplastic follicles are seen scattered in a background of normal follicles in a "sprinkling-like" fashion (fig. 7-56) (255); and the rarer cases in which there is

diffuse tumor involvement of the whole thyroid gland, without formation of grossly discernible nodules ("diffuse" or "multinodular" form). The latter are aggressive tumors, with a prevalence of multicentricity, extrathyroid extension, nodal metastases, vascular invasion, and distant metastases to lung and bone (256–258).

Careful search for papillae in cases with an appearance consistent with FVPTC usually demonstrates a few scattered representatives. It has been suggested that if these tumors were to be exhaustively sampled, all would contain foci with a clear-cut papillary configuration. This may be true, but it is important to remember that identification of papillae is not a requisite for the diagnosis of this variant; as a matter of fact, if papillae are easily found, the tumor should not be diagnosed as the follicular variant.

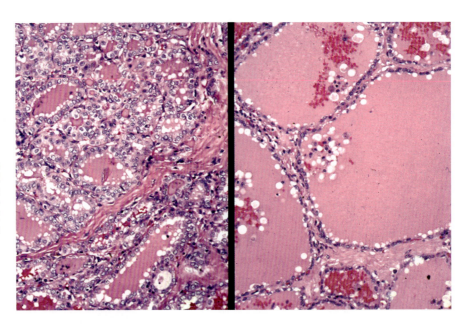

Figure 7-54

FOLLICULAR AND MACROFOLLICULAR VARIANTS

The neoplastic follicles on the left side are small and compact, whereas those on the right are markedly dilated. Nuclear changes of the papillary carcinoma type are present in both areas.

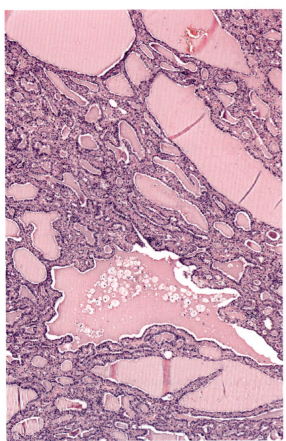

Figure 7-55

FOLLICULAR AND MACROFOLLICULAR VARIANTS

This PTC is composed of different sized follicles (some cystic) and lacks papillae.

Support for the interpretation that this tumor belongs to the papillary family of thyroid neoplasms derives from several sources: 1) some of these tumors are accompanied by multicentric foci within the thyroid gland that have a conventional papillary architecture (227); 2) the natural history of these tumors matches closely that of conventional PTC, particularly in regard to the high incidence of cervical lymph node involvement (8,259,260); 3) these nodal metastases often have a papillary configuration (8,246); 4) the types of keratin expressed by the tumor cells match those of papillary rather than follicular carcinoma (261–263); and finally, 5) their molecular profile is closer to that of conventional PTC than that of follicular carcinoma (but see chapter 19). To summarize our views about the "infiltrative" form of FVPTC, it is a tumor that looks and behaves like a conventional PTC in all regards except for the fact that it makes follicles instead of papillae.

FVPTC is easily recognizable as malignant, and just as easily recognizable as belonging to the PTC family. The situation is considerably more complex and controversial with the "encapsulated form" of FVPTC. A description of this variant follows, preceded by the comment that, as expected, there are examples of FVPTC that are somewhere between these two extremes. These tumors, which have been referred to as "partially encapsulated" or "well-circumscribed"

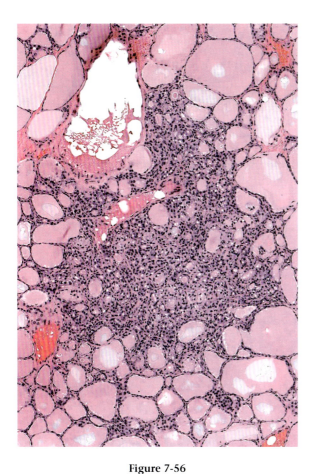

Figure 7-56

FOLLICULAR VARIANT

The admixture of cellular tumor foci scattered in a background of larger follicles results in a "sprinkling" appearance.

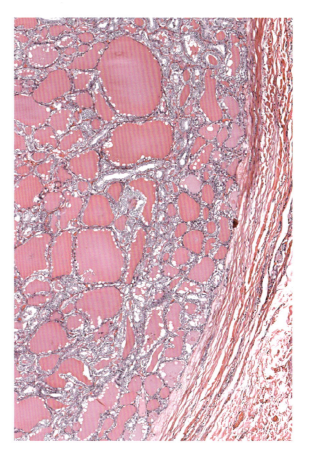

Figure 7-57

ENCAPSULATED FOLLICULAR VARIANT

The tumor is surrounded by a continuous intact capsule.

are closer in behavior to the "encapsulated" than the "infiltrative" type (264).

Encapsulated Follicular Variant of PTC and the "Uncertain Malignant Potential (UMP)" Concept

The *encapsulated follicular variant of PTC* (EFVPTC) combines the features of two variants. As the name indicates, this is an encapsulated neoplasm (with or without capsular or vascular invasion) with the cytoarchitectural features of FVPTC (figs. 7-45, 7-57, 7-58) (265). For diagnosis, these features need to be displayed prominently throughout the neoplasm. Many immunohisto-chemical markers have been tested as potential aids in the differentiation of EFVPTC from other benign and malignant follicular tumors. These include HBME-1, CK19, galectin-3, CD57, and several others (266). These markers are usually positive in the EFVPTC and negative in the follicular neoplasms, but they also tend to stain the abnormal follicular epithelium of Hashimoto thyroiditis, a feature that limits considerably their use, particularly when the thyroiditis is associated with nodular hyperplasia. Of these markers, HBME-1 seems to be the one offering the best differential staining potential, but we have not found these immunostains particularly useful and rarely employ them in our diagnostic work.

The overall prognosis of patients with EFVPTC is excellent, especially if there is no evidence of capsular or blood vessel invasion. Baloch et al. (267), however, reported five cases of this tumor type associated with bone metas-tases. In two cases, the primary was discovered following the detection of the bone metastases;

Table 7-1

NOMENCLATURE PROPOSAL FOR WELL-DIFFERENTIATED THYROID TUMORS WITH A FOLLICULAR PATTERN OF GROWTH

		Capsular Invasion		
		Present	Questionable	Absent
PTC-Type Nuclear Changes	Present	PC-FV[a]	PC-FV	PC-FV
	Questionable	WDCa-NOS	WDT-UMP	WDT-UMP
	Absent	FC	FT-UMP	FA

[a]PC-FV = papillary carcinoma, follicular variant; WDCa-NOS = well-differentiated carcinoma, not otherwise specified; WDT-UMP = well-differentiated tumor of uncertain malignant potential; FC = follicular carcinoma; FA = follicular adenoma.

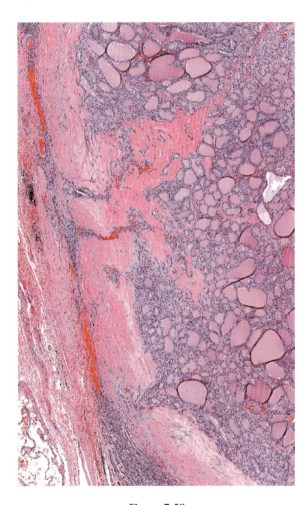

Figure 7-58

ENCAPSULATED FOLLICULAR VARIANT

This tumor shows areas of total capsular interruption and therefore qualifies as a minimally invasive carcinoma.

in the other three cases, there was evidence of blood vessel invasion.

Sometimes, an encapsulated nodule with a follicular pattern of growth exhibiting capsular or vascular invasion (and therefore malignant) has some features suggestive of PTC (such as clear nuclei or darkly staining colloid) but lacks others. In such instances, assignment to a follicular carcinoma as opposed to a FVPTC category becomes extremely subjective and is probably an unwarranted exercise. It may be instead preferable to simply designate such tumors *well-differentiated carcinoma, not otherwise specified*, as recommended in the consensus document of the Chernobyl group of thyroid pathologists (Table 7-1) (268).

A related and equally difficult diagnostic dilemma arises when some of the cytologic features of PTC are found focally within a lesion that otherwise appears to be a benign follicular lesion, i.e., a hyperplastic nodule or a follicular adenoma. Closer examination of the process may allow its placement into one of the following three categories: 1) a sharply outlined focus of typical PTC (usually of the conventional but sometimes of the follicular variant type) within a lesion that appears otherwise benign, with no areas of transition between them. This rare phenomenon should probably be interpreted as a PTC arising in either a hyperplastic nodule or a follicular adenoma (248); 2) a focus with an appearance consistent with a PTC (usually of the follicular variant rather than the conventional type) that merges with areas that on low power

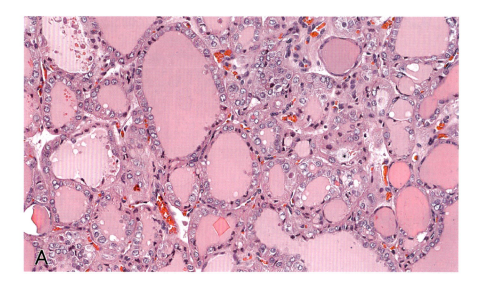

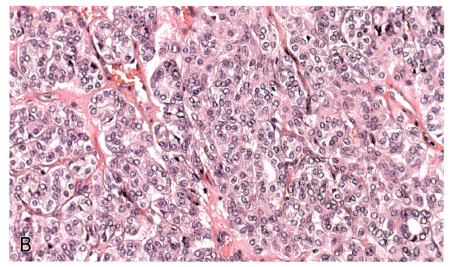

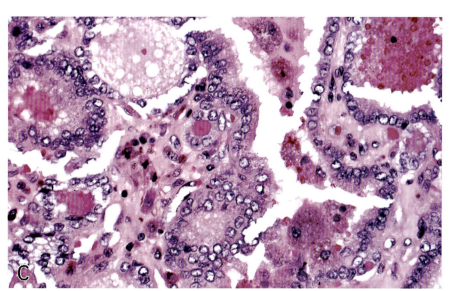

Figure 7-59

WELL-DIFFERENTIATED (FOLLICULAR) TUMOR OF UNCERTAIN MALIGNANT POTENTIAL

A: The nuclei are vesicular and slightly overlapping, but the changes are too subtle and focal to justify a diagnosis of carcinoma.

B: A well-differentiated tumor with "incomplete" nuclear changes, not sufficient for a diagnosis of carcinoma.

C: This focus with over-lapping clear nuclei occupied only a minute portion of a lesion having otherwise the typical features of a benign follicular nodule.

greatly resemble a hyperplastic nodule or a follicular neoplasm but in which high magnification reveals numerous foci of transition. The presence in some of the benign-looking follicles of nuclear features similar to those present in the more typical foci should probably be interpreted as an extreme manifestation of the FVPTC, in which the tumor resembles a hyperplastic or neoplastic follicular process; and 3) a lesion with the overall features of a hyperplastic nodule or a follicular adenoma in which occasional follicles (isolated or in clusters) are lined by follicular cells with clear nuclei, some of which approach a ground-glass appearance (fig. 7-59). This, the most common of the three scenarios, remains a source of interminable argument. The two basic choices for a pathologist when encountering such a lesion are to place it into either a benign or a malignant category by making an arbitrary and subjective estimate of the severity of the changes, or to place it into an intermediate category of its own, thus following the trend that has been established in recent times for analogous situations in other sites (such as uterine smooth muscle tumors, ovarian serous tumors, urothelial tumors, prostatic lesions, cutaneous melanocytic tumors, and others). Thyroid lesions have been traditionally handled following the first of these two approaches, i.e., the benign versus malignant paradigm, even though all the intraobserver and interobserver studies that have been done have shown an unacceptably low level of concordance (269–272), and most clinicopathologic studies have failed to show a statistically significant difference in outcome (273).

The alternative approach, first articulated through a consensus statement by the Chernobyl Pathologists Group, has resulted in the introduction of two new categories: *well-differentiated tumor of uncertain malignant potential (WDT-UMP)* and *follicular tumor of uncertain malignant potential* (FT-UMP). The WDT-UMP is an encapsulated tumor composed of well-differentiated follicular cells with questionable PTC-type nuclear changes, no blood vessel invasion, and capsular invasion that is either absent or questionable. The FT-UMP is an encapsulated tumor composed of well-differentiated follicular cells with questionable capsular invasion, no blood vessel invasion, and no PTC-type nuclear changes. The feature of concern in this tumor is

that capsular involvement by tumor extends to the edge of the capsule and cannot be explained by an irregular tumor/capsule interaction or by tumor trapped by fibrosis on the inner aspect of the capsule (Table 7-1; figs. 7-60, 7-61).

These two conditions do not represent two new specific tumor entities. They are certainly not, as supported by the continuous range they exhibit at the morphologic, immunohistochemical, and molecular genetic levels (274–277). The alternative is, rather, a pragmatic attempt to avoid the word "carcinoma," with all of its formidable therapeutic and psychological implications, for lesions that behave in a favorable fashion following a conservative approach (such as a lobectomy) in the overwhelming majority of the cases, while at the same time rendering the pathologist less exposed to the risk of a medicolegal action.

A spirited argument has developed about the issue in recent years, with various experts taking opposing viewpoints (278–282). Our own position, lucidly articulated by Renshaw and Gould (279), is that a problem exists with the use of the current manichean approach for what represents points along a continuum, and that the easiest way to handle it is to accept the existence of an atypical, uncertain or intermediate category, whether one calls it "atypical thyroid nodule," "atypical adenoma," or "well-differentiated tumor of uncertain malignant potential." We prefer the latter, always followed by an explanatory note along these lines: "Tumors with this set of morphologic features behave in a favorable way in the overwhelming majority of the cases. Although they may conceivably represent the earliest recognizable change along the lines of a well-differentiated carcinoma, at this stage they are essentially of no clinical significance and can be treated similarly to follicular adenomas."

A somewhat analogous situation exists with Hashimoto thyroiditis, in which one or several small foci may be present having a morphological appearance either diagnostic or questionable of PTC. If the former, the term PTC (or mPTC if smaller than 1cm) in Hashimoto thyroiditis would be appropriate: if the latter, one could pick any of the ambiguous terms just listed in the previous paragraph or go for yet another appellation that has been recently proposed, i.e., follicular epithelial dysplasia (280).

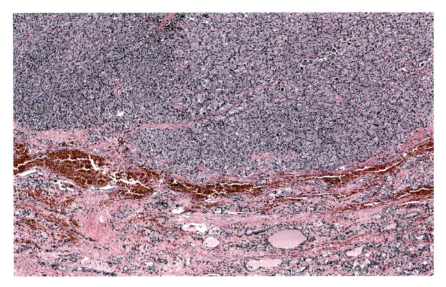

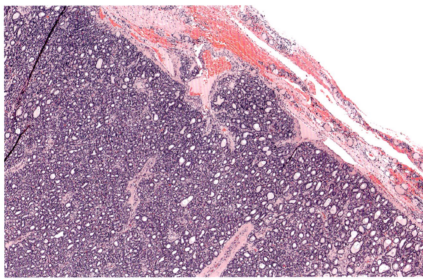

Figure 7-60

WELL-DIFFERENTIATED (FOLLICULAR) TUMOR OF UNCERTAIN MALIGNANT POTENTIAL

Top: The tumor penetrates into the capsule, but a thin peripheral rim remains.
Bottom: Intracapsular "bumpy" appearance of the outer aspect of a nodule.

Our proposal is similar to others that have been increasingly accepted in other organ systems, employing various terminologies but having an essentially analogous meaning. The better known examples are serous tumor of borderline malignancy (ovary), smooth muscle tumor of unknown or uncertain malignant potential (STUMP) (uterus), melanocytic tumor of uncertain malignant potential (skin), papillary neoplasm of low malignant potential (bladder), and indolent lesion of epithelial origin (IDLE) (a variety of sites) (283,284). To quote the latter authors: "Changing the terminology for some of the lesions currently referred to as cancer will allow physicians to shift medico-legal options and low physicians to shift medico-legal options and perceive risk to reflect the evolving understanding of biology, be more judicious about when a biopsy should be done, and organize studies and registries that offer observation or less invasive approaches for indolent disease" (284).

Solid/Trabecular Variant

It is not unusual for PTC to exhibit foci of solid and/or trabecular growth (figs. 7-62, 7-63). Such foci are more common in pediatric tumors, in the diffuse sclerosing variant, and in the papillary microcarcinoma type. The term *solid/trabecular variant* should be used when all, or nearly all, of a tumor not belonging to any of the other variants has a solid and/or trabecular appearance.

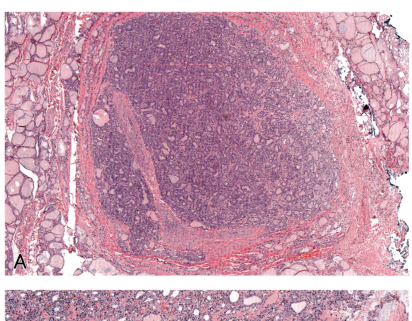

Figure 7-61

WELL-DIFFERENTIATED (FOLLICULAR) TUMOR OF UNCERTAIN MALIGNANT POTENTIAL

A–C: Partially permeated capsules. It is debatable whether the intracapsular tumor focus present in in C also represents vascular invasion.

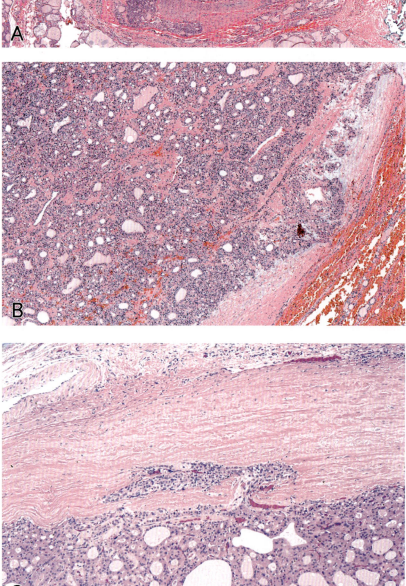

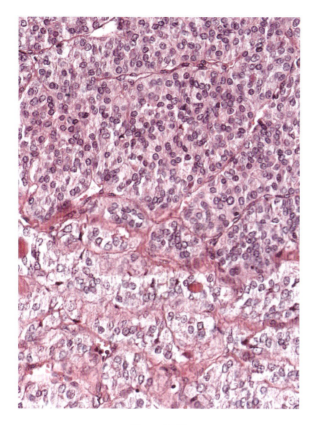

Figure 7-62

WELL-DIFFERENTIATED (FOLLICULAR) TUMOR OF UNCERTAIN MALIGNANT POTENTIAL

This tumor was placed in the uncertain malignant potential category because of the "incomplete" nuclear features.

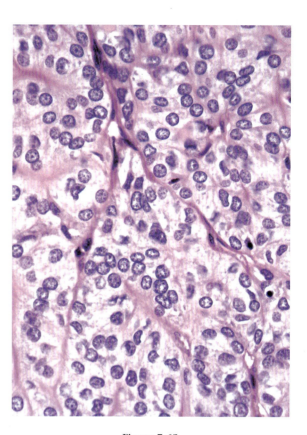

Figure 7-63

WELL-DIFFERENTIATED (FOLLICULAR) TUMOR OF UNCERTAIN MALIGNANT POTENTIAL

"Incomplete" nuclear features.

When thus defined, this variant is rare, and it should not be overdiagnosed as poorly differentiated or undifferentiated carcinoma. Diagnostic clues for this variant include the presence of irregular fibrous and fibrohyaline trabeculae within the tumor, an occasional psammoma body, and clusters of lymphocytes in or around the tumor. An absolute requirement for diagnosis is that the typical nuclear features of PTC must be retained. When this is the case, the tumor behavior is associated with a slightly higher frequency of distant metastases and less favorable prognosis than classic PTC, but not nearly as bad as that of poorly differentiated papillary carcinoma (285).

Diffuse Sclerosing Variant

The *diffuse sclerosing variant*, originally described by Vickery et al. (249), is characterized by the following features: 1) diffuse involvement of one or (more commonly) both lobes;

2) numerous small papillary formations located within intrathyroidal cleft-like spaces, probably representing lymph vessels; 3) extensive squamous metaplasia; 4) large number of psammoma bodies; 5) marked inflammatory infiltration; and 6) prominent fibrosis (figs. 7-64–7-68) (286). The inflammatory component is represented by an admixture of B and T lymphocytes, plasma cells, Langerhans cells, and other S-100 protein-positive cells (278,287–289).

Of these features, widespread lymphatic permeation is the most important because it probably conditions the other morphologic findings as well as tumor behavior. Other features of the tumor are analogous to those of conventional PTC.

When compared with conventional PTC, this variant exhibits: 1) similar prevalence in women; 2) greater incidence of cervical lymph node involvement; 3) greater incidence of pulmonary

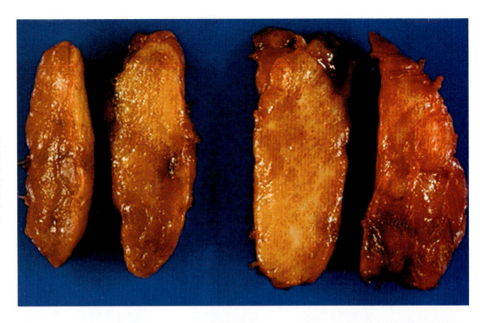

Figure 7-64

DIFFUSE SCLEROSING VARIANT

The outer aspect and cut surface of both thyroid lobes are involved by PTC of the diffuse sclerosing variant. The diffuse pattern of growth and the fibrosing features are evident throughout.

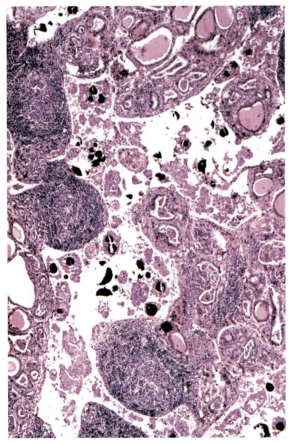

Figure 7-65

DIFFUSE SCLEROSING VARIANT

Massive dilatation of vessels due to packing by tumor cells is accompanied by prominent lymphoid follicles.

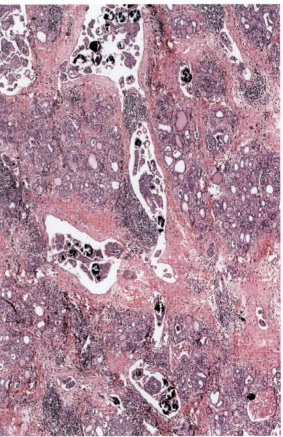

Figure 7-66

DIFFUSE SCLEROSING VARIANT

The vascular involvement by tumor is accompanied by diffuse fibrosis.

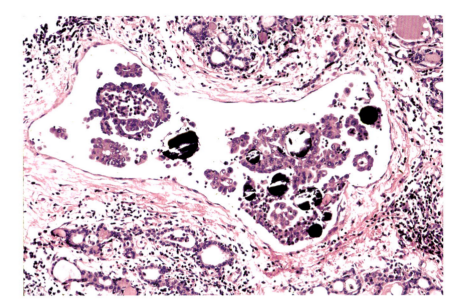

Figure 7-67

DIFFUSE SCLEROSING VARIANT

The intravascular nests of tumor cells contain numerous psammoma bodies.

metastases; and 4) lesser probability of disease-free survival on follow-up. Distant metastases in unusual places such as brain have been reported (290).

An interesting clinical observation is that there is often a delay in diagnosis, probably explainable by the fact that the diffuse glandular enlargement simulates thyroiditis clinically and on thyroid scan (291). It is also interesting that, despite the high incidence of pulmonary metastases, the tumor death rate is extremely low (287,291–295). It is possible that the young age of most patients with this variant counterbalances the adverse clinical significance of the other findings (293).

In one series, a "dominant" tumor nodule was found in over half of the cases (fig. 7-69) (291). This finding may indicate that this variant, like its conventional counterpart, begins as a single tumor mass and that its subsequent configuration is the result of early widespread permeation of intrathyroid lymph vessels, as originally proposed by Lindsay (247). The clinicopathologic features of this variant justify the performance of a total or near-total thyroidectomy followed by the administration of radioactive iodine as treatment.

Oncocytic and Warthin-Like Variants

The *oncocytic variant* of PTC combines the nuclear features of PTC with the cytoplasmic features of an oncocytic neoplasm. The oncocytic variant may exhibit papillary, follicular, or solid/

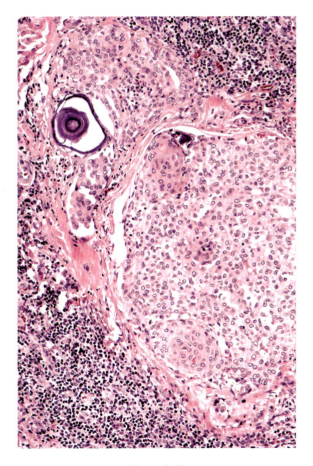

Figure 7-68

DIFFUSE SCLEROSING VARIANT

Extensive squamous metaplasia and a prominent psammoma body are seen.

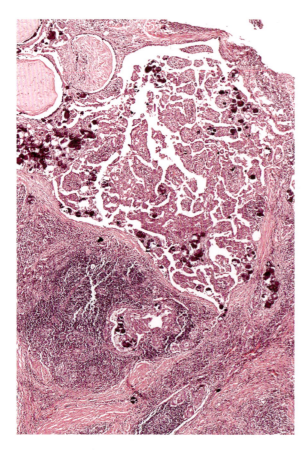

Figure 7-69

DIFFUSE SCLEROSING VARIANT

Massive vascular involvement, prominent lymphoid follicles, extensive fibrosis, and scattered psammoma bodies are seen. All the distinguishing features of the diffuse sclerosing variant are present. It is possible that the large tumor nodule is the "parent" tumor which later spread to the rest of the gland.

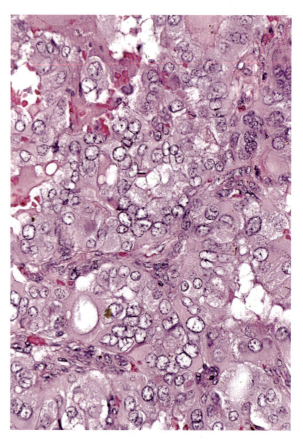

Figure 7-70

ONCOCYTIC VARIANT

Because of the nuclear features, this tumor type should be regarded as a PTC with oncocytic change of the tumor cells rather than an oncocytoma with a papillary pattern of growth.

trabecular patterns of growth, and thus combine the features of two or more variants (such as the oncocytic follicular variant) (figs. 7-70, 7-71).

The main differential diagnosis (especially for those tumors having a follicular pattern of growth) is with benign and malignant oncocytic follicular tumors, i.e., Hürthle cell adenomas and carcinomas. The distinction is based almost entirely on the nuclear features which, if present, place the tumor into the PTC category (296). Such nuclear features, however, are often not as overt in the oncocytic variant as they are in conventional PTC. This becomes particularly evident in PTC combining oncocytic and nononcocytic components, the latter featuring fully developed nuclear abnormalities while the former

exhibiting them in a much subtler fashion (fig. 7-53). The claim has been made that, as a group, oncocytic PTC is more aggressive than classic PTC, but it is possible that some series contain an admixture of oncocytic PTCs and oncocytic neoplasms of non-PTC type (297,298).

The *Warthin-like variant* of PTC is probably closely related to the oncocytic variant of this tumor, as supported by its molecular genetic profile (299). The pattern of growth is overtly papillary, the nuclei are of PTC type, the cytoplasm is granular and eosinophilic, and the stroma is packed with lymphocytes (sometimes including lymphoid follicles with germinal centers) (figs. 7-72–7-74). The overall appearance is reminiscent of the salivary gland neoplasm known as Warthin tumor (300). The prognosis

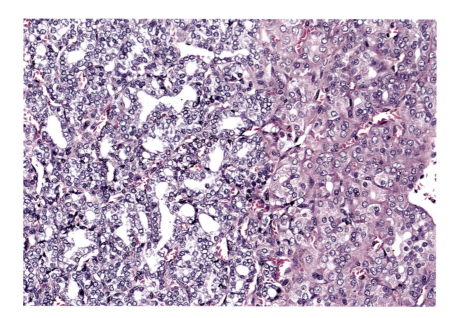

Figure 7-71

ONCOCYTIC VARIANT

Oncocytic features are prominent in half of this papillary carcinoma and absent in the other half.

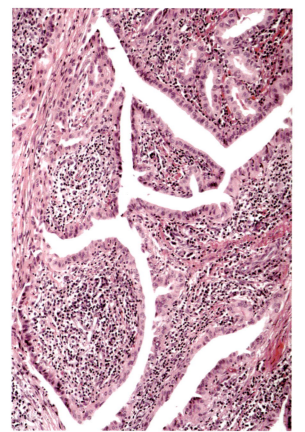
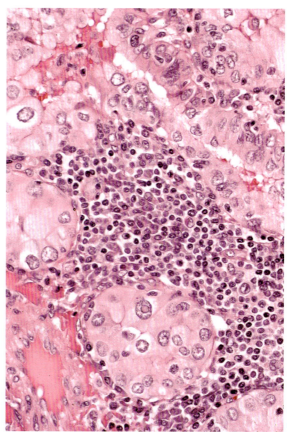

Figure 7-72

WARTHIN-LIKE VARIANT

Left: Bland papillae are lined by oncocytic follicular cells and accompanied by a heavy lymphoid infiltrate.
Right: On high power, both the oncocytic character of the follicular cells and the heavy lymphoid infiltrate are evident. Note the prominent nuclear pseudoinclusion.

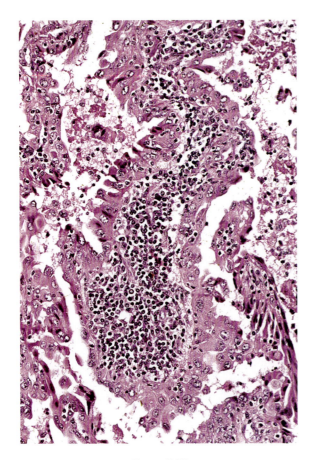

Figure 7-73

WARTHIN-LIKE VARIANT

This oncocytic papillary tumor resembles its better known homonym in the salivary gland.

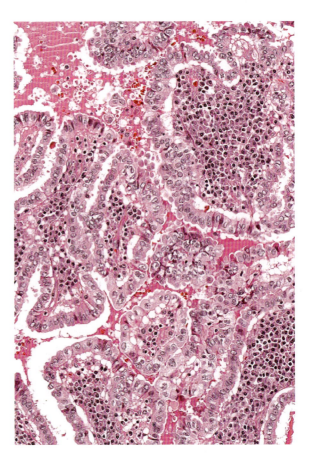

Figure 7-74

PAPILLARY CARCINOMA WITH WARTHIN AND TALL CELL FEATURES

The existence of cases like this suggest that Warthin-like tumor is a subset of the tall cell variant of papillary carcinoma.

seems to be just as good or even better than that of classic PTC (299,300).

Tall and Columnar Cell Variants

Hawk and Hazard (204) first proposed the existence of the *tall cell variant* of PTC and found that it made up about 10 percent of all cases in their material. This variant tends to occur in older patients, but it can also be seen in young adults and children (301). Most are of large size (usually over 5 cm). The pattern of growth is usually highly papilliferous, and the papillae are often overly elongated, cord-like, and running side-to-side in a regimented fashion (figs. 7-75, 7-76). Extrathyroid extension and multicentricity are frequent, and there is a greater incidence of vascular invasion than in conventional PTC (304).

The papillae are partially or entirely covered by cells whose heights are at least two times their widths (fig. 7-76B,C) (305). These cells often have abundant acidophilic ("pink") cytoplasm that approaches, but does not attain, the appearance of oncocytes, an admittedly subtle distinction. Mitotic figures are found easily (in striking contrast to conventional PTC), and the nuclei have typical PTC-type features (249). Some of the better-developed nuclear pseudoinclusions that we have seen have been in this variant. Flint et al. (205) found no difference in DNA content, chromatin texture, or nuclear size or shape between the tall cell variant and conventional PTC.

The behavior of the tall cell variant of PTC is more aggressive than that of conventional PTC (239,306). Because several unfavorable features

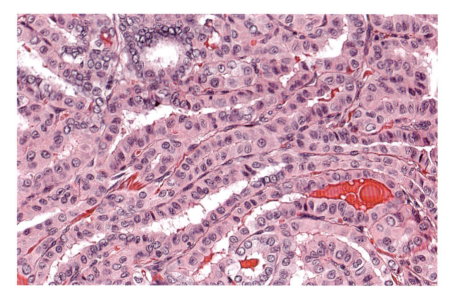

Figure 7-75

TALL CELL VARIANT

The tumor cells are "tall," their cytoplasm is oncocytic, and the pattern of growth is that of highly packed, regimented papillae.

Figure 7-76

TALL CELL VARIANT

A: The regimented papillae are obvious.

B: In another example, the tall shape of the cells, the oncocytic quality of their cytoplasm, and the nuclear changes are evident.

C: Several prominent nuclear pseudo-inclusions are present in this tumor.

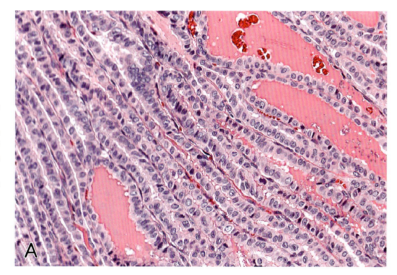

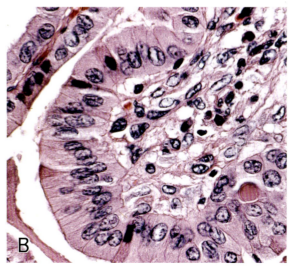

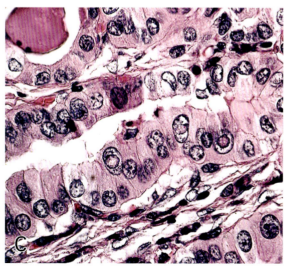

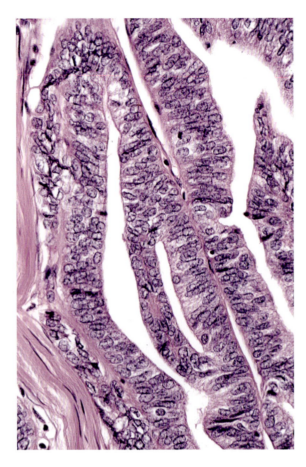

Figure 7-77

COLUMNAR CELL CARCINOMA

There is stratification of the hyperchromatic nuclei, which lack the features of those seen in PTC and its variants.

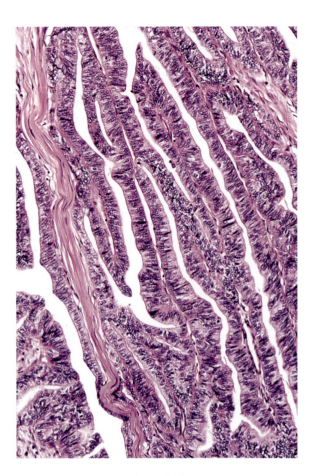

Figure 7-78

COLUMNAR CELL CARCINOMA

Markedly enlarged papillae are lined by pseudostratified epithelium.

converge in this variant (e.g., advanced age, large tumor size, and mitotic activity), it is not easy to discern how much each contributes to this worsened outlook (307,308). This apparently higher degree of aggressiveness of the tall cell variant has also been observed in papillary microcarcinoma (309), but not in the very rare cases that have been reported in children (310).

There is yet no consensus as to what percentage of the tumor needs to be composed of tall cells in order to be placed into the tall cell variant category. Some authors believe, though, that even a content of 10 percent tall cells endows PTC with a greater degree of aggressiveness (311).

Columnar cell carcinoma differs from both the conventional and the tall cell forms of PTC because of the presence of prominent nuclear

stratification (fig. 7-77) (312–315). In addition, the nuclei may lack the typical features of PTC (315,316). The cytoplasm tends to be very clear, to the point of exhibiting subnuclear vacuolation resembling that seen in secretory endometrium. There is also a resemblance to colonic epithelium, a finding of possible pathogenetic significance in view of the immunoreactivity for CDX2 that has been detected in this entity (figs. 7-78, 7-79) (317).

The behavior of columnar cell carcinoma is variable. Early reports emphasized their aggressiveness (318,319), but tumors from more recent series have shown a more indolent behavior, especially if small, well-circumscribed or encapsulated, and occurring in young females (312,314,320).

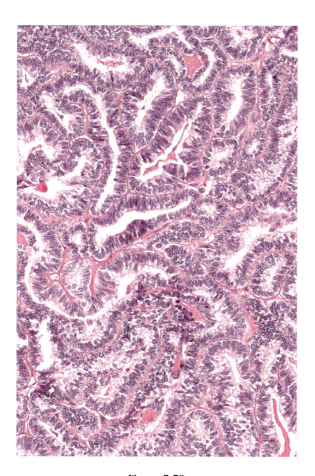

Figure 7-79

COLUMNAR CELL CARCINOMA

The pattern of growth of this tumor has been likened to that of colonic and endometrial adenocarcinomas.

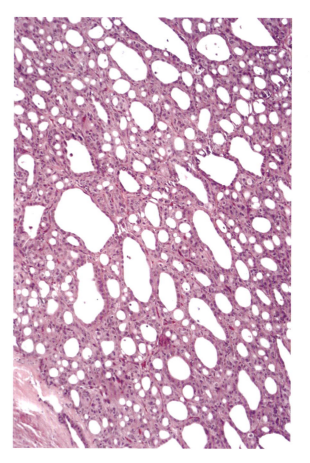

Figure 7-80

CRIBRIFORM/MORULAR VARIANT

Low-power view shows a prominent cribriform pattern.

It is not clear what the relationship is between the tall and columnar variants. Cases combining features of both types have been reported (321, 322). Parenthetically, cases combining features of tall cell variant of PTC and Hürthle cell carcinoma have also been reported (323).

The suggestion that P-glycoprotein (the central mediator of in vitro tumor multidrug resistance) is hyperexpressed in the tall cell variant of PTC has been advanced by Axiotis et al. (324). Others have found common expression of this marker both in benign and malignant conditions (325).

Two other variants, *oncocytic papillary tumors* and *PTC with clear cell changes*, the latter being an inconsequential morphologic variation of PTC, are discussed in chapters 10 and 11, respectively.

A curiosity perhaps worth mentioning before concluding this section is that there exists in the breast a primary tumor with morphologic (but only morphologic) features that recapitulate closely those of the tall cell variant of PTC (326,327).

Cribriform/Morular Variant

This fairly new entity, the *cribriform/morular variant*, is regarded by some as yet another variant of PTC and by others as a distinct category of thyroid carcinoma. It occurs in a sporadic form or as an extraintestinal component of the familial adenomatous polyposis syndrome, of which it may be the initial clinical manifestation (328–331). It is seen almost exclusively in females. Isolated cases have been reported in children (332). The sporadic form is solitary, larger, and accompanied by less fibrosis (333).

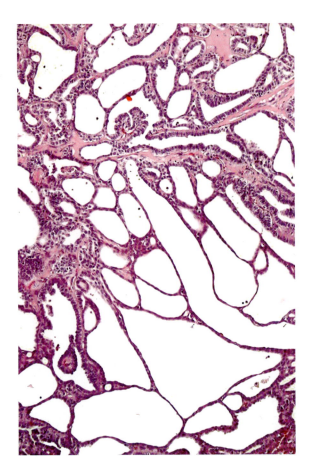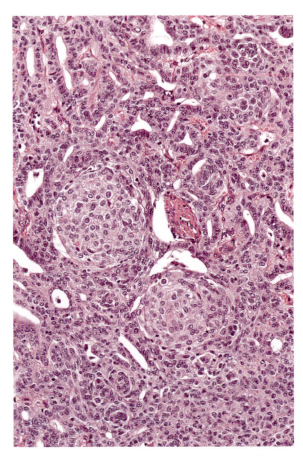

Figure 7-81

CRIBRIFORM/MORULAR VARIANT

Left: There is great variability in the size and shape of the cystic spaces. A few inconspicuous morulae are seen.
Right: The morular formations predominate over the cribriform areas.

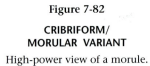

Figure 7-82

CRIBRIFORM/ MORULAR VARIANT

High-power view of a morule.

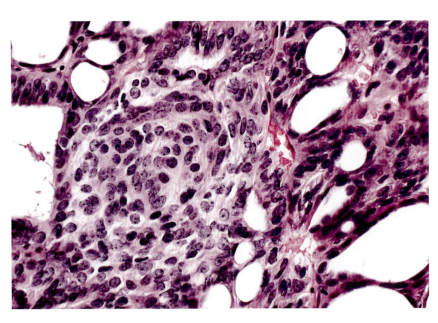

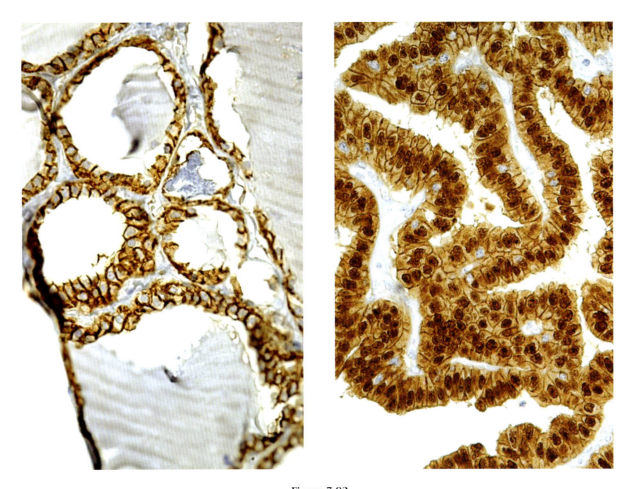

Figure 7-83

CRIBRIFORM/ MORULAR VARIANT

Left: In the normal thyroid gland, beta-catenin is restricted to the cell membrane of the follicular cells.
Right: In the papillary carcinoma there is cytoplasmic and nuclear accumulation of beta-catenin.

The tumor is usually encapsulated and shows an intimate admixture of cribriform, follicular, papillary, trabecular, and solid patterns of growth, with round squamoid structures known as morules. Cribriform areas formed by anastomosing bars and arches of cells unaccompanied by intervening stroma are present (figs. 7-80–7-82). The papillae are lined by cells of columnar shape, and intraluminal colloid is scanty. The trabecular areas resemble those of hyalinizing trabecular adenoma. The nuclei are not particularly clear, but they exhibit varying numbers of grooves and pseudoinclusions. The morules contain optically clear nuclei different from those of conventional PTC but similar to nuclei seen in morule-containing tumors of other sites (334).

These tumors result from the accumulation of biotin, which appears ultrastructurally as perinuclear aggregates of microfilaments (335). They are positive for CD10, CK19, p53, BCL-2, and estrogen receptor-beta, and are thought to develop as a result of a mutation in exon 3 of the beta-catenin gene, which is manifested by cytoplasmic and nuclear accumulation of beta-catenin (fig. 7-83) (336–338). Focal neuroendocrine differentiation has been described in some cases (334) and poorly differentiated features in others (339). Capsular or blood vessel invasion is usually present. Some cases are very aggressive, with distant metastases and death (326).

REFERENCES

1. Lieberman PH, Foote FW Jr, Schottenfeld D. A study of the pathology of thyroid cancer, 1930-1960. Clin Bull (MSKCC) 1972;2:7-12.

2. Hofstädter F. Frequency and morphology of malignant tumors of the thyroid before and after the introduction of iodine-prophylaxis. Virchows Arch A Pathol Anat Histol 1980;385:263-70.

3. Williams ED, Doniach I, Bjarnason O, Michie W. Thyroid cancer in an iodine rich area: a histopathological study. Cancer 1977;39:215-22.

4. Calandra DB, Shah KH, Lawrence AM, Paloyan E. Total thyroidectomy in irradiated patients. A twenty-year experience in 206 patients. Ann Surg 1985;202:356-60.

5. Hempelmann LH, Hall WJ, Phillips M, Cooper RA, Ames WR. Neoplasms in persons treated with x-rays in infancy: fourth survey in 20 years. J Natl Cancer Inst 1975;55:519-30.

6. Schneider AB, Pinsky S, Bekerman C, Ryo UY. Characteristics of 108 thyroid cancers detected by screening in a population with a history of head and neck irradiation. Cancer 1980;46:1218-27.

7. Wilson SD, Komorowski R, Cerletty J, Majewski JT, Hooper M. Radiation-associated thyroid tumors: extent of operation and pathology technique influence the apparent incidence of carcinoma. Surgery 1983;94:663-9.

8. Carcangiu ML, Zampi G, Pupi A, Castagnoli A, Rosai J. Papillary carcinoma of the thyroid. A clinicopathologic study of 241 cases treated at the University of Florence, Italy. Cancer 1985;55:805-28.

9. Bakri K, Shimaoka K, Rao U, Tsukada Y. Adenosquamous carcinoma of the thyroid after radiotherapy for Hodgkin's disease. A case report and review. Cancer 1983;52:465-70.

10. Block MA, Miller MJ, Horn RC Jr. Carcinoma of the thyroid after external radiation to the neck in adults. Am J Surg 1969;118:764-9.

11. Hawkins MM, Kingston JE. Malignant thyroid tumours following childhood cancer. Lancet 1988;2:804.

12. McDougall IR, Coleman CN, Burke JS, Saunders W, Kaplan HS. Thyroid carcinoma after high-dose external radiotherapy for Hodgkin's disease: report of three cases. Cancer 1980;45:2056-60.

13. Tang TT, Holcenberg JS, Duck SC, Hodach AE, Oechler HW, Camitta BM. Thyroid carcinoma following treatment for acute lymphoblastic leukemia. Cancer 1980;46:1572-6.

14. Vane D, King DR, Boles ET Jr. Secondary thyroid neoplasms in pediatric cancer patients: increased risk with improved survival. J Pediatr Surg 1984;19:855-60.

15. Mazzaferri EL, Young RL, Oertel JE, Kemmerer WT, Page CP. Papillary thyroid carcinoma: the impact of therapy in 576 patients. Medicine (Baltimore) 1977;56:171-96.

16. Williams D. Radiation carcinogenesis: lessons from Chernobyl. Oncogene 2008;27:S9-18.

17. LiVolsi VA. Papillary thyroid carcinoma: an update. Mod Pathol 2011;24:S1-9.

18. LiVolsi VA, Abrosimov AA, Bogdanova T, et al. The Chernobyl thyroid cancer experience: pathology. Clin Oncol (R Coll Radiol) 2011;23:261-7.

19. Thomas GA, Tronko MD, Tsyb AF, Tuttle RM. What have we learnt from Chernobyl? What have we still to learn? Clin Oncol (R Coll Radiol) 2011;23:229-33.

20. Tuttle RM, Becker DV. The Chernobyl accident and its consequences: update at the millennium. Semin Nucl Med 2000;30:133-40.

21. Doniach I. Aetiological consideration of thyroid carcinoma. In: Smithers DW, ed. Tumours of the thyroid gland. Edinburgh: E & S Livingstone; 1970:66-7.

22. Farbota LM, Calandra DB, Lawrence AM, Paloyan E. Thyroid carcinoma in Graves' disease. Surgery 1985;98:1148-52.

23. Meissner WA, Adler A. Papillary carcinoma of the thyroid: a study of the pathology of two hundred twenty-six cases. Arch Pathol 1958;66:518-25.

24. Miller M, Chodos RB, Olen E, Klinck GH. Thyroid carcinoma occurring in Graves' disease. Arch Intern Med 1966;117:432-5.

25. Rieger R, Pimpl W, Money S, Rettenbacher L, Galvan G. Hyperthyroidism and concurrent thyroid malignancies. Surgery 1989;106:6-10.

26. Shapiro SJ, Friedman NB, Perzik SL, Catz B. Incidence of thyroid carcinoma in Graves' disease. Cancer 1970;26:1261-70.

27. Filetti S, Belfiore A, Amir SM, et al. The role of thyroid-stimulating antibodies of Graves' disease in differentiated thyroid cancer. N Engl J Med 1988;318:753-9.

28. Chesky VE, Hellwig CA, Welch JW. Cancer of the thyroid associated with Hashimoto's disease: an analysis of forty-eight cases. Am Surg 1962;28:678-85.

29. Ott RA, Calandra DB, McCall A, Shah KH, Lawrence AM, Paloyan E. The incidence of thyroid carcinoma in patients with Hashimoto's thyroiditis and solitary cold nodules. Surgery 1985;98:1202-6.

30. Segal K, Ben-Bassat M, Avraham A, Har-El G, Sidi J. Hashimoto's thyroiditis and carcinoma of the thyroid gland. Int Surg 1985;70:205-9.

31. Lote K, Andersen K, Nordal E, Brennhovd IO. Familial occurrence of papillary thyroid carcinoma. Cancer 1980;46:1291-7.

32. Narita T, Takagi K. Ataxia-telangiectasia with dysgerminoma of right ovary, papillary carcinoma of thyroid, and adenocarcinoma of pancreas. Cancer 1984;54:1113-6.

33. Larraza-Hernandez O, Albores-Saavedra J, Benavides G, Krause LG, Perez-Merizaldi JC, Ginzo A. Multiple endocrine neoplasia. Pituitary adenoma, multicentric papillary thyroid carcinoma, bilateral carotid body paraganglioma, parathyroid hyperplasia, gastric leiomyoma, and systemic amyloidosis. Am J Clin Pathol 1982;78:527-32.

34. Hedman I, Tisell LE. Associated hyperparathyroidism and nonmedullary thyroid carcinoma: the etiologic role of radiation. Surgery 1984;95:392-7.

35. Albores-Saavedra J, Durán ME. Association of thyroid carcinoma and chemodectoma. Am J Surg 1968;116:887-90.

36. Plail RO, Bussey HJ, Glazer G, Thomson JP. Adenomatous polyposis: an association with carcinoma of the thyroid. Br J Surg 1987;74:377-80.

37. Lever EG, Refetoff S, Straus FH 2nd, Nguyen M, Kaplan EL. Coexisting thyroid and parathyroid disease—are they related? Surgery 1983;94:893-900.

38. Franssila KO. Is the differentiation between papillary and follicular thyroid carcinoma valid? Cancer 1973;32:853-64.

39. Hawk WA, Hazard JB. The many appearances of papillary carcinoma of the thyroid. Cleve Clin Q 1976;43:207-15.

40. Mazzaferri EL, Young RL. Papillary thyroid carcinoma: a 10 year follow-up report of the impact of therapy in 576 patients. Am J Med 1981;70:511-8.

41. Sierk A, Askin FB, Reddick RL, Thomas CG Jr. Pediatric thyroid cancer. Pediatr Pathol 1990;10:877-93.

42. Woolner LB, Beahrs OH, Black BM, McConahey WM, Keating FR Jr. Classification and prognosis of thyroid carcinoma: a study of 885 cases observed in a thirty year period. Am J Surg 1961;102:354-87.

43. Cady B, Sedgwick CE, Meissner WA, Bookwalter JR, Romagosa V, Werber J. Changing clinical, pathologic, therapeutic, and survival patterns in differentiated thyroid carcinoma. Ann Surg 1976;184:541-53.

44. Crile G Jr. Changing end results in patients with papillary carcinoma of the thyroid. Surg Gynecol Obstet 1971;132:460-8.

45. Hay ID. Nodal metastases from papillary thyroid carcinoma. Lancet 1986;2:1283.

46. Mazzaferri EL. Papillary thyroid carcinoma: factors influencing prognosis and current therapy. Semin Oncol 1987;14:315-32.

47. Mizukami Y, Michigishi T, Nonomura A, et al. Autonomously functioning (hot) nodule of the thyroid gland. A clinical and histopathologic study of 17 cases. Am J Clin Pathol 1994;101:29-35.

48. Hay ID. Papillary thyroid carcinoma. Endocrinol Metab Clin North Am 1990;19:545-76.

49. Tscholl-Ducommun J, Hedinger CE. Papillary thyroid carcinomas. Morphology and prognosis. Virchows Arch A Pathol Anat Histol 1982;396:19-39.

50. Frauenhoffer CM, Patchefsky AS, Cobanoglu A. Thyroid carcinoma: a clinical and pathologic study of 125 cases. Cancer 1979;43:2414-21.

51. Thompson AD, Pasieka JL, Kneafsey P, DiFrancesco LM. Hypopigmentation of a papillary carcinoma arising in a black thyroid. Mod Pathol 1999;12:1181-5.

52. Vestfrid MA. Papillary carcinoma of the thyroid gland with lipomatous stroma: report of a peculiar histological type of thyroid tumour. Histopathology 1986;10:97-100.

53. LiVolsi V. Papillary neoplasms of the thyroid. Pathologic and prognostic features. Am J Clin Pathol 1992;97:426-34.

54. Fischer AH, Bond JA, Taysavang P, Battles OE, Wynford-Thomas D. Papillary thyroid carcinoma oncogene (RET/PTC) alters the nuclear envelope and chromatin structure. Am J Pathol 1998;153:1443-50.

55. Albores-Saavedra J, Altamirano-Dimas M, Alcorta-Anguizola B, Smith M. Fine structure of human papillary thyroid carcinoma. Cancer 1971;28:763-74.

56. Johannessen JV, Gould VE, Jao W. The fine structure of human thyroid cancer. Hum Pathol 1978;9:385-400.

57. Chan JK, Saw D. The grooved nucleus. A useful diagnostic criterion of papillary carcinoma of the thyroid. Am J Surg Pathol 1986;10:672-9.

58. Scopa CD, Melachrinou M, Saradopoulou C, Merino MJ. The significance of the grooved nucleus in thyroid lesions. Mod Pathol 1993;6:691-4.

59. Asioli S, Bussolati G. Emerin immunohistochemistry reveals diagnostic features of nuclear membrane arrangement in thyroid lesions. Histopathology 2009;54:571-9.

60. Hinrichs BH, Kinsella MD, Lawson D, Cohen C, Siddiqui MT. Emerin immunohistochemistry: a useful ancillary test for the identification of papillary thyroid carcinoma. Lab Invest 2012;92:145A (abstract).

61. Papotti M, Manazza AD, Chiarle R, Bussolati G. Confocal microscope analysis and tridimensional reconstruction of papillary thyroid carcinoma nuclei. Virchows Arch 2004;444:350-5.

62. Baloch ZW, LiVolsi VA. Etiology and significance of the optically clear nucleus. Endocr Pathol 2002;13:289-99.

63. DeLellis RA. Orphan Annie eye nuclei: a historical note. Am J Surg Pathol 1993;17:1067-8.

64. Gray A, Doniach I. Morphology of the nuclei of papillary carcinoma of the thyroid. Br J Cancer 1969;23:49-51.

65. Carcangiu ML, Zampi G, Rosai J. Papillary thyroid carcinoma: a study of its many morphologic expressions and clinical correlates. Pathol Annu 1985;20(Pt. 1):1-44.

66. Ip YT, Dias Filho MA, Chan JK. Nuclear inclusions and pseudoinclusions: friends or foes of the surgical pathologist? Int J Surg Pathol 2010;18:465-81.

67. Naganuma H, Murayama H, Ohtani N, et al. Optically clear nuclei in papillary carcinoma of the thyroid: demonstration of one of the fixation artifacts and its practical usefulness. Pathol Int 2000;50:113-8.

68. Rosai J, Kuhn E, Carcangiu ML. Pitfalls in thyroid tumour pathology. Histopathology 2006;49:107-20.

69. Yamashita T, Hosoda Y, Kameyama K, Aiba M, Ito K, Fujimoto Y. Peculiar nuclear clearing composed of microfilaments in papillary carcinoma of the thyroid. Cancer 1992;70:2923-8.

70. Okamoto Y, Kashima K, Daa T, Yokoyama S, Nakayama I, Noguchi S. Morule with biotin-containing intranuclear inclusions in thyroid carcinoma. Pathol Int 1995;45:573-9.

71. Vergilio J, Baloch ZW, LiVolsi VA. Spindle cell metaplasia of the thyroid arising in association with papillary carcinoma and follicular adenoma. Am J Clin Pathol 2002;117:199-204.

72. Matoso A, Easley SE, Mangray S, Jacob R, DeLellis RA. Spindle cell foci in the thyroid gland: an immunohistochemical analysis. Appl Immunohistochem Mol Morphol 2011;19:400-7.

73. Woenckhaus C, Cameselle-Teijeiro J, Ruiz-Ponte C, Abdulkader I, Reyes-Santías R, Sobrinho-Simões M. Spindle cell variant of papillary thyroid carcinoma. Histopathology 2004;45:424-7.

74. Papi G, Corrado S, LiVolsi VA. Primary spindle cell lesions of the thyroid gland; an overview. Am J Clin Pathol 2006;125:S95-123.

75. Yoshida A, Kamma H, Asaga T, et al. Proliferative activity in thyroid tumors. Cancer 1992;69:2548-52.

76. Lee TK, Myers RT, Marshall RB, Bond MG, Kardon B. The significance of mitotic rate: a retrospective study of 127 thyroid carcinomas. Hum Pathol 1985;16:1042-6.

77. Asioli S, Erickson LA, Sebo TJ, et al. Papillary thyroid carcinoma with prominent hobnail features: a new aggressive variant of moderately differentiated papillary carcinoma. A clinicopathologic, immunohistochemical, and molecular study of eight cases. Am J Surg Pathol 2010;34:44-52.

78. Asioli S, Erickson LA, Righi A, Lloyd RV. Papillary thyroid carcinoma with hobnail features: histopathologic criteria to predict aggressive behavior. Hum Pathol 2013;44:320-8.

79. Lino-Silva LS1, Domínguez-Malagón HR, Caro-Sánchez CH, Salcedo-Hernández RA. Thyroid gland papillary carcinomas with "micropapillary pattern," a recently recognized poor prognostic finding: clinicopathologic and survival analysis of 7 cases. Hum Pathol 2012;43:1596-600.

80. Lubitz CC, Economopoulos KP, Pawlak AC, et al. Hobnail variant of papillary thyroid carcinoma: an institutional case series and molecular profile. Thyroid 2014;24:958-65.

81. Tunio GM, Hirota S, Nomura S, Kitamura Y. Possible relation of osteopontin to development of psammoma bodies in human papillary thyroid cancer. Arch Pathol Lab Med 1998;122:1087-90.

82. Johannessen JV, Sobrinho-Simões M. The origin and significance of thyroid psammoma bodies. Lab Invest 1980;43:287-96.

83. Klinck GH, Winship T. Psammoma bodies and thyroid cancer. Cancer 1959;12:656-62.

84. Patchefsky AS, Hoch WS. Psammoma bodies in diffuse toxic goiter. Am J Clin Pathol 1972;57:551-6.

85. Hunt JL, Barnes EL. Non-tumor-associated psammoma bodies in the thyroid. Am J Clin Pathol 2003;119:90-4.

86. Satoh Y, Sakamoto A, Yamada K, Kasai N. Psammoma bodies in metastatic carcinoma to the thyroid. Mod Pathol 1990;3:267-70.

87. Koperek O, Asari R, Niederle B, Kaserer K. Desmoplastic stromal reaction in papillary thyroid microcarcinoma. Histopathology 2011;58:919-24.

88. Chan JK, Carcangiu ML, Rosai J. Papillary carcinoma of thyroid with exuberant nodular fasciitis-like stroma. Report of three cases. Am J Clin Pathol 1991;95:309-14.

89. Mizukami Y, Nonomura A, Matsubara F, Michigishi T, Ohmura K, Hashimoto T. Papillary carcinoma of the thyroid gland with fibromatosis-like stroma. Histopathology 1992;20:355-7.

90. Terayama K, Toda S, Yonemitsu N, Koike N, Sugihara H. Papillary carcinoma of the thyroid with exuberant nodular fasciitis-like stroma. Virchows Arch 1997;431:291-5.

91. Mizukami Y, Kurumaya H, Kitagawa T, et al. Papillary carcinoma of the thyroid gland with fibromatosis-like stroma: a case report and review of the literature. Mod Pathol 1995;8:366-70.

92. Naganuma H, Iwama N, Nakamura Y, et al. Papillary carcinoma of the thyroid gland forming a myofibroblastic nodular tumor: report of two cases and review of the literature. Pathol Int 2002;52:54-8.

93. Michal M, Chlumska A, Fakan F. Papillary carcinoma of thyroid with exuberant nodular fasciitis-like stroma. Histopathology 1992;21:577-9.

94. Toti P, Tanganelli P, Schürfeld K, et al. Scarring in papillary carcinoma of the thyroid: report of two new cases with exuberant nodular fasciitis-like stroma. Histopathology 1999;35:418-22.

95. Ostrowski MA, Asa SL, Chamberlain D, Moffat FL, Rotstein LE. Myxomatous change in papillary carcinoma of the thyroid. Surg Pathol 1989;2:249-56.

96. Kondo T, Nakazawa T, Murata S, Katoh R. Stromal elastosis in papillary thyroid carcinomas. Hum Pathol 2005;36:474-9.

97. Pinto A, Nose V. Localized amyloid in thyroid: are we missing it? Adv Anat Pathol 2013;20:61-7.

98. Akslen LA, LiVolsi VA. Prognostic significance of histologic grading compared with subclassification of papillary thyroid carcinoma. Cancer 2000;88:1902-8.

99. Lucas SD, Karlsson-Parra A, Nilsson B, et al. Tumor-specific deposition of immunoglobulin G and complement in papillary thyroid carcinoma. Hum Pathol 1996;27:1329-35.

100. Kamma H, Fujii K, Ogata T. Lymphocytic infiltration in juvenile thyroid carcinoma. Cancer 1988;62:1988-93.

101. Selzer G, Kahn LB, Albertyn L. Primary malignant tumors of the thyroid gland: a clinicopathologic study of 254 cases. Cancer 1977;40:1501-10.

102. Schröder S, Schwarz W, Rehpenning W, Löning T, Böcker W. Dendritic/Langerhans cells and prognosis in patients with papillary thyroid carcinomas. Immunocytochemical study of 106 thyroid neoplasms correlated to follow-up data. Am J Clin Pathol 1988;89:295-300.

103. Hilly O, Koren R, Raz R, et al. The role of S100-positive dendritic cells in the prognosis of papillary thyroid carcinoma. Am J Clin Pathol 2013;139:87-92.

104. Guiter GE, DeLellis RA. Multinucleate giant cells in papillary thyroid carcinoma. A morphologic and immunohistochemical study. Am J Clin Pathol 1996;106:765-8.

105. Hommell-Fontaine J, Borda A, Ragage F, Berger N, Decaussin-Petrucci M. Nonconventional papillary thyroid carcinomas with pleomorphic tumor giant cells: a diagnostic pitfall with anaplastic carcinoma. Virchows Arch 2010;456:661-70.

106. Rivera M, Ricarte-Filho J, Patel S, et al. Encapsulated thyroid tumors of follicular cell origin with high grade features (high mitotic rate/tumor necrosis): a clinicopathologic and molecular study. Hum Pathol 2010;41:172-80.

107. Sobrinho-Simões M. Hail to the histologic grading of papillary thyroid carcinoma? Cancer 2000;88:1766-8.

108. McConahey WM, Hay ID, Woolner LB, van Heerden JA, Taylor WF. Papillary thyroid cancer treated at the Mayo Clinic, 1946 through 1970: initial manifestations, pathologic findings, therapy, and outcome. Mayo Clin Proc 1986;61:978-96.

109. Beaumont A, Ben Othman S, Fragu P. The fine structure of papillary carcinoma of the thyroid. Histopathology 1981;5:377-88.

110. Johannessen JV, Sobrinho-Simões M, Finseth I, Pilström L. Papillary carcinomas of the thyroid have pore-deficient nuclei. Int J Cancer 1982;30:409-11.

111. Echeverría OM, Hernández-Pando R, Vázquez-Nin GH. Ultrastructural, cytochemical, and immunocytochemical study of nuclei and cytoskeleton of thyroid papillary carcinoma cells. Ultrastruct Pathol 1998;22:185-97.

112. Permanetter W, Nathrath WB, Löhrs U. Immunohistochemical analysis of thyroglobulin and keratin in benign and malignant thyroid tumours. Virchows Arch A Pathol Anat Histopathol 1982;398:221-8.

113. Stanta G, Carcangiu ML, Rosai J. The biochemical and immunohistochemical profile of thyroid neoplasia. Pathol Annu 1988;23(Pt. 1):129-57.

114. Cheung CC, Ezzat S, Freeman JL, Rosen IB, Asa SL. Immunohistochemical diagnosis of papillary thyroid carcinoma. Mod Pathol 2001;14:338-42.

115. Buley ID, Gatter KC, Heryet A, Mason DY. Expression of intermediate filament proteins in normal and diseased thyroid glands. J Clin Pathol 1987;40:136-42.

116. Henzen-Logmans SC, Mullink H, Ramaekers FC, Tadema T, Meijer CJ. Expression of cytokeratins and vimentin in epithelial cells of normal and pathologic thyroid tissue. Virchows Arch A Pathol Anat Histopathol 1987;410:347-54.

117. Viale G, Dell'Orto P, Coggi G, Gambacorta M. Coexpression of cytokeratins and vimentin in normal and diseased thyroid glands. Lack of diagnostic utility of vimentin immunostaining. Am J Surg Pathol 1989;13:1034-40.

118. Wilson NW, Pambakian H, Richardson TC, Stokoe MR, Makin CA, Heyderman E. Epithelial markers in thyroid carcinoma: an immunoperoxidase study. Histopathology 1986;10:815-29.

119. Bejarano PA, Nikiforov YE, Swenson ES, Biddinger PW. Thyroid transcription factor-1, thyroglobulin, cytokeratin 7, and cytokeratin 20 in thyroid neoplasms. Appl Immunohistochem Mol Morphol 2000;8:189-94.

120. Raphael SJ, Apel RL, Asa SL. Brief report: detection of high-molecular-weight cytokeratins in neoplastic and non-neoplastic thyroid tumors using microwave antigen retrieval. Mod Pathol 1995;8:870-2.

121. Miettinen M, Kovatich AJ, Kärkkäinen P. Keratin subsets in papillary and follicular thyroid lesions. A paraffin section analysis with diagnostic implications. Virchows Arch 1997;431:407-13.

122. Liberman E, Weidner N. Papillary and follicular neoplasms of the thyroid gland. Differential immunohistochemical staining with high-molecular-weight keratin and involucrin. Appl Immunohistochem Mol Morphol 2000;8:42-8.

123. Kragsterman B, Grimelius L, Wallin G, Werga P, Johansson H. Cytokeratin 19 expression in papillary thyroid carcinoma. Appl Immunohistochem Mol Morphol 1999;7:181-5.

124. Schelfhout LJ, Van Muijen GN, Fleuren GJ. Expression of keratin 19 distinguishes papillary thyroid carcinoma from follicular carcinomas and follicular thyroid adenoma. Am J Clin Pathol 1989;92:654-8.

125. Beesley MF, McLaren KM. Cytokeratin 19 and galectin-3 immunohistochemistry in the differential diagnosis of solitary thyroid nodules. Histopathology 2002;41:236-43.

126. Erkiliç S, Koçer NE. The role of cytokeratin 19 in the differential diagnosis of true papillary carcinoma of thyroid and papillary carcinoma-like changes in Graves' disease. Endocr Pathol 2005;16:63-6.

127. Lloyd RV. Distinguishing benign from malignant thyroid lesions: galectin 3 as the latest candidate. Endocr Pathol 2001;12:255-7.

128. Nasr MR, Mukhopadhyay S, Zhang S, Katzenstein AL. Immunohistochemical markers in diagnosis of papillary thyroid carcinoma: utility of HBME1 combined with CK19 immunostaining. Mod Pathol 2006;19:1631-7.

129. Casey MB, Lohse CM, Lloyd RV. Distinction between papillary thyroid hyperplasia and papillary thyroid carcinoma by immunohistochemical staining for cytokeratin 19, galectin-3, and HBME-1. Endocr Pathol 2003;14:55-60.

130. Mehrotra P, Okpokam A, Bouhaidar R, et al. Galectin-3 does not reliably distinguish benign from malignant thyroid neoplasms. Histopathology 2004;45:493-500.

131. Sahoo S, Hoda SA, Rosai J, DeLellis RA. Cytokeratin 19 immunoreactivity in the diagnosis of papillary thyroid carcinoma: a note of caution. Am J Clin Pathol 2001;116:696-702.

132. McLaren KM, Cossar DW. The immunohistochemical localization of S100 in the diagnosis of papillary carcinoma of the thyroid. Hum Pathol 1996;27:633-6.

133. Unger P, Ewart M, Wang BY, Gan L, Kohtz DS, Burstein DE. Expression of p63 in papillary thyroid carcinoma and in Hashimoto's thyroiditis: a pathobiologic link? Hum Pathol 2003;34:764-9.

134. Yamamoto Y, Izumi K, Otsuka H. An immunohistochemical study of epithelial membrane antigen, cytokeratin, and vimentin in papillary thyroid carcinoma. Recognition of lethal and favorable prognostic types. Cancer 1992;70:2326-33.

135. Keen CE, Szakacs S, Okon E, Rubin JS, Bryant BM. CA125 and thyroglobulin staining in papillary carcinomas of thyroid and ovarian origin is not completely specific for site of origin. Histopathology 1999;34:113-7.

136. Miettinen M, Kärkkäinen P. Differential reactivity of HBME-1 and CD15 antibodies in benign and malignant thyroid tumours. Preferential reactivity with malignant tumours. Virchows Arch 1996;429:213-9.

137. Jennings TA, Boguniewicz AB, Sheehan CE, Figge J. Involucrin selectively stains papillary thyroid carcinoma. Appl Immunohistochem 1998;6:55-61.

138. Poblete MT, Nualart F, del Pozo M, Perez JA, Figueroa CD. Alpha 1-antitrypsin expression in human thyroid papillary carcinoma. Am J Surg Pathol 1996;20:956-63.

139. Lai ML, Rizzo N, Liguori C, Zucca G, Faa G. Alpha-1-antichymotrypsin immunoreactivity in papillary carcinoma of the thyroid gland. Histopathology 1998;33:332-6.

140. Rocha AS, Risberg B, Magalhães J, et al. The p75 neurotrophin receptor is widely expressed in conventional papillary thyroid carcinoma. Hum Pathol 2006;37:562-8.

141. Inoue H, Oshimo K, Miki H, Kawano M, Monden Y. Immunohistochemical study of estrogen receptors and the responsiveness to estrogen in papillary thyroid carcinoma. Cancer 1993;72:1364-8.

142. Tanda F, Cossu A, Bosincu L, Manca A, Ibba M, Massarelli G. Intercellular adhesion molecule-1 (ICAM-1) immunoreactivity in well-differentiated thyroid papillary carcinomas. Mod Pathol 1996;9:53-6.

143. Katoh R, Iida Y, Suzuki K, Kawaoi A, Muramatsu A. Immunohistochemical and immunoelectron microscopical localization of procollagen III peptide in papillary carcinoma of thyroid. Endocr Pathol 1992;3:129-33.

144. Maiorano E, Ciampolillo A, Viale G, et al. Insulin-like growth factor 1 expression in thyroid tumors. Appl Immunohistochem Mol Morphol 2000;8:110-9.

145. Resnick MB, Schacter P, Finkelstein Y, Kellner Y, Cohen O. Immunohistochemical analysis of p27/kip1 expression in thyroid carcinoma. Mod Pathol 1998;11:735-9.

146. Erickson LA, Yousef OM, Jin L, Lohse CM, Pankratz VS, Lloyd RV. p27kip1 expression distinguishes papillary hyperplasia in Graves' disease from papillary thyroid carcinoma. Mod Pathol 2000;13:1014-9.

147. El Demellawy D, Nasr AL, Babay S, Alowami S. Diagnostic utility of CD56 immunohistochemistry in papillary carcinoma of the thyroid. Pathol Res Pract 2009;205:303-9.

148. El Demellawy D, Nasr A, Alowami S. Application of CD56, P63 and CK19 immunohistochemistry in the diagnosis of papillary carcinoma of the thyroid. Diagn Pathol 2008;3:5.

149. Chan JK, Tse CC. Mucin production in metastatic papillary carcinoma of the thyroid. Hum Pathol 1988;19:195-200.

150. Alves P, Soares P, Fonseca E, Sobrinho-Simões M. Papillary thyroid carcinoma overexpresses fully and underglycosylated mucins together with native and sialylated simple mucin antigens and histo-blood group antigens. Endocr Pathol 1999;10:315-24.

151. Damiani S, Fratamico F, Lapertosa G, Dina R, Eusebi V. Alcian blue and epithelial membrane antigen are useful markers in differentiating benign from malignant papillae in thyroid lesions. Virchows Arch A Pathol Anat Histopathol 1991;419:131-5.

152. Kuhn E, Teller L, Piana S, Rosai J, Merino MJ. Different clonal origin of bilateral papillary thyroid carcinoma, with a review of the literature. Endocr Pathol 2012;23:101-7.

153. Bansal M, Gandhi M, Ferris RL, et al. Molecular and histopathologic characteristics of multifocal papillary thyroid carcinoma. Am J Surg Pathol 2013;37:1586-91.

154. Russell WO, Ibanez ML, Clark RL, White EC. Thyroid carcinoma. Classification, intraglandular dissemination and clinicopathological study based upon whole organ sections of 80 glands. Cancer 1963;16:1425-60.

155. Katoh R, Sasaki J, Kurihara H, Suzuki K, Iida Y, Kawaoi A. Multiple thyroid involvement (intraglandular metastasis) in papillary thyroid carcinoma. A clinicopathologic study of 105 consecutive patients. Cancer 1992;70:1585-90.

156. Cady B, Sedgwick CE, Meissner WA, Wool MS, Salzman FA, Werber J. Risk factor analysis in differentiated thyroid cancer. Cancer 1979;43:810-20.

157. Cody HS 3rd, Shah JP. Locally invasive, well-differentiated thyroid cancer. 22 years' experience at Memorial Sloan-Kettering Cancer Center. Am J Surg 1981;142:480-3.

158. Tang W, Kakudo K, Nakamura MD Y, et al. Parathyroid gland involvement by papillary carcinoma of the thyroid gland. Arch Pathol Lab Med 2002;126:1511-4.

159. Hale RJ, Merchant W, Hasleton PS. Polypoidal intra-oesophageal thyroid carcinoma: a rare cause of dysphagia. Histopathology 1990;17:475-6.

160. Tsumori T, Nakao K, Miyata M, et al. Clinicopathologic study of thyroid carcinoma infiltrating the trachea. Cancer 1985;56:2843-8.

161. Shin DH, Mark EJ, Suen HC, Grillo HC. Pathologic staging of papillary carcinoma of the thyroid with airway invasion based on the anatomic manner of extension to the trachea: a clinicopathologic study based on 22 patients who underwent thyroidectomy and airway resection. Hum Pathol 1993;24:866-70.

162. Grebe SK, Hay ID. Thyroid cancer nodal metastases: biologic significance and therapeutic considerations. Surg Oncol Clin N Am 1996;5:43-63.

163. Frazell EL, Foote FW Jr. Papillary thyroid carcinoma: pathological findings in cases with and without clinical evidence of cervical node involvement. Cancer 1955;8:1165-6.

164. Chung YJ, Lee JS, Park SY, et al. Histomorphological factors in the risk prediction of lymph node metastasis in papillary thyroid carcinoma. Histopathology 2013;62:578-88.

165. Jung YY, Lee CH, Park SY, et al. Characteristic tumor growth patterns as novel histomorphologic predictors for lymph node metastasis in papillary thyroid carcinoma. Hum Pathol 2013;44:2620-7.

166. Noguchi M, Kumaki T, Taniya T, Miyazaki I. Bilateral cervical lymph node metastases in well-differentiated thyroid cancer. Arch Surg 1990;125:804-6.

167. Fukui Y, Yamakawa T, Taniki T, Numoto S, Miki H, Monden Y. Sentinel lymph node biopsy in patients with papillary thyroid carcinoma. Cancer 2001;92:2868-74.

168. Wallace MP, Betsill WL. Papillary carcinoma of the thyroid gland seen as lateral neck cyst. Arch Otolaryngol 1984;110:408-11.

169. al-Talib RK, Wilkins BS, Theaker JM. Cystic metastasis of papillary carcinoma of the thyroid—an unusual presentation. Histopathology 1992;20:176-8.

170. Estevez S, Bosisio FM. Dilated high endothelial venules in lymph nodes simulating metastatic thyroid carcinoma. Int J Surg Pathol 2013;21:142-3.

171. Harness JK, Thompson NW, Sisson JC, Beierwaltes WH. Proceedings: differentiated thyroid carcinomas. Treatment of distant metastases. Arch Surg 1974;108:410-9.

172. Hoie J, Stenwig AE, Kullmann G, Lindegaard M. Distant metastases in papillary thyroid cancer. A review of 91 patients. Cancer 1988;61:1-6.

173. Schlumberger M, Tubiana M, De Vathaire F, et al. Long-term results of treatment of 283 patients with lung and bone metastases from differentiated thyroid carcinoma. J Clin Endocrinol Metab 1986;63:960-7.

174. Samaan NA, Schultz PN, Haynie TP, Ordonez NG. Pulmonary metastasis of differentiated thyroid carcinoma: treatment results in 101 patients. J Clin Endocrinol Metab 1985;60:376-80.

175. Gamboa-Dominguez A, Tenorio-Villalvazo A. Metastatic follicular variant of papillary thyroid carcinoma manifested as a primary renal neoplasm. Endocr Pathol 1999;10:256-268.

176. Pucci A, Suppo M, Lucchesi G, et al. Papillary thyroid carcinoma presenting as a solitary soft tissue arm metastasis in an elderly hyperthyroid patient. Case report and review of the literature. Virchows Arch 2006;448:857-61.

177. Alcaraz I, Cerroni L, Rutten A, Kutzner H, Requena L. Cutaneous metastases from internal malignancies: a clinicopathologic and immunohistochemical review. Am J Dermatopathol 2012;34:347-93.

178. Tahmasebi FC, Farmer P, Powell SZ, et al. Brain metastases from papillary thyroid carcinomas. Virchows Arch 2013;462:473-8.

179. Hamming JF, van de Velde CJ, Goslings BM, et al. Preoperative diagnosis and treatment of metastases to the regional lymph nodes in papillary carcinoma of the thyroid gland. Surg Gynecol Obstet 1989;169:107-14.

180. Hutter RV, Frazell EL, Foote FW Jr. Elective radical neck dissection: an assessment of its use in the management of papillary thyroid cancer. CA Cancer J Clin 1970;20:87-93.

181. Noguchi S, Murakami N. The value of lymph-node dissection in patients with differentiated thyroid cancer. Surg Clin North Am 1987;67:251-61.

182. Clark OH. Total thyroidectomy: the treatment of choice for patients with differentiated thyroid cancer. Ann Surg 1982;196:361-70.

183. Harness JK, Thompson NW, McLeod MK, Eckhauser FE, Lloyd RV. Follicular carcinoma of the thyroid gland: trends and treatment. Surgery 1984;96:972-80.

184. Maheshwari YK, Hill CS Jr, Haynie TP 3rd, Hickey RC, Samaan NA. I-131 therapy in differentiated thyroid carcinoma: M.D. Anderson Hospital experience. Cancer 1981;47:664-71.

185. Cohn KH, Bäckdahl M, Forsslund G, et al. Biologic considerations and operative strategy in papillary thyroid carcinoma: arguments against the routine performance of total thyroidectomy. Surgery 1984;96:957-71.

186. Crile G Jr, Antunez AR, Esselstyn CB Jr, Hawk WA, Skillern PG. The advantages of subtotal thyroidectomy and suppression of TSH in the primary treatment of papillary carcinoma of the thyroid. Cancer 1985;55:2691-7.

187. Schroder DM, Chambors A, France CJ. Operative strategy for thyroid cancer. Is total thyroidectomy worth the price? Cancer 1986;58:2320-8.

188. Starnes HF, Brooks DC, Pinkus GS, Brooks JR. Surgery for thyroid carcinoma. Cancer 1985;55:1376-81.

189. Vickery AL Jr, Wang CA, Walker AM. Treatment of intrathyroidal papillary carcinoma of the thyroid. Cancer 1987;60:2587-95.

190. Cady B. Papillary carcinoma of the thyroid. Semin Surg Oncol 1991;7:81-6.

191. Zimmerman D, Hay ID, Gough IR, et al. Papillary thyroid carcinoma in children and adults: long-term follow-up of 1039 patients conservatively treated at one institution during three decades. Surgery 1988;104:1157-66.

192. Sisson JC, Giordano TJ, Jamadar DA, et al. 131-I treatment of micronodular pulmonary metastases from papillary thyroid carcinoma. Cancer 1996;78:2184-92.

193. Samaan NA, Schultz PN, Ordonez NG, Hickey RC, Johnston DA. A comparison of thyroid carcinoma in those who have and have not had head and neck irradiation in childhood. J Clin Endocrinol Metab 1987;64:219-23.

194. Hay ID, Bergstralh EJ, Goellner JR, Ebersold JR, Grant CS. Predicting outcome in papillary thyroid carcinoma: development of a reliable prognostic scoring system in a cohort of 1779 patients surgically treated at one institution during 1940 through 1989. Surgery 1993;114:1050-7.

195. Crile G Jr, Hazard JB. Relationship of the age of the patient to the natural history and prognosis of carcinoma of the thyroid. Ann Surg 1953;138:33-8.

196. Lindsay S. Carcinoma of the thyroid gland. A clinical and pathologic study of 293 patients at the University of California Hospital. Springfield, IL: Charles C. Thomas; 1960.

197. Schindler AM, van Melle G, Evequoz B, Scazziga B. Prognostic factors in papillary carcinoma of the thyroid. Cancer 1991;68:324-30.

198. Collini P, Mattavelli F, Pellegrinelli A, Barisella M, Ferrari A, Massimino M. Papillary carcinoma of the thyroid gland of childhood and adolescence: morphologic subtypes, biologic behavior and prognosis: a clinicopathologic study of 42 sporadic cases treated at a single institution during a 30-year period. Am J Surg Pathol 2006;30:1420-6.

199. Simpson WJ, McKinney SE, Carruthers JS, Gospodarowicz MK, Sutcliffe SB, Panzarella T. Papillary and follicular thyroid cancer. Prognostic factors in 1,578 patients. Am J Med 1987;83:479-88.

200. Huang BY, Hseuh C, Chao TC, Lin KJ, Lin JD. Well-differentiated thyroid carcinoma with concomitant Hashimoto's thyroiditis present with less aggressive clinical stage and low recurrence. Endocr Pathol 2011;22:144-9.

201. Matsubayashi S, Kawai K, Matsumoto Y, et al. The correlation between papillary thyroid carcinoma and lymphocytic infiltration in the thyroid gland. J Clin Endocrinol Metab 1995;80:3421-4.

202. Hofstädter F, Unterkircher S. [Histologic criteria for the prognosis of malignant struma.] Pathologe 1980;1:79-85. [German]

203. Mai KT, Perkins DG, Yazdi HM, Commons AS, Thomas J, Meban S. Infiltrating papillary thyroid carcinoma: review of 134 cases of papillary carcinoma. Arch Pathol Lab Med 1998;122:166-71.

204. Yamashita H, Noguchi S, Murakami N, et al. Extracapsular invasion of lymph node metastasis. A good indicator of disease recurrence and poor prognosis in patients with thyroid microcarcinoma. Cancer 1999;86:842-9.

205. McCormack KR. Bone metastases from thyroid carcinoma. Cancer 1966;19:181-4.

206. Smith SA, Hay ID, Goellner JR, Ryan JJ, McConahey WM. Mortality from papillary thyroid carcinoma. A case-control study of 56 lethal cases. Cancer 1988;62:1381-8.

207. Lang BH, Lo CY, Chan WF, Lam KY, Wan KY. Staging systems for papillary thyroid carcinoma: a review and comparison. Ann Surg 2007;245:366-78.

208. Bai Y, Zhou G, Nakamura M, et al. Survival impact of psammoma body, stromal calcification, and bone formation in papillary thyroid carcinoma. Mod Pathol 2009;22:887-94.

209. Vickery AL Jr. Thyroid papillary carcinoma. Pathological and philosophical controversies. Am J Surg Pathol 1983;7:797-807.

210. LiVolsi VA, Baloch ZW. Determining the diagnosis and prognosis of thyroid neoplasms: do special studies help? Hum Pathol 1999;30:885-6.

211. DeLellis RA, Lloyd RV, Heitz PU, Eng C. Pathology and genetics of tumours of endocrine organs, Lyon: IARC Press; 2004:64.

212. Hazard JB. Small papillary carcinoma of the thyroid. A study with special reference to so-called nonencapsulated sclerosing tumor. Lab Invest 1960;9:86-97.

213. Klinck GH, Winship T. Occult sclerosing carcinoma of the thyroid. Cancer 1955;8:701-6.

214. Hubert JP Jr, Keirnan PD, Beahrs OH, McConahey WM, Woolner LB. Occult papillary carcinoma of the thyroid. Arch Surg 1980;115:394-8.

215. Bondeson L, Ljungberg O. Occult papillary thyroid carcinoma in the young and the aged. Cancer 1984;53:1790-2.

216. Pacini F. Thyroid microcarcinoma. Best Pract Res Clin Endocrinol Metab 2012;26:421-9

217. Lang W, Borrusch H, Bauer L. Occult carcinomas of the thyroid. Evaluation of 1,020 sequential autopsies. Am J Clin Pathol 1988;90:72-6.

218. Sampson RJ, Oka H, Key CR, Buncher CR, Iijima S. Metastases from occult thyroid carcinoma. An autopsy study from Hiroshima and Nagasaki, Japan. Cancer 1970;25:803-11.

219. Yamamoto Y, Maeda T, Izumi K, Otsuka H. Occult papillary carcinoma of the thyroid. A study of 408 autopsy cases. Cancer 1990;65:1173-9.

220. Yamashita H, Nakayama I, Noguchi S, et al. Minute carcinoma of the thyroid and its development to advanced carcinoma. Acta Pathol Jpn 1985;35:377-83.

221. Fink A, Tomlinson G, Freeman JL, Rosen IB, Asa SL. Occult micropapillary carcinoma associated with benign follicular thyroid disease and unrelated thyroid neoplasms. Mod Pathol 1996;9:816-20.

222. Soares P, Celestino R, Gaspar da Rocha A, Sobrinho-Simões M. Papillary thyroid microcarcinoma: how to diagnose it and how to manage this epidemics? Int J Surg Pathol 2014;22:113-9.

223. Harach HR, Franssila KO, Wasenius VM. Occult papillary carcinoma of the thyroid. A "normal" finding in Finland. A systematic autopsy study. Cancer 1985;56:531-8.

224. Poli F, Trezzi R, Rosai J. Images in pathology. Single thyroid follicle involved by papillary carcinoma: partially classic and partially oncocytic. Int J Surg Pathol 2009;17:272-3.

225. Böcker W, Schröder S, Dralle H. Minimal thyroid neoplasia. Recent Results Cancer Res 1988;106:131-8.

226. Gikas PW, Labow SS, DiGiulio W, Finger JE. Occult metastasis from occult papillary carcinoma of the thyroid. Cancer 1967;20:2100-4.

227. Rosai J, Zampi G, Carcangiu ML. Papillary carcinoma of the thyroid. A discussion of its several morphologic expressions, with particular emphasis on the follicular variant. Am J Surg Pathol 1983;7:809-17.

228. Allo MD, Christianson W, Koivunen D. Not all "occult" papillary carcinomas are "minimal." Surgery 1988;104:971-6.

229. Patchefsky AS, Keller IB, Mansfield CM. Solitary vertebral column metastasis from occult sclerosing carcinoma of the thyroid gland: report of a case. Am J Clin Pathol 1970;53:596-601.

230. Strate SM, Lee EL, Childers JH. Occult papillary carcinoma of the thyroid with distant metastases. Cancer 1984;54:1093-100.

231. Piana S, Ragazzi M, Tallini G, et al. Papillary thyroid microcarcinoma with fatal outcome: evidence of tumor progression in lymph node metastases: report of 3 cases, with morphological and molecular analysis. Hum Pathol 2013;44:556-65.

232. Londero SC, Krogdahl A, Bastholt L, et al. Papillary thyroid microcarcinoma in Denmark 1996-2008: a national study of epidemiology and clinical significance. Thyroid 2013;23:1159-64.

233. Bernstein J, Virk RK, Hui P, et al. Tall cell variant of papillary thyroid microcarcinoma: clinicopathologic features with BRAF(V600E) mutational analysis. Thyroid 2013;23:1525-31.

234. Min HS, Choe G, Kim SW, et al. S100A4 expression is associated with lymph node metastasis in papillary microcarcinoma of the thyroid. Mod Pathol 2008;21:748-55.

235. Chow SM, Law SC, Chan JK, Au SK, Yau S, Lau WH. Papillary microcarcinoma of the thyroid-prognostic significance of lymph node metastasis and multifocality. Cancer 2003;98:31-40.

236. Hay ID, Grant CS, van Heerden JA, Goellner JR, Ebersold JR, Bergstralh EJ. Papillary thyroid microcarcinoma: a study of 535 cases observed in a 50-year period. Surgery 1992;112:1139-46.

237. Rosai J, LiVolsi VA, Sobrinho-Simões M, Williams ED. Renaming papillary microcarcinoma of the thyroid gland: the Porto proposal. Int J Surg Pathol 2003;11:249-51.

238. Rosario PW. Papillary microtumor or papillary microcarcinoma of the thyroid? A prospective analysis of the Porto Proposal. Int J Surg Pathol 2013;21:639-40.

239. Hawk WA, Hazard JB. The many appearances of papillary carcinoma of the thyroid. Comparison with the common form of papillary carcinoma by DNA and morphometric analysis. Cleve Clin Q 1976;43:207-15.

240. Schröder S, Böcker W, Dralle H, Kortman KB, Stern C. The encapsulated papillary carcinoma of the thyroid. A morphologic subtype of the papillary thyroid carcinoma. Cancer 1984;54:90-3.

241. Meissner WA, Warren S. Tumors of the thyroid gland. Atlas of Tumor Pathology, 2nd Series, Fascicle 4. Washington, DC: Armed Forces Institute of Pathology; 1969:50-2.

242. Evans HL. Encapsulated papillary neoplasms of the thyroid. A study of 14 cases followed for a minimum of 10 years. Am J Surg Pathol 1987;11:592-7.

243. Oyama T, Ishida T, Ishii K, et al. Encapsulated papillary carcinoma of the thyroid gland: clinicopathological and cytofluorometric study in comparison with non-encapsulated papillary carcinoma. Acta Pathol Jpn 1993;43:516-21.

244. Chan JK, Tsang WY. Endocrine malignancies that may mimic benign lesions. Semin Diagn Pathol 1995;12:45-63.

245. Eloy C, Santos J, Soares P, Sobrinho-Simões M. Intratumoural lymph vessel density is related to presence of lymph node metastases and separates encapsulated from infiltrative papillary thyroid carcinoma. Virchows Arch 2011;459:595-605.

246. Chen KT, Rosai J. Follicular variant of thyroid papillary carcinoma: a clinicopathologic study of six cases. Am J Surg Pathol 1977;1:123-30.

247. Gupta S, Ajise O, Dultz L, et al. Follicular variant of papillary thyroid cancer: encapsulated, nonencapsulated, and diffuse: distinct biologic and clinical entities. Arch Otolaryngol Head Neck Surg. 2012;138:227-33.

248. Mazzaferri EL, Oertel JE. The pathology and prognosis of thyroid cancer. In: Kaplan EL, ed. Surgery of the thyroid and parathyroid glands, Vol. 6, Clinical surgery international. Edinburgh: Churchill Livingstone; 1983:22-3.

249. Vickery AL Jr, Carcangiu ML, Johannessen JV, Sobrinho-Simões M. Papillary carcinoma. Semin Diagn Pathol 1985;2:90-100.

250. Bell CD, Coire C, Treger T, Volpe R, Baumal R, Fornasier VL. The 'dark nucleus' and disruptions of follicular architecture: possible new histological aids for the diagnosis of the follicular variant of papillary carcinoma of the thyroid. Histopathology 2001;39:33-42.

251. Giorgadze TA, Baloch ZW, Pasha T, Zhang PJ, Livolsi VA. Lymphatic and blood vessel density in the follicular patterned lesions of thyroid. Mod Pathol 2005;18:1424-31.

252. Albores-Saavedra J, Gould E, Vardaman C, Vuitch F. The macrofollicular variant of papillary thyroid carcinoma: a study of 17 cases. Hum Pathol 1991;22:1195-205.

253. Lugli A, Terracciano LM, Oberholzer M, Bubendorf L, Tornillo L. Macrofollicular variant of papillary carcinoma of the thyroid: a histologic, cytologic, and immunohistochemical study of 3 cases and review of the literature. Arch Pathol Lab Med 2004;128:54-8.

254. Nakamura T, Moriyama S, Nariya S, Sano K, Shirota H, Kato R. Macrofollicular variant of papillary thyroid carcinoma. Pathol Int 1998;48:467-70.

255. Vanzati A, Mercalli F, Rosai J. The "sprinkling" sign in the follicular variant of papillary thyroid carcinoma: a clue to the recognition of this entity. Arch Pathol Lab Med 2013;137:1707-9.

256. Sobrinho-Simões M, Soares J, Carneiro F, Limbert E. Diffuse follicular variant of papillary carcinoma of the thyroid: report of eight cases of a distinct aggressive type of thyroid tumor. Surg Pathol 1990;3:189-203.

257. Mizukami Y, Nonomura A, Michigishi T, Ohmura K, Noguchi M, Ishizaki T. Diffuse follicular variant of papillary carcinoma of the thyroid. Histopathology 1995;27:575-7.

258. Ivanova R, Soares P, Castro P, Sobrinho-Simões M. Diffuse (or multinodular) follicular variant of papillary thyroid carcinoma: a clinicopathologic and immunohistochemical analysis of ten cases of an aggressive form of differentiated thyroid carcinoma. Virchows Arch 2002;440:418-24.

259. Evans HL Follicular neoplasms of the thyroid. A study of 44 cases followed for a minimum of 10 years, with emphasis on differential diagnosis. Cancer 1984;54:533-40.

260. Zidan J, Karen D, Stein M, Rosenblatt E, Basher W, Kuten A. Pure versus follicular variant of papillary thyroid carcinoma: clinical features, prognostic factors, treatment, and survival. Cancer 2003;97:1181-5.

261. Miettinen M, Franssila K, Lehto VP, Paasivuo R, Virtanen I. Expression of intermediate filament proteins in thyroid gland and thyroid tumors. Lab Invest 1984;50:262-70.

262. Yagi Y, Yagi S, Saku T. The localization of cytoskeletal proteins and thyroglobulin in thyroid microcarcinoma in comparison with clinically manifested thyroid carcinoma. Cancer 1985;56:1967-71.

263. Baloch ZW, Abraham S, Roberts S, LiVolsi VA. Differential expression of cytokeratins in follicular variant of papillary carcinoma: an immunohistochemical study and its diagnostic utility. Hum Pathol 1999;30:1166-71.

264. Vivero M, Kraft S, Barletta JA. Risk stratification of follicular variant of papillary thyroid carcinoma. Thyroid 2013;23:273-9.

265. Rosai J. The encapsulated follicular variant of papillary thyroid carcinoma: back to the drawing board. Endocr Pathol 2010;21:7-11.

266. Khan A, Baker SP, Patwardhan NA, Pullman JM. CD57 (Leu-7) expression is helpful in diagnosis of the follicular variant of papillary thyroid carcinoma. Virchows Arch 1998;432:427-32.

267. Baloch ZW, LiVolsi VA. Encapsulated follicular variant of papillary thyroid carcinoma with bone metastases. Mod Pathol 2000;13:861-5.

268. Williams ED. Two proposals regarding the terminology of thyroid tumors (Guest Editorial). Int J Surg Pathol 2000;8:181-3.

269. Elsheikh TM, Asa SL, Chan JK, et al. Interobserver and intraobserver variation among experts in the diagnosis of thyroid follicular lesions with borderline nuclear features of papillary carcinoma. Am J Clin Pathol 2008;130:736-44.

270. Hirokawa M, Carney JA, Goellner JR, et al. Observer variation of encapsulated follicular lesions of the thyroid gland. Am J Surg Pathol 2002;26:1508-14.

271. Lloyd RV, Erickson LA, Casey MB, et al. Observer variation in the diagnosis of follicular variant of papillary thyroid carcinoma. Am J Surg Pathol 2004;28:1336-40.

272. Wallander M, Layfield LJ, Jarboe E, et al. Follicular variant of papillary carcinoma: reproducibility of histologic diagnosis and utility of HBME-1 immunohistochemistry and BRAF mutational analysis as diagnostic adjuncts. Appl Immunohistochem Mol Morphol 2010;18:231-5.

273. Widder S, Guggisberg K, Khalil M, Pasieka JL. A pathologic re-review of follicular thyroid neoplasms: the impact of changing the threshold for the diagnosis of the follicular variant of papillary thyroid carcinoma. Surgery 2008;144:80-5.

274. Min HS, Choe G, Kang GH, Park SH, Park SY. Immunohistochemical and molecular characteristics of follicular patterned thyroid nodules with incomplete papillary thyroid carcinoma-like nuclei. Lab Invest 2009;89:118A (Abstract).

275. Papotti M, Rodriguez J, De Pompa R, Bartolazzi A, Rosai J. Galectin-3 and HBME-1 expression in well-differentiated thyroid tumors with follicular architecture of uncertain malignant potential. Mod Pathol 2005;18:541-6.

276. Fusco A, Chiappetta G, Hui P, et al. Assessment of RET/PTC oncogene activation and clonality in thyroid nodules with incomplete morphological evidence of papillary carcinoma: a search for the early precursors of papillary cancer. Am J Pathol 2002;160:2157-67.

277. Hofman V, Lassalle S, Bonnetaud C, et al. Thyroid tumours of uncertain malignant potential: frequency and diagnostic reproducibility. Virchows Arch 2009;455:21-33.

278. Chan JK. Strict criteria should be applied in the diagnosis of encapsulated follicular variant of papillary thyroid carcinoma. Am J Clin Pathol 2002;117:16-8.

279. Renshaw AA, Gould EW. Why there is the tendency to "overdiagnose" the follicular variant of papillary thyroid carcinoma. Am J Clin Pathol 2002;117:19-21.

280. Chui MH, Cassol CA, Asa SL, Mete O. Follicular epithelial dysplasia of the thyroid: morphological and immunohistochemical characterization of a putative preneoplastic lesion to papillary thyroid carcinoma in chronic lymphocytic thyroiditis. Virchows Arch 2013;462:557-63.

281. Hunt JL, Dacic S, Barnes EL, Bures JC. Encapsulated follicular variant of papillary thyroid carcinoma. Am J Clin Pathol 2002;118:602-3.

282. LiVolsi VA, Baloch ZW. Follicular-patterned tumors of the thyroid: the battle of benign vs. malignant vs. so-called uncertain. Endocr Pathol 2011;22:184-9.

283. Chui MH, Cassol CA, Asa SL, Mete O. Follicular epithelial dysplasia of the thyroid: morphological and immunohistochemical characterization of a putative preneoplastic lesion to papillary thyroid carcinoma in chronic lymphocytic thyroiditis. Virchows Arch 2013;462:557-63.

284. Esserman LJ, Thompson IM, Reid B, et al. Addressing overdiagnosis and overtreatment in cancer: a prescription for change. Lancet Oncol 2014;15:e234-42.

285. Nikiforov YE, Erickson LA, Nikiforova MN, Caudill CM, Lloyd RV. Solid variant of papillary thyroid carcinoma: incidence, clinical-pathologic characteristics, molecular analysis, and biologic behavior. Am J Surg Pathol 2001;25:1478-84.

286. Thompson LD, Wieneke JA, Heffess CS. Diffuse sclerosing variant of papillary thyroid carcinoma: a clinicopathologic and immunophenotypic analysis of 22 cases. Endocr Pathol 2005;16:331-48.

287. Gómez-Morales M, Alvaro T, Muñoz M, et al. Diffuse sclerosing papillary carcinoma of the thyroid gland: immunohistochemical analysis of the local host immune response. Histopathology 1991;18:427-33.

288. Schröder S, Bay V, Dumke K, et al. Diffuse sclerosing variant of papillary thyroid carcinoma. S-100 protein immunocytochemistry and prognosis. Virchows Arch A Pathol Anat Histopathol 1990;416:367-71.

289. Gómez-Morales M, Alvaro T, Muñoz M, et al. Diffuse sclerosing papillary carcinoma of the thyroid gland: immunohistochemical analysis of the local host immune response. Histopathology 1991;18:427-33.

290. Imamura Y, Kasahara Y, Fukuda M. Multiple brain metastases from a diffuse sclerosing variant of papillary carcinoma of the thyroid. Endocr Pathol 2000;11:97-108.

291. Carcangiu ML, Bianchi S. Diffuse sclerosing variant of papillary thyroid carcinoma. Clinicopathologic study of 15 cases. Am J Surg Pathol 1989;13:1041-9.

292. Chan JK, Tsui MS, Tse CH. Diffuse sclerosing variant of papillary carcinoma of the thyroid: a histological and immunohistochemical study of three cases. Histopathology 1987;11:191-201.

293. Fujimoto Y, Obara T, Ito Y, Kodama T, Aiba M, Yamaguchi K. Diffuse sclerosing variant of papillary carcinoma of the thyroid. Cancer 1990;66:2306-12.

294. Mizukami Y, Nonomura A, Michigishi T, et al. Diffuse sclerosing variant of papillary carcinoma of the thyroid. Report of three cases. Acta Pathol Jpn 1990;40:676-82.

295. Soares J, Limbert E, Sobrinho-Simões M. Diffuse sclerosing variant of papillary thyroid carcinoma. A clinicopathologic study of 10 cases. Pathol Res Pract 1989;185:200-6.

296. Berho M, Suster S. The oncocytic variant of papillary carcinoma of the thyroid: a clinicopathologic study of 15 cases. Hum Pathol 1997;28:47-53.

297. Herrera MF, Hay ID, Wu PS, et al. Hürthle cell (oxyphilic) papillary thyroid carcinoma: a variant with more aggressive biologic behavior. World J Surg 1992;16:669-74.

298. Beckner ME, Heffess CS, Oertel JE. Oxyphilic papillary thyroid carcinomas. Am J Clin Pathol 1995;103:280-7.

299. D'Antonio A, De Chiara A, Santoro M, Chiappetta G, Losito NS. Warthin-like tumour of the thyroid gland: RET/PTC expression indicates it is a variant of papillary carcinoma. Histopathology 2000;36:493-8.

300. Baloch ZW, LiVolsi VA. Warthin-like papillary carcinoma of the thyroid. Arch Pathol Lab Med 2000;124:1192-5.

301. Apel RL, Asa SL, LiVolsi VA. Papillary Hürthle cell carcinoma with lymphocytic stroma. "Warthin-like tumor" of the thyroid. Am J Surg Pathol 1995;19:810-4.

302. Ludvíková M, Ryska A, Korabecná M, Rydlová M, Michal M. Oncocytic papillary carcinoma with lymphoid stroma (Warthin-like tumour) of the thyroid: a distinct entity with favorable prognosis. Histopathology 2001;39:17-24.

303. Collini P, Massimino M, Mattavelli F, Barisella M, Pellegrinelli A, Rosai J. Papillary thyroid carcinoma, tall cell variant, in children: report of three cases retrieved at a single institution during a 30-year experience and with a long follow-up. Int J Surg Pathol 2014 [In Press].

304. Ostrowski ML, Merino MJ. Tall cell variant of papillary thyroid carcinoma: a reassessment and immunohistochemical study with comparison to the usual type of papillary carcinoma of the thyroid. Am J Surg Pathol 1996;20:964-74.

305. Tscholl-Ducommun J, Hedinger CE. Papillary thyroid carcinomas. Morphology and prognosis. Virchows Arch A Pathol Anat Histol 1982;396:19-39.

306. Ito Y, Hirokawa M, Fukushima M, et al. Prevalence and prognostic significance of poor differentiation and tall cell variant in papillary carcinoma in Japan. World J Surg 2008;32:1535-43.

307. Johnson TL, Lloyd RV, Thompson NW, Beierwaltes WH, Sisson JC. Prognostic implications of the tall cell variant of papillary thyroid carcinoma. Am J Surg Pathol 1988;12:22-7.

308. Michels JJ, Jacques M, Henry-Amar M, Bardet S. Prevalence and prognostic significance of tall cell variant of papillary thyroid carcinoma. Hum Pathol 2007;38:212-9.

309. Ganly I, Ibrahimpasic T, Rivera M, et al. Prognostic implications of papillary thyroid carcinoma with tall cell features. Lab Invest 2012; 92:144A (Abstract).

310. Collini P, Massimino M, Mattavelli F, Barisella M, Pellegrinelli A, Rosai J. Tall cell variant of papillary thyroid carcinoma in children. Report of three cases with long-term follow-up from a single institution. Int J Surg Pathol 2014. [In press]

311. Dettmer MS, Schmitt A, Steiner H, Moch H, Komminoth P, Perren A. Tall cell variant of papillary thyroid carcinoma—How many tall cells are needed? Lab Invest 2012;92:143A (Abstract).

312. Chen JH, Faquin WC, Lloyd RV, Nosé V. Clinicopathological and molecular characterization of nine cases of columnar cell variant of papillary thyroid carcinoma. Mod Pathol 2011;24:739-49.

313. LiVolsi VA. Papillary carcinoma tall cell variant (TCV): a review. Endocr Pathol 2010;21:12-5.

314. Wenig BM, Thompson LD, Adair CF, Shmookler B, Heffess CS. Thyroid papillary carcinoma of columnar cell type: a clinicopathologic study of 16 cases. Cancer 1998;82:740-53.

315. Evans HL. Columnar-cell carcinoma of the thyroid. A report of two cases of an aggressive variant of thyroid carcinoma. Am J Clin Pathol 1986;85:77-80.

316. Sobrinho-Simões M, Nesland JM, Johannessen JV. Columnar-cell carcinoma. Another variant of poorly differentiated carcinoma of the thyroid. Am J Clin Pathol 1988;89:264-7.

317. Enriquez ML, Baloch ZW, Montone KT, Zhang PJ, LiVolsi VA. CDX2 expression in columnar cell variant of papillary thyroid carcinoma. Am J Clin Pathol 2012;137:722-6.

318. LiVolsi VA. Surgical pathology of the thyroid. In: Major problems in pathology; Vol 22 [series]. Philadelphia: WB Saunders; 1990.

319. Gaertner EM, Davidson M, Wenig BM. The columnar cell variant of thyroid papillary carcinoma. Case report and discussion of an unusually aggressive thyroid papillary carcinoma. Am J Surg Pathol 1995;19:940-7.

320. Evans HL. Encapsulated columnar-cell neoplasms of the thyroid. A report of four cases suggesting a favorable prognosis. Am J Surg Pathol 1996;20:1205-11.

321. Akslen LA, Varhaug JE. Thyroid carcinoma with mixed tall-cell and columnar-cell features. Am J Clin Pathol 1990;94:442-5.

322. Shimizu M, Hirokawa M, Manabe T. Tall cell variant of papillary thyroid carcinoma with foci of columnar cell component. Virchows Arch 1999;434:173-5.

323. Baloch ZW, Mandel S, LiVolsi VA. Combined tall cell carcinoma and Hürthle cell carcinoma (collision tumor) of the thyroid. Arch Pathol Lab Med 2001;125:541-3.

324. Axiotis C, Merino MJ, Campo E, LaPorte N, Neumann R. P-glycoprotein is expressed in thyroid carcinomas but not in benign conditions Lab Invest 1991;64:31A (Abstract).

325. Loy TS, Gelven PL, Mullins D, Diaz-Arias AA. Immunostaining for P-glycoprotein in the diagnosis of thyroid carcinomas. Mod Pathol 1992;2:200-4.

326. Eusebi V, Damiani S, Ellis IO, Azzopardi JG, Rosai J. Breast tumor resembling the tall cell variant of papillary thyroid carcinoma: report of 5 cases. Am J Surg Pathol 2003;27:1114-8.

327. Cameselle-Teijeiro J, Abdulkader I, Barreiro-Morandeira F, et al. Breast tumor resembling the tall cell variant of papillary thyroid carcinoma: a case report. Int J Surg Pathol 2006;14:79-84.

328. Cameselle-Teijeiro J, Chan JK. Cribriform-morular variant of papillary carcinoma: a distinctive variant representing the sporadic counterpart of familial adenomatous polyposis-associated thyroid carcinoma? Mod Pathol 1999;12:400-11.

329. Harach HR, Williams GT, Williams ED. Familial adenomatous polyposis associated thyroid carcinoma: a distinct type of follicular cell neoplasm. Histopathology 1994;25:549-61.

330. Cetta F, Toti P, Petracci M, et al. Thyroid carcinoma associated with familial adenomatous polyposis. Histopathology 1997;31:231-6.

331. Soravia C, Sugg SL, Berk T, et al. Familial adenomatous polyposis-associated thyroid cancer: a clinical, pathological, and molecular genetics study. Am J Pathol 1999;154:127-35.

332. Rossi ED, Revelli L, Martini M, et al. Cribriform-morular variant of papillary thyroid carcinoma in an 8-year-old girl: a case report with immunohistochemical and molecular testing. Int J Surg Pathol 2012;20:629-32.

333. Kovacs CM, Nose V. Cribriform morular variant of papillary thyroid carcinoma: morphological characteristics of an unusual tumor that distinguish the inherited and sporadic subtypes. Lab Invest 2012; 92:147-8A (Abstract).

334. Cameselle-Teijeiro J, Menasce LP, Yap BK, et al. Cribriform-morular variant of papillary thyroid carcinoma: molecular characterization of a case with neuroendocrine differentiation and aggressive behavior. Am J Clin Pathol 2009; 131:134-42.

335. Kameyama K, Mukai M, Takami H, Ito K. Cribriform-morular variant of papillary thyroid carcinoma: ultrastructural study and somatic/germline mutation analysis of the APC gene. Ultrastruct Pathol 2004;28:97-102.

336. Xu B, Yoshimoto K, Miyauchi A, et al. Cribriform-morular variant of papillary thyroid carcinoma: a pathological and molecular genetic study with evidence of frequent somatic mutations in exon 3 of the beta-catenin gene. J Pathol 2003;199:58-67.

337. Nakatani Y, Masudo K, Nozawa A, et al. Biotin-rich, optically clear nuclei express estrogen receptor-beta: tumors with morules may develop under the influence of estrogen and aberrant beta-catenin expression. Hum Pathol 2004;35:869-74.

338. Lovitch SB, Faquin W, Nose V. Cribriform-morular variant of thyroid carcinoma: distinct immunohistochemical profile from other papillary thyroid carcinoma variants. Lab Invest 2009;89:117A (Abstract).

339. Nakazawa T, Celestino R, Machado JC, et al. Cribriform-morular variant of papillary thyroid carcinoma displaying poorly differentiated features. Int J Surg Pathol 2013;21:379-89.

8 POORLY DIFFERENTIATED THYROID CARCINOMA

Some carcinomas composed of follicular cells do not fit easily into any of the traditional categories, i.e., follicular, papillary, Hürthle cell, medullary, and undifferentiated (anaplastic). It is our belief (1) and that of other authors (2,3) that many of these tumors occupy both morphologically and behaviorally an intermediate place between the well-differentiated follicular and papillary carcinomas on one side and the undifferentiated (anaplastic) carcinomas on the other. It is arguable whether they represent independent tumor entities or higher grades of one or another of the conventional types (4). We favor the latter interpretation and therefore acknowledge that, by incorporating them into the conventional classification of thyroid tumors, we are introducing grading criteria into a scheme that is largely based on other parameters (see chapter 4). We believe that this approach is justifiable because of the reasonably distinctive morphologic appearance of its prototypic representative, which we have designated *insular carcinoma*, and because of the important prognostic connotations of the concept.

INSULAR CARCINOMA

Definition. *Insular carcinoma* is the term that was proposed in 1984 for a morphologically distinctive form of poorly differentiated carcinoma arising from follicular cells (5). It is probably the same tumor type described by Langhans (6) in 1907 as wuchernde Struma (proliferating goiter) (fig. 8-1).

General Considerations. Insular carcinoma was initially viewed by the World Health Organization (WHO) Committee as a morphologic variant of follicular carcinoma (7). We believe that this interpretation is correct for most, but not all, cases of this entity. In some instances, we have seen it coexisting with, or developing after, a typical papillary carcinoma of either the conventional or the follicular variant type. In other instances, we have found that the architectural progression from a conventional

papillary to an insular pattern was paralleled by a gradual change in the nuclear appearance, from the typical ground-glass nuclei of papillary carcinoma to the smaller and hyperchromatic forms with irregularly shaped ("convoluted") nuclei that are characteristic of some insular carcinomas (fig. 8-2). From a prognostic standpoint, we believe that it is much more important to identify the tumor as being poorly differentiated than try to decide whether it belongs to the follicular or papillary group, a task that in some instances may be impossible.

General and Clinical Features. Insular carcinoma seems to be more common in some parts of the world than in others. The cases originally reported were largely from central Italy, where they constituted approximately 4 percent of all the thyroid carcinomas seen at one institution (5). The figure is even higher (6.7 percent) in the mountainous areas of northern Italy (7). In Paraguay, carcinomas with an insular pattern comprise a high percentage of all thyroid malignancies (A. Rolón, personal communication, 1990), at least in times past. By contrast, in the United States, this tumor is rare (less than 2 percent), although there is no question about its existence (8,9).

Insular carcinoma is slightly more common in women than men, and the mean age at the time of the initial diagnosis is 55 years (5). It can also present in adolescents and children, as well as in the elderly (9). Exceptionally, it develops against a background of diffuse hyperplasia (Graves disease) (10). It can occur any place where thyroid tissue is present, including the mediastinum (11).

Gross Findings. The tumor is solid and grayish white, and often exhibits foci of necrosis (figs. 8-3–8-5). Most tumors show invasive margins, and extrathyroid extension may be observed. Others are partially or completely encapsulated (10,12).

Microscopic Findings. The most distinctive histologic feature of insular carcinoma is the

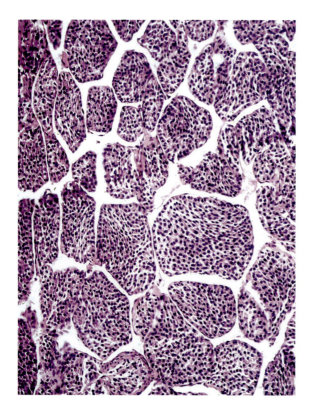 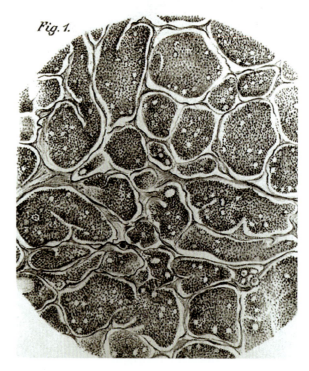

Figure 8-1

POORLY DIFFERENTIATED CARCINOMA (INSULAR TYPE)

Left: The typical nesting appearance is accentuated by artifactual retraction from the stroma.
Right: Reproduction of Figure 1 from Langhans' original article on wuchernde Struma (6). The microscopic similarities are striking.

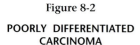

Figure 8-2

POORLY DIFFERENTIATED CARCINOMA

The nuclei of this tumor are small, with very irregular contours ("convoluted"), suggesting a histogenetic relationship with papillary carcinoma.

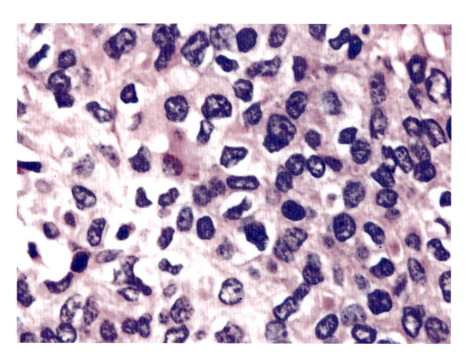

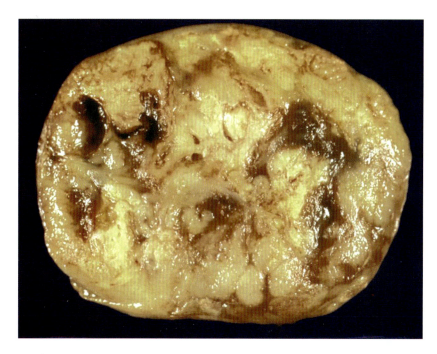

Figure 8-3

POORLY DIFFERENTIATED CARCINOMA (INSULAR TYPE)

Grossly, the tumor is unusually well circumscribed. The cut surface shows areas of necrosis and hemorrhage.

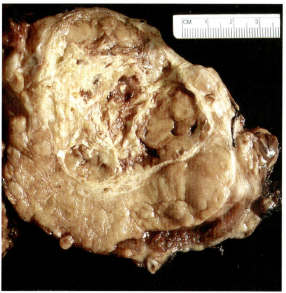

Figure 8-4

POORLY DIFFERENTIATED CARCINOMA (INSULAR TYPE)

This tumor is invasive, with tan-colored solid nests bulging on the surface and large necrotic foci.

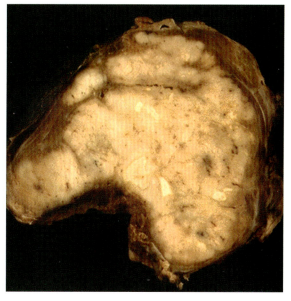

Figure 8-5

POORLY DIFFERENTIATED CARCINOMA (INSULAR TYPE)

The tumor replaced most of the thyroid gland and has an invasive pattern of growth. There are multiple foci of necrosis.

presence of well-defined round or oval-shaped nests (insulae), composed of a monotonous population of small cells with scant cytoplasm and round hyperchromatic nuclei, sometimes with wrinkled ("convoluted") nuclear mem-

branes (fig. 8-2). The insular pattern is sometimes accentuated by an artifactual retraction from the stroma, in a carcinoid-like fashion (figs. 8-6–8-8). The predominant pattern of

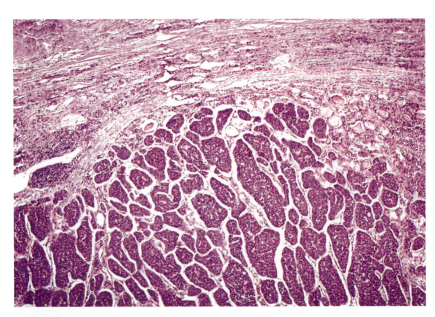

Figure 8-6

POORLY DIFFERENTIATED CARCINOMA (INSULAR TYPE)

Low-power view of a typical insular carcinoma invading the surrounding gland. There is a striking resemblance to carcinoid and other neuroendocrine tumors.

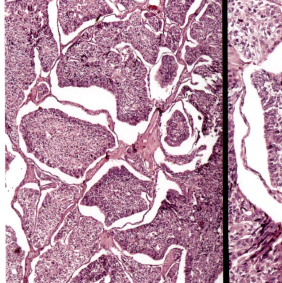

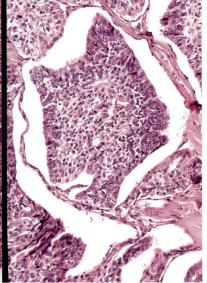

Figure 8-7

POORLY DIFFERENTIATED CARCINOMA (INSULAR TYPE)

The carcinoid-like appearance of this insular carcinoma, partially due to artifactual refraction from the stroma, may result in a misdiagnosis.

growth is solid, but microfollicles are commonly encountered, some of which contain dense colloid (figs. 8-8, 8-9). This appearance has been likened to that of primordial follicular cells in the early stages of fetal thyroid development (13). Mitoses are nearly always present but in a widely variable number (fig. 8-10).

The pattern of growth is usually infiltrative (but see under Gross Findings), and blood vessel invasion is common. Foci of necrosis are frequent. When small, these foci tend to be located in the center of the insulae, whereas the larger ones spare the insulae situated around blood vessels, thus leading to the so-called perithelio-matous appearance (fig. 8-11).

Immunohistochemical Findings. The tumor cells are positive for keratin, thyroglobulin, and thyroid transcription factor (TTF)-1, and negative for calcitonin and chromogranin (fig. 8-12). They usually overexpress p53 (in contrast with well-differentiated follicular and papillary carcinomas), and have a high MIB-1 staining ratio (15 percent or more) (14). E-cadherin loss is a common feature (15). Focal reactivity for somatostatin and synaptophysin has also been described (5,16).

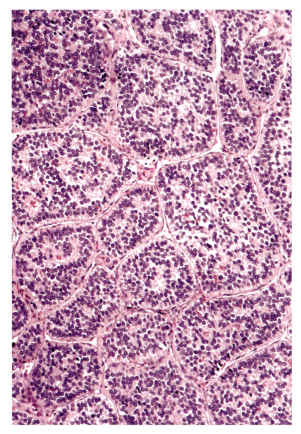

Figure 8-8

POORLY DIFFERENTIATED CARCINOMA (INSULAR TYPE)

The prototypical appearance of insular carcinoma is that of individual insulae made up of uniform small round cells.

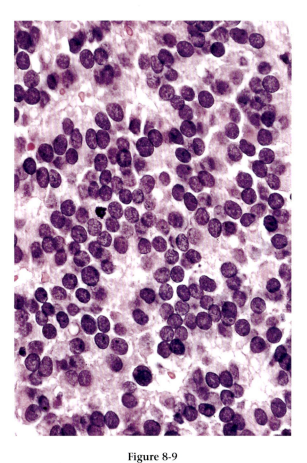

Figure 8-9

POORLY DIFFERENTIATED CARCINOMA (INSULAR TYPE)

High-power view shows a monotonous population of small round cells with highly hyperchromatic nuclei.

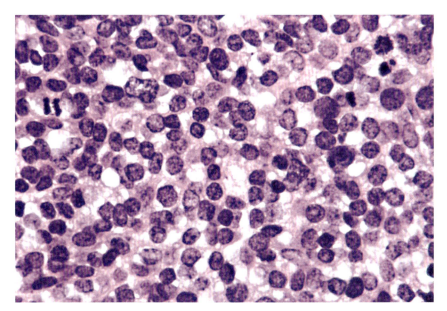

Figure 8-10

POORLY DIFFERENTIATED CARCINOMA (INSULAR TYPE)

High cellularity, nuclear hyperchromasia, and mitotic activity are present. In the past, tumors with this appearance were regarded as a subtype of undifferentiated (anaplastic) carcinoma.

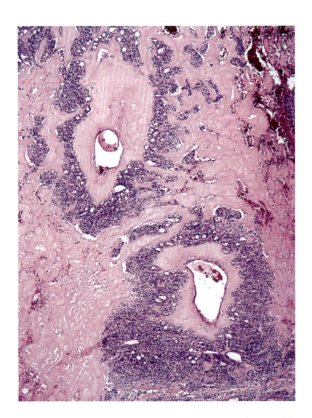 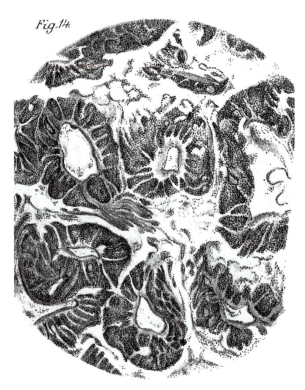

Figure 8-11

POORLY DIFFERENTIATED CARCINOMA (INSULAR TYPE)

Left: The extensive tumor necrosis accompanied by preservation of the tumor cells surrounding the vessels results in a so-called peritheliomatous appearance.

Right: Reproduction of Figure 14 from Langhans' original article on wuchernde Struma (6), showing a markedly similar microscopic appearance on low-power examination.

Figure 8-12

POORLY DIFFERENTIATED CARCINOMA (INSULAR TYPE)

The immunostain for thyroglobulin is more intense in the neoplastic microfollicles than in the solid areas.

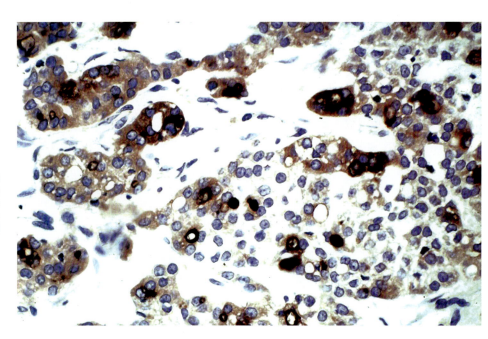

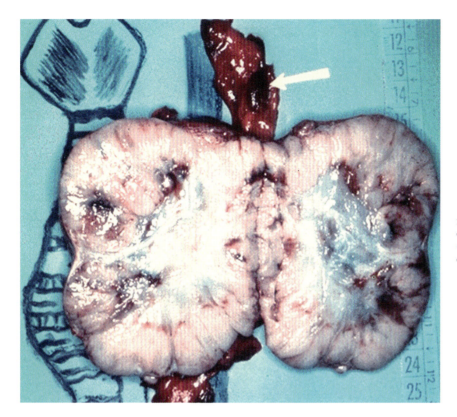

Figure 8-13

POORLY DIFFERENTIATED CARCINOMA (INSULAR TYPE)

Massive cervical lymph node metastasis from a poorly differentiated (insular) carcinoma. (Courtesy of Dr. P. Rolón, Asunción, Paraguay.)

Molecular Genetic Findings. See chapter 19.

Cytologic Findings. See chapter 20.

Differential Diagnosis. This tumor can be confused with medullary carcinoma and other neuroendocrine neoplasms because of its carcinoid-like insular configuration, and it may be overdiagnosed as undifferentiated (anaplastic) carcinoma when the pattern of growth is solid throughout. It is likely that many of the thyroid neoplasms formerly designated as the compact subtype of anaplastic carcinoma belong to this category (17,18).

Spread and Metastases. Metastases are common, both to regional lymph nodes and by the hematogenous route to distant sites (particularly lung and bone) (fig. 8-13) (19,20).

Treatment and Prognosis. The primary treatment of insular carcinoma is surgical and consists of total thyroidectomy, usually in conjunction with cervical lymph node dissection. In contrast to anaplastic carcinoma, insular carcinoma often concentrates radioiodide and is therefore a candidate for ^{131}I therapy (21).

Pure insular carcinoma is a more aggressive tumor than either well-differentiated follicular or well-differentiated papillary carcinoma (22).

This was already obvious in the original series of Carcangiu et al. (5), in which 14 of 25 patients died as the result of the tumor, and 7 were alive but with persistent or recurrent disease at the time of the last follow-up. This has been confirmed in subsequent series (9,23–25).

A related and still controversial issue concerns the possible prognostic significance of insular carcinoma when it appears as a focal feature in what is otherwise a well-differentiated follicular or papillary neoplasm, or one of their variants. A few authors claim that this finding is of no clinical significance (26), but most published series and our personal observations suggest otherwise (27,28). Johnson et al. (29) retrospectively identified five cases with insular features. Four tumors were greater than 7 cm; three of these showed extrathyroid extension with lung and/or bone metastases at presentation, and the fourth caused lung metastasis 3 years after initial diagnosis. Yamashita et al. (30) found that of their patients 50 years of age or older with follicular carcinoma, the incidence of distant metastases at initial presentation was 10 percent in those without an insular component and 83 percent in those in which that component was

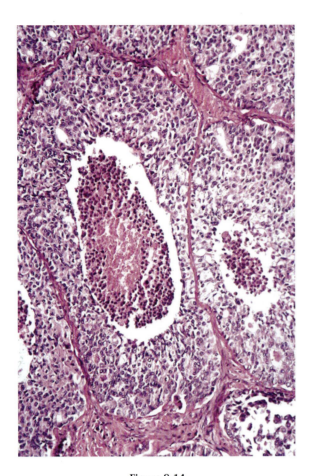

Figure 8-14

POORLY DIFFERENTIATED CARCINOMA

The central necrosis in the tumor nests results in an appearance similar to that of the breast tumor known as comedocarcinoma.

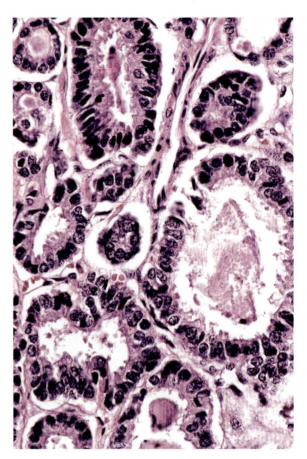

Figure 8-15

HIGH-GRADE FOLLICULAR CARCINOMA

The nuclear hyperchromasia and pleomorphism are those of an aggressive tumor (indeed, it proved fatal), but this lesion does not belong to the poorly differentiated category because the predominant pattern of growth is follicular rather than solid or trabecular.

present. We have had on several occasions the opportunity of reviewing the slides of the initial operation on patients with recurrent or metastatic thyroid carcinomas initially diagnosed as conventional follicular or papillary carcinoma, and finding in them foci of insular carcinomas that had been overlooked or dismissed.

OTHER POORLY DIFFERENTIATED CARCINOMAS

Some thyroid carcinomas share with insular carcinoma the presence of well-defined tumor nests, a predominantly solid growth pattern, mitotic activity, and necrosis, but are composed of larger cells, both in terms of nuclear size and cytoplasmic volume (fig. 8-14). The group is heterogeneous, in the sense that

some members have nuclear features similar to those of papillary carcinoma, others have an architectural configuration consistent with a follicular carcinoma, and still others have oncocytic cytoplasmic features (figs. 8-15, 8-16). (3,31,32). On occasion, a remarkably complex appearance results from the intimate admixture within the same tumor of follicular, papillary, oncocytic, and clear cell foci, some of which exhibit prominent nesting. As in the case of insular carcinoma, we feel that it is more important to emphasize their poorly differentiated nature (with its implication of more aggressive behavior) than to make the difficult and sometimes futile attempt to place them into one conventional category or another.

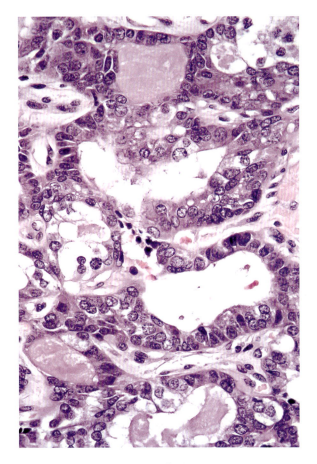

Figure 8-16

HIGH-GRADE PAPILLARY CARCINOMA

This papillary carcinoma has high-grade nuclear features but does not qualify as poorly differentiated because of the absence of solid/trabecular areas.

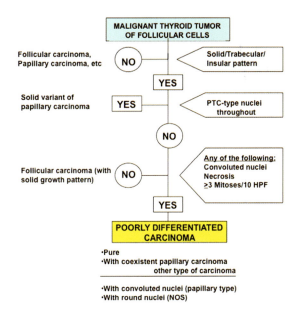

Figure 8-17

DIAGNOSTIC CRITERIA FOR POORLY DIFFERENTIATED THYROID CARCINOMAS

STI = solid/trabecular/insular; PTC = papillary thyroid carcinoma; PD = poorly differentiated. (Modified from fig. 1 from Volante M, Collin P, Nikiforov YE, et al. Poorly differentiated thyroid carcinoma: the Turin proposal for the use of uniform diagnostic criteria and an algorithmic diagnostic approach. Am J Surg Pathol 2007;31:1259.)

Some authors have attempted a grading system for such tumors but within the confines of the papillary or follicular categories, or by using criteria somewhat different from the ones we are advocating (33–40). For instance, Hiltzick et al. (41) defined poorly differentiated carcinomas on the basis of mitoses (5 or more per 10 high-power fields) or necrosis, independently of the pattern of growth. We think it is important not to equate the tumor microscopic grade with the degree of differentiation, while acknowledging that there is clearly a correlation between the two (42). In any event, the main message is that the tumor differentiation/tumor grading overrides considerations based on the standard binary classification scheme (follicular versus papillary) for prognostic and therapeutic purposes. It is our strong suspicion that a high proportion of the tumors classified as either papillary or follicular carcinomas that behave in an unexpectedly aggressive fashion, even when occurring in low-risk populations (such as patients under 40 years), belong to this category (37).

In an attempt to standardize the microscopic diagnosis of poorly differentiated thyroid carcinoma, a group of pathologists interested in the subject met in Turin, Italy, in 2006 to propose the use of uniform diagnostic criteria ("the Turin proposal") (fig. 8-17) (43). Those criteria were: 1) the presence of a solid/trabecular/insular pattern of growth; 2) the absence of the nuclear features of papillary carcinoma; and 3) the presence of at least one of the following features: convoluted nuclei, mitotic activity of 3 or more mitoses per 10 high-power fields, and tumor necrosis. This was accompanied by an algorithmic approach for practical use of the system. A validation of this proposal has already been published, based on the combined study of a large number of cases from the United States and Italy (7,44). Rare poorly differentiated carcinomas having an encapsulated appearance are associated with a better prognosis than those with invasive edges, regardless whether they are defined as poorly differentiated carcinomas on the basis of the Turin criteria or the more restrictive ones (mitosis and/or necrosis) proposed by the Memorial Sloan-Kettering authors (45).

REFERENCES

1. Rosai J. Poorly differentiated thyroid carcinoma: introduction to the issue, its landmarks, and clinical impact. Endocr Pathol 2004;15:293-6.

2. Sobrinho-Simões M. Poorly differentiated carcinomas of the thyroid. Endocr Pathol 1996;7:99-102.

3. Volante M, Rapa I, Papotti M. Poorly differentiated thyroid carcinoma: diagnostic features and controversial issues. Endocr Pathol 2008;19:150-5.

4. Tallini G. Poorly differentiated thyroid carcinoma. Are we there yet? Endocr Pathol 2011;22:190-4.

5. Carcangiu ML, Zampi G, Rosai J. Poorly differentiated ("insular") thyroid carcinoma. A reinterpretation of Langhans' "wuchernde Struma." Am J Surg Pathol 1984;8:655-68.

6. Langhans T. Über die epithelialen formen der malignen Struma. Virchows Arch Pathol Anat Physiol Klin Med 1907;189:69-188.

7. Hedinger CE, Williams ED, Sobin LH. Histological classification of thyroid tumors. WHO International classification of tumours, 2nd ed. Berlin: Springer-Verlag; 1988.

8. Flynn SD, Forman BH, Stewart AF, Kinder BK. Poorly differentiated ("insular") carcinoma of the thyroid gland: an aggressive subset of differentiated thyroid neoplasms. Surgery 1988;104:963-70.

9. Hassoun AA, Hay ID, Goellner JR, Zimmerman D. Insular thyroid carcinoma in adolescents: a potentially lethal endocrine malignancy. Cancer 1997;79:1044-8.

10. Foroughi F, Saadat N, Salehian MT, Beneshti S. Encapsulated insular carcinoma of the thyroid arising in Graves disease: report of a case and review of the literature. Int J Surg Pathol 2012;20:636-9.

11. Dominguez-Malagon H, Guerrero-Medrano J, Suster S. Ectopic poorly differentiated (insular) carcinoma of the thyroid. Report of a case presenting as an anterior mediastinal mass. Am J Clin Pathol 1995;104:408-12.

12. Mizukami Y, Nonomura A, Michigishi T, et al Poorly differentiated ('insular') carcinoma of the thyroid. Pathol Int 1995;45:663-8.

13. Papotti M, Botto Micca F, Favero A, Palestini N, Bussolati G. Poorly differentiated thyroid carcinomas with primordial cell component. A group of aggressive lesions sharing insular, trabecular, and solid patterns. Am J Surg Pathol 1993;17:291-301.

14. Martyniak A, Nose V. Does p53 and MIB-1 immunostaining help in the diagnosis of poorly differentiated thyroid carcinoma using the Turin criteria? Lab Invest 2009;89:118A (Abstract).

15. Rocha AS, Soares P, Fonseca E, Cameselle-Teijeiro J, Oliveira MC, Sobrinho-Simões M. E-cadherin loss rather than beta-catenin alterations is a common feature of poorly differentiated thyroid carcinomas. Histopathology 2003;42:580-7.

16. Satoh F, Umemura S, Yasuda M, Osamura RY. Neuroendocrine marker expression in thyroid epithelial tumors. Endocr Pathol 2001;12:291-9.

17. Meissner WA, Warren S. Tumors of the thyroid gland. Atlas of Tumor Pathology, 2nd Series, Fascicle 4. Washington, DC: Armed Forces Institute of Pathology; 1969.

18. Rosai J, Saxén EA, Woolner L. Undifferentiated and poorly differentiated carcinoma. Semin Diagn Pathol 1985;2:123-36.

19. Pittas AG, Adler M, Fazzari M, et al. Bone metastases from thyroid carcinoma: clinical characteristics and prognostic variables in one hundred forty-six patients. Thyroid 2000;10:261-8.

20. Tickoo SK, Pittas AG, Adler M, et al. Bone metastases from thyroid carcinoma: a histopathologic study with clinical correlates. Arch Pathol Lab Med 2000;124:1440-7.

21. Justin EP, Seabold JE, Robinson RA, Walker WP, Gurll NJ, Hawes DR. Insular carcinoma: a distinct thyroid carcinoma with associated iodine-131 localization. J Nucl Med 1991;32:1358-63.

22. Siironen P, Hagström J, Mäenpää HO, et al. Anaplastic and poorly differentiated thyroid carcinoma: therapeutic strategies and treatment outcome of 52 consecutive patients. Oncology 2010;79:400-8.

23. Pellegriti G, Giuffrida D, Scollo C, et al. Long-term outcome of patients with insular carcinoma of the thyroid: the insular histotype is an independent predictor of poor prognosis. Cancer 2002;95:2076-85.

24. Volante M, Landolfi S, Chiusa L, et al. Poorly differentiated carcinomas of the thyroid with trabecular, insular, and solid patterns: a clinicopathologic study of 183 patients. Cancer 2004;100:950-7.

25. Nishida T, Katayama S, Tsujimoto M, Nakamura J, Matsuda H. Clinicopathological significance of poorly differentiated thyroid carcinoma. Am J Surg Pathol 1999;23:205-11.

26. Ashfaq R, Vuitch F, Delgado R, Albores-Saavedra J. Papillary and follicular thyroid carcinomas with an insular component. Cancer 1994;73:416-23.

27. Sasaki A, Daa T, Kashima K, Yokoyama S, Nakayama I, Noguchi S. Insular component as a risk factor of thyroid carcinoma. Pathol Int 1996;46:939-46.

28. Decaussin M, Bernard MH, Adeleine P, et al. Thyroid carcinomas with distant metastases: a review of 111 cases with emphasis on the prognostic significance of an insular component. Am J Surg Pathol 2002;26:1007-15.

29. Johnson MW, Hunnicutt JW, Bilbao JE, Bassion S. Poorly differentiated thyroid carcinoma with focal insular pattern: clinicopathologic correlation. Am J Clin Pathol 1990;94:497-8A. (Abstract)

30. Yamashita H, Noguchi Y, Noguchi S, et al. Significance of an insular component in follicular thyroid carcinoma with distant metastasis at initial presentation. Endocr Pathol 2005;16:41-8.

31. Sobrinho-Simões M, Sambade C, Fonseca E, Soares P. Poorly differentiated carcinomas of the thyroid gland: a review of the clinicopathologic features of a series of 28 cases of a heterogeneous, clinically aggressive group of thyroid tumors. Int J Surg Pathol 2002;10:123-31.

32. Dettmer M, Schmitt A, Steinert H, Moch H, Kominoth P, Perren A. Poorly differentiated oncocytic thyroid carcinoma—diagnostic implications and outcome. Histopathology 2012;60:1045-51.

33. Cabanne F, Gérard-Marchant R, Heimann R, Williams ED. [Malignant tumors of the thyroid gland. Problems of histopathologic diagnosis. Apropos of 692 lesions collected by the Thyroid Cancer Cooperative Group of the O.E.R.T.C.] Ann Anat Pathol (Paris) 1974;19:129-48. [French]

34. Harach HR, Franssila KO. Thyroglobulin immunostaining in follicular thyroid carcinoma: relationship to the degree of differentiation and cell type. Histopathology 1988;13:43-54.

35. McConahey WM, Hay ID, Woolner LB, van Heerden JA, Taylor WF. Papillary thyroid cancer treated at the Mayo Clinic, 1946 through 1970: initial manifestations, pathologic findings, therapy, and outcome. Mayo Clin Proc 1986;61:978-96.

36. Mueller-Gaertner HW, Brzac HT, Rehpenning W. Prognostic indices for tumor relapse and tumor mortality in follicular thyroid carcinoma. Cancer 1991;67:1903-11.

37. Rosen IB, Bowden J, Luk SC, Simpson JA. Aggressive thyroid cancer in low-risk age population. Surgery 1987;102:1075-80.

38. Sakamoto A, Kasai N, Sugano H. Poorly differentiated carcinoma of the thyroid. A clinicopathologic entity for a high-risk group of papillary and follicular carcinomas. Cancer 1983;52:1849-55.

39. Simpson WJ, McKinney SE, Carruthers JS, Gospodarowicz MK, Sutcliffe SB, Panzarella T. Papillary and follicular thyroid cancer. Prognostic factors in 1,578 patients. Am J Med 1987;83:479-88.

40. Tscholl-Ducommun J, Hedinger CE. Papillary thyroid carcinomas. Morphology and prognosis. Virchows Arch A Pathol Anat Histol 1982;396:19-39.

41. Hiltzik D, Carlson DL, Tuttle RM, et al. Poorly differentiated thyroid carcinomas defined on the basis of mitosis and necrosis: a clinicopathologic study of 58 patients. Cancer 2006;106:1286-95.

42. Gnemmi V, Renaud F, Do Cao C, et al. Poorly differentiated thyroid carcinomas: application of the Turin proposal provides prognostic results similar to those from the assessment of high-grade features. Histopathology 2014;64:263-73.

43. Volante M, Collini P, Nikiforov YE, et al. Poorly differentiated thyroid carcinoma: the Turín proposal for the use of uniform diagnostic criteria and an algorithmic diagnostic approach. Am J Surg Pathol 2007;31:1256-64.

44. Asioli S, Erickson LA, Righi A, et al. Poorly differentiated carcinoma of the thyroid: validation of the Turín proposal and analysis of IMP3 expression. Mod Pathol 2010;23:1269-78.

45. Rivera M, Ricarte-Filho J, Patel S, et al. Encapsulated thyroid tumors of follicular cell origin with high grade features (high mitotic rate/tumor necrosis): a clinicopathologic and molecular study. Hum Pathol 2010;41:172-80.

9 UNDIFFERENTIATED (ANAPLASTIC) THYROID CARCINOMA

Undifferentiated (anaplastic) thyroid carcinoma is a highly malignant tumor that appears partially or totally undifferentiated with standard light microscopic techniques but in which some evidence of epithelial differentiation is found on morphologic, immunohistochemical, or ultrastructural grounds. Other terms that have been used to designate this tumor and related entities include *pleomorphic carcinoma, sarcomatoid carcinoma, metaplastic carcinoma*, and *carcinosarcoma*.

CLINICAL FEATURES

Undifferentiated thyroid carcinoma is characteristically a tumor of elderly individuals. In most series, the mean age at the time of the initial diagnosis is between 60 and 65 years. Few patients present below the age of 50 years, and such a diagnosis should therefore be suspect when made in a young patient; however, exceptions do occur. Isolated cases have been reported at the age of 37 years (1), 30 years (2), 26 years (3), and 22 years (4). As with most other thyroid tumors, undifferentiated carcinoma is most common in women. Most reported series quote a ratio of men to women of 1:3 to 1:4.

The clinical presentation is remarkably constant, with few cases departing from the classic description of a rapidly enlarging neck mass in the thyroid region. This is associated in about half of the cases with compression signs, such as dyspnea, dysphagia, and hoarseness. The duration is characteristically short, ranging from a few weeks to a few months. Occasionally, patients first present with symptoms or signs related to distant metastatic involvement, such as in skin (5), bowel (6), or bone (personal observation), but even in these patients, there is usually clinical evidence of a thyroid mass. In one reported case, the patient presented with hyperthyroidism, presumably as a result of necrosis of the normal thyroid gland and release of thyroid hormone (7). A history of preexistent nodular or diffuse enlargement of the thyroid gland is given in some cases because undifferentiated thyroid carcinoma nearly always engrafts itself on an abnormal gland.

Physical examination reveals nodular thyroid enlargement in almost every case, and this is usually of considerable magnitude. In about half of the cases, there is clinical evidence of extension beyond the thyroid gland, and in approximately one third, there is cervical lymph node enlargement resulting from metastatic disease.

Undifferentiated carcinoma is invariably cold on radioactive iodine scan, both in the primary site and in metastatic foci, and remains so even after the residual non-neoplastic thyroid gland has been removed. Areas of uptake in the metastatic deposits are indicative of the presence of a better-differentiated component. Euthyroidism is the rule in patients with undifferentiated carcinoma, even when most of the gland has been destroyed by tumor.

GROSS FINDINGS

Undifferentiated carcinoma is usually large and widely invasive on gross inspection (figs. 9-1–9-3). The consistency is highly variable and the appearance variegated, reflecting the common presence of necrotic and hemorrhagic foci. In most instances, the tumor replaces most of the thyroid gland and, in many instances, violates the thyroid capsule, spreading into the soft tissues of the neck. Areas with a granular appearance and firm consistency and those suggesting the residue of a capsule should be sought because they may provide the evidence for a preexisting papillary or follicular carcinoma, respectively. Occasionally, metaplastic cartilage or bone is seen grossly (fig. 9-4).

MICROSCOPIC FINDINGS

The microscopic appearance of undifferentiated carcinoma shows considerable variation from case to case and sometimes even within the same case. Three major morphologic patterns exist, allowing for transitions and intermediate forms among them. These patterns are

177

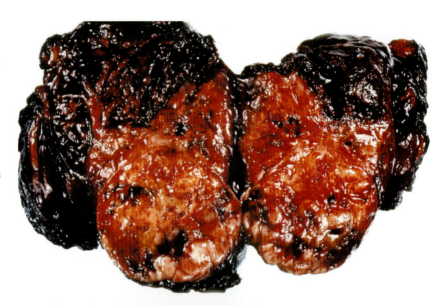

Figure 9-1

UNDIFFERENTIATED (ANAPLASTIC) CARCINOMA

Large invasive tumor with areas of necrosis and hemorrhage.

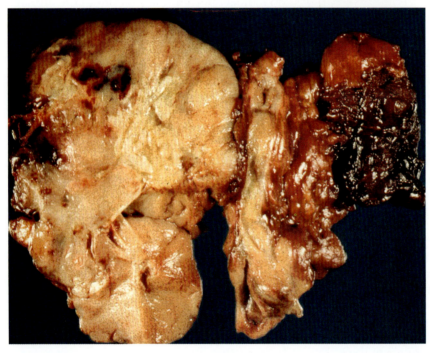

Figure 9-2

UNDIFFERENTIATED (ANAPLASTIC) CARCINOMA

The tumor involves a whole thyroid lobe and most of the contralateral lobe.

descriptively designated squamoid, spindle cell, and giant cell (1).

The *squamoid* (or *malpighian*) *pattern* is so named because of its morphologic similarity to nonkeratinizing squamous cell carcinoma of other organs, such as lung or cervix. The appearance in these areas is unmistakably epithelial because of the formation of distinct tumor nests of irregular configuration (figs. 9-5, 9-6). Pleomorphism is moderate, and giant cells are generally absent. The cytoplasm is abundant

and acidophilic. In rare instances, squamous pearls are seen in the center of the islands. In these cases, the appearance is epidermoid (squamous) rather than merely squamoid. Small foci of mucin accumulation are sometimes demonstrated in these areas by the use of the Mayer mucicarmine or other mucin stains.

The *spindle cell pattern* is best described as sarcoma-like since it is indistinguishable from a true sarcoma morphologically. Sometimes the appearance is reminiscent of fibrosarcoma

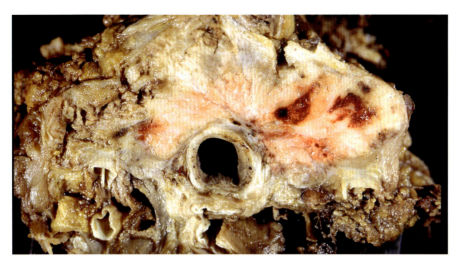

Figure 9-3

UNDIFFERENTIATED (ANAPLASTIC) CARCINOMA

There is massive extrathyroidal spread, with encircling of the trachea, which still has an open lumen.

Figure 9-4

UNDIFFERENTIATED (ANAPLASTIC) CARCINOMA

This tumor is uncharacteristically well circumscribed and has a homogeneous cut surface. A portion of the residual thyroid gland is visible in the upper pole. There are foci of necrosis and hemorrhage in the lower edge of the figure. The whitish area near the center represents neoplastic cartilage.

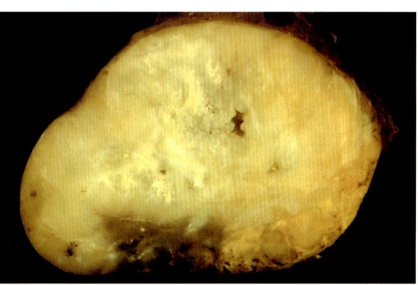

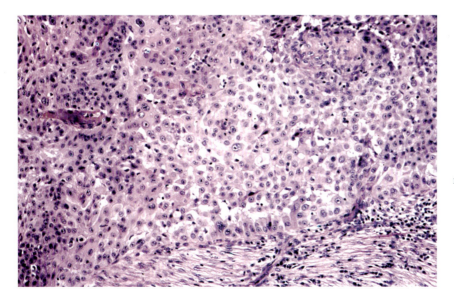

Figure 9-5

UNDIFFERENTIATED (ANAPLASTIC) CARCINOMA

The tumor cells have a squamoid appearance.

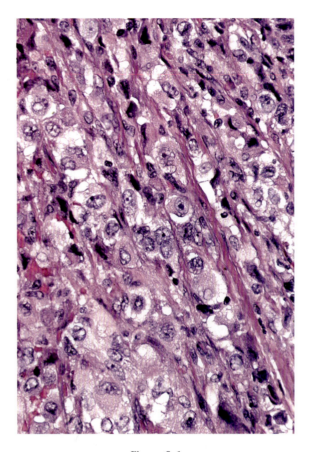

Figure 9-6

UNDIFFERENTIATED (ANAPLASTIC) CARCINOMA

The tumor cells are large and epithelioid, with an abundant acidophilic cytoplasm consistent with squamoid change.

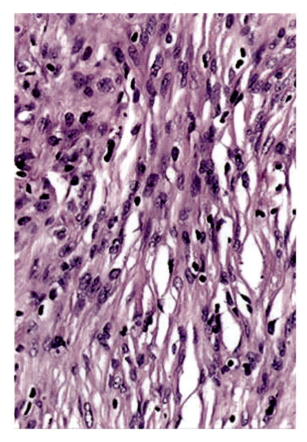

Figure 9-7

UNDIFFERENTIATED (ANAPLASTIC) CARCINOMA

The spindle shape of the tumor cells simulates the appearance of a sarcoma.

due to a fascicular arrangement and heavy deposition of collagen fibers (fig. 9-7). In most instances, however, the marked degree of nuclear pleomorphism, scattered giant tumor cells, storiform pattern of growth, and inflammatory infiltrate give the tumor an appearance similar to that exhibited by the tumor formerly known as the storiform-pleomorphic form of malignant fibrous histiocytoma and now more commonly designated as pleomorphic sarcoma, not otherwise specified (fig. 9-8). These cellular areas alternate with extensive areas of necrosis and sclerohyaline deposition. The necrotic foci tend to have sharply angulated outlines and to be surrounded by a palisading of tumor cells, resulting in an appearance similar to that seen in some malignant tumors of the central and peripheral nervous systems, notably glioblastoma multiforme. Areas of myxoid change may be

present; when abundant, there is a resemblance to myxofibrosarcoma of soft tissues.

Vascularization is generally prominent in the spindle cell variant. Sometimes the vessels are branching, with a "staghorn" or antler-like appearance, similar to that seen in hemangiopericytoma. In other instances, the appearance of angiosarcoma (malignant hemangioendothelioma) is simulated by the formation of freely connecting spaces lined by tumor cells. A characteristic formation often seen in the spindle cell areas is caused by the permeation of the wall of large vessels by neoplastic cells, sometimes resulting in polypoid subendothelial growth (fig. 9-9). Some of these structures stand out in a sea of necrotic or hyalinized tissue.

The *giant cell pattern* is characterized by a degree of pleomorphism that is substantially greater than that seen in association with the

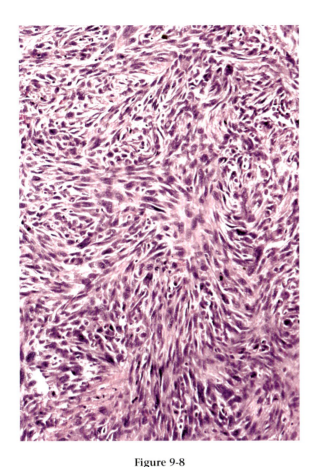

Figure 9-8

UNDIFFERENTIATED (ANAPLASTIC) CARCINOMA

The storiform pattern of this tumor results in a malignant fibrous histocytoma-like appearance.

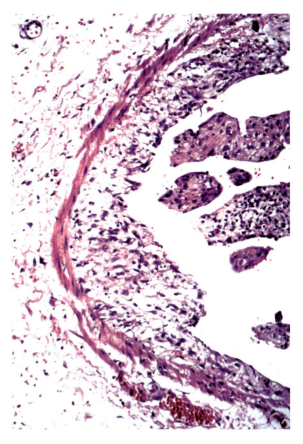

Figure 9-9

UNDIFFERENTIATED (ANAPLASTIC) CARCINOMA

Invasion of a large vein by the tumor, which spreads along the subendothelial layer and protrudes into the lumen.

other patterns (figs. 9-10, 9-11). This is due to the presence of numerous tumor giant cells with bizarre (sometimes multiple) hyperchromatic nuclei, abundant amphophilic and somewhat granular cytoplasm, and a plump (round or oval) shape. Variations include giant cells with homogeneous (nongranular), deeply acidophilic cytoplasm and others with variously sized, round, acidophilic, intracytoplasmic hyaline globules. The tumor giant cells may be the only element present, but more often they are interspersed with smaller mononuclear tumor cells that have otherwise similar morphologic features. The pattern of growth in these areas is usually solid, but on occasion, an artifactual separation of the cells leads to the formation of alveolar (pseudoglandular) or pseudovascular structures. The latter are particularly notable in areas where the highly vascular nature of the

tumor has led to the accumulation of red blood cells within these cavities.

A scattering of inflammatory cells is often present among the tumor cells, especially in the giant cell and squamoid patterns. When it is heavy and rich in neutrophils, the tumor resembles the soft tissue tumor formerly known as the inflammatory variant of malignant fibrous histiocytoma. In these areas, the giant tumor cells may contain numerous (possibly phagocytosed) neutrophils in their cytoplasm (fig. 9-12).

Features common to all three patterns are high mitotic activity, large foci of necrosis, and a marked degree of invasiveness, both within the gland and in the extrathyroid structures. Malignant cells grow between residual follicles or destroy them in their path. They invade adipose tissue and skeletal muscle, and sometimes even ulcerate through the skin. On occasion,

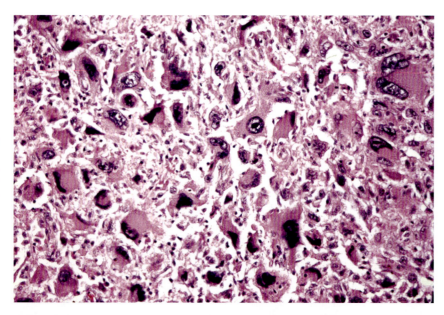

Figure 9-10

UNDIFFERENTIATED (ANAPLASTIC) CARCINOMA

The tumor is largely composed of bizarre giant cells. These should not be confused with non-neoplastic osteoclast-like multinucleated giant cells, which are present in about 10 percent of the cases.

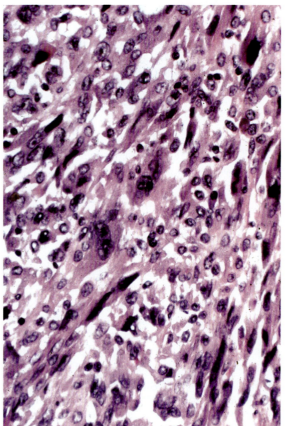

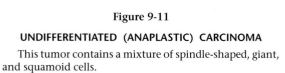

Figure 9-11

UNDIFFERENTIATED (ANAPLASTIC) CARCINOMA

This tumor contains a mixture of spindle-shaped, giant, and squamoid cells.

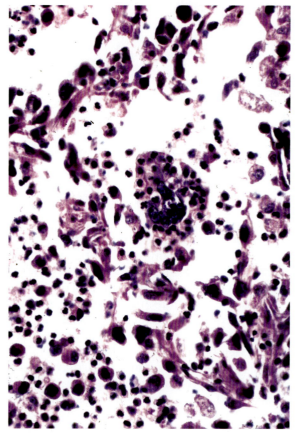

Figure 9-12

UNDIFFERENTIATED (ANAPLASTIC) CARCINOMA

The tumor cells are admixed with a heavy inflammatory infiltrate. The cytoplasm of a giant tumor cell is packed with neutrophils.

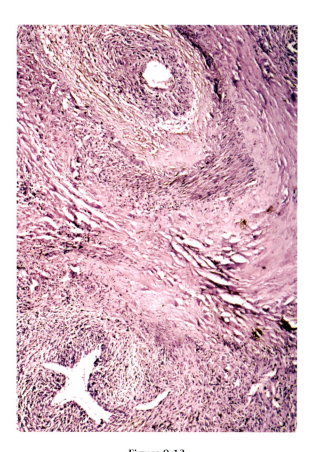

Figure 9-13

UNDIFFERENTIATED (ANAPLASTIC) CARCINOMA

Two large blood vessels show prominent tumor invasion of their wall, but their lumen remains open.

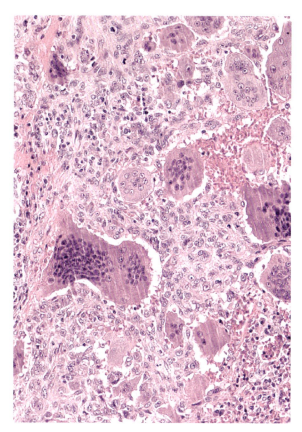

Figure 9-14

UNDIFFERENTIATED (ANAPLASTIC) CARCINOMA

The osteoclast-like multinucleated cells within the tumor represent non-neoplastic elements.

they penetrate inside skeletal muscle fibers in a manner analogous to that seen more commonly in carcinoma of the breast (8). Blood vessel invasion in the form of tumor thrombi (as opposed to the infiltration of the vessel wall described above) (figs. 9-9, 9-13) is a common finding.

As mentioned, transitions and admixtures between the three major patterns are often seen. The most common is between the spindle cell and giant cell patterns, but sometimes foci indistinguishable from sarcoma blend with those that have a clear-cut epithelial configuration.

Multinucleated cells with an appearance indistinguishable from osteoclasts (and therefore substantially different from the previously described tumor giant cells) are scattered among the neoplastic elements in about 10 percent of the cases (9,10). These cells have numerous (up to 100 or more) nuclei devoid of atypical features that never undergo mitotic division (fig. 9-14).

Ultrastructurally and immunohistochemically, they lack epithelial features. Instead, they express markers characteristic of cells of monocytic or histiocytic lineage (11). This finding suggests that these osteoclast-like elements are non-neoplastic, derived from blood-borne or indigenous monocytes or histiocytes, and formed as a result of cellular fusion. The phenomenon is analogous to that sometimes seen in carcinoma of breast and other organs (12) and may result in an appearance simulating an aneurysmal bone cyst (11).

In about 5 percent of undifferentiated carcinomas, the mesenchymal-like component of the tumor exhibits heterologous features, such as neoplastic skeletal muscle, cartilage, or bone (figs. 9-15, 9-16) (13–15). This may occur in association with any of the major basic patterns but is more common with the spindle cell type. Some authors use the term *carcinosarcoma* for this particular occurrence (16), but we do not believe

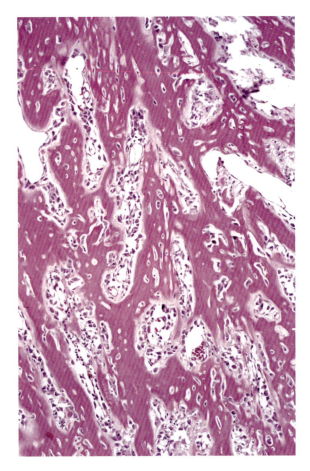

Figure 9-15

UNDIFFERENTIATED (ANAPLASTIC) CARCINOMA

Extensive osseous metaplasia.

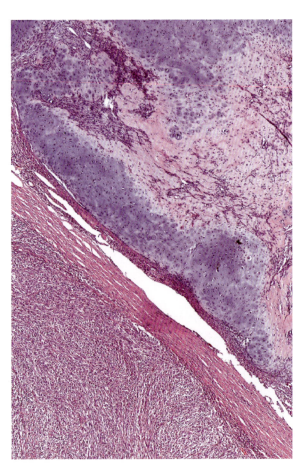

Figure 9-16

UNDIFFERENTIATED (ANAPLASTIC) CARCINOMA

A portion of the tumor shows a cartilaginous type of differentiation.

that a sharp separation from the larger group of undifferentiated carcinomas is warranted on either clinical or histogenetic grounds.

The microscopic appearance of the metastases generally recapitulates that of the primary tumor. No microscopic grading of undifferentiated carcinoma has been attempted or seems feasible. By definition, all representatives of this tumor type belong to the highest category of any grading system.

IMMUNOHISTOCHEMICAL FINDINGS

The immunohistochemical profile of undifferentiated carcinoma is somewhat related to the pattern of growth. In the squamoid and other epithelial-appearing foci, there is strong and consistent expression of both high and low molecular weight keratins (fig. 9-17) (17). Spindle and giant cell foci generally lack high molecular weight keratins but show reactivity for the low molecular weight forms of this marker in a variable number of cases (fig. 9-18). The incidence of positivity has ranged from 47 to 100 percent in the reported series (1,17–22). The positivity is often in the form of individual cells or cell clusters (23). Many of the tumor cells coexpress vimentin, especially in the spindle cell areas (19,21).

Staining for epithelial membrane antigen (EMA) recapitulates the pattern described for high molecular weight keratin, in the sense that the more epithelial-looking tumors are the only ones likely to exhibit positivity. Thus, the diagnostic utility of this marker is limited (20,24). Similarly, the basal cell marker p63 is expressed in undifferentiated carcinoma, although its diagnostic utility remains unclear (25,26).

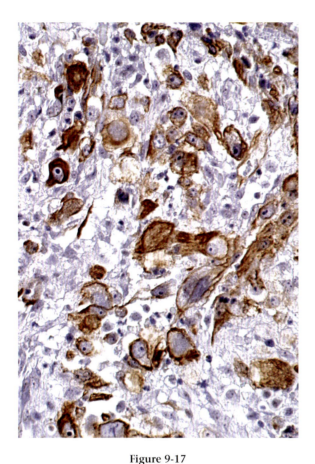

Figure 9-17

UNDIFFERENTIATED (ANAPLASTIC) CARCINOMA

The tumor cells of this undifferentiated carcinoma of squamoid type stain strongly for pankeratin.

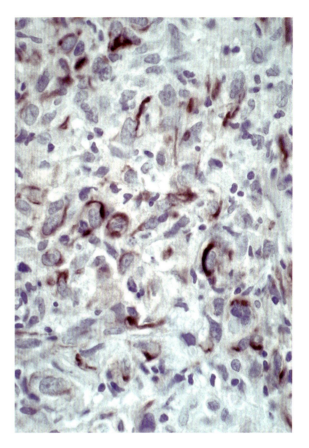

Figure 9-18

UNDIFFERENTIATED (ANAPLASTIC) CARCINOMA

Immunohistochemical positivity for low molecular weight keratin (Cam 5.2) is seen in many of the mesenchymal-like tumor cells.

Carcinoembryonic antigen (CEA) is positive in some of the more squamoid examples of undifferentiated carcinoma. This is usually limited to the center of the tumor nests (fig. 9-19) (1,20).

Intense positivity for laminin (a component of basal lamina) has been found by Miettinen and Virtanen (27) in scattered tumor cells; however, neoplasms lacking a distinct compartmentalization of tumor cells also lacked pericellular laminin. Rare cases of undifferentiated thyroid carcinoma show immunoreactivity for beta-human chorionic gonadotropin (HCG) and for the transcription factor PAX8 (see below; 28,29). Another novel finding is the expression of the epithelial-mesenchymal transition markers Slug and Twist, associated with the absence of e-cadherin (30).

Conflicting results have been obtained when staining these tumors for thyroglobulin and other thyroid hormone-related markers, such as thyroxine and triiodothyronine. Carcangiu et al. (1) did not encounter convincing positivity for thyroglobulin in any of the tumors they examined. Other authors reported reactivity ranging from 9 to 71 percent (18,31–36). In most cases, however, the reaction was described as weak, focal, and restricted to a few tumor cells. The interpretation of this stain is subject to two important pitfalls: 1) entrapment of non-neoplastic follicles and isolated follicular cells and 2) release of thyroglobulin from the entrapped follicles, with secondary diffusion into the cytoplasm of the tumor cells, a phenomenon analogous to that seen in other sites (fig. 9-20) (37,38). In our experience and that of others (38,39), thyroglobulin is of little use in the evaluation of undifferentiated carcinoma.

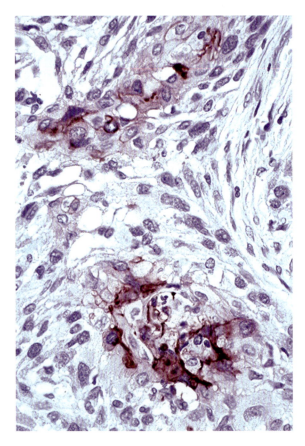

Figure 9-19

UNDIFFERENTIATED (ANAPLASTIC) CARCINOMA

Focal immunoreactivity for carcinoembryonic antigen (CEA) is evident in the necrotic and inflamed areas of an undifferentiated carcinoma with a squamoid pattern of growth.

In the few instances in which we have found convincing tumor positivity, this was restricted to the residual better-differentiated components, which were already clearly identifiable on morphologic grounds. Similarly, thyroid transcript factor (TTF)-1 is present in only a few cases (17). Among the other transcription factors that regulate follicular cell differentiation, only PAX8 has been reported to be variably expressed in a substantial number of undifferentiated carcinomas, making it a potentially useful marker (28,40).

Another controversial marker in this context is calcitonin. Occasional cases of undifferentiated carcinoma are immunohistochemically reactive for this hormone, but we believe that most of them are recognizable as anaplastic variants of medullary carcinoma on morphologic grounds. Our own findings (1) and those of others (20,38,41) have failed to support the surprising claim (42) that most undifferentiated carcinomas are calcitonin positive and therefore related to medullary carcinoma. It seems to us that all the available evidence concerning undifferentiated carcinoma indicates otherwise.

We conclude that low molecular weight keratin is the most useful marker for the evaluation of undifferentiated carcinoma. It may not indicate the follicular origin of the tumor and is not even entirely pathognomonic of its epithelial nature, but if it is present in a substantial number of tumor cells in the absence of vascular markers, it constitutes strong supporting evidence for the diagnosis, probably the strongest that can be marshaled with available techniques.

Undifferentiated carcinomas typically have a high proliferative rate, with a labeling index for MIB-1 (Ki-67) often greater than 50 percent, much higher than that of differentiated thyroid carcinomas. Several studies have analyzed the immunohistochemical reactivity for proteins that regulate the cell cycle (p53, p27, p21, cyclinD1) and apoptosis (BCL-2) (43–47). Since many undifferentiated carcinomas have *TP53* mutations that inactivate the gene, the mutated p53 protein, which cannot be effectively degraded, accumulates in the nucleus. Widespread nuclear immunoreactivity is typical, and although it does not help in the distinction of undifferentiated carcinoma from other high-grade tumors, it can distinguish them from thyroid tumors that are better differentiated. *TP53* mutations are rare in differentiated carcinomas (papillary or follicular). In tumors in which undifferentiated carcinoma is associated with a residual differentiated component, the mutations and immunohistochemical reactivity segregate with the high-grade, undifferentiated areas (43,48–50). The pattern of immunoreactivity for the other markers may also be useful, since, unlike most differentiated thyroid carcinomas, the cell cycle inhibitors p27 and p21 have markedly reduced expression in undifferentiated tumors (44,45,47). Cyclin D1 is often strongly expressed (51), while BCL-2 expression is usually absent (43).

ULTRASTRUCTURAL FINDINGS

Epithelial differentiation in the form of specialized cell junctions of zonula adherens type and arrays of microvilli projecting into intercellular

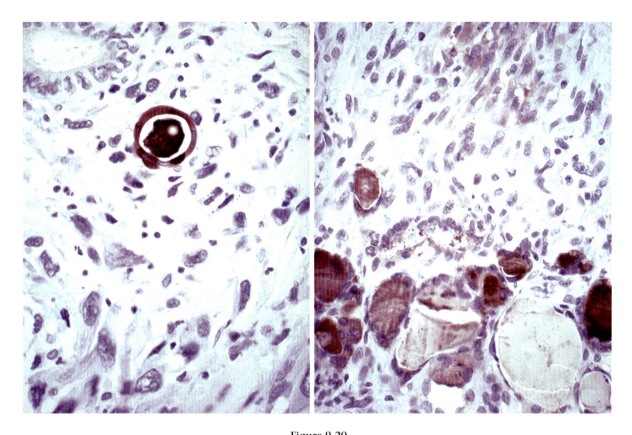

Figure 9-20

UNDIFFERENTIATED (ANAPLASTIC) CARCINOMA

Left: In this field, an entrapped thyroglobulin-positive non-neoplastic follicle is surrounded by unreactive tumor cells.

Right: Apparent focal positivity for thyroglobulin is evident in the malignant tumor cells (upper third) surrounding entrapped follicles (lower third). This is probably the result of thyroglobulin diffusion from the latter, followed by nonspecific absorption by the tumor cells.

spaces have been described in the cells of undifferentiated carcinoma by several authors (figs. 9-21–9-23) (1,52–55). Such features may not necessarily be present, however, presumably because of total dedifferentiation of the neoplasm. In the series of Carcangiu et al. (1), they were detected in only four of seven cases.

The nuclei are large, with clumped chromatin and prominent nucleoli. The cytoplasm is abundant. Usually it has a primitive appearance that consists of ribosomes, scattered mitochondria, and vesicles of granular endoplasmic reticulum. Randomly distributed cytoplasmic filaments of intermediate thickness (11 nm) are found in some cases. Judging from the immunohistochemical results, we assume that some of these filaments are composed of vimentin and others of keratin. Occasionally, they form huge whorls that fill most of the cytoplasm. These corre-

spond to the cells that have a homogeneous, deeply acidophilic cytoplasm with lateralization of the nucleus by light microscopy, i.e., a rhabdoid appearance.

Membrane-bound, highly electron-dense cytoplasmic granules are frequently present. Their irregular size and shape suggest a lysosomal nature. Granules clearly identifiable as secretory, neuroendocrine or otherwise, are absent. Focal basal lamina deposition may be detected.

MICROSCOPIC TYPES

Traditionally, undifferentiated carcinomas have been divided into three types: spindle cell, giant cell or pleomorphic, and small cell. The first two are discussed in the section on microscopic findings but not as separate types. We view them instead as two morphologic manifestations of the same tumor that can be

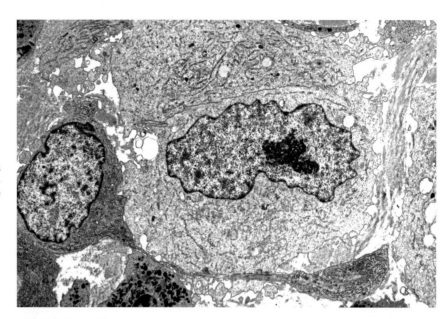

Figure 9-21

UNDIFFERENTIATED (ANAPLASTIC) CARCINOMA

Electron micrograph shows a tumor cell with primitive-appearing cytoplasm and scarce organelles.

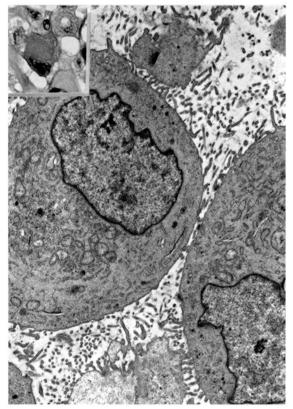

Figure 9-22

UNDIFFERENTIATED (ANAPLASTIC) CARCINOMA

This electron micrograph shows retention of microvilli and an abundance of intracytoplasmic intermediate filaments in the tumor cells. The latter results in a hyaline appearance at the light microscopic level (inset). (Courtesy of Dr. R. Erlandson, New York, NY.)

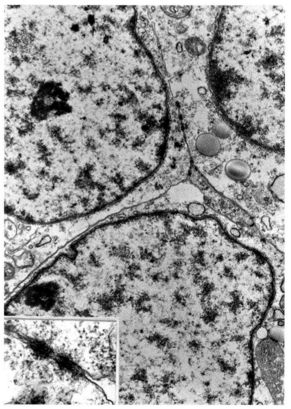

Figure 9-23

UNDIFFERENTIATED (ANAPLASTIC) CARCINOMA

Ultrastructurally, the tumor cells appear extremely primitive, but a few specialized cell junctions are present, as highlighted in the inset. (Courtesy of Dr. R. Erlandson, New York, NY.)

seen singly or in combination. We have added a squamoid pattern, which we believe to be as distinctive, albeit not as common, as the others, and which, although undifferentiated, has an unmistakable epithelial appearance at the morphologic, immunohistochemical, and ultrastructural levels (1).

The wisdom of grouping the latter pattern with the other two could be questioned, especially because, in other organs in which this situation occurs, this practice is not followed. In the lung, for instance, undifferentiated but clearly epithelial tumors are designated large cell undifferentiated carcinomas; tumors with a predominant component of tumor giant cells are known as giant cell carcinomas; and carcinomas that are mostly composed of spindle cells or contain heterologous mesenchymal tissues are variously designated spindle cell, sarcomatoid, or metaplastic. Perhaps the best argument for keeping the thyroid tumors under discussion in a single category is the commonly observed merging of patterns and their essentially identical natural history. The issue raised by undifferentiated small cell carcinoma is very different. In the past it has been regarded as a distinctive form of undifferentiated carcinoma, and even subdivided into diffuse and compact subtypes (56). Currently, it is accepted that nearly all thyroid tumors reported in the old literature as diffuse small cell undifferentiated carcinomas represent malignant lymphomas instead (57–62).

As far as the compact subtype is concerned, it is a heterogeneous group. Some, probably most, tumors in this category are variants of medullary carcinoma with a prominent nesting pattern, predominance of small cells, and scanty or no amyloid (see chapter 12). Others are examples of poorly differentiated (insular) carcinoma in which follicles are scanty or absent (see chapter 8) (63). Others are analogous in all respects to small cell carcinoma of the lung and, as such, usually exhibit evidence of neuroendocrine differentiation (see chapter 12). Yet another type has recently been described as having a basaloid appearance and being possibly related histogenetically to solid cell nests (64).

It could be argued that because the aforementioned malignant tumors are epithelial, mostly undifferentiated (at least by conventional techniques), and composed of small cells, it is accurate to call them small cell carcinomas. It is obvious, however, that their natural histories and associations are so different from those of bona fide undifferentiated carcinoma that placing them into the same category would be highly misleading. We believe that the use of the term undifferentiated small cell carcinoma without a qualifier should be avoided.

Additional thyroid tumors that we would include into the generic category of undifferentiated carcinomas are the exceptionally rare *rhabdoid tumor* (65–67) and *lymphoepithelioma-like carcinoma* (68,69). The latter, in contrast with its most common counterpart in the nasopharynx, has not shown evidence of Epstein-Barr virus participation (69).

MOLECULAR AND CYTOLOGIC FINDINGS

See chapters 19 and 20.

DIFFERENTIAL DIAGNOSIS

The differential diagnosis of undifferentiated carcinoma includes a long list of entities, depending on the pattern of growth they may exhibit. True sarcoma can be primary in the thyroid gland or can reach the gland through direct invasion or metastatic spread from a soft tissue site. As already indicated, undifferentiated carcinoma may simulate a variety of soft tissue sarcomas, including fibrosarcoma, malignant fibrous histiocytoma, myxofibrosarcoma, malignant hemangiopericytoma, and angiosarcoma (malignant hemangioendothelioma). Features favoring the diagnosis of undifferentiated carcinoma are the presence of recognizable epithelial foci, immunohistochemical positivity for keratin, and ultrastructural presence of desmosomes and microvilli. In general, the diagnosis of undifferentiated carcinoma should be favored in the presence of any pleomorphic malignant tumor that seems to arise in the thyroid gland, especially if the patient is elderly and if there is evidence of a residual better-differentiated epithelial neoplasm in the gland, even if no clear-cut evidence of epithelial differentiation is found by any technique. Under these circumstances, the diagnosis of "undifferentiated malignant tumor, consistent with carcinoma" is justified. The only possible exception to this is angiosarcoma, a tumor discussed in chapter 13.

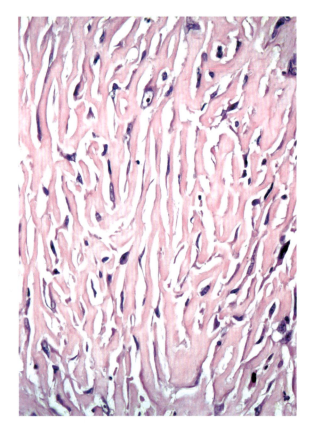

Figure 9-24

**PAUCICELLULAR VARIANT OF
UNDIFFERENTIATED (ANAPLASTIC) CARCINOMA**

The scanty atypia of the tumor cells and the heavy hyaline background may result in a mistaken diagnosis of Riedel thyroiditis.

The solid variant of papillary thyroid carcinoma retains the nuclear features of the more conventional types of papillary carcinoma, mitotic activity is minimal, and pleomorphism is not pronounced. Poorly differentiated carcinoma of the insular type has a nesting arrangement, uniformity in size and shape of the small round tumor cells, focal microfollicular differentiation, and immunohistochemical positivity for thyroglobulin.

Diagnostic confusion is more likely to arise with the spindle cell and pleomorphic variants of medullary carcinoma (70,71). The latter is particularly prone to misinterpretation because of the presence of bizarre cellular forms with monstrous nuclei. In most instances, however, these features are accompanied by areas with a more conventional appearance. Stains for calcitonin and chromogranin, ideally supplemented by an electron microscopic examination, will point to the correct diagnosis.

Malignant lymphoma still constitutes the most common source of diagnostic error. The cells of malignant lymphoma are more evenly distributed, smaller, more uniform in size, and have a rounder shape than those of undifferentiated carcinoma. Intraluminal packing of entrapped follicles by tumor cells is a common feature (58). Stains for CD45 are generally positive, whereas keratin is invariably negative. The adjacent thyroid gland is likely to exhibit changes of Hashimoto thyroiditis.

In metastatic tumors, multiple nodules are usually present, and their margins are likely to be sharper. Most of them exhibit a lesser degree of pleomorphism than undifferentiated thyroid carcinoma.

The so-called paucicellular variant of undifferentiated thyroid carcinoma can simulate the fibrous variant of Riedel thyroiditis, a sclerosing inflammatory process, because of the massive deposition of fibrohyaline stroma and scantiness of tumor cells (figs. 9-24, 9-25). A useful clue in this situation is that the blood vessels within the undifferentiated carcinoma will often show clearly malignant cells in their wall (fig. 9-25) (72,73).

SPREAD AND METASTASES

There are few tumors in the human body that tend to spread through all routes as quickly as undifferentiated thyroid carcinoma. Extrathyroid extension is the rule at the time of initial diagnosis. The tumor grows luxuriantly in the soft tissues of the neck, surrounds and invades the major vessels and nerves of the region, and spreads into the larynx, trachea, and esophagus (fig. 9-3) (74). Cases with prominent tracheal invasion may masquerade as primary tumors of this organ (75). Metastases to regional lymph nodes are common, although they are usually overshadowed by the massiveness of the primary growth; in contrast to other types of thyroid malignancy, they rarely are the first clinical manifestation of the disease. Blood-borne distant metastases are also frequent; the most common sites are adrenal gland, lung, bone, and gastrointestinal tract (figs. 9-26, 9-27).

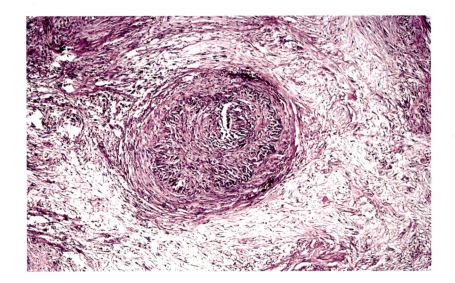

Figure 9-25

PAUCICELLULAR VARIANT OF UNDIFFERENTIATED (ANAPLASTIC) CARCINOMA

The presence of viable tumor cells in the wall of this vessel allows the identification of the tumor.

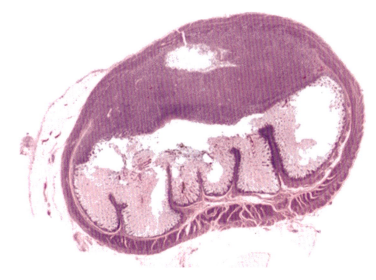

Figure 9-26

UNDIFFERENTIATED (ANAPLASTIC) CARCINOMA.

Top: Metastasis of undifferentiated thyroid carcinoma to the wall of the bowel.

Bottom: Multiple metastases of undifferentiated thyroid carcinoma to the stomach. Most show an ulcerated center (inset) (Top and bottom courtesy of Dr. C. Siderides, Stamford, CT.)

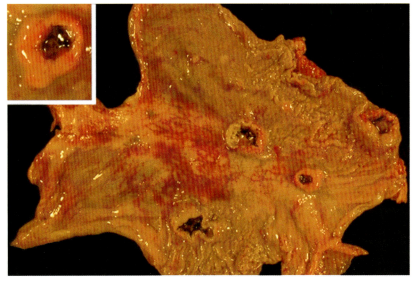

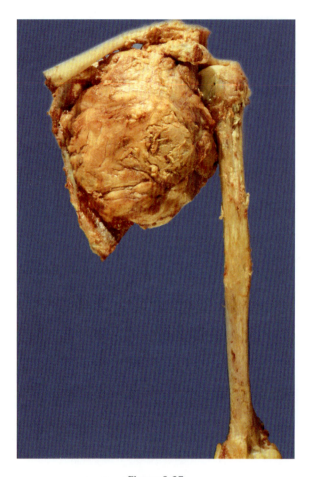

Figure 9-27

UNDIFFERENTIATED (ANAPLASTIC) CARCINOMA

A massive bone metastasis is centered in the scapula. This was the initial presentation of this thyroid tumor. (Courtesy of Dr. J. J. Segura, San José, Costa Rica.)

TREATMENT AND PROGNOSIS

Surgical excision is the first line of therapy, although in most cases the tumor is so widespread that total removal is impossible. It is more likely to be effective for the small undifferentiated tumors found incidentally in an otherwise well-differentiated neoplasm, but unfortunately this is rare. Suppression of thyroid function and administration of ^{131}I are of no value. Postoperative radiation therapy is generally administered but has proved ineffective in most cases. Many chemotherapeutic agents have been tried, singly or in combination. Initial tumor regression can be obtained with some regularity, and this may render a previously inoperable tumor amenable to surgical excision; however, in nearly all cases, the tumor quickly recurs and kills the patient. Currently, the best chances for cure, however slim, are obtained with a combination of surgery, radiation therapy, and multidrug chemotherapy (76–79).

Undifferentiated thyroid carcinoma is fatal in nearly all cases (80,81). In the series of Carcangiu et al. (1), all patients died as a result of tumor in weeks or months, the longest survival time being 2.5 years. In the series of Venkatesh et al. (22), the mean survival period was 7.2 to 10.0 months.

Unrestrained tumor growth in the neck is most often the cause of death, with widespread distant metastatic involvement accounting for the others. Casterline et al. (82) reviewed 10 series of undifferentiated carcinomas in a search for patients who had survived for 2 or more years after initial diagnosis. Only 14 were found among 420, i.e., 3.3 percent of the total. The real percentage is probably even lower, because some of these series were probably contaminated with malignant lymphomas and other tumor types (63,83). Nevertheless, indisputable cases of long-term cure of clinically obvious undifferentiated thyroid carcinoma exist. We have seen a case in which the patient was alive and well 8 years after the removal of an undifferentiated carcinoma that had spread to the soft tissues of the neck and metastasized to the lung. The best available survival figures are those reported by Aldinger et al. (76), with 4 survivors among 14 patients who had a combination of surgery, radiation therapy, and chemotherapy. The follow-up was short, however, and in most cases, the undifferentiated carcinoma was small. Small tumor size is said to be a favorable sign (74). It has also been claimed that the survival time is a little longer if there is residual well-differentiated tumor, if there is no evidence of extrathyroid extension, and if the patient is under 60 years old (84), but in most series, no significant difference has been noted (85–87).

NOSOLOGIC CONSIDERATIONS

A significant number of undifferentiated carcinomas are topographically and probably causally associated with a preexisting well-differentiated thyroid tumor or, more rarely, with a poorly differentiated (including insular) carcinoma (figs. 9-28, 9-29) (52,88,89). The admixture

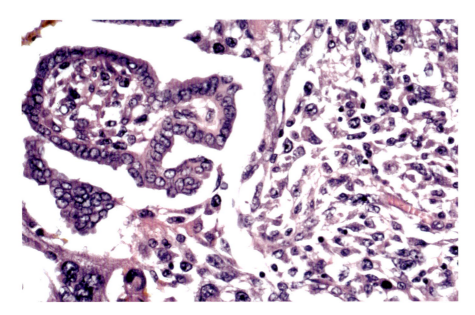

Figure 9-28

PAPILLARY CARCINOMA WITH UNDIFFERENTIATED (ANAPLASTIC) TRANSFORMATION

The two components are sharply segregated.

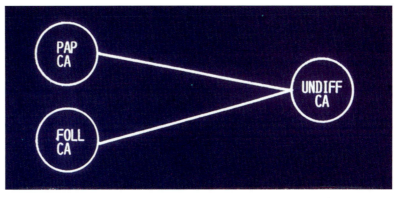

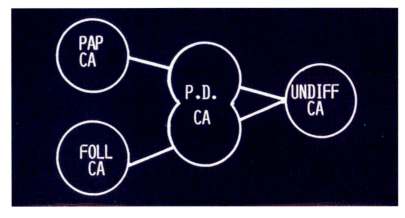

Figure 9-29

POSSIBLE RELATIONSHIP AMONG MAJOR TYPES OF CARCINOMA COMPOSED OF FOLLICULAR CELLS

Top: Well-differentiated (papillary and follicular) carcinomas can undergo a transformation into undifferentiated carcinoma in an abrupt fashion, without recognizable intermediate steps.

Bottom: Well-differentiated carcinomas of either type can progress to poorly differentiated carcinoma, and the latter may evolve into an undifferentiated carcinoma. The more atypical the tumor, the more difficult (and the less significant) the nature and very presence of a well-differentiated component becomes.

can be seen in the initial pathologic specimen, or the higher grade tumor may develop months or years after the removal of a well-differentiated neoplasm. The incidence of this occurrence in undifferentiated carcinoma varies from 8.5 percent (87) to 80 percent (90). The lower fig-ures probably represent underestimates, either because the sampling was not thorough or because the undifferentiated or poorly differentiated component was so extensive that it totally obliterated the other. It may be that all undifferentiated carcinomas arise in association with a well-differentiated tumor, as some authors have suggested (90). Occasionally, well-differentiated, poorly differentiated, and undifferentiated patterns coexist in metastatic foci. More rarely, the higher-grade transformation supervenes only in a local recurrence or metastasis of a well-differentiated tumor (91).

All major types of thyroid carcinoma of follicular cell derivation are susceptible to this change (figs. 9-28, 9-29). In some series, the follicular tumors greatly predominate (46,90), whereas in others there is a preponderance of papillary carcinoma, including the Warthin tumor-like variant (4,92,93). It is not clear whether this represents a true difference, perhaps geographically based, or is simply the result of variations in diagnostic criteria.

There is no relationship between the type of well-differentiated carcinoma and the pattern of undifferentiated carcinoma that it may give rise to, except between papillary carcinoma and the squamoid or squamous type of undifferentiated carcinoma (94) and specifically between the tall cell variant of papillary carcinoma and the spindle cell form of squamous cell carcinoma, an association that can be present in several guises (95,96). Fortunately, the probability of an anaplastic transformation occurring in any of the well-differentiated thyroid neoplasms is very low, probably not higher than 1 or 2 percent.

It has been suggested that anaplastic transformation may be induced in these tumors by the administration of radioactive iodine (97,98) or external radiation therapy. Kapp et al. (99) found 60 cases of this association. Regardless of whether the radiation is related causally to the transformation, the event is so rare that it should not interfere with the administration of radiation therapy if this is necessary to control unresectable, locally recurrent, or metastatic well-differentiated thyroid carcinomas (76). On the other hand, this potential danger should be kept in mind when considering prophylactic administration of ^{131}I after surgical removal of a papillary carcinoma, especially because the benefit of this approach is far from proven.

Another antecedent mentioned in some series of undifferentiated carcinomas is a history of longstanding goiter. The incidence quoted is around 40 percent in most series but substantially higher in others (76,100). Perhaps related to this is the observation that undifferentiated carcinoma has a higher incidence in areas of endemic goiter and that its frequency in those areas has decreased with the introduction of iodine prophylaxis (101).

An interesting model for human undifferentiated thyroid carcinoma is represented by a thyroid tumor induced in mice by sustained stimulation of the gland with endogenous thyrotropic hormone-secreting tumors. One such tumor, originally thyrotropic hormone dependent, able to trap ^{131}I, and composed of papillary or follicular structures, became transformed after 7 years of serial transplantation into a pure sarcomatoid growth, one line with and the other without osteoclast-like giant cells (102).

Another animal model that is relevant to the issue of histogenesis of undifferentiated thyroid carcinoma is that described by Greenburg and Hay (103). The authors showed that follicular epithelium from normal rat thyroid gland growing in tridimensional collagen gels moved into the matrix, acquired mesenchymal-like morphologic and immunohistochemical features, and lost immunoreactivity for thyroglobulin.

REFERENCES

1. Carcangiu ML, Steeper T, Zampi G, Rosai J. Anaplastic thyroid carcinoma. A study of 70 cases. Am J Clin Pathol 1985;83:135-58.

2. Shoumacher P, Metz R, Bey P, Chesneau AM. Anaplastic carcinoma of the thyroid gland. Eur J Cancer 1977;13:381-3.

3. Pichardo-Lowden A, Durvesh S, Douglas S, Todd W, Bruno M, Goldenberg D. Anaplastic thyroid carcinoma in a young woman: a rare case of survival. Thyroid 2009;19:775-9.

4. Albores Saavedra J, Alcántara Vázquez A, Meza Chávez L, de la Garza T, Rodriguez Martinez HA. Carcinoma anaplásico de células fusiformes y gigantes del tiroides: estudio de 63 casos. Prensa Med Mex 1972;37:421-6.

5. Barr R, Dann F. Anaplastic thyroid carcinoma metastatic to skin. J Cutan Pathol 1974;1:201-6.

6. Phillips DL, Benner KG, Keeffe EB, Traweek ST. Isolated metastasis to small bowel from anaplastic thyroid carcinoma. With a review of extra-abdominal malignancies that spread to the bowel. J Clin Gastroenterol 1987;9:563-7.

7. Oppenheim A, Miller M, Anderson GH Jr, Davis B, Slagle T. Anaplastic thyroid cancer presenting with hyperthyroidism. Am J Med 1983;75:702-4.

8. Slatkin DN, Pearson J. Intramyofiber metastases in skeletal muscle. Hum Pathol 1976;7:347-9.

9. Hashimoto H, Koga S, Watanabe H, Enjoji M. Undifferentiated carcinoma of the thyroid gland with osteoclast-like giant cells. Acta Pathol Jpn 1980;30:323-34.

10. Silverberg SG, DeGiorgi LS. Osteoclastoma-like giant cell tumor of the thyroid. Report of a case with prolonged survival following partial excision and radiotherapy. Cancer 1973;31:621-5.

11. Gaffey MJ, Lack EE, Christ ML, Weiss LM. Anaplastic thyroid carcinoma with osteoclast-like giant cells. A clinicopathologic, immunohistochemical, and ultrastructural study. Am J Surg Pathol 1991;15:160-8.

12. Agnantis NT, Rosen PP. Mammary carcinoma with osteoclast-like giant cells. A study of eight cases with follow-up data. Am J Clin Pathol 1979; 72:383-9.

13. Blasius S, Edel G, Grünert J, Böcker W, Schmid KW. Anaplastic thyroid carcinoma with osteosarcomatous differentiation. Pathol Res Pract 1994;190:507-10.

14. Carda C, Ferrer J, Vilanova M, Peydró A, Llombart-Bosch A. Anaplastic carcinoma of the thyroid with rhabdomyosarcomatous differentiation: a report of two cases. Virchows Arch 2005;446:46-51.

15. Olthof M, Persoon AC, Plukker JT, van der Wal JE, Links TP. Anaplastic thyroid carcinoma with rhabdomyoblastic differentiation: a case report with a good clinical outcome. Endocr Pathol 2008;19:62-5.

16. Donnell CA, Pollock WJ, Sybers WA. Thyroid carcinosarcoma. Arch Pathol Lab Med 1987;111:1169-72.

17. Miettinen M, Franssila KO. Variable expression of keratins and nearly uniform lack of thyroid transcription factor 1 in thyroid anaplastic carcinoma. Hum Pathol 2000;31:1139-45.

18. Hurlimann J, Gardiol D, Scazziga B. Immunohistology of anaplastic thyroid carcinoma. A study of 43 cases. Histopathology 1987;11:567-80.

19. Miettinen M, Franssila K, Lehto VP, Paasivuo R, Virtanen I. Expression of intermediate filament proteins in thyroid gland and thyroid tumors. Lab Invest 1984;50:262-70.

20. Ordóñez NG, el-Naggar AK, Hickey RC, Samaan NA. Anaplastic thyroid carcinoma. Immunocytochemical study of 32 cases. Am J Clin Pathol 1991;96:15-24.

21. Tötsch M, Dobler G, Feichtinger H, Sandbichler P, Ladurner D, Schmid KW. Malignant hemangioendothelioma of the thyroid. Its immunohistochemical discrimination from undifferentiated thyroid carcinoma. Am J Surg Pathol 1990;14:69-74.

22. Venkatesh YS, Ordóñez NG, Schultz PN, Hickey RC, Goepfert H, Samaan NA. Anaplastic carcinoma of the thyroid. A clinicopathologic study of 121 cases. Cancer 1990;66:321-30.

23. Kobayashi S, Yamadori I, Ohmori M, Kurokawa T, Umeda M. Anaplastic carcinoma of the thyroid with osteoclast-like giant cells. An ultrastructural and immunohistochemical study. Acta Pathol Jpn 1987;37:807-15.

24. Cuevas-Alvarez E, Forteza-Vila J. Carcinoma anaplásico de tiroides. Estudio inmunohistoquímico de 15 casos. Patología 1991;24:287-95.

25. Preto A, Reis-Filho JS, Ricardo S, Soares P. P63 expression in papillary and anaplastic carcinomas of the thyroid gland: lack of an oncogenetic role in tumorigenesis and progression. Pathol Res Pract 2002;198:449-54.

26. Kim YW, Do IG, Park YK. Expression of the GLUT1 glucose transporter, p63 and p53 in thyroid carcinomas. Pathol Res Pract 2006;202:759-65.

27. Miettinen M, Virtanen I. Expression of laminin in thyroid gland and thyroid tumors: an immunohistologic study. Int J Cancer 1984;34:27-30.

28. Bishop JA, Sharma R, Westra WH. PAX8 immunostaining of anaplastic thyroid carcinoma: a reliable means of discerning thyroid origin for undifferentiated tumors of the head and neck. Hum Pathol 2011;42:1873-7.

29. Becker N, Chernock RD, Nussenbaum B, Lewis JS Jr. Prognostic significance of β-human chorionic gonadotropin and PAX8 expression in anaplastic thyroid carcinoma. Thyroid 2014;24:319-26.

30. Buehler D, Hardin H, Shan W, Rehrauer W, Chen H, Lloyd RV. Expression of epithelial-mesenchymal transition regulators slug and twist in thyroid carcinomas. Lab Invest 2012;92:142-3A (abstract).

31. Albores-Saavedra J, Nadji M, Civantos F, Morales AR. Thyroglobulin in carcinoma of the thyroid: an immunohistochemical study. Hum Pathol 1983;14:62-6.

32. Böcker W, Dralle H, Husselmann H, Bay B, Brassow M. Immunohistochemical analysis of thyroglobulin synthesis in thyroid carcinomas. Virchows Arch A Pathol Anat Histol 1980;385:187-200.

33. Burt A, Goudie RB. Diagnosis of primary thyroid carcinoma by immunohistological demonstration of thyroglobulin. Histopathology 1979;3:279-86.

34. Kawaoi A, Okano T, Nemoto N, Shiina T, Shikata T. Simultaneous detection of thyroglobulin (Tg), thyroxine (T4), and triiodothyronine (T3) in nontoxic thyroid tumors by the immunoperoxidase method. Am J Pathol 1982;108:39-49.

35. Lo Gerfo P, LiVolsi V, Colacchio D, Feind C. Thyroglobulin production by thyroid cancers. J Surg Res 1978;24:1-6.

36. Shvero J, Gal R, Avidor I, Hadar T, Kessler E. Anaplastic thyroid carcinoma. A clinical, histologic and immunohistochemical study. Cancer 1988;62:319-25.

37. Eusebi V, Bondi A, Rosai J. Immunohistochemical localization of myoglobin in nonmuscular cells. Am J Surg Pathol 1984;8:51-5.

38. LiVolsi VA, Brooks JJ, Arendash-Durand B. Anaplastic thyroid tumors. Immunohistology. Am J Clin Pathol 1987;87:434-42.

39. Ryff-de Lèche A, Staub JJ, Kohler-Faden R, Müller-Brand J, Heitz PU. Thyroglobulin production by malignant thyroid tumors. An immunocytochemical and radioimmunoassay study. Cancer 1986;57:1145-53.

40. Nonaka D, Tang Y, Chiriboga L, Rivera M, Ghossein R. Diagnostic utility of thyroid transcription factors Pax8 and TTF-2 (FoxE1) in thyroid epithelial neoplasms. Mod Pathol 2008;21:192-200.

41. Wilson NW, Pambakian H, Richardson TC, Stokoe MR, Makin CA, Heyderman E. Epithelial markers in thyroid carcinoma: an immunoperoxidase study. Histopathology 1986;10:815-29.

42. Nieuwenhuijzen Kruseman AC, Bosman FT, van Bergen Henegouw JC, Cramer-Knijnenburg G, Brutel de la Riviere G. Medullary differentiation of anaplastic thyroid carcinoma. Am J Clin Pathol 1982;77:541-7.

43. Pilotti S, Collini P, Del Bo R, Cattoretti G, Pierotti MA, Rilke F. A novel panel of antibodies that segregates immunocytochemically poorly differentiated carcinoma from undifferentiated carcinoma of the thyroid gland. Am J Surg Pathol 1994;18:1054-64.

44. Erickson LA, Jin L, Wollan PC, Thompson GB, van Heerden J, Lloyd RV. Expression of p27kip1 and Ki-67 in benign and malignant thyroid tumors. Mod Pathol 1998;11:169-74.

45. Tallini G, García-Rostán G, Herrero A, et al. Downregulation of p27KIP1 and Ki67/Mib1 labeling index support the classification of thyroid carcinoma into prognostically relevant categories. Am J Surg Pathol 1999;23:678-85.

46. Wang HM, Huang YW, Huang JS, et al. Anaplastic carcinoma of the thyroid arising more often from follicular carcinoma than papillary carcinoma. Ann Surg Oncol 2007;14:3011-8.

47. Saltman B, Singh B, Hedvat CV, Wreesmann VB, Ghossein R. Patterns of expression of cell cycle/apoptosis genes along the spectrum of thyroid carcinoma progression. Surgery 2006;140:899-905.

48. Donghi R, Longoni A, Pilotti S, Michieli P, Della Porta G, Pierotti MA. Gene p53 mutations are restricted to poorly differentiated and undifferentiated carcinomas of the thyroid gland. J Clin Invest 1993;91:1753-60.

49. Dobashi Y, Sugimura H, Sakamoto A, et al. Stepwise participation of p53 gene mutation during dedifferentiation of human thyroid carcinomas. Diagn Mol Pathol 1994;3:9-14.

50. Quiros RM, Ding HG, Gattuso P, Prinz RA, Xu X. Evidence that one subset of anaplastic thyroid carcinomas are derived from papillary carcinomas due to BRAF and p53 mutations. Cancer 2005;103:2261-8.

51. Wang S, Lloyd RV, Hutzler MJ, Safran MS, Patwardhan NA, Khan A. The role of cell cycle regulatory protein, cyclin D1, in the progression of thyroid cancer. Mod Pathol 2000;13:882-7.

52. Fisher ER, Gregorio R, Shoemaker R, Horvat B, Hubay C. The derivation of so-called "giant-cell" and "spindle-cell" undifferentiated thyroidal neoplasms. Am J Clin Pathol 1974;61:680-9.

53. Hayashi Y, Tokuoka S. Anaplastic carcinoma of the thyroid gland. An ultrastructural study of four cases. Acta Pathol Jpn 1979;29:119-33.

54. Jao W, Gould VE. Ultrastructure of anaplastic (spindle and giant cell) carcinoma of the thyroid. Cancer 1975;35:1280-92.

55. Newland JR, Mackay B, Hill CS Jr, Hickey RC. Anaplastic thyroid carcinoma: an ultrastructural study of 10 cases. Ultrastruct Pathol 1981;2:121-9.

56. Meissner WA, Phillips MJ. Diffuse small-cell carcinoma of the thyroid. Arch Pathol 1962;74:291-7.

57. Burke JS, Butler JJ, Fuller LM. Malignant lymphomas of the thyroid: a clinical pathologic study of 35 patients including ultrastructural observations. Cancer 1977;39:1587-602.

58. Compagno J, Oertel JE. Malignant lymphoma and other lymphoproliferative disorders of the thyroid gland. A clinicopathologic study of 245 cases. Am J Clin Pathol 1980;74:1-11.

59. Heimann R, Vannineuse A, De Sloover C, Dor P. Malignant lymphomas and undifferentiated small cell carcinoma of the thyroid: a clinicopathological review in the light of the Kiel classification for malignant lymphomas. Histopathology 1978;2:201-13.

60. Rayfield EJ, Nishiyama RH, Sisson JC. Small cell tumors of the thyroid. Cancer 1971;28:1023-30.

61. Schmid KW, Kroll M, Hofstadter F, Ladurner D. Small cell carcinoma of the thyroid. A reclassification of cases originally diagnosed as small cell carcinomas of the thyroid. Pathol Res Pract 1986;181:540-3.

62. Wolf BC, Sheahan K, DeCoste D, Variakojis D, Alpern HD, Haselow RE. Immunohistochemical analysis of small cell tumors of the thyroid gland: an Eastern Cooperative Oncology Group study. Hum Pathol 1992;23:1252-61.

63. Carcangiu ML, Zampi G, Rosai J. Poorly differentiated ("insular") thyroid carcinoma. A reinterpretation of Langhans' "wuchernde Struma." Am J Surg Pathol 1984;8:655-68.

64. Cruz J, Eloy C, Aragüés JM, Vinagre J, Sobrinho-Simões M. Small-cell (basaloid) thyroid carcinoma: a neoplasm with a solid cell nest histogenesis? Int J Surg Pathol 2011;19:620-6.

65. Chetty R, Govender D. Follicular thyroid carcinoma with rhabdoid phenotype. Virchows Arch 1999;435:133-6.

66. Lai ML, Faa G, Serra S, et al. Rhabdoid tumor of the thyroid gland: a variant of anaplastic carcinoma. Arch Pathol Lab Med 2005;129:e55-7.

67. Albores-Saavedra J, Sharma S. Poorly differentiated follicular thyroid carcinoma with rhabdoid phenotype: a clinicopathologic, immunohistochemical and electron microscopic study of two cases. Mod Pathol 2001;14:98-104.

68. Dominguez-Malagon H, Flores-Flores G, Vilchis JJ. Lymphoepithelioma-like anaplastic thyroid carcinoma: report of a case not related to Epstein-Barr virus. Ann Diagn Pathol 2001;5:21-4.

69. Shek TW, Luk IS, Ng IO, Lo CY. Lymphoepithelioma-like carcinoma of the thyroid gland: lack of evidence of association with Epstein-Barr virus. Hum Pathol 1996;27:851-3.

70. Kakudo K, Miyauchi A, Ogihara T, et al. Medullary carcinoma of the thyroid. Giant cell type. Arch Pathol Lab Med 1978;102:445-7.

71. Mendelsohn G, Baylin SB, Bigner SH, Wells SA Jr, Eggleston JC. Anaplastic variants of medullary thyroid carcinoma: a light microscopic and immunohistochemical study. Am J Surg Pathol 1980;4:333-41.

72. Canos JC, Serrano A, Matias-Guiu X. Paucicellular variant of anaplastic thyroid carcinoma: report of two cases. Endocr Pathol 2001;12:157-61.

73. Wan SK, Chan JK, Tang SK. Paucicellular variant of anaplastic thyroid carcinoma. A mimic of Riedel's thyroiditis. Am J Clin Pathol 1996;105:388-93.

74. Nel CJ, van Heerden JA, Goellner JR, et al. Anaplastic carcinoma of the thyroid: a clinicopathologic study of 82 cases. Mayo Clin Proc 1985;60:51-8.

75. Banville NM, Timon CI, Bermingham NJ, Toner ME. Anaplastic and squamous thyroid carcinoma masquerading as primary mucosal squamous cell carcinoma of the trachea: morphologic and immunohistochemical findings. Lab Invest 2009;89:245A (abstract).

76. Aldinger KA, Samaan NA, Ibanez M, Hill CS Jr. Anaplastic carcinoma of the thyroid: a review of 84 cases of spindle and giant cell carcinoma of the thyroid. Cancer 1978;41:2267-75.

77. Kim JH, Leeper RD. Treatment of anaplastic giant and spindle cell carcinoma of the thyroid gland with combination Adriamycin and radiation therapy. A new approach. Cancer 1983;52:954-7.

78. Giuffrida D, Gharib H. Anaplastic thyroid carcinoma: current diagnosis and treatment. Ann Oncol 2000;11:1083-9.

79. Ito K, Hanamura T, Murayama K, et al. Multimodality therapeutic outcomes in anaplastic thyroid carcinoma: improved survival in subgroups of patients with localized primary tumors. Head Neck 2012;34:230-7.

80. McIver B, Hay ID, Giuffrida DF, et al. Anaplastic thyroid carcinoma: a 50-year experience at a single institution. Surgery 2001;130:1028-34.

81. Smallridge RC, Copland JA. Anaplastic thyroid carcinoma: pathogenesis and emerging therapies. Clin Oncol (R Coll Radiol) 2010;22:486-97.

82. Casterline PF, Jaques DA, Blom H, Wartofsky L. Anaplastic giant cell and spindle-cell carcinoma of the thyroid: a different therapeutic approach. Cancer 1980;45:1689-92.

83. Ain KB. Anaplastic thyroid carcinoma: behavior, biology, and therapeutic approaches. Thyroid 1998;8:715-26.

84. Kebebew E, Greenspan FS, Clark OH, Woeber KA, McMillan A. Anaplastic thyroid carcinoma. Treatment outcome and prognostic factors. Cancer 2005;103:1330-5.

85. Hutter RV, Tollefsen HR, De Cosse JJ, Foote FW Jr, Frazell EL. Spindle and giant cell metaplasia in papillary carcinoma of the thyroid. Am J Surg 1965;110:660-8.

86. Tallroth E, Wallin G, Lundell G, Lowhagen T, Einhorn J. Multimodality treatment in anaplastic giant cell thyroid carcinoma. Cancer 1987;60:1428-31.

87. Wychulis AR, Beahrs OH, Woolner LB. Papillary carcinoma with associated anaplastic carcinoma in the thyroid gland. Surg Gynecol Obstet 1965;120:28-34.

88. Harada T, Ito K, Shimaoka K, Hosoda Y, Yakumaru K. Fatal thyroid carcinoma. Anaplastic transformation of adenocarcinoma. Cancer 1977;39:2588-96.

89. Spires JR, Schwartz MR, Miller RH. Anaplastic thyroid carcinoma. Association with differentiated thyroid cancer. Arch Otolaryngol Head Neck Surg 1988;114:40-4.

90. Nishiyama RH, Dunn EL, Thompson NW. Anaplastic spindle-cell and giant-cell tumors of the thyroid gland. Cancer 1972;30:113-27.

91. Al-Qsous W, Miller ID. Anaplastic transformation in lung metastases of differentiated papillary thyroid carcinoma: an autopsy case report and review of the literature. Ann Diagn Pathol 2010;14:41-3.

92. Lam KY, Lo CY, Wei WI. Warthin tumor-like variant of papillary thyroid carcinoma: a case with dedifferentiation (anaplastic changes) and aggressive biological behavior. Endocr Pathol 2005;16:83-9.

93. Woolner LB, Beahrs OH, Black BM, McConahey WM, Keating FR Jr. Classification and prognosis of thyroid carcinomas. Am J Surg 1961; 102:354-87.

94. Katoh R, Sakamoto A, Kasai N, Yagawa K. Squamous differentiation in thyroid carcinoma with special reference to histogenesis of squamous cell carcinoma of the thyroid. Acta Pathol Jpn 1989;39:306-12.

95. Bronner MP, LiVolsi VA. Spindle cell squamous carcinoma of the thyroid: An unusual anaplastic tumor associated with tall cell papillary cancer. Mod Pathol 1991;4:637-43.

96. Gopal PP, Montone KT, Baloch Z, Tuluc M, LiVolsi V. The variable presentations of anaplastic spindle cell squamous carcinoma associated with tall cell variant of papillary thyroid carcinoma. Thyroid 2011;21:493-9.

97. Baker HW. Anaplastic thyroid cancer twelve years after radioiodine therapy. Cancer 1969; 23:885-90.

98. Crile G Jr, Wilson DH. Transformation of low grade papillary carcinoma of the thyroid to an anaplastic carcinoma after treatment with radioiodine. Surg Gynecol Obstet 1959;108:355-60.

99. Kapp DS, LiVolsi VA, Sanders MM. Anaplastic carcinoma following well-differentiated thyroid cancer: etiological considerations. Yale J Biol Med 1982;55:521-8.

100. Jereb B, Stjernswärd J, Lowhagen T. Anaplastic giant-cell carcinoma of the thyroid. A study of treatment and prognosis. Cancer 1975; 35:1293-5.

101. Hofstadter F. Frequency and morphology of malignant tumours of the thyroid before and after the introduction of iodine prophylaxis. Virchows Arch A Pathol Anat Histol 1980;385:263-70.

102. Ueda G, Furth J. Sarcomatoid transformation of transplanted thyroid carcinoma. Similarity to anaplastic human thyroid carcinoma. Arch Pathol 1967;83:3-12.

103. Greenburg G, Hay ED. Cytoskeleton and thyroglobulin expression change during transformation of thyroid epithelium to mesenchyme-like cells. Development 1988;102:605-22.

10 THYROID TUMORS WITH ONCOCYTIC (HÜRTHLE CELL) FEATURES

Thyroid tumors in which 75 percent or more of the cells have the appearance of oncocytes are placed into the *oncocytic (Hürthle cell)* category. Obviously, this is an arbitrary decision since follicular adenomas, follicular carcinomas, and papillary carcinomas exist in which 30, 40, or 50 percent of the cells are oncocytic, indicating that we are dealing with a spectrum rather than two distinct groups (figs. 10-1, 10-2). In practice, such a precise quantitative evaluation is rare since most thyroid neoplasms are either composed entirely or almost entirely of oncocytes or feature them in small, inconspicuous clusters. Notably, oncocytic and nononcocytic follicular cells may coexist in the same follicle (1).

GENERAL CONSIDERATIONS

Terminology and Identification of Oncocytic Cells. The subject of thyroid neoplasms composed of oncocytes is one of the most controversial in

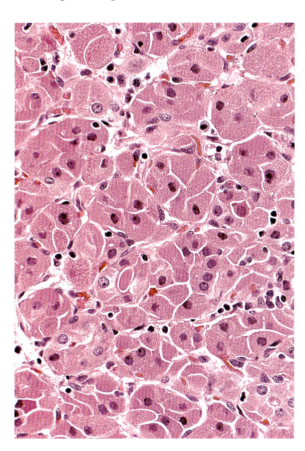

Figure 10-1

ONCOCYTIC TUMOR

This thyroid tumor is entirely composed of oncocytic follicular cells.

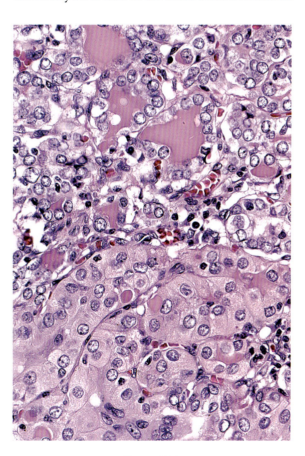

Figure 10-2

PAPILLARY CARCINOMA WITH ONCOCYTIC FEATURES

There is an admixture of oncocytic and nononcocytic cells.

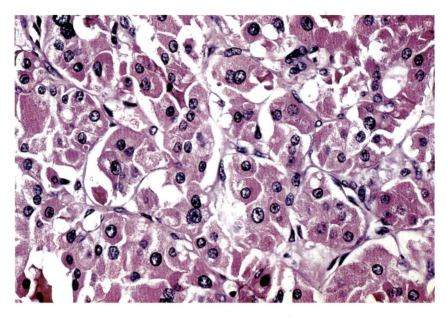

Figure 10-3

ONCOCYTES

The abundant cytoplasm of these follicular cells is packed with eosinophilic granules.

thyroid pathology. This controversy involves several related issues that should be discussed individually (2,3).

The follicular cells crowded with mitochondria that characterize the tumors described in this chapter have been variously designated *Hürthle cells, Askanazy cells, oxyphilic cells, large cells*, and *oncocytes* (4–6). It has been repeatedly pointed out that "Hürthle cell" is a misnomer. The cells that Hürthle described in the thyroid gland of dogs were probably C-cells (5,7), whereas Askanazy (5) provided instead a very accurate and pictorially beautiful demonstration of the cells discussed in this chapter. The term oxyphilic cell suffers from a lack of specificity. It has the same meaning as acidophilic cell, and therefore, could be applied to many cell types in addition to those that are the subject of this section. The designation large cell is too generic. The term oncocyte is probably the most appropriate, and is certainly the most widely used (8,9). Although etymologically oncocyte simply means "swollen cell," its use is restricted in the thyroid gland and other sites to the cell under discussion. We have chosen to use it in this section, with the understanding that the designation *Hürthle cell neoplasm* is too entrenched (especially among American clinicians and surgeons) to be expunged easily.

The identification of a cell as an oncocyte was initially based on the presence of abundant granular acidophilic cytoplasm (fig. 10-3). Only later did special (supravital) stains, such as Janus green, and ultrastructural and enzyme histochemical studies reveal that this granularity was due to the presence of a large number of mitochondria (10). Since acidophilic cytoplasmic granularity rarely is due to a richness in granular endoplasmic reticulum (ergastoplasm), some authors have suggested that granular acidophilic follicular cells (and their tumors) be divided on the basis of their ultrastructural appearance into mitochondrion-rich and ergastoplasm-rich, and that only the former be equated with oncocytes. This seems an impractical and potentially confusing policy, and we have not followed it in this section. Other authors thought it was important to distinguish between mitochondrion-rich cells and oncocytes. Tremblay and Pearse (10) stated that only in the latter is the accumulation of mitochondria so extreme as to result in the loss of cell polarity. Others have used the same distinction, pointing out that in oncocytes, but not in other nononcocytic mitochondria-rich cells, mitochondria accumulate preferentially in the basal portion of the cell, displacing the endoplasmic reticulum to its apical part (11).

The validity of distinctions too subtle to be reproducible may be questioned. It is important, however, to recognize that some cells, including some neoplastic thyroid cells, like those of tall cell papillary carcinoma, are rich in mitochondria. They feature a distinctive "oncocytoid" appearance, but they do not qualify as oncocytic cells because the accumulation of mitochondria is not extreme and the cell maintains its polarity. The term "mitochondria rich" can thus be used in a descriptive sense but not as synonym for "oncocytic" (10).

The cytoplasmic acidophilia must be granular for the cell to be defined as oncocytic. Diffuse or fibrillary acidophilia is usually due to the accumulation of cytoplasmic filaments and therefore represents an unrelated phenomenon (12). Although neoplastic C-cells also undergo oncocytic change, the term oncocyte, when applied to the thyroid gland without a qualifier, refers to a variant of follicular cell. As such, this cell possesses an intact thyroid-stimulating hormone receptor-adenylate cyclase system, even in the neoplastic state (13).

Nature of the Oncocyte. The molecular alterations leading to the accumulation of mitochondria that defines an oncocyte have been investigated in the thyroid gland, as well as in other organs (2). Most of the work has been carried out on tumors, both because of their relevance and because it is easier to analyze them than to study non-neoplastic cells that occur singly or in small groups. Many of the studies have focused on mitochondrial DNA, i.e., the remnant of the DNA of the aerobic bacteria that colonized the primitive eukaryotic cell that was unable to utilize oxygen to produce energy. In humans, this DNA encodes 13 respiratory chain subunits that are crucial for the efficiency of oxidative phosphorylation. Mitochondrial DNA is an obvious candidate, also considering that the accumulation of mitochondria is a characteristic feature of many mitochondrial encephalomyopathies, a class of neuromuscular degenerative disorders with defined mitochondrial DNA alterations (2).

The increased amount of mitochondrial DNA (14) is often associated with somatic mitochondrial DNA alterations, including both small mutations (point mutations or insertion/deletions of a few nucleotides) and large deletions (14–16). In particular, the "common mtDNA deletion," often reported in cancer and ageing and consisting of a 4977bp stretch of lost mitochondrial DNA, is present with increased frequency and represents a higher proportion of mitochondrial DNA molecules in neoplastic than in non-neoplastic oncocytic cells (15,16). These mitochondrial DNA abnormalities, however, occur also in many other tumors that do not have oncocytic features (16). Because of the properties of mitochondrial DNA, which include a high mutation rate, the coexistence of several DNA variants in the mitochondria of a single cell, and the presence of a critical proportion of mutated mitochondrial DNA molecules necessary for a deficit to become apparent (i.e., the threshold effect), it has been difficult to demonstrate that these DNA alterations cause a cell to become an oncocyte (17). A series of studies conducted in the last few years has shown that the biochemical, metabolic, and phenotypic (i.e., accumulation of mitochondria) alterations of oncocytic cells are induced by defects in the mitochondrial DNA that encode for respiratory chain subunits, almost always those of the NADH dehydrogenase (ND, complex I of the respiratory chain), both in thyroid and extrathyroid oncocytic lesions (18–20).

Alterations of nuclear genes that code for mitochondrial proteins also cause mitochondrial dysfunction. Missense mutations of *GRIM19* (also termed *NDUFA13*), a nuclear gene coding a subunit of the respiratory complex I, have been found at the somatic level in oncocytic follicular and papillary carcinomas and as a germline mutation in one patient who developed an oncocytic variant of papillary carcinoma and multiple benign oncocytic thyroid nodules (21). If these complex I subunits are missing or defective, the respiratory chain complex may not properly assemble, resulting in impaired oxidative phosphorylation. Mutations of respiratory chain subunits and induction of a pro-tumorigenic "pseudohypoxic" state, mediated by increased levels of hypoxia-inducible factors, occur in paraganglioma and pheochromocytoma, where succinate dehydrogenase (SDH, complex II of the respiratory chain) subunits encoded by the nuclear DNA are defective (22). Hypoxia-inducible factors, of which Hif1α is the most studied, are responsible for the physiologic response to tissue hypoxia, which includes enhanced angiogenesis and induction of molecules that promote glycolysis.

Pseudohypoxia is believed to play a significant role in the development of several tumors, notably renal cell carcinoma, which is characterized by the loss of the von Hippel–Lindau tumor suppressor protein (pVHL) that is essential for Hif1α degradation. Recent studies have shown that in the case of oncocytic cells, the pathogenic lesions involving complex I result in the accumulation of Krebs cycle metabolites that instead of increasing Hif1α levels destabilize it (23). As a consequence, the cell with a complex I mutation cannot react to the pseudohypoxic condition, and is unable to overcome the mitochondrial defect by inducing angiogenesis or with more efficient glycolysis. The only solution is thus to increase the mass of (defective) mitochondria. This is exactly what happens, and the cell becomes oncocytic (23). Even the increased mitochondrial mass does not fully compensate for the defect. Since in oncocytic cells there is no Hif1α stabilization, glycolysis is not enhanced, there is no angiogenesis, and the blood supply to the tumor is poor (23). This explains the notorious tendency of oncocytic cells (in the thyroid and elsewhere) to undergo infarction. It also explains the reduced viability, slow proliferation, and generally benign behavior of many oncocytic lesions.

Oncocytoma as a Tumor Entity. The prevalent view at present is that thyroid tumors composed of oncocytic follicular cells should not be placed into a special category but rather classified on the basis of their architectural and nuclear features (independent of the presence and degree of oncocytic transformation) into follicular adenoma, follicular carcinoma, papillary carcinoma, or poorly differentiated carcinoma, using the criteria outlined in the respective chapters, followed by the qualifier *oncocytic variant* (7,24). The implication of this position is that the oncocytic change is a secondary event that has no effect on the natural history of the disease. Although we largely agree with this approach, we believe that tumors made up of this cell type have gross, microscopic, behavioral, cytogenetic, and conceivably, etiopathogenetic features that set them apart from their nononcocytic counterparts and justify discussing them in a separate section (6,15,25). A similar approach is taken in most other organs in which this phenomenon occurs, such as salivary gland and kidney.

Mechanisms for Oncocytic Change in Tumors. Sobrinho-Simões et al. (26) have proposed a highly original and appealing theory in an attempt to explain the relationship between onco-

cytic change and tumor development. It is based on the belief that the molecular alterations that lead to the development of a tumor containing oncocytes are of a possibly related, but independent, nature: those that render the follicular cell oncocytic and those that render it neoplastic, the issue being which comes first and which comes later. In Sobrinho-Simões' scheme, both sequences occur. In the first, a (non-neoplastic) thyroid follicular cell becomes oncocytic, and in a second step it becomes neoplastic. In the second sequence, a follicular cell gives rise to a tumor of one type or another, and in a second step some of the cells of that tumor become oncocytic. In the first scenario, all tumor cells are oncocytic since they all originate from a single oncocyte, the end result being a "true oncocytoma," whereas in the second scenario, the oncocytic change is partial because if affects only a portion of the tumor cell population, the end result being a tumor of one type or another "with oncocytic features" (26,27).

Alterations of mitochondria and oxidative metabolism promote tumor development in several ways that may affect apoptosis, the production of reactive oxygen species, the level and stability of hypoxia-inducible factors, and the occurrence of aerobic glycolysis (so called Warburg effect). However, if one of the pathogenic mitochondrial DNA mutations that affect complex I causing oncocytic change accumulates beyond a certain threshold, the cell cannot sustain the metabolic impairment and tumor growth is decreased. This is again consistent with reduced proliferation and a benign behavior for most oncocytic lesions (28).

The relationship between oxidative phosphorylation, cell metabolism, and cancer development is very complex. It is an area of active investigation, but to date, there is no proof that specific mitochondrial DNA mutations have a direct tumorigenic role (17–28).

Malignancy of Oncocytomas. It has been suggested by some that all thyroid oncocytic neoplasms should be regarded as malignant or potentially malignant and treated accordingly. Most authors, ourselves included, have taken a radically different view. Not only do we believe in the existence of both benign and malignant forms of this neoplasm, but maintain that the former predominate over the latter (6).

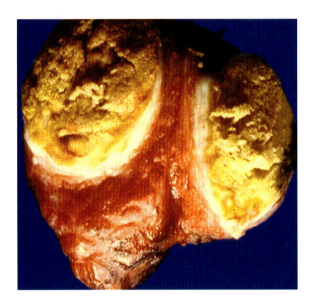

Figure 10-4

ONCOCYTIC NEOPLASM WITH MASSIVE INFARCT

The infarct in this tumor resulted from a fine-needle aspiration procedure. The entire tumor has a grumous appearance and is extremely friable.

ONCOCYTIC ADENOMA
(HÜRTHLE CELL ADENOMA)

Definition. *Oncocytic adenoma* is a benign thyroid neoplasm composed exclusively or predominantly (over 75 percent) of oncocytes. Synonyms include *follicular adenoma of oxyphilic cell type, Hürthle cell adenoma* (perhaps the most widely used), and *benign oncocytoma*.

Gross Findings. The tumor is completely encapsulated, round or oval, and usually solitary. In one large series, 20 percent were multiple. Some occurred in families, suggesting the existence of a germline mutation (29). The most distinctive gross feature of oncocytic adenoma (and oncocytic lesions in general) is the brown color of the cut surface, which directly correlates with the richness in mitochondria and is thought to be due to the cytochrome present in these organelles.

The tumor tends to be homogeneously solid, although secondary changes in the form of calcification, hemorrhage, cystic change, and central scarring are as likely to be present as in other forms of follicular adenoma. Sometimes, the entire tumor undergoes massive infarct-type necrosis, a type of complication to which oncocytomas of other organs (e.g., salivary glands) are also prone. This necrosis

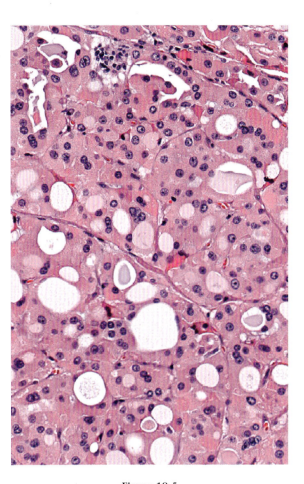

Figure 10-5

ONCOCYTIC NEOPLASM

The tumor is composed of solid and microfollicular areas.

may develop spontaneously or be induced by the performance of a fine-needle biopsy (30). At the gross level, this dramatic event results in a friable, grumous, deep brown mass with a bulging cut surface (fig. 10-4)

Microscopic Findings. This tumor shares most of the features of follicular adenoma of ordinary type (see chapter 5). The pattern of growth is usually follicular (fig. 10-5). It can also be trabecular or solid, but if either of these two patterns predominates, the index of suspicion for malignancy should rise. The intrafollicular colloid tends to be basophilic, in stark contrast with the deep red colloid often seen in the lumens of the neoplastic follicles present in the follicular variant of papillary carcinoma.

In the center of the follicle, round calcified bodies with concentric laminations that

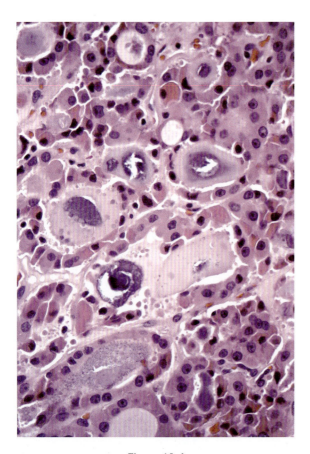

Figure 10-6

ONCOCYTIC NEOPLASM

The intraluminal colloid has a characteristic basophilic stain.

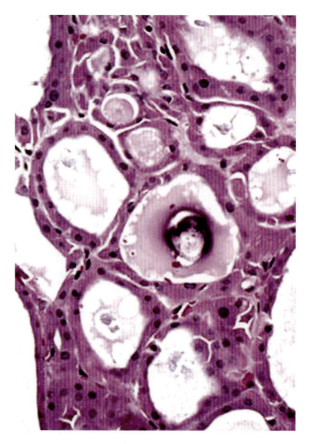

Figure 10-7

ONCOCYTIC NEOPLASM

A psammoma body-like formation is present in the lumen of a follicle. Because of the intraluminal location, this finding is not indicative of the presence of a papillary carcinoma.

resemble psammoma bodies are common. The main differences between these structures and true psammoma bodies as seen in papillary carcinoma lies in their intraluminal position and their basophilia (figs. 10-6, 10-7). Under these circumstances, their presence is of no diagnostic significance. They should be disregarded even when secondary changes or the tumor hypercellularity obscures their original intraluminal site (fig. 10-8). It is common for these formations to cluster in one portion of the tumor while being scanty or absent in others.

The nuclei of the tumor cells of oncocytic adenomas tend to be vesicular and uniform; however, they often feature marked nuclear atypia in the form of scattered, enlarged hyperchromatic forms, sometimes reaching giant dimensions (fig. 10-9). This change is not indicative of

malignancy; it is also seen in non-neoplastic thyroid disorders associated with oncocytic change, such as Hashimoto thyroiditis. When the tumor cells are round or polygonal, the nuclei tend to be centrally located. When the cells acquire a columnar shape, the nuclei may be centrally located or at the apical side. This results in a peg-like configuration and suggests an inversion of cell polarity (fig. 10-10).

Variations in the appearance of the cytoplasm relate to shape (round, vesicular, or columnar), size (usually larger than nononcocytic cells, but see Oncocytic Carcinoma), and degree of granularity. Most commonly, this granularity is uniformly distributed throughout the cytoplasm (see fig. 10-3). When the granularity within the cell is focal, either the oncocytic change itself is focal or part of it has undergone a secondary

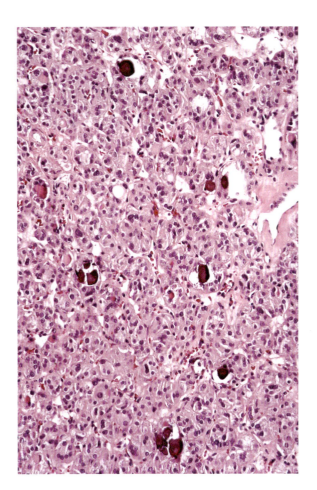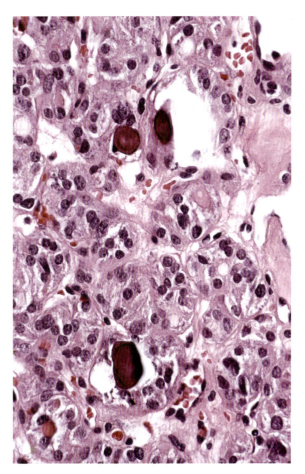

Figure 10-8

ONCOCYTIC NEOPLASM

Left: Clusters of psammoma body-like structures are seen in this oncocytic tumor. It is likely that most, if not all, of these are within tiny follicular lamina and therefore are of no significance for the diagnosis of papillary carcinoma.

Right: The high-power view shows the intraluminal location of the psammoma body-like round structures.

vesicular swelling of the mitochondria. The latter phenomenon, which results in progressive clearing of the originally oncocytic areas, is discussed in chapter 11.

As already stated, infarct-type necrosis may be present, sometimes involving the entire neoplasm (figs. 10-4, 10-11). This is probably a reflection of the greater sensitivity to anoxia of the abnormal mitochondria that characterize the condition.

The shadows of necrotic oncocytes are sometimes identified, particularly when arranged in a follicular pattern (fig. 10-11). This development is probably the result of the increased intratumoral pressure from the edema and hemorrhage induced by fine-needle aspiration.

Support for this interpretation was obtained by examining an oncocytic neoplasm with focal capsular invasion in which the entire tumor underwent necrosis after fine-needle aspiration except for the extracapsular component, presumably because it had not been subjected to the pressure increase (fig. 10-12) (personal observation). It seems that this event may supervene in either benign or malignant oncocytic tumors as long as a fibrous capsule (whether complete or incomplete) is present. The tumor cells at the periphery of the lesion remain viable and appear entrapped within the thickened capsule. This change can be particularly striking in adenomas that have undergone some degree of secondary cystic change with undulations of the capsule.

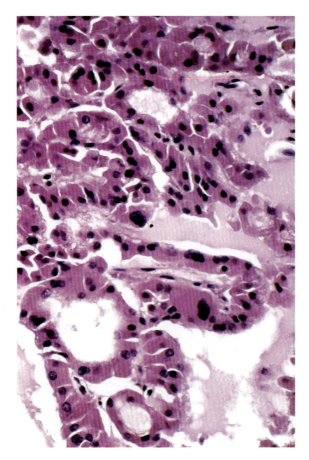

Figure 10-9

ONCOCYTIC NEOPLASM

Bizarre huge nuclei in an oncocytoma. They are not an indicator of malignancy.

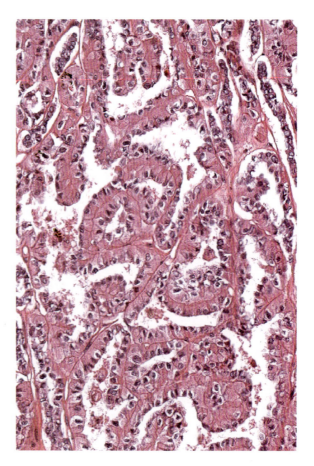

Figure 10-10

ONCOCYTIC NEOPLASM

Randomly oriented septa simulate papillae. Nuclear polarization is seen.

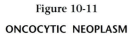

Figure 10-11

ONCOCYTIC NEOPLASM

Massive tumor necrosis following a fine-needle aspiration procedure. The shadow of the follicles can still be recognized.

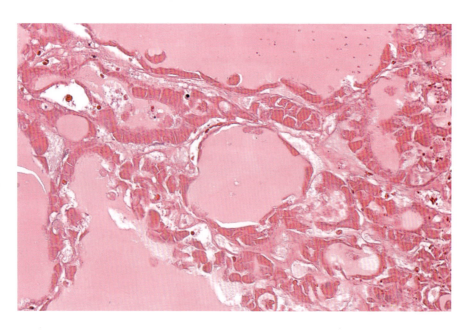

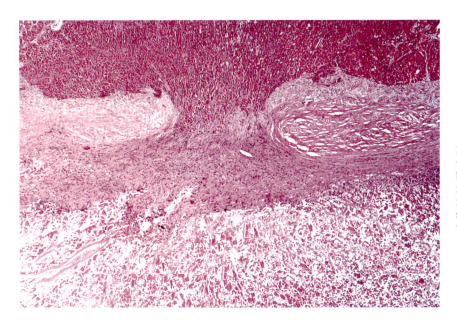

Figure 10-12

ONCOCYTIC CARCINOMA

The tumor is necrotic (lower half) except in the area invading the capsule and growing beyond. This suggests that the necrosis is induced by increased intratumoral pressure which spares the invasive portion of the tumor.

Other tissue reactions to fine-needle aspiration that cause diagnostic difficulties include the irregular growth of proliferating follicles along the needle tract through the capsule and the vaguely pseudoangiosarcomatous appearance that may develop as the result of hemorrhage and thrombosis, with subsequent organization (30–33).

Immunohistochemical Findings. Immunoreactivity for thyroglobulin is present (34), but is generally of a lesser degree than in ordinary follicular cells. The more pronounced the mitochondrial accumulation, the less intense the reactivity for thyroglobulin. Some reactivity, however, usually remains. This is true even in tumors that have undergone extensive necrosis, whether spontaneously or following a fine-needle aspiration procedure, a finding of significance in demonstrating the thyroid lineage of both primary and metastatic necrotic tumor masses (35).

Positivity for pankeratin is also diminished in oncocytic tumors when compared with that exhibited by their nononcocytic counterparts. The outstanding exception is cytokeratin (CK)14, which is said to specifically stain oncocytic cells (36). Reactivity for thyroid transcription factor (TTF)-1 is expressed in a fashion similar to that seen in nononcocytic follicular cells. Nuclear and cytoplasmic positivity for S-100 protein is the rule (37). There is also strong expression of glucose transporter 4 (GLUT-4) (38) and of E2F-1 transcription factor (39).

Johnson et al. (34) found consistent expression of carcinoembryonic antigen (CEA) by benign and malignant oncocytic tumors, a somewhat surprising finding that has not been confirmed in other studies (40) or in our own experience. In one series, galectin-3 and HBME-1 were found to be positive in 95.1 percent and 53.0 percent of the oncocytic tumors, respectively (41), but their usefulness in distinguishing benign from malignant forms is limited. The same seems true for the proliferative index (as measured with Ki-67) (42), and cell cycle regulatory proteins (p27kip1, cyclins D1 and E) (43).

Immunohistochemical techniques for the demonstration of the mitochondria themselves are now available. They are based on the use of monoclonal antibodies against mitochondrial-related antigens, especially mitochondrial enzymes (such as cytochrome C oxidase, complex IV of the mitochondrial respiratory chain) (fig. 10-13) (44,45). Consistent with its role in the pathogenesis of oncocytic change, the reduction or loss of expression of complex I subunits (e.g., NDUFS4) and of complex I enzyme activity, is a common feature in oncocytic cells both in the thyroid gland and the kidney (20,23,46).

Ultrastructural Findings. The distinctive feature of the cells of oncocytic adenoma is the packing of the cytoplasm by mitochondria (fig. 10-14). In the most advanced stages of this process, few other organelles remain. Some of the mitochondria have a normal appearance; they are

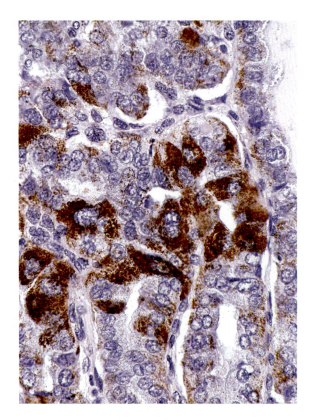

Figure 10-13

PAPILLARY CARCINOMA WITH
FOCAL ONCOCYTIC FEATURES

The oncocytic component of the tumor is clearly seen with an immunohistochemical stain for mitochondrial antigen.

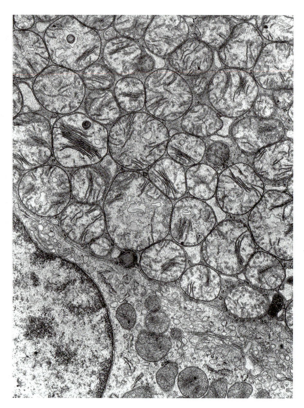

Figure 10-14

ONCOCYTIC ADENOMA

Ultrastructurally, the cytoplasm of a tumor cell is packed with abnormal mitochondria and few residual organelles. Several abnormalities of these mitochondria are observed, including the formation of myelin figures. The tumor cell present in the lower third of the photograph has mitochondria with a more normal appearance. (Courtesy of Dr. R. Erlandson, New York, NY.)

provided with a large number of inner membranes and a matrix of high density. In most instances, however, marked abnormalities of size, shape, and content are observed, and there may be an increase in the number, size, and pleomorphism of the intramitochondrial dense bodies (fig. 10-15) (12). Some mitochondria appear dilated, with distortion and eventual disappearance of the cristae. When this secondary change becomes prominent, the organelles acquire a round vesicular shape and may no longer be recognizable as mitochondria. This is the ultrastructural equivalent of the progressive clearing of the cytoplasm seen at the light microscopic level.

Ultrastructural abnormalities of mitochondria in the thyroid gland are not restricted to oncocytomas or, for that matter, to oncocytes (47). The presence of distinct smooth-surfaced cells interspersed with cells with many microvilli is a distinctive feature of oncocytic neoplasms when examined under the scanning electron microscope (12).

Molecular Genetic Findings. Oncocytic follicular adenoma and carcinoma share a common tumorigenic pathway, like their nononcocytic counterparts. There are no molecular tests that can distinguish an oncocytic adenoma from an oncocytic carcinoma, and the main genetic alterations found in adenomas are mentioned below with those of oncocytic carcinomas. If we exclude the molecular defects responsible for the accumulation of mitochondria discussed in the previous paragraphs, the genetic alterations that occur in nononcocytic follicular adenomas are also generally found in oncocytic adenomas. These are discussed in chapter 19.

Cytologic Findings. See chapter 20.

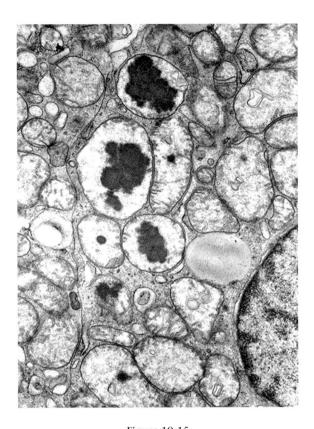

Figure 10-15

ONCOCYTIC ADENOMA

The mitochondria are dilated and show diminution in the number of cristae; several of them have large, irregularly shaped, and pleomorphic intramitochondrial bodies. (Courtesy of Dr. R. Erlandson, New York, NY.)

Treatment and Prognosis. We believe that the surgical procedure for oncocytic adenoma does not need to be more extensive than that employed for conventional follicular adenoma. This seems to be the consensus, even among groups that had previously advocated a more aggressive approach (48).

In most reported series, conservative surgical excision of oncocytic adenoma has resulted in permanent cure. There were no instances of recurrence or metastasis in any of the 27 cases reported by Horn (follow-up time not specified) (49); the 34 cases reported by Bronner and LiVolsi (mean follow-up time, 10.4 years) (40); the 34 cases reported by Bondeson et al. (follow-up time 2 to 20 years) (50); the 26 patients reported by Caplan et al. (follow-up time 2 to 22 years) (51); the 32 cases reported by Gerken et al. (follow-up time, 2 to 27 years) (52); the 71 patients reported by Gosain and Clark (follow-up time, 675 patient years) (53); the 90 cases reported by Carcangiu et al. (follow-up time 5 to 26 years) (54); or the 59 cases studied by Erickson et al. (follow-up time, 7.8 years) (55). In two other series, however, the results were strikingly different. The first, from Switzerland, recorded the development of recurrence in the form of carcinoma in 5 of 30 patients operated for oncocytic adenoma (56). In the second series, more widely quoted, Thompson et al. (57) recorded metastases in 3 of 4 cases that they had diagnosed as adenomas, this being the basis for their proposed radical approach to the treatment of oncocytic thyroid neoplasms. We have no explanation for this startling experience, other than that advanced by pathologists from the same institution who reviewed these cases years later: that the sampling of those tumors might have been inadequate (4). Interestingly, a subsequent report from the same group listed 23 additional cases of oncocytic adenoma, none of which gave rise to metastases (48).

ONCOCYTIC CARCINOMA (HÜRTHLE CELL CARCINOMA)

Definition. *Oncocytic carcinoma*, also termed *Hürthle cell carcinoma*, is a malignant thyroid neoplasm composed exclusively or predominantly (over 75 percent) of oncocytes.

General Features. Oncocytic carcinomas account for 2 to 3 percent of all thyroid carcinomas and approximately 20 percent of follicular carcinomas (3). In one series, a third of the patients had associated nonmalignant thyroid diseases (58).

Clinical Features. Oncocytic carcinomas are most common in women; however, this predominance is not as pronounced as for oncocytic adenomas (ratio of women to men of 2:1 versus 8:1), a fact to remember in the differential diagnosis (54,58). The mean age at the time of initial diagnosis is about 55 years (i.e., a decade older than for benign oncocytic tumors) (54,58). The clinical presentation does not differ from that of other malignant follicular tumors.

Oncocytic carcinomas do not take up radioactive iodine. They therefore appear as cold nodules on a thyroid scintigram, and metastases may not be detectable with this technique.

Gross Findings. Oncocytic carcinomas usually are larger than their benign counterparts, but the size range is wide (58–60). They share

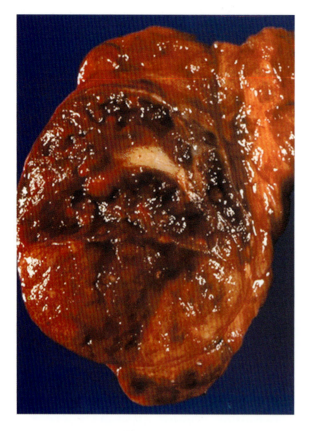

Figure 10-16

ONCOCYTIC CARCINOMA

At the gross level, the tumor is mostly encapsulated, but several foci of invasion of the capsule are appreciated. The cut surface has the characteristic brown color of this tumor type and exhibits foci of hemorrhage and necrosis.

with oncocytic adenomas a characteristic light brown color and a predominantly solid appearance (figs. 10-16, 10-17). Multiplicity is rare. Secondary degenerative features in the form of necrosis, hemorrhage, and central scarring are more common than in the adenoma.

The boundaries of the tumor vary depending on the subtype. In minimally invasive neoplasms, a complete capsule surrounds the tumor so that the distinction from adenoma at the gross level becomes impossible. In widely invasive tumors, the capsule is violated by tumor masses, or is absent. It is characteristic for this tumor type to invade the surrounding thyroid gland in the form of sharply outlined nodules that connect with each other and with the main tumor mass. Sometimes these nodules are so distinct that they are misinterpreted at the gross level (and even microscopically) as separate neoplasms or as evidence of nodular hyperplasia.

Microscopic Findings. The cytologic features of oncocytic carcinomas resemble those of oncocytic adenomas in many ways, so that it becomes impossible in most cases to decide whether a given oncocytic tumor is benign or malignant on cytologic grounds alone. Some differences exist, however, at least at a statistical level. In many oncocytic carcinomas, the amount of cytoplasm is less abundant than in adenomas, resulting in a greater nuclear to cytoplasmic ratio. More of the tumor cells are tall cuboidal

Figure 10-17

ONCOCYTIC CARCINOMA

This large tumor has a variegated cut surface, with areas of hemorrhage and necrosis.

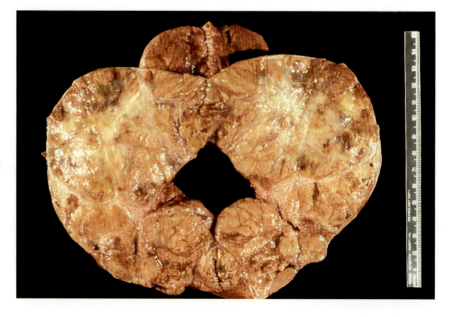

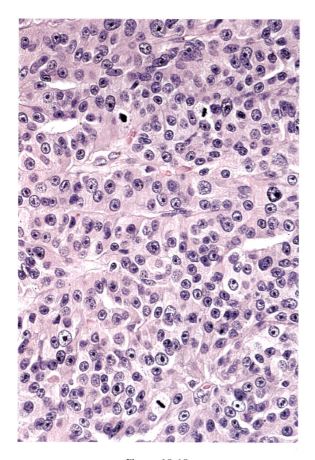

Figure 10-18

ONCOCYTIC CARCINOMA

The pattern of growth is predominantly solid. Several mitoses are present. Note the prominent nucleoli.

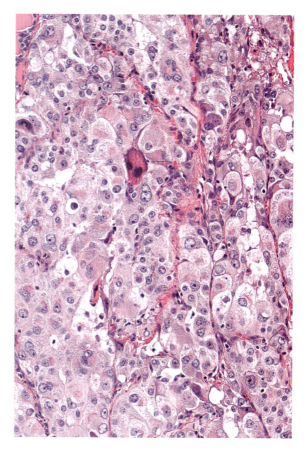

Figure 10-19

ONCOCYTIC CARCINOMA

This tumor grows mainly in a trabecular fashion.

or columnar, as opposed to round or polygonal. The appearance of the nuclei varies as well: scattered bizarre hyperchromatic forms are seen, as in the adenomas, but there is a tendency for increased mitotic activity and for all the nuclei to be more hyperchromatic.

Architecturally, most tumors have a solid/trabecular pattern of growth, as opposed to the predominantly follicular pattern of adenomas (figs. 10-18, 10-19). Sometimes the cells group in well-defined nests or insulae. Exceptionally, the stroma shows extensive myxoid changes (61).

Although a careful evaluation of the cytologic and architectural features described above is important, it cannot be overemphasized that the feature that overrides all of the others in terms of diagnostic importance is invasion. Its presence identifies an oncocytic neoplasm as malignant, and, when this is the case, the degree of this invasion determines whether the carcinoma is to be regarded as minimally invasive or widely invasive.

Minimally Invasive. This type of carcinoma is sometimes also designated *encapsulated* because it features a fibrous capsule similar to that of an adenoma. The capsule, however, is invaded at one or more points by the tumor (fig. 10-20). In addition, blood vessels lying within the capsule are invaded as well in most instances, hence the alternative designation *angioinvasive carcinoma*. The criteria used to decide whether capsular or vascular invasion exists are the same as those used for conventional follicular carcinoma (see chapter 6) and are not repeated here. In our experience, the phenomenon of blood vessel invasion by thyroid tumors is expressed in a more florid fashion (both in terms of number of vessels involved and degree of tumor infiltration) in

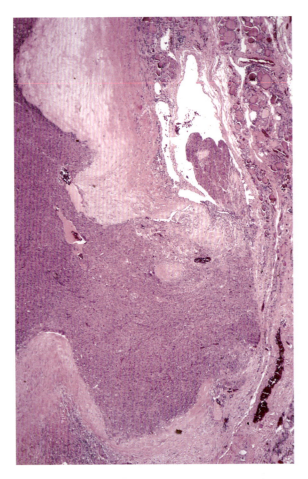

Figure 10-20

ONCOCYTIC CARCINOMA

There is obvious capsular and vascular invasion.

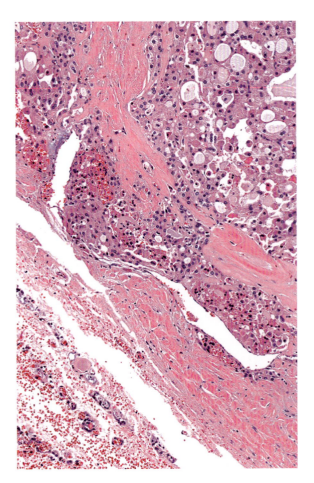

Figure 10-21

ONCOCYTIC CARCINOMA

A capsular vessel is extensively involved by tumor.

oncocytic carcinoma than in follicular carcinoma of nononcocytic type (figs. 10-20, 10-21).

Widely Invasive. Whereas tumors in the previous category are wholly encapsulated and the question is whether this capsule is invaded or not, in the widely invasive type, the invasion is obvious and the difficulty (although obviously not an important one) is to determine whether there is a capsule at all. It is rare for the invasive component to be accompanied by the prominent desmoplastic reaction commonly seen with papillary carcinoma. Instead, it often presents in the form of compact nodules or cords that may be separated by residual follicles (fig. 10-22). Vascular permeation is more common and widespread than in the minimally invasive form.

Oncocytic carcinomas with a solid/trabecular/insular pattern of growth, if associated with mi-

totic activity or necrosis, fulfill the so-called Turin criteria for poorly differentiated carcinomas, and it is reasonable to designate them as such (62).

Immunohistochemical and Ultrastructural Findings. In oncocytic carcinomas these features are not significantly different from those described for oncocytic adenomas. Oncocytic carcinomas show greater p53 expression and less BCL-2 expression than oncocytic adenomas, but it is doubtful whether the differences are of a degree or consistency such as to be diagnostically useful (63–68)

Molecular Genetic Findings. Apart from the molecular alterations that cause the accumulation of mitochondria discussed in the previous paragraphs, the genetic alterations observed in nononcocytic neoplasms are also observed in the corresponding oncocytic variants. *RAS*

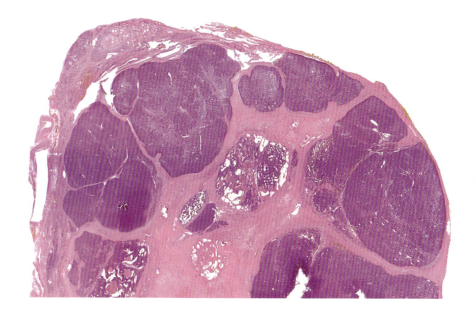

Figure 10-22

ONCOCYTIC CARCINOMA

The characteristic pattern of infiltration of oncocytic carcinoma seen here may be misinterpreted as nodular hyperplasia.

mutations and *PAX8/PPARγ* occur in follicular oncocytic tumors (although they are usually detected less frequently) (69–71), and *BRAF* mutations occur in papillary carcinomas with oncocytic features (72). Some studies have identified *RET/PTC* in many oncocytic follicular adenomas and carcinomas (73), but the relevance of this observation is disputable since *RET/PTC* was detected using highly sensitive methods that may reflect a very low rearrangement level or tumor heterogeneity (74,75). One study reported *RET/PTC* in about 35 percent of both oncocytic follicular adenomas and carcinomas, and associated the presence of the rearrangement with a solid pattern of growth (76). In another study, no *RET/PTC* rearrangement was found in 19 oncocytic follicular carcinomas and 8 follicular adenomas (71).

Oncocytic follicular adenoma and carcinoma share a common tumorigenic pathway, but similar to their nononcocytic counterparts, there are no molecular tests that can distinguish between the two. Few oncocytic neoplasms have been analyzed by conventional karyotyping, and usually only in series dealing with the general cytogenetic features of thyroid tumors (77). While there are no specific chromosomal abnormalities, both oncocytic adenomas and oncocytic follicular carcinomas commonly show polyploidy and aneuploidy, with numerical chromosomal changes (gains more frequently than losses) that involve whole chromosomes or chromosome arms. This finding is anticipated by the abnormal nuclear features detected morphologically. Aneuploidy, initially identified by cytometric measurement of DNA content (78–82), often has a higher prevalence than in the corresponding nononcocytic follicular adenomas and carcinomas, and has been confirmed by comparative genomic hybridization and fluorescence in situ hybridization (FISH) (83–86). The same pattern observed in nononcocytic follicular neoplasms, with a sequential acquisition of chromosomal changes that starts with trisomy 7, has been described in oncocytic tumors, but the higher prevalence of aneuploidy indicates that numerical chromosomal alterations are favored in the latter (86). It has been speculated that the large number of mitochondria disrupt normal chromosomal segregation and predispose the cell to selective chromosomal gain or losses (83). Genomic DNA gains corresponding to chromosomes 5, 7, 12, and 17 are those more commonly identified, while chromosomal unbalance with DNA loss is found at several sites including chromosomes 2 and 22 (71,83–86). An in depth analysis of chromosomal DNA alterations, mutations, and gene expression indicates that the molecular profile of oncocytic carcinoma (and adenoma) is clearly different from that of conventional follicular and papillary carcinomas (71).

Aneuploidy, as determined by cytometric DNA content analysis of histologically malignant tumors, has been linked to invasion, metastases, and clinically aggressive behavior in most studies (78–80,82). The most impressive results in this regard are those of Rainwater et al. (82): in a series of 37 oncocytic carcinomas, none of the patients with diploid or polyploid carcinomas died, but 11 of the 19 patients (58 percent) with aneuploid carcinomas did. A high number of chromosomal gains detected by comparative genomic hybridization, specifically those on chromosome 12q, 19q, and 20p, have been associated with recurrence in oncocytic carcinomas (85). Loss of chromosome 22 has been associated with poor prognosis (84). There is no convincing evidence, however, that cytometric DNA content analysis, comparative genomic hybridization, or FISH add much to the diagnostic conclusions derived from the pathologic evaluation; they cannot be currently used to either document or rule out malignancy. Specifically, and despite some statements to the contrary (81), there does not appear to be any unfavorable prognostic significance for abnormal DNA content in histologically benign oncocytic neoplasms (78–80).

Among cases of familial nonmedullary thyroid carcinoma there are patients that develop oncocytic tumors. The trait, inherited as an autosomal dominant character, has been linked to the predisposing locus TCO (thyroid carcinoma with oxyphilia) mapped at 19p13.2 (87), but the causative gene has not been identified (17). Patients are young, with a mean age of about 20 years, and present clinically with goiter. The nodules show adenomatous features, with variable degrees of oncocytic change, and sometimes with a hyalinizing trabecular pattern. The carcinomas that develop in these patients are papillary, with oncocytic features, but an oncocytic follicular carcinoma has also been described (88).

Cytologic Findings. See chapter 20.

Differential Diagnosis. The appearance of thyroid nodules largely or entirely composed of oncocytes is so distinctive that the problem of cell type recognition hardly arises. Difficulties instead exist regarding the basic nature of the mass. These possibilities include the following. *Oncocytic hyperplastic nodule* is viewed as a "dominant" manifestation of nodular hyperplasia (adenomatoid goiter) (described in chapter 17).

Follicular adenoma, oncocytic variant (*Hürthle cell adenoma*), described in the previous section, is a possibility when generally multiple oncocytic follicular nodules are surrounded by a thick fibrohyaline capsule (and therefore qualify as neoplasms) and exhibit foci of capsular pseudoinvasion, in a patient with Hashimoto thyroiditis.

Follicular carcinoma, oncocytic variant, is the type usually meant when the term *Hürthle cell carcinoma* without a qualifier is used. Like its nononcocytic counterpart, the pattern of growth can be follicular, solid/trabecular, or (pseudo)papillary, the common denominator being the oncocytic cytoplasm and the lack of papillary carcinoma-type nuclei (see below).

Papillary carcinoma, oncocytic variant (*oncocytic papillary carcinoma*) has been approached in an inconsistent fashion in the literature, so that when an author writes about papillary Hürthle cell carcinoma, the reader is often left uncertain whether he is referring to an oncocytic variant of follicular carcinoma that makes papillae or to an oncocytic variant of papillary carcinoma. In cases of this sort, we feel that the distinction should be primarily based on the nuclear appearance, according to the following scheme: if the nuclei are large, pleomorphic, hyperchromatic, with prominent centrally located nucleoli and a variable number of mitoses, but lack longitudinal grooves, pseudoinclusions, or overlapping, the tumor should be placed in the category of oncocytic follicular carcinoma. If, on the other hand, the nuclei have irregular contours, an optically clear appearance, longitudinal grooves, pseudoinclusions, overlapping, no mitoses, and nucleoli displaced peripherally against the nuclear membrane, it should be regarded as an oncocytic variant of papillary carcinoma. These papillary carcinomas with oncocytic features are usually euploid (82) (unlike conventional oncocytic follicular adenomas and carcinomas), and may harbor *BRAF* mutations or *RET/PTC* rearrangement (72). Unfortunately, most papers dealing with Hürthle cell tumors have failed to make this distinction by ignoring this set of criteria, the article by Berho et al. (89) being an outstanding exception. It is also fair to say that the distinction here advocated based on the nuclear features is more easily made in a textbook than in real life.

Medullary carcinoma, oncocytic variant (*oncocytic medullary carcinoma*) is described in chapter 12.

Oncocytic parathyroid carcinoma (90,91) is described in chapter 26.

Spread and Metastasis. Direct spread into the perithyroidal soft tissues is more common in oncocytic carcinoma than in conventional follicular carcinoma. This is probably also true for distant metastases. The most common sites are lung and bone, followed by regional lymph nodes (92). The latter are more frequent than for conventional follicular carcinoma but substantially less so than for papillary carcinoma (59). Some of these metastases occur very late in the course of the disease (up to 10 years or more), emphasizing the need for long-term follow-up (92). Most of the tumor implants found in the neck of patients with oncocytic carcinomas are not lymph node metastases but the result of the invasion of venous blood vessels (93).

Treatment and Prognosis. It is generally agreed that widely invasive oncocytic carcinomas should be treated by total or near-total thyroidectomy (94,95). Most minimally invasive tumors are also treated in this fashion (95), but there is no available evidence that doing so produces better results than performing a more conservative operation. Adjunctive therapeutic modalities, such as suppression, radioactive iodine, or external irradiation, are of little or no value. Significantly, a review of recurrent cases of thyroid carcinoma that have not responded to radioactive iodine showed that the majority display oncocytic or "oncocytoid" features (Sobrinho-Simões, personal communication, 2012).

The overall 5-year survival rate for patients with oncocytic carcinoma ranges between 50 and 60 percent in most series. It is directly dependent on the degree of invasiveness and is therefore substantially better for those with minimally invasive rather than widely invasive tumors (92). Obviously, blood-borne metastases impact greatly on survival (54). Interestingly, this is also true for regional nodal metastases, whereas this parameter bears no prognostic significance in papillary carcinoma (96). In multivariant analysis, older patient age and larger tumor size predict worse survival (97). In a univariant analysis of another large series, major vascular invasion, tumor size (over 4 cm), presence of mitoses, and a solid/trabecular pattern of growth correlated with a decreased recurrence-free survival rate (98,99). Yet another

microscopic feature shown to be associated with an unfavorable prognosis in (poorly differentiated) oncocytic carcinoma is a small/medium size of the tumor cells (99).

A difficult and still unresolved issue is whether oncocytic carcinomas are more malignant than follicular carcinomas of nononcocytic type having a similar size and degree of invasiveness. Some series suggest that this might be the case (100), whereas others have shown no statistically significant differences (101). The poor response to radioactive iodine and the older age of the patients, compared with nononcocytic follicular carcinoma, may explain the presumably worse outcome for those with oncocytic tumors (100,102).

PAPILLARY ONCOCYTIC NEOPLASMS

As already stated, most oncocytic thyroid neoplasms exhibit follicular, trabecular, and/or solid patterns of growth. For this reason, they are regarded by most as a subtype of follicular neoplasms. In some of these tumors, particularly those with a macrofollicular pattern of growth, the septa separating the follicles are very thin, so that when cut tangentially, they simulate papillae. This feature has no diagnostic significance (fig. 10-23).

There are, however, rare oncocytic neoplasms that exhibit a papillary configuration throughout, a feature that is analogous in all regards to that seen in papillary carcinoma. These papillae are lined by a single layer of oncocytic cells of either cuboidal or columnar shape (fig. 10-24) (103). The nuclei, although vesicular, usually lack a well-developed ground-glass appearance. Some of these tumors are invasive and seem to behave similarly to conventional papillary carcinoma, i.e., they have a tendency for regional lymph node involvement. Their long-term behavior is said to be comparable to that of their nononcocytic counterparts (58), but our own (limited) experience suggests that they may behave more aggressively (104). In reported series of papillary carcinomas, the incidence of the oncocytic type has ranged from 1.1 to 11.3 percent. This probably reflects differences in diagnostic criteria (105). We suspect that the higher figures derive from the inclusion of other types of papillary carcinoma. For these invasive papillary neoplasms exhibiting true oncocytic features, we prefer the

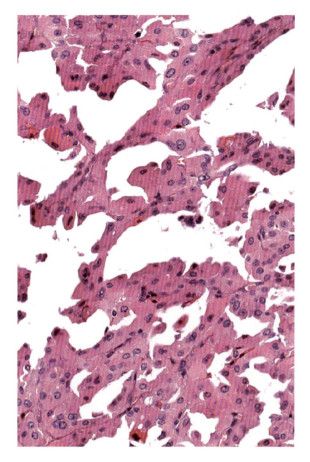

Figure 10-23

ONCOCYTOMA

The pseudopapillae result from tangential sectioning of intratumoral septa.

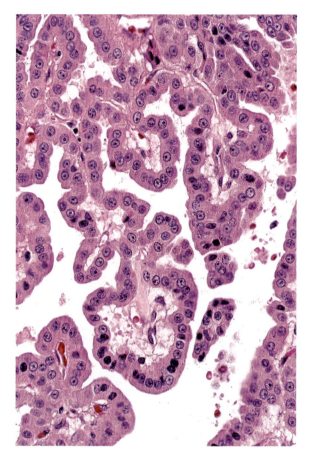

Figure 10-24

ONCOCYTIC CARCINOMA WITH PAPILLARY PATTERN OF GROWTH

The nuclear features of the papillary family of neoplasms are absent (compare to fig. 10-25).

designation *oncocytic papillary carcinoma* (or *papillary carcinoma, oncocytic variant*) (fig. 10-25). Other oncocytic papillary neoplasms are totally encapsulated and exhibit no signs of either capsular or vascular invasion (102). The position of these lesions in the classification scheme of thyroid neoplasia remains controversial. Some authors have regarded them as *encapsulated papillary carcinomas of oncocytic type*. Conversely, they could be viewed as *oncocytic follicular adenomas with papillary hyperplasia*, by use of reasoning similar to that applied to nononcocytic follicular adenomas. We favor the latter interpretation because we have found no documentation of metastases in our series or in those of others (102–106). We recommend that these tumors be provisionally designated with the noncommittal term *encapsulated papillary oncocytic neoplasm (EPONs)*, a suggestion that has been followed by others (101). A conservative surgical approach seems justified in view of the above findings.

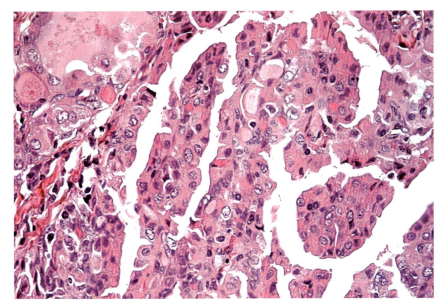

Figure 10-25

PAPILLARY CARCINOMA: ONCOCYTIC VARIANT

The pattern of growth is papillary, and the nuclei lining the papillae have papillary carcinoma-type features.

REFERENCES

1. Poli F, Trezzi R, Rosai J. Images in pathology. Single thyroid follicle involved by papillary carcinoma: partially classic and partially oncocytic. Int J Surg Pathol 2009;17:272-3.
2. Tallini G. Oncocytic tumours. Virchows Arch 1998;433:5-12.
3. Máximo V, Rios E, Sobrinho-Simões M. Oncocytic lesions of the thyroid, kidney, salivary glands, adrenal cortex, and parathyroid glands. Int J Surg Pathol 2014;22:33-6.
4. Flint A, Lloyd RV. Hürthle-cell neoplasms of the thyroid gland. Pathol Annu 1990;25(Pt 1):37-52.
5. Hamperl H. Benign and malignant oncocytoma. Cancer 1962;15:1019-27.
6. Tallini G, Carcangiu ML, Rosai J. Oncocytic neoplasms of the thyroid gland. Acta Pathol Jpn 1992;42:305-15.
7. Hedinger CE, Williams ED, Sobin LH. Histological typing of thyroid tumours. WHO International histological classification of tumours, 2nd ed. Berlin: Springer-Verlag; 1988.
8. Chang A, Harawi SJ. Oncocytes, oncocytosis, and oncocytic tumors. Pathol Annu 1992;27(Pt 1):263-304.
9. Lloyd RV. Oncocytic tumors of the thyroid gland. Adv Anat Pathol 1997;4:306-10.
10. Tremblay G, Pearse AG. Histochemistry of oxidative enzyme systems in the human thyroid, with special reference to Askanazy cells. J Pathol Bacteriol 1960;80:353-8.
11. Tsybrovskyy O, Rössmann-Tsybrovskyy M. Oncocytic versus mitochondrion-rich follicular thyroid tumours: should we make a difference? Histopathology 2009;55:665-82.
12. Nesland JM, Sobrinho-Simões MA, Holm R, Sambade MC, Johannessen JV. Hürthle-cell lesions of the thyroid: a combined study using transmission electron microscopy, scanning electron microscopy, and immunocytochemistry. Ultrastruct Pathol 1985;8:269-90.
13. Clark OH, Gerend PL. Thyrotropin receptor-adenylate cyclase system in Hürthle cell neoplasms. J Clin Endocrinol Metab 1985;61:773-8.
14. Tallini G, Ladanyi M, Rosai J, Jhanwar SC. Analysis of nuclear and mitochondrial DNA alterations in thyroid and renal oncocytic tumors. Cytogenet Cell Genet 1994;66:253-9.
15. Máximo V, Sobrinho-Simões M. Hürthle cell tumours of the thyroid. A review with emphasis on mitochondrial abnormalities with clinical relevance. Virchows Arch 2000;437:107-15.
16. Máximo V, Soares P, Lima J, Cameselle-Teijeiro J, Sobrinho-Simões M. Mitochondrial DNA somatic mutations (point mutations and large deletions) and mitochondrial DNA variants in human thyroid pathology: a study with emphasis on Hürthle cell tumors. Am J Pathol 2002;160:1857-65.
17. Gasparre G, Bonora E, Tallini G, Romeo G. Molecular features of thyroid oncocytic tumors. Mol Cell Endocrinol 2010;321:67-76.
18. Bonora E, Porcelli AM, Gasparre G, et al. Defective oxidative phosphorylation in thyroid oncocytic carcinoma is associated with pathogenic mitochondrial DNA mutations affecting complexes I and III. Cancer Res 2006;66:6087-96.

19. Gasparre G, Porcelli AM, Bonora E, et al. Disruptive mitochondrial DNA mutations in complex I subunits are markers of oncocytic phenotype in thyroid tumors. Proc Natl Acad Sci U S A 2007;104:9001-6.

20. Mayr JA, Meierhofer D, Zimmermann F, et al. Loss of complex I due to mitochondrial DNA mutations in renal oncocytoma. Clin Cancer Res 2008;14:2270-5.

21. Máximo V, Botelho T, Capela J, et al. Somatic and germline mutation in GRIM-19, a dual function gene involved in mitochondrial metabolism and cell death, is linked to mitochondrion-rich (Hurthle cell) tumours of the thyroid. Br J Cancer 2005;92:1892-8.

22. Favier J, Giménez-Roqueplo AP. Pheochromocytomas: the (pseudo)-hypoxia hypothesis. Best Pract Res Clin Endocrinol Metab 2010;24:957-68.

23. Porcelli AM, Ghelli A, Ceccarelli C, et al. The genetic and metabolic signature of oncocytic transformation implicates HIF1alpha destabilization. Hum Mol Genet 2010;19:1019-32.

24. Mete O, Asa SL. Oncocytes, oxyphils, Hürthle, and Askanazy cells: morphological and molecular features of oncocytic thyroid nodules. Endocr Pathol 2010;21:16-24.

25. Wakely PE Jr. Oncocytic and oncocyte-like lesions of the head and neck. Ann Diagn Pathol 2008;12:222-30.

26. Sobrinho-Simões M, Máximo V, Castro IV, et al. Hürthle (oncocytic) cell tumors of thyroid: etiopathogenesis, diagnosis and clinical significance. Int J Surg Pathol 2005;13:29-35.

27. Máximo V, Lima J, Prazeres H, Soares P, Sobrinho-Simões M. The biology and the genetics of Hürthle cell tumors of the thyroid. Endocr Relat Cancer 2012; 19:R131-47.

28. Gasparre G, Kurelac I, Capristo M, el al. A mutation threshold distinguishes the antitumorigenic effects of the mitochondrial gene MTND1, an oncojanus function. Cancer Res 2011;71:6220-9.

29. Katoh R, Harach HR, Williams ED. Solitary, multiple, and familial oxyphil tumours of the thyroid gland. J Pathol 1998;186:292-9.

30. Kini SR. Post-fine-needle biopsy infarction of thyroid neoplasms: a review of 28 cases. Diagn Cytopathol 1996;15:211-20.

31. Axiotis CA, Merino MJ, Ain K, Norton JA. Papillary endothelial hyperplasia in the thyroid following fine-needle aspiration. Arch Pathol Lab Med 1991;115:240-2.

32. Baloch ZW, LiVolsi VA. Post fine-needle aspiration histologic alterations of thyroid revisited. Am J Clin Pathol 1999;112:311-6.

33. Roh JL. Intrathyroid hemorrhage and acute upper airway obstruction after fine needle apiration of the thyroid gland. Laryngoscope 2006;116:154-6.

34. Johnson TL, Lloyd RV, Burney RE, Thompson NW. Hürthle cell thyroid tumors. An immunohistochemical study. Cancer 1987;59:107-12.

35. Judkins AR, Roberts SA, Livolsi VA. Utility of immunohistochemistry in the evaluation of necrotic thyroid tumors. Hum Pathol 1999;30:1373-6.

36. Santeusanio G, D'Alfonso V, Iafrate E, et al. Antibodies to cytokeratin 14 specifically identify oncocytes (Hürthle cells) in thyroid lesions and tumors. Appl Immunohistochem 1997;5:223-8.

37. Abu-Alfa AK, Straus FH 2nd, Montag AG. An immunohistochemical study of thyroid Hürthle cells and their neoplasms: the roles of S-100 and HMB-45 proteins. Mod Pathol 1994;7:529-32.

38. Schönberger J, Rüschoff J, Grimm D, et al. Glucose transporter 1 gene expression is related to thyroid neoplasms with an unfavorable prognosis: an immunohistochemical study. Thyroid 2002;12:747-54.

39. Volante M, Croce S, Pecchioni C, Papotti M. E2F-1 transcription factor is overexpressed in oxyphilic thyroid tumors. Mod Pathol 2002;15:1038-43.

40. Bronner MP, LiVolsi VA. Oxyphilic (Askanazy/Hürthle cell) tumors of the thyroid. Microscopic features predict biologic behavior. Surg Pathol 1988;1:137-50.

41. Volante M, Bozzalla-Cassione F, DePompa R, et al. Galectin-3 and HBME-1 expression in oncocytic cell tumors of the thyroid. Virchows Arch 2004;445:183-8.

42. Tretiakova MS, Papotti M, Bussolati G. Proliferative activity of oxyphilic (Hürthle) cells in reactive and neoplastic thyroid lesions. Endocr Pathol 1999;10:173-9.

43. Maynes LJ, Hutzler MJ, Patwardhan NA, Wang S, Khan A. Cell cycle regulatory proteins p27(kip), cyclins Dl and E and proliferative activity in oncocytic (Hürthle cell) lesions of the thyroid. Endocr Pathol 2000;11:331-40.

44. Ortmann M, Vierbuchen M, Koller G, Fisher R. Renal oncocytoma. I. Cytochrome c oxidase in normal and neoplastic renal tissue as detected by immunohistochemistry: a valuable aid to distinguish oncocytomas from renal cell carcinomas. Virchows Arch B Cell Pathol Incl Mol Pathol 1988;56:165-73.

45. Papotti M, Torchio B, Grassi L, Favero A, Bussolati G. Poorly differentiated oxyphilic (Hürthle cell) carcinomas of the thyroid. Am J Surg Pathol 1996;20:686-94.

46. Zimmermann FA, Mayr JA, Neureiter D, et al. Lack of complex I is associated with oncocytic thyroid tumours. Br J Cancer 2009;100:1434-7.

47. Matias C, Moura Nunes JF, Sobrinho LG, Soares J. Giant mitochondria and intramitochondrial inclusions in benign thyroid lesions. Ultrastruct Pathol 1991;15:221-9.

48. McLeod MK, Thompson NW. Hürthle cell neoplasms of the thyroid. Otolaryngol Clin North Am 1990;23:441-52.

49. Horn RC Jr. Hürthle cell tumors of the thyroid. Cancer 1954;7:234-44.

50. Bondeson L, Bondeson AG, Ljungberg O, Tibblin S. Oxyphil tumors of the thyroid: follow-up of 42 surgical cases. Ann Surg 1981;194:677-80.

51. Caplan RH, Abellera RM, Kisken WA. Hürthle cell tumors of the thyroid gland. A clinicopathologic review and long-term follow-up. JAMA 1984;251:3114-7.

52. Gerken K, Nuñez C, Broughan T, Esselstyn C, Sebek B. Clinical outcome of Hürthle cell tumors of the thyroid [Abstract]. Am J Clin Pathol 1988;90:498A.

53. Gosain AK, Clark OH. Hürthle cell neoplasms. Malignant potential. Arch Surg 1984;119:515-9.

54. Carcangiu ML, Bianchi S, Savino D, Voynick IM, Rosai J. Follicular Hürthle cell neoplasms of the thyroid gland. Cancer 1991;68:1944-53.

55. Erickson LA, Jin L, Goellner JR, et al. Pathologic features, proliferative activity, and cyclin D1 expression in Hürthle cell neoplasms of the thyroid. Mod Pathol 2000;13:186-92.

56. Ruchti C, Komor J, König MP. [Thyroid macrocellular tumors (so-called Hürthle cell tumors).] Helv Chir Acta 1976;43:129-32. [German]

57. Thompson NW, Dunn EL, Batsakis JG, Nishiyama RH. Hürthle cell lesions of the thyroid gland. Surg Gynecol Obstet 1974;139:555-60.

58. Watson RG, Brennan MD, Goellner JR, van Heerden JA, McConahey WM, Taylor WF. Invasive Hürthle cell carcinoma of the thyroid: natural history and management. Mayo Clin Proc 1984;59:851-5.

59. González-Cámpora R, Herrero-Zapatero A, Lerma E, Sanchez F, Galera H. Hürthle cell and mitochondrion-rich cell tumors. A clinicopathologic study. Cancer 1986;57:1154-63.

60. Samulski TD, Bai S, LiVolsi VA, Montone K, Baloch Z. Malignant potential of small oncoytic follicular carcinoma/Hürthle cell carcinoma: an institutional experience. Histopathology 2013;63:568-73.

61. Kuma S, Hirokawa M, Miyauchi A, Kakudo K. Oncocytic thyroid carcinoma with extensive myxoid stroma. Histopathology 2003;42:514-6.

62. Asioli S, Righi A, Volante M, Chiusa L, Lloyd RV, Bussolati G. Cell size as a prognostic factor in oncocytic poorly differentiated carcinomas of the thyroid. Hum Pathol 2014;45:1489-95.

63. Müller-Höcker J. Immunoreactivity of p53, Ki-67, and Bcl-2 in oncocytic adenomas and carcinomas of the thyroid gland. Hum Pathol 1999;30:926-33.

64. Kohli A, Baker SP, Patwardhan NA, Khan A. Expression of BCL-2 and p53 on oncocytic (Hürthle cell) tumors of the thyroid: an immunohistochemical study. Endocr Pathol 1998;9:117-23.

65. Oestreicher-Kedem Y, Halpern M, Roizman P, et al. Diagnostic value of galectin-3 as a marker for malignancy in follicular patterned thyroid lesions. Head Neck 2004;26:960-6.

66. Saleh HA, Jin B, Barnwell J, Alzohaili O. Utility of immunohistochemical markers in differentiating benign from malignant follicular-derived thyroid nodules. Diagn Pathol 2010;5:9.

67. Herrmann ME, LiVolsi VA, Pasha TL, Roberts SA, Wojcik EM, Baloch ZW. Immunohistochemical expression of galectin-3 in benign and malignant thyroid lesions. Arch Pathol Lab Med 2002;126:710-3.

68. Nascimento MC, Bisi H, Alves VA, Longatto-Filho A, Kanamura CT, Medeiros-Neto G. Differential reactivity for galectin-3 in Hürthle cell adenomas and carcinomas. Endocr Pathol 2001;12:275-9.

69. Nikiforova MN, Lynch RA, Biddinger PW, et al. RAS point mutations and PAX8-PPAR gamma rearrangement in thyroid tumors: evidence for distinct molecular pathways in thyroid follicular carcinoma. J Clin Endocrinol Metab 2003;88:2318-26.

70. Sahin M, Allard BL, Yates M, et al. PPAR gammastaining as a surrogate for PAX8/PPAR gamma fusion oncogene expression in follicular neoplasms: clinicopathological correlation and histopathological diagnostic value. J Clin Endocrinol Metab 2005;90:463-8.

71. Ganly I, Ricarte Filho J, Eng S, et al. Genomic dissection of Hürthle cell carcinoma reveals a unique class of thyroid malignancy. J Clin Endocrinol Metab 2013;98:E962-72.

72. Trovisco V, Vieira de Castro I, Soares P, et al. BRAF mutations are associated with some histological types of papillary thyroid carcinoma. J Pathol 2004;202:247-51.

73. Chiappetta G, Toti P, Cetta F, et al. The RET/PTC oncogene is frequently activated in oncocytic thyroid tumors (Hürthle cell adenomas and carcinomas), but not in oncocytic hyperplastic lesions. J Clin Endocrinol Metab 2002;87:364-9.

74. Zhu Z, Ciampi R, Nikiforova MN, Gandhi M, Nikiforov YE. Prevalence of RET/PTC rearrangements in thyroid papillary carcinomas: effects of the detection methods and genetic heterogeneity. J Clin Endocrinol Metab 2006;91:3603-10.

75. Rhoden KJ, Unger K, Salvatore G, et al. RET/papillary thyroid cancer rearrangement in nonneoplastic thyrocytes: follicular cells of Hashimoto's thyroiditis share low-level recombination events with a subset of papillary carcinoma. J Clin Endocrinol Metab 2006;91:2414-23.

76. de Vries MM, Celestino R, Castro P, et al. RET/PTC rearrangement is prevalent in follicular Hürthle cell carcinomas. Histopathology 2012;61:833-43.

77. Jenkins RB, Hay ID, Herath JF, et al. Frequent occurrence of cytogenetic abnormalities in sporadic nonmedullary thyroid carcinoma. Cancer 1990;66:1213-20.

78. Bondeson L, Azavedo E, Bondeson AG, Caspersson T, Ljungberg O. Nuclear DNA content and behavior of oxyphil thyroid tumors. Cancer 1986;58:672-5.

79. Bronner MP, Clevenger CV, Edmonds PR, Lowell DM, McFarland MM, LiVolsi VA. Flow cytometric analysis of DNA content in Hürthle cell adenomas and carcinomas of the thyroid. Am J Clin Pathol 1988;89:764-9.

80. el-Naggar AK, Batsakis JG, Luna MA, Hickey RC. Hürthle cell tumors of the thyroid. A flow cytometric DNA analysis. Arch Otolaryngol Head Neck Surg 1988;114:520-1.

81. Flint A, Davenport RD, Lloyd RV, Beckwith AL, Thompson NW. Cytophotometric measurements of Hürthle cell tumors of the thyroid gland. Correlation with pathologic features and clinical behavior. Cancer 1988;61:110-3.

82. Rainwater LM, Farrow GM, Hay ID, Lieber MM. Oncocytic tumours of the salivary gland, kidney, and thyroid: nuclear DNA patterns studied by flow cytometry. Br J Cancer 1986;53:799-804.

83. Tallini G, Hsueh A, Liu S, Garcia-Rostan G, Speicher MR, Ward DC. Frequent chromosomal DNA unbalance in thyroid oncocytic (Hürthle cell) neoplasms detected by comparative genomic hybridization. Lab Invest 1999;79:547-55.

84. Erickson LA, Jalal SM, Goellner JR, et al. Analysis of Hürthle cell neoplasms of the thyroid by interphase fluorescence in situ hybridization. Am J Surg Pathol 2001;25:911-7.

85. Wada N, Duh QY, Miura D, Brunaud L, Wong MG, Clark OH. Chromosomal aberrations by comparative genomic hybridization in Hürthle cell thyroid carcinomas are associated with tumor recurrence. J Clin Endocrinol Metab 2002;87:4595-601.

86. Dettori T, Frau DV, Lai ML, et al. Aneuploidy in oncocytic lesions of the thyroid gland: diffuse accumulation of mitochondria within the cell is associated with trisomy 7 and progressive numerical chromosomal alterations. Genes Chromosomes Cancer 2003;38:22-31.

87. Canzian F, Amati P, Harach HR, et al. A gene predisposing to familial thyroid tumors with cell oxyphilia maps to chromosome 19p13.2. Am J Hum Genet 1998;63:1743-8.

88. Harach HR, Lesueur F, Amati P, et al. Histology of familial thyroid tumours linked to a gene mapping to chromosome 19p13.2. J Pathol 1999;189:387-93.

89. Berho M, Suster S. The oncocytic variant of papillary carcinoma of the thyroid: a clinicopathologic study of 15 cases. Hum Pathol 1997;28:47-53.

90. Obara T, Fujimoto Y, Yamaguchi K, Takanashi R, Kino I, Sasaki Y. Parathyroid carcinoma of the oxyphil cell type. A report of two cases, light and electron microscopic study. Cancer 1985;55:1482-9.

91. Wolpert HR, Vickery AL Jr, Wang CA. Functioning oxyphil cell adenomas of the parathyroid gland. A study of 15 cases. Am J Surg Pathol 1989;13:500-4.

92. Tollefsen HR, Shah JP, Huvos AG. Hürthle cell carcinoma of the thyroid. Am J Surg 1975;130:390-4.

93. Bishop JA, Wu G, Tufano RP, Westra WH. Histological patterns of locoregional recurrence in Hürthle cell carcinoma of the thyroid gland. Thyroid 2012;22:690-4.

94. Gundry SR, Burney RE, Thompson NW, Lloyd R. Total thyroidectomy for Hürthle cell neoplasm of the thyroid. Arch Surg 1983;118:529-32.

95. McLeod MK, Thompson NW. Hürthle cell neoplasms of the thyroid. Otolaryngol Clin North Am 1990;23:441-52.

96. Stojadinovic A, Ghossein RA, Hoos A, et al. Hürthle cell carcinoma: a critical histopathologic appraisal. J Clin Oncol 2001;19:2616-25.

97. Lopez-Penabad L, Chiu AC, Hoff AO, et al. Prognostic factors in patients with Hürthle cell neoplasms of the thyroid. Cancer 2003;97:1186-94.

98. Ghossein RA, Hiltzik DH, Carlson DL, et al. Prognostic factors of recurrence in encapsulated Hurthle cell carcinoma of the thyroid gland: a clinicopathologic study of 50 cases. Cancer 2006;106:1669-76.

99. Asioli S, Righi A, Volante M, Chiusa L, Lloyd RV, Bussolati G. Cell size as a prognostic factor in oncocytic poorly differentiated carcinomas of the thyroid. Hum Pathol 2014;45:1489-95

100. Schröder S, Pfannschmidt N, Dralle H, Arps H, Böcker W. The encapsulated follicular carcinoma of the thyroid. A clinicopathologic study of 35 cases. Virchows Arch A Pathol Anat Histopathol 1984;402:259-73.

101. Evans HL, Vassilopoulou-Sellin R. Follicular and Hürthle cell carcinomas of the thyroid: a comparative study. Am J Surg Pathol 1998;22:1512-20.

102. Phitayakorn R, McHenry CR. Follicular and Hürthle cell carcinoma of the thyroid gland. Surg Oncol Clin N Am 2006;15:603-23, ix-x.

103. Mai KT, Elmontaser G, Perkins DG, Thomas J, Stinson WA. Benign Hürthle cell adenoma with papillary architecture: a benign lesion mimicking oncocytic papillary carcinoma. Int J Surg Pathol 2005;13:37-41.

104. Barbuto D, Carcangiu ML, Rosai J. Papillary Hürthle cell neoplasms of the thyroid gland. A study of 20 cases [Abstract]. Mod Pathol 1990;3:7A.

105. Sobrinho-Simões MA, Nesland JM, Holm R, Sambade MC, Johannessen JV. Hürthle cell and mitochondrion-rich papillary carcinomas of the thyroid gland: an ultrastructural and immunocytochemical study. Ultrastruct Pathol 1985;8:131-42.

106. Woodford RL, Nikiforov YE, Hunt JL, et al. Encapsulated papillary oncocytic neoplasms of the thyroid: morphologic, immunohistochemical, and molecular analysis of 18 cases. Am J Surg Pathol 2010;34:1582-90.

11 THYROID TUMORS WITH CLEAR CELL, SQUAMOUS, AND MUCINOUS FEATURES

TUMORS WITH CLEAR CELL FEATURES

General Considerations

Tumors with *clear cell features* are those thyroid neoplasms in which 75 percent or more of the tumor cells show marked cytoplasmic clearing (a change totally unrelated to the nuclear clearing associated with papillary carcinoma). Older classification schemes of thyroid tumors often include a category of clear cell carcinoma, implying the existence of a distinctive type of thyroid neoplasm that is always malignant. We believe that neither assumption is correct. Instead, we view cytoplasmic clear changes in follicular cells as a secondary event that results from a variety of mechanisms and occurs in almost any of the major tumor types (1). This situation is not substantially different from that in other organs. In the lung, for instance, the belief in the existence of a clear cell carcinoma existed for many years; it was later convincingly shown that clear cell changes occur in any of the major types of lung carcinoma and that these changes, albeit morphologically spectacular, have no significant impact on the natural history of the tumor (2).

There are several mechanisms by which a follicular cell acquires a clear cytoplasmic appearance when examined in hematoxylin and eosin (H&E)-stained sections. The most important are the following:

Cytoplasmic Vesicles. At the ultrastructural level, these are membrane-bound structures of fairly uniform diameter that contain electron-lucent material. Although the appearance of most is nondescript, the presence of distorted residual cristae in some suggests that, in most instances, these vesicles are massively dilated mitochondria. Others represent dilated secretory vesicles or are derived from the endoplasmic reticulum or Golgi apparatus (3–7).

When the cytoplasmic clearing is due to vesicle accumulation, the cells appear clear in the H&E-stained specimens but still retain a fine granularity, which could be graphically depicted as having the appearance of a washed-out oncocyte. The nucleus is usually centrally located and has smooth contours. The cell membrane is sharply outlined, a feature shared by most other types of follicular clear cells.

Glycogen. This type of clear cell tends to be larger than the preceding type, and the clearing is more complete. Instead of a fine granularity, empty cytoplasm is seen with an appearance that has been compared to that of a vegetable cell. The glycogen, which tends to be scattered throughout the cytoplasm, is demonstrated with the periodic acid–Schiff (PAS) reaction with diastase control, by other glycogen stains, or by ultrastructural examination. The nucleus is usually centrally located and has smooth contours, as in the preceding type.

Lipid. This type of alteration, which may occur in association with glycogen particles, presents in its fully developed form as an accumulation of cytoplasmic vesicles that are small to medium sized, and that typically indent the centrally located nucleus. This results in an appearance similar to that of a lipoblast or a spongiocyte from the fasciculata layer of the adrenal cortex. The lipid present in these vacuoles is demonstrated with oil red O or other fat stains in wet (nonparaffin-embedded) formalin-fixed tissue or by ultrastructural examination.

Thyroglobulin. Under some conditions, thyroglobulin accumulates in the cytoplasm in the form of small or large membrane-bound aggregates. Most of these formations have a homogeneous or granular acidophilic appearance, but others have a very light staining quality; i.e., they appear clear on H&E-stained sections. When the aggregates are small, the nucleus retains its central position and may acquire indentations similar to those formed as a result of cytoplasmic lipid accumulation. When large, the aggregates displace the nucleus laterally and distort it in such a way as to create a signet-ring cell configuration.

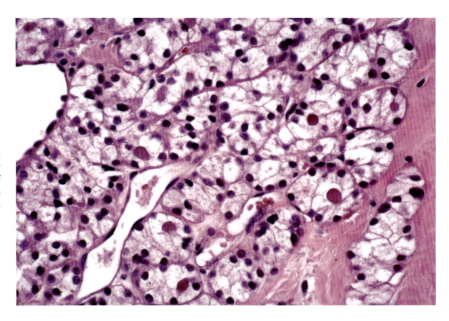

Figure 11-1

ONCOCYTOMA WITH CLEAR CELL FEATURES

Most primary thyroid tumors with cytoplasmic clear cell changes are the result of secondary alterations of Hürthle cell tumors (mitochondrial swelling).

Mucin. If the cytoplasmic clearing seen in the follicular cells has a slight basophilic quality, the probability that this is due to the accumulation of mucosubstances should be considered and further investigated with mucin stains such as Alcian blue. The source of the mucin deposition, which is sometimes accompanied by a similar deposition extracellularly, is not easily apparent. Thyroglobulin is a glycoprotein and the number of acidic groups in it can range widely; it is therefore possible that some instances of clear cell thyroid tumors of mucinous type are related to the accumulation of highly acidic forms of thyroglobulin.

Tumor Types

Primary thyroid tumors in which clear cell changes have been documented include the following types:

Oncocytic Neoplasms. There is probably no type of thyroid follicular cell that is more prone to undergo secondary clear changes than the oncocyte, whether neoplastic or not. The change can be observed in any thyroid disorder in which oncocytes occur, such as Hashimoto thyroiditis, nodular hyperplasia, and benign and malignant oncocytic tumors. The mechanism is apparently the same in all of them, and is related to vesicular swelling of mitochondria. In the oncocytic neoplasms, the change may be focal or extensive. The oncocytes and the clear cells are segregated in nests or closely in-

termingled (fig. 11-1). Sometimes, transitional forms between these two cell types are evident. The most spectacular of these is the tall cuboidal or columnar cell in which the basal cytoplasm is oncocytic and the apical cytoplasm is clear (fig. 11-2) (9). Parenthetically, this change also occurs in oncocytic neoplasms of other sites, such as salivary glands.

The reasons for the mitochondrial swelling are unknown. Some authors have suggested that the vesicular cytoplasmic formation may be induced by thyroid-stimulating hormone overstimulation of these cells (10), but this hypothesis remains unsubstantiated.

This type of clear cell change occurs in both benign and malignant oncocytic tumors. The criteria for distinguishing them are the same as for oncocytic (or, for that matter, follicular) tumors in general; however, there is a disproportionately high number of malignant cases (80 percent in one series [2]) among the oncocytic tumors with clear cell changes compared with oncocytic neoplasms in general. The finding of clear cell changes in an oncocytic neoplasm should therefore heighten the suspicion of carcinoma and lead to a careful search for confirmatory evidence.

Follicular Neoplasms. This group represents the prototypic example of a clear cell thyroid tumor, and the one generally referred to when described as *clear cell tumor, clear cell carcinoma, hypernephroid tumor,* and *parastruma* (fig. 11-3)

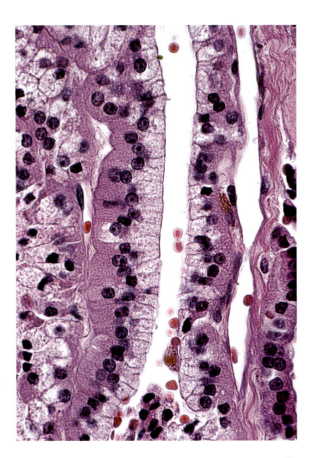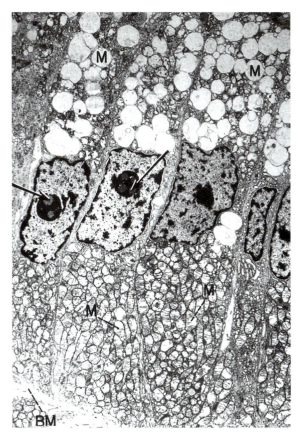

Figure 11-2

BIPHASIC ONCOCYTIC-CLEAR CELL TUMOR

The lower half of the cytoplasm of these cells is oncocytic, whereas the upper half is clear, as a consequence of the swelling of the many mitochondria present. (Left: light microscopy; right: electron microscopy.) (Right; fig. 6 from Dickersin GR, Vickery AL Jr, Smith SB. Papillary carcinoma of the thyroid, oxyphil cell type, "clear cell" variant: a light- and electron-microscopic study. Am J Surg Pathol 1980;4:505.)

(11–13). Some thyroid tumors have been included in the category of atypical adenoma just because their cytoplasm was clear (14).

The criteria for malignancy are the same as for follicular tumors in general, i.e., capsular or blood vessel invasion. When thus defined, both benign and malignant forms are identified, with the latter predominating (1). In some instances, scattered follicles of nondescript appearance are seen among those composed of clear cells. The pattern of growth is usually follicular, but it may be solid or trabecular (fig. 11-4). It is possible that some of the tumors that are entirely composed of clear cells represent oncocytic neoplasms in which the cytoplasmic clearing proceeded to its ultimate expression. This is suggested by the fact that, ultrastructurally, the change is due, in most cases, to vesicles that appear similar to those of clear cell oncocytomas. In other instances, the change is the result of glycogen accumulation or dilatation of granular endoplasmic reticulum (fig. 11-5) (3).

There is immunoreactivity for thyroglobulin in most cells, but it is usually mild to moderate. In general, the more clear the cell, the less prominent the thyroglobulin staining (15). Although the existence of benign clear cell follicular tumors of the thyroid gland with the features described above is now widely accepted, the index of suspicion for malignancy should be raised if this clear cell change is widespread or combined with oncocytic features.

Although a small to moderate number of glycogen granules are occasionally detected in

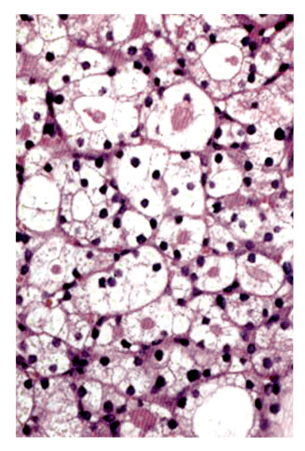

Figure 11-3

CLEAR CELL TUMOR

The cytoplasmic clearing is not complete since there is residual fine granularity. This is a useful feature in the differential diagnosis with metastatic renal cell carcinoma.

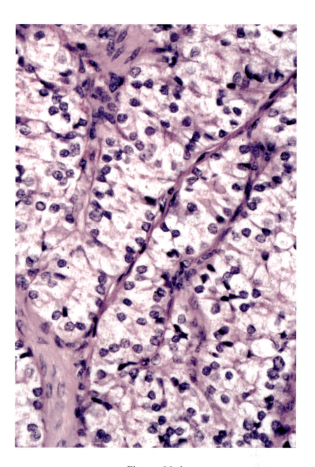

Figure 11-4

CLEAR CELL TUMOR

This case is similar to that shown in figure 11-3, except that the pattern of growth is trabecular rather than follicular.

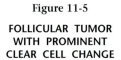

Figure 11-5

FOLLICULAR TUMOR WITH PROMINENT CLEAR CELL CHANGE

The clear cell change seen in this electron micrograph is due to marked dilatation of the cisternae of the granular endoplasmic reticulum. This is an unusual occurrence. (Courtesy of Dr. R. Erlandson, New York, NY.)

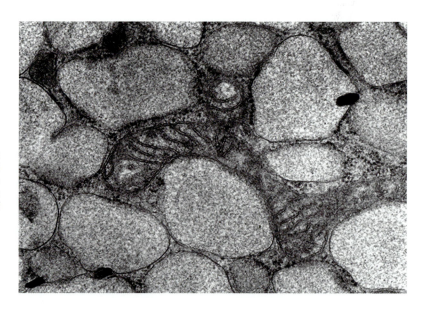

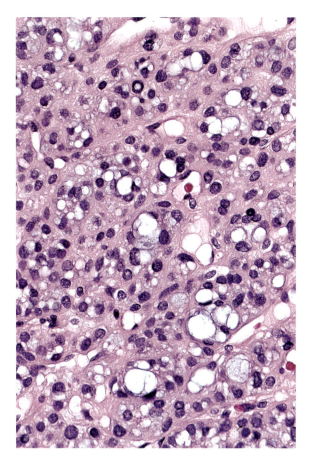

Figure 11-6

FOLLICULAR ADENOMA WITH SIGNET RING CELLS

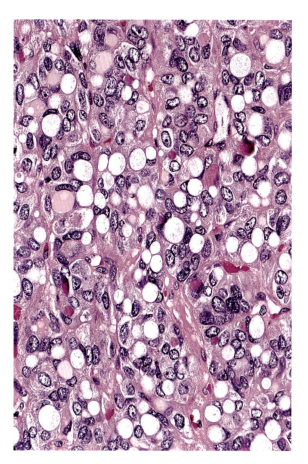

Figure 11-7

SIGNET RING FOLLICULAR ADENOMA

Most of the spaces look empty, while others have a pale acidophilic quality. The latter are immunoreactive for thyroglobulin.

the cytoplasm of follicular clear cells by special stains or electron microscopy, glycogen-rich clear cell follicular adenomas are very rare (13). Before such a diagnosis is considered, the more likely alternative of a metastatic clear cell carcinoma (particularly from the kidney) should be ruled out.

Signet Ring Follicular Adenoma and Carcinoma. These tumors are characterized by cells that exhibit a large cytoplasmic vacuole that displaces the nucleus laterally, leading to a signet ring configuration (16). In H&E-stained sections, the content of the cytoplasmic vacuole may appear clear, homogeneously acidophilic, basophilic, or granular. The nucleus may retain its original round or oval shape, but more often it acquires a semilunar shape, which heightens the resemblance of the cell to a signet ring (figs. 11-6, 11-7). Usually these cells alternate with others having a

more conventional appearance. Ultrastructurally, the vacuoles represent either intracellular lumens bordered by microvilli or distended vesicles which may contain mucin (fig. 11-8) (12).

A variant is the follicular adenoma in which the intracytoplasmic vacuoles are small and the nucleus remains centrally located. This may represent an early stage of the cell destined to become a signet ring cell. In these tumors, the stroma tends to be hyaline and is occasionally peppered with fine particles of calcium salts.

Immunohistochemical studies have shown that these cytoplasmic vacuoles, whether small or large, are strongly reactive for thyroglobulin (fig. 11-9). Interestingly, they may also be positive for mucin stains, a fact that has led to the alternative designations *signet ring cell mucinous*

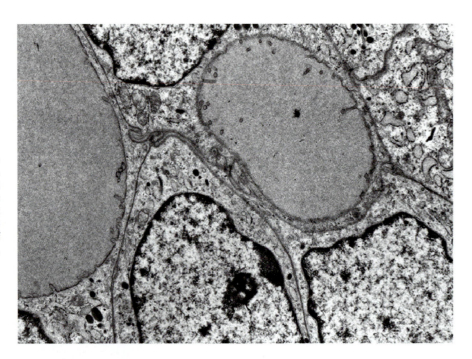

Figure 11- 8

FOLLICULAR NEOPLASM WITH CLEAR CELL AND SIGNET RING FEATURES

The intracytoplasmic lumens containing finely granular material consistent with colloid are visible in this electron micrograph. Short microvilli are projecting into the lumens. (Courtesy of Dr. R. Erlandson, New York, NY.)

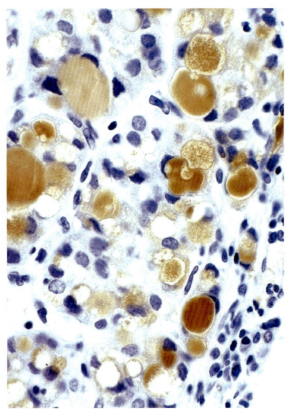

Figure 11-9

SIGNET RING FOLLICULAR ADENOMA

Strong intracytoplasmic immunoreactivity for thyroglobulin is evident.

adenoma (17) and *mucin-producing microfollicular adenoma* (18). It has been suggested that the mucin reactivity is due to the presence of protein-polysaccharide complexes derived from the partial degradation of thyroglobulin (19) and that the intracellular accumulation of thyroglobulin results from an inability of the cell to excrete it, perhaps due to a deletion in one or more of the many proteins needed to carry out this complex task. This interpretation is analogous to that advanced for neoplastic signet ring cells in other tumors, such as adenocarcinoma, malignant lymphoma, and plasmacytoma.

Lipid-Rich Follicular Adenoma and Carcinoma. In lipid-rich follicular adenoma, so rare as to represent a pathologic curiosity, the cytoplasm contains numerous lipid vacuoles (20–22). This should not be confused with adenolipoma, in which islands of mature adipose tissue alternate with the neoplastic epithelial cells (see chapter 15). A case of lipid-rich follicular carcinoma has been described in a patient with McCune-Albright syndrome (23).

Papillary Thyroid Carcinoma. In our experience, clear cell change is a rare event in this tumor type, but Meissner and Adler (24) reported its occurrence in 28 percent of their 226 cases. This marked discrepancy is probably due to a difference in threshold criteria. It is not unusual for the

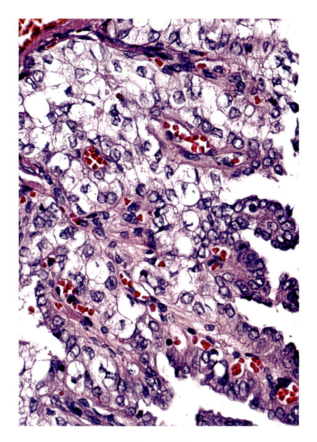

Figure 11-10

PAPILLARY CARCINOMA WITH CLEAR CELL FEATURES

The cytoplasmic clearing is more pronounced in the deep portion of the tumor.

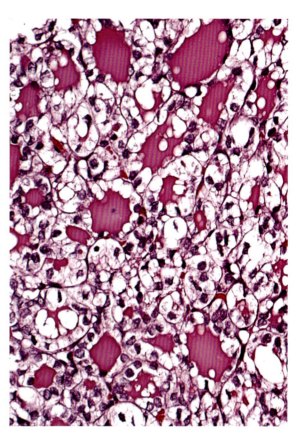

Figure 11-11

FOLLICULAR VARIANT OF PAPILLARY CARCINOMA WITH PROMINENT CYTOPLASMIC CLEAR CELL FEATURES

The colloid has a dark red staining quality.

cells of papillary thyroid carcinoma to have a pale staining quality, but not sufficient in our opinion to place them in a clear cell category. True cytoplasmic clearing seems to be more common in the follicular variant of papillary carcinoma than in the more conventional form (figs. 11-10–11-12) (1). In most instances, the cause of clearing is the accumulation of glycogen; in others, the change is the result of vesicle formation (1). The latter was the case in the spectacular example of clear cell papillary carcinoma reported by Variakojis et al. (25). There is no evidence that papillary carcinomas exhibiting clear cell change behave differently from those lacking this feature.

Undifferentiated Carcinoma. In rare instances, thyroid tumors with an undifferentiated (anaplastic) appearance feature extensive clear cell changes (fig. 11-13) (1,26). This was true for 7 of the 130 anaplastic carcinomas reported by

Woolner et al. (27). Some of these tumors have squamoid features, as is also the case for undifferentiated thyroid carcinomas in general (28). Glycogen accumulation is the most common cause for the clear cell change in this group.

Clear Cell Medullary Carcinoma. This exceptionally rare tumor is discussed in more detail in chapter 12 (29).

Other Conditions

Non-neoplastic disorders, such as dyshormonogenetic goiter, Hashimoto thyroiditis, and nodular hyperplasia, have an appearance analogous to that of the respective entities they represent, except for the clear cell change (figs.11-14–11-16). Metastatic clear cell carcinoma, particularly from kidney, is discussed in chapter 16. Metastatic signet ring carcinoma, particularly from stomach or breast, has nuclei

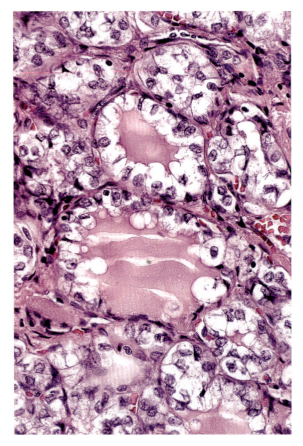

Figure 11-12

**FOLLICULAR VARIANT OF PAPILLARY
CARCINOMA WITH CLEAR CELL FEATURES**

The cytoplasmic clearing is very pronounced, and the nuclei are of the papillary carcinoma type.

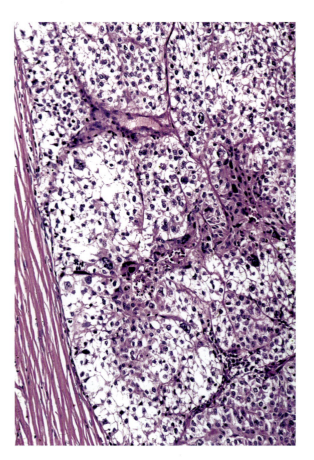

Figure 11-13

**UNDIFFERENTIATED (ANAPLASTIC) CARCINOMA
WITH CLEAR CELL FEATURES.**

The nonclear portion of the tumor has squamoid features.

that are clearly malignant looking, a pattern of growth that is interfollicular, mucin stains that are strongly positive, and absent thyroglobulin and thyroid transcription factor (TTF)-1 immunoreactivity.

Parathyroid adenoma and carcinoma have usually smaller cells, a prominent nesting pattern, and a better-developed capillary network. The endothelial cells of these vessels are very hyperplastic and mitotically active, useful diagnostic clues. Most patients have serum abnormalities of calcium, phosphorus, and circulating parathyroid hormone. Immunohistochemically, these tumors are reactive for parathyroid hormone and negative for thyroglobulin and TTF-1.

Clear cell salivary gland tumors, particularly mucoepidermoid carcinoma, are also in the differential diagnosis. Interestingly, a case of clear cell follicular thyroid adenoma ectopically located in the submandibular region has been reported (30).

TUMORS WITH SQUAMOUS FEATURES

There is a large variety of thyroid neoplasms that exhibit focal or extensive *squamous differentiation*. Most have been discussed elsewhere in this Fascicle, but they are listed here in a single section for comparative and differential diagnostic purposes.

Papillary Carcinoma. Squamous metaplasia is common in papillary thyroid carcinoma (reported in 20 to 40 percent of the cases). The squamous component has a well-differentiated appearance, analogous to that seen in so-called adenoacanthomas of the endometrium and other organs.

Mucoepidermoid Carcinoma. *Mucoepidermoid carcinoma* is a rare malignant thyroid neoplasm exhibiting a combination of squamous and mucin-secreting features (31). Most patients are women, and the age of presentation in the reported cases ranges from 10 to 57 years (32–36). Grossly, the tumors are well-

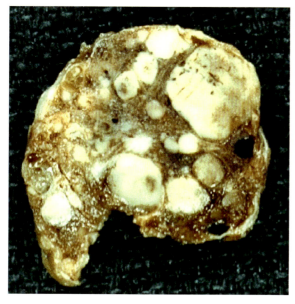

Figure 11-14

NODULAR HYPERPLASIA WITH CLEAR CELL CHANGE

The clear cell-containing nodules are variously sized, whitish gray, and well circumscribed.

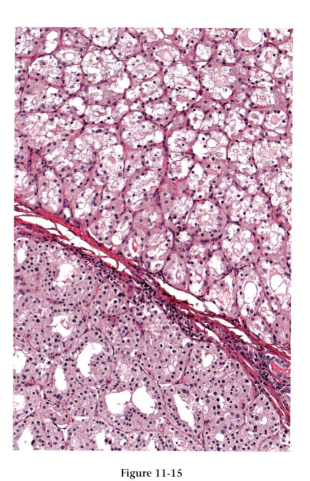

Figure 11-15

NODULAR HYPERPLASIA WITH CLEAR CELL COMPONENT

The two components are sharply separated from each other.

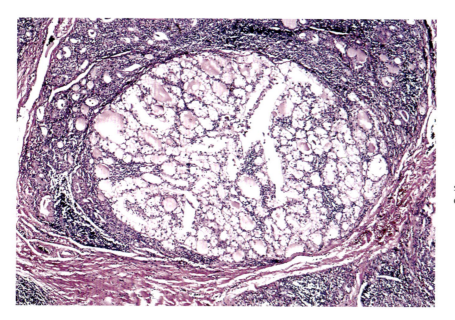

Figure 11-16

FOCAL CLEAR CELL CHANGE IN NODULAR HYPERPLASIA

The clear cell component is sharply outlined and displays oncocytic features.

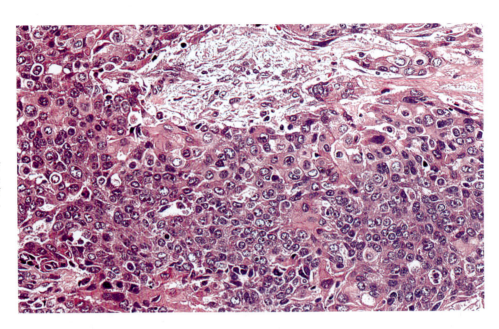

Figure 11-17

MUCOEPIDERMOID CARCINOMA

The pattern of growth is solid. There is a predominance of squamous and intermediate cells.

circumscribed but not encapsulated and often show prominent cystic formations (31). Microscopically, the squamous areas are arranged in solid sheets with horny pearl formation, while the mucinous cells often line duct-like structures, which exceptionally are ciliated (21,37). A close intermingling of the two components is the rule (fig. 11-17). The stroma is markedly fibrotic, and psammoma bodies are present in several of the reported cases. The mucinous material is positive with Mayer mucicarmine and Alcian blue stains.

Immunohistochemically, the tumor cells are positive for keratin and polyclonal carcinoembryonic antigen (CEA), the latter antigen predominating in the duct-like elements. Although thyroglobulin was negative in the original series, subsequent studies have shown that it is often expressed (31,36,38). Neuroendocrine markers, including calcitonin, are absent. Marked abnormalities of the cadherin/catenin complex have been documented, of a type rarely, if ever, observed in papillary carcinoma of either classic or diffuse sclerosing type (39).

Lymph node metastases to the neck are common. Distant metastases or death from this tumor, however, is rare.

The origin of mucoepidermoid carcinoma of the thyroid gland remains controversial. It has been suggested that the tumor arises from intrathyroidal solid cell nests, i.e., from vestiges of the ultimobranchial body (32,33,40,41). The other possibility, which we and others favor, is that this tumor is of metaplastic follicular cell derivation, a possibility supported by the identification of TTF-1, TTF-2, PAX8, Na-I symporter, and thyroid peroxidase mRNA (31,42,43). Some features suggest that mucoepidermoid carcinoma is histogenetically related to papillary carcinoma, a tumor well known for its tendency to undergo squamous metaplastic changes (see chapter 7). Although the *BRAF* mutations typical of papillary carcinoma have not been detected in mucoepidermoid carcinoma (44), the tumor shares with papillary carcinoma the common presence of prominent fibrosis and psammoma bodies, and the tendency for regional nodal metastases. Furthermore, it has been reported in association with papillary carcinoma of the classic, tall cell, and follicular variant types (32,36,43,45). Some of the reported cases of mucoepidermoid carcinoma (with or without concomitant papillary carcinoma) exhibit undifferentiated (anaplastic) areas (46), and others contain areas with an insular pattern of growth (32). It is unclear whether the translocation t(11;19) associated with *MECTI-MAML2* gene fusion identified in mucoepidermoid carcinomas of salivary and bronchial glands is also present in mucoepidermoid carcinoma of the thyroid (47).

Sclerosing Mucoepidermoid Carcinoma with Eosinophilia. The descriptive term *sclerosing mucoepidermoid carcinoma with eosinophilia* (SMECE) has been proposed for a

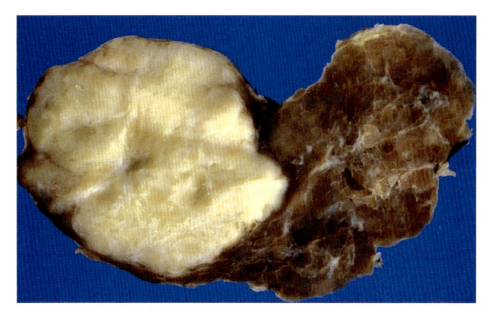

Figure 11-18

SCLEROSING MUCOEPIDERMOID CARCINOMA WITH EOSINOPHILIA

The tumor has an unusually well-circumscribed appearance. The dense fibrosis that is characteristic of this entity is appreciated. The tumor is arising in a fibrous variant of Hashimoto thyroiditis.

Figure 11-19

SCLEROSING MUCOEPIDERMOID TUMOR WITH EOSINOPHILIA

Eosinophils and other inflammatory cells are numerous. There is also extensive fibrosis. The prominence of the nucleolus and the tissue eosinophilia are important diagnostic clues to the development of a malignancy in fibrous Hashimoto thyroiditis.

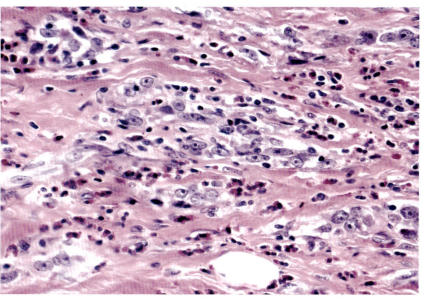

morphologically distinctive, generally low-grade malignant neoplasm arising in thyroid glands affected by Hashimoto thyroiditis, often of the fibrous type (48). At the gross level, the tumor is white, homogeneous, firm, and either poorly or well circumscribed (fig. 11-18). Microscopically, strands and small nests of squamoid tumor cells that exhibit mild to moderate nuclear pleomorphism, distinct nucleoli, and pale cytoplasm are seen infiltrating an abundant, dense fibrohyaline stroma (fig. 11-19). Foci of definite squamous differentiation and pools of mucin are often present. Some of the tumors contain nests of

clear cells, secondary to the accumulation of cytoplasmic glycogen (49).

The tumor cells are consistently immunoreactive for keratin and inconstantly positive for TTF-1, but (in contrast to mucoepidermoid carcinoma) not for thyroglobulin (49). Stains for mucin are focally positive in the squamoid islands. There is also strong positivity for p63 (50). A striking feature of the tumor is the heavy infiltration of the stroma and many of the tumor islands by mature eosinophils (fig. 11-20). Extrathyroidal extension occurs, as well as perineurial and vascular permeation. Some cases have resulted

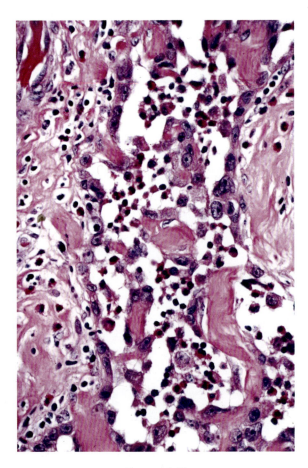

Figure 11-20

**SCLEROSING MUCOEPIDERMOID
TUMOR WITH EOSINOPHILIA**

The disaggregation of the tumor cells by the eosinophils results in an angiosarcoma-like appearance.

in regional lymph node metastases, which microscopically may simulate Hodgkin lymphoma (51). Distant metastases are rare (52).

The exact position of this tumor type in the scheme of thyroid malignancies remains to be determined. It shares many features with mucoepidermoid carcinoma, of which it may simply represent a variant. Other features of this tumor, however, and its constant association with Hashimoto thyroiditis, justify a separate description.

In regard to histogenesis, an origin from the benign squamous nests that are often found in Hashimoto thyroiditis (particularly its fibrous variant) is suggested by the close intermingling and occasional merging with these structures. The marked tissue eosinophilia (sometimes designated as *tumor-associated tissue eosinophilia*

[TATE]) is analogous to that sometimes occurring in carcinomas of other sites, including oral cavity, vulva, and cervix, and thought to be the result of the secretion of eosinophil chemotactic factors by the tumor cells. Interestingly, most of these tumors show evidence of squamous differentiation (53).

Squamous Cell and Undifferentiated Carcinomas. The term *squamous cell carcinoma* has been applied in the literature to primary malignant thyroid neoplasms with obvious squamous differentiation and marked cytologic atypia. It is rare in its pure form. When associated with mucin production, it has been designated *adenosquamous carcinoma* (54). In most cases, the squamous component merges with undifferentiated areas, so that the tendency has been to place the tumor into the undifferentiated (anaplastic) category. A residual component of papillary carcinoma is sometimes found in these neoplasms (fig. 11-21) (55).

Immunohistochemically, squamous cell carcinoma of the thyroid gland is consistently positive for cytokeratin (CK)19 and CK7, occasionally positive for CK18, and negative for CK1, CK4, CK6, CK10/13, and CK 20 (56). Its cytokeratin profile is different from that of the tumor described in the next section (56).

Carcinoma with Thymus-Like Differentiation. The unusual intrathyroid or perithyroidal *carcinoma with thymus-like differentiation* (CASTLE) is characterized by a lobular pattern of growth, lymphocytic infiltration, and occasional perivascular space formation. It is thought to arise from thymic or related branchial pouch derivatives (see chapter 15). Most of these tumors have squamoid features, and a few exhibit obvious squamous differentiation.

Follicular Neoplasms. In contrast to papillary carcinoma, the occurrence of squamous metaplasia in follicular neoplasms of either benign or malignant type is extremely rare. One such case, developing in a follicular carcinoma, was reported as *adenoacanthoma* (see chapter 6) (57).

Medullary Carcinoma. A squamous variety of this tumor is described in chapter 12.

Secondary Carcinoma. The thyroid gland can be involved by direct extension of squamous cell carcinoma of pharynx, larynx, trachea, esophagus, or adjacent metastatic lymph nodes, or colonized through blood-borne metastases by squamous cell carcinoma of distant sites, particularly lung (see chapter 16). The distinction from primary thyroid squamous cell carcinoma often requires the integration of clinical, endoscopic, radiographic, and pathologic data (58).

Non-Neoplastic Conditions. Epithelial nests of squamoid or squamous appearance are seen in a variety of non-neoplastic conditions, of which Hashimoto thyroiditis (especially its fibrous variant) is the most common (59). They also appear in other types of thyroiditis, in the atrophic and fibrotic gland accompanying myxedema, and in nodular hyperplasia (adenomatoid goiter). The nests are solid or cystic, and are sometimes accompanied by mucin deposition.

These tumors are invariably positive immunohistochemically for keratin and often for CEA (60). Some are also reactive for thyroglobulin, whereas others contain or are surrounded by clusters of C-cells (61,62). The source of these structures is probably varied. Some (perhaps most) represent metaplastic follicles. Others may be remnants of either the third or fourth branchial pouches (in which case they may have the appearance of thymic nests), or the fifth pouch, which corresponds to the ultimobranchial body (in which case they may contain C-cells). The solid and cystic formations that occur with great frequency in the neonatal thyroid gland are probably of branchial pouch derivation (38), the latter also probably the source of the gross cystic formations occasionally seen in Hashimoto thyroiditis (63).

TUMORS WITH MUCINOUS FEATURES

It was often assumed in the past that if a thyroid neoplasm was positive for mucin stains (in the sense of epithelial glycoproteins), this meant that it was of metastatic nature, and that mucin positivity in a tumor present in another site (e.g., lymph node or lung) ruled out a thyroid origin for it. Both assumptions have proven incorrect.

The types and number of primary thyroid neoplasms in which epithelial mucosubstances have been detected is substantial (64). Thyroglobulin is a sialic acid–containing glycoprotein and the mucin detectable in the follicular lumen or cytoplasm of some follicular-derived thyroid tumors by Mayer mucicarmine, Alcian blue, or other conventional mucin stains may therefore

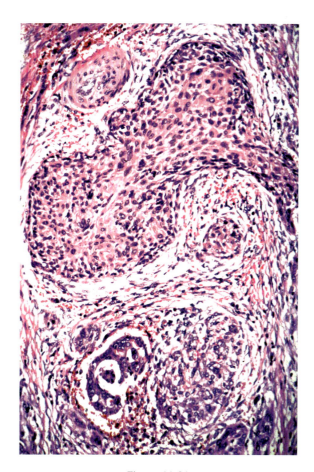

Figure 11-21

**PAPILLARY CARCINOMA WITH
EXTENSIVE SQUAMOUS METAPLASIA**

The squamous areas show a moderate degree of atypia. Tumors with this appearance behave more aggressively than conventional papillary thyroid carcinoma but less so than undifferentiated (anaplastic) carcinomas.

be an abnormal form of this substance or related polysaccharides (65,66). Specific types of thyroid neoplasms that may contain variable amounts of mucin are described below.

Signet Ring Follicular Adenoma and Carcinoma. The intracellular thyroglobulin that accumulates in *signet ring follicular adenoma,* a rare variant of follicular adenoma, is often mucin-positive, usually weakly but sometimes strongly (fig. 11-22) (65–69). This is also true for the even rarer malignant counterpart of this tumor, *signet ring follicular carcinoma.*

Mucoepidermoid Carcinoma and Sclerosing Mucoepidermoid Carcinoma with Eosinophilia. The mucin deposition in these tumors is

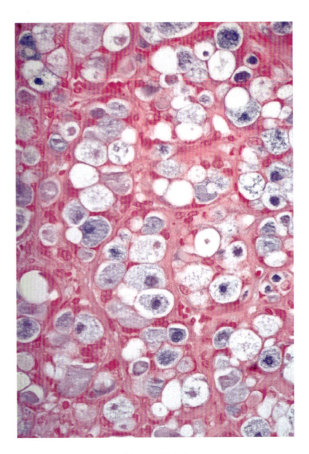

Figure 11-22

SIGNET RING FOLLICULAR ADENOMA

The presence of acidic mucin is made evident in this signet ring adenoma by the strong intracytoplasmic positivity for Alcian blue.

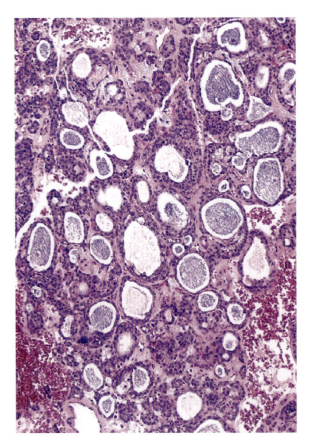

Figure 11-23

FOLLICULAR ADENOMA WITH MUCIN PRODUCTION

The intraluminal content of this follicular adenoma is granular and basophilic, indicative of the presence of acidic mucosubstances. Mucin stains were strongly positive.

accompanied by squamous metaplasia. They are discussed in other portions of this chapter.

Mucinous Carcinoma. There are a few cases of *mucinous* or *mucin-producing* (*adeno*)*carcinoma* of the thyroid gland in the literature (70–75). Postulated sources for this tumor include metaplastic follicles and ultimobranchial body remnants, in particular, the mucin-containing follicles normally grouped in the C-cell area of the gland (76,77). Some of these tumors are probably closely related to mucoepidermoid carcinoma, but their exact place in the scheme of thyroid neoplasia is still uncertain. Analysis of the individual case reports supports the position that mucinous carcinoma is not a distinct entity but rather a heterogeneous group of tumors sharing the feature of mucin secretion (figs. 11-23, 11-24).

Papillary Carcinoma. It has been shown that *papillary thyroid carcinoma* metastatic to cervical lymph nodes exhibits intracytoplasmic mucin positivity in 17 percent of cases (78). An even higher percentage was recorded by Mlynek et al. (64) in their study of primary papillary carcinomas.

The presence and significance of mucins in this tumor type has also been investigated by searching for the mucin genes and their products (the various MUC proteins) with reverse transcriptase polymerase chain reaction (RT-PCR) evaluation and immunohistochemistry. There is some suggestion that MUC1 and MUC4 are expressed more commonly in papillary carcinoma and that their overexpression is related to tumor aggressiveness, but the results obtained by the various investigators have been conflicting (79–81). The diagnostic

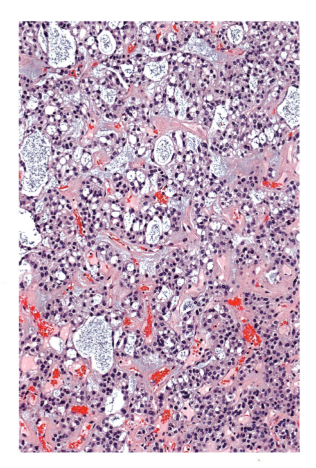

Figure 11-24

FOLLICULAR ADENOMA WITH MUCIN PRODUCTION

The mucinous material is entirely intraluminal, suggesting a relationship with thyroglobulin. This change is more common in follicular carcinomas than in follicular adenomas.

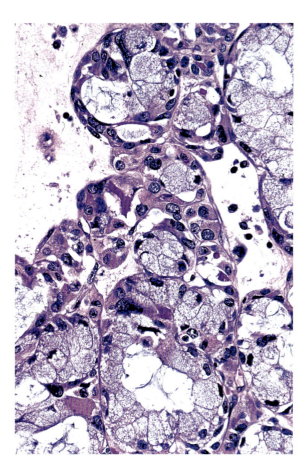

Figure 11-25

ONCOCYTIC (HÜRTHLE) CELL TUMOR WITH MUCIN PRODUCTION

There is an intimate admixture of oncocytes and mucin-secreting cells.

and prognostic value of these determinations remains doubtful at present (82,83).

Oncocytic (Hürthle Cell) Carcinoma. Spectacular examples of mixed mucus-secreting and *oncocytic carcinoma* of the thyroid gland have been reported (fig. 11-25) (84).

Poorly Differentiated Carcinoma. A few cases of *poorly differentiated carcinoma* with extensive mucin deposition are on record (85,86).

Undifferentiated Carcinoma. Some otherwise typical *undifferentiated carcinomas* show focal mucin positivity, almost always in intimate admixture with squamoid or squamous foci (see chapter 9) (87).

Medullary Carcinoma. In about 10 percent of cases of *medullary carcinoma,* positivity for mucin is found in the cytoplasm of the tumor cells (see chapter 12) (88,89). Also, mixed *medullary-mucinous (amphicrine) carcinomas* of the thyroid gland have been reported (90).

Secondary Carcinoma. A variety of mucin-producing adenocarcinomas metastasize to the thyroid gland. Those arising from the gastrointestinal tract and breast are the most common, but they can also originate in lung, pancreas, ovary, and other sites (see chapter 16) (91)

Myxoid Stromal Changes. Some thyroid tumors contain extracellular myxoid material composed of hyaluronic acid and related acid mucopolysaccharides. This is regarded as a nonspecific finding of probable degenerative nature, which on occasion is prominent but not of clinical significance. It can be seen in follicular and Hürthle cell tumors of both benign and malignant types, as well as non-neoplastic conditions such as nodular hyperplasia (92,93).

A variation on the theme that may have some diagnostic significance is the focal extracellular myxoid change limited to the interphase between the peripheral edge of a follicular neoplasm and the inner aspect of the fibrous capsule that surrounds it. Although not pathognomonic, it is our impression that this change is more commonly seen in minimally invasive follicular carcinomas than in follicular adenomas, and that it may represent a warning sign of the beginning of capsular invasion by the tumor.

REFERENCES

1. Carcangiu ML, Sibley RK, Rosai J. Clear cell change in primary thyroid tumors. A study of 38 cases. Am J Surg Pathol 1985;9:705-22.
2. Katzenstein AL, Prioleau PG, Askin FB. The histologic spectrum and significance of clear-cell change in lung carcinoma. Cancer 1980;45:943-7.
3. Ishimaru Y, Fukuda S, Kurano R, Miura K, Tajiri J, Maeda K. Follicular thyroid carcinoma with clear cell change showing unusual ultrastructural features. Am J Surg Pathol 1988;12:240-6.
4. Mochizuki M, Saito K, Kanazawa K. Benign follicular thyroid nodule composed of signet-ring-like cells with PAS-negative thyroglobulin accumulation in dilated rough endoplasmic reticulums. Acta Pathol Jpn 1992;42:111-4.
5. Sobel HJ, Lamovec J, Us-Krasovec M, Zitnik V. Benign clear cell thyroid tumor with "balloon cell" change: evidence suggesting its pathogenesis. Ultrastruct Pathol 1993;17:469-75.
6. Nishimura R, Noguchi M, Tsujimoto M, et al. Thyroid clear cell adenoma with marked dilation of membranous structures: electron-microscopic study. Ultrastruct Pathol 2001;25:361-6.
7. Tsybrovskyy O, Rossman-Tsybrovskyy M. Oncocytic versus mitochondrion-rich follicular thyroid tumors. Should we make a difference? Histopathology 2009;55:665-82.
8. Batsakis JG, Nishiyama RH, Schmidt RW. "Sporadic goiter syndrome": a clinicopathologic analysis. Am J Clin Pathol 1963;39:241-51.
9. Dickersin GR, Vickery AL Jr, Smith SB. Papillary carcinoma of the thyroid oxyphil cell type, "clear cell" variant. Am J Surg Pathol 1980;4:501-9.
10. Kniseley RM, Andrews GA. Transformation of thyroidal carcinoma to clear-cell type. Am J Clin Pathol 1956;26:1427-38.

11. Harach HR, Virgili E, Soler G, Zusman SB, Saravia-Day E. Cytopathology of follicular tumours of the thyroid with clear cell change. Cytopathology 1991;2:125-35.
12. Schröder S, Böcker W. Clear-cell carcinomas of thyroid gland: a clinicopathological study of 13 cases. Histopathology 1986;10:75-89.
13. Stoll W, Lietz H. Zur Kenntnis und Problematik des hellzelligen Adenomes in der Schilddrüse. Virchows Arch [A] 1973;361:163-73.
14. Hazard JB, Kenyon R. Atypical adenoma of the thyroid. Arch Pathol 1954;58:554-63.
15. Civantos F, Albores-Saavedra J, Nadji M, Morales AR. Clear cell variant of thyroid carcinoma. Am J Surg Pathol 1984;8:187-92.
16. Schröder S, Böcker W. Signet-ring-cell thyroid tumors. Follicle cell tumors with arrest of folliculogenesis. Am J Surg Pathol 1985;9:619-29.
17. Gherardi G. Signet ring cell 'mucinous' thyroid adenoma: a follicle cell tumour with abnormal accumulation of thyroglobulin and a peculiar histochemical profile. Histopathology 1987;11:317-26.
18. Rigaud C, Peltier F, Bogomoletz WV. Mucin producing microfollicular adenoma of the thyroid. J Clin Pathol 1985;38:277-80.
19. Mendelsohn G. Signet-ring-simulating microfollicular adenoma of the thyroid. Am J Surg Pathol 1984;8:705-8.
20. Schröder S, Hüsselmann H, Böcker W. Lipid-rich cell adenoma of the thyroid gland. Report of a peculiar thyroid tumour. Virchows Arch A Pathol Anat Histopathol 1984;404:105-8.
21. Ranaldi R, Goteri G, Bearzi I. Lipid-rich adenoma of the thyroid. Pathol Res Pract 1993;189:1101-6; discussion 1106-7.

22. Chetty R. Thyroid follicular adenoma composed of lipid-rich cells. Endocr Pathol 2011;22:31-4.

23. Yang GC, Yao JL, Feiner HD, Roses DF, Kumar A, Mulder JE. Lipid-rich follicular carcinoma of the thyroid in a patient with McCune-Albright syndrome. Mod Pathol 1999;12:969-73.

24. Meissner WA, Adler A. Papillary carcinoma of the thyroid; a study of the pathology of two hundred twenty-six cases. Arch Pathol 1958;66:518-25.

25. Variakojis D, Getz ML, Paloyan E, Straus FH. Papillary clear cell carcinoma of the thyroid gland. Hum Pathol 1975;6:384-90.

26. Wassef M, Monteil JP, Bourgeon F, Le Charpentier Y. [Undifferentiated clear cell thyroid carcinoma. Diagnostic interest of ultrastructural study (author's transl).] Ann Pathol 1981;1:95-8. [French]

27. Woolner LB, Beahrs OH, Black BM, McConahey WM, Keating FR Jr. Classification and prognosis of thyroid carcinoma. A study of 885 cases observed in a thirty year period. Am J Surg 1961;102:354-87.

28. Fisher ER, Kim WS. Primary clear cell thyroid carcinoma with squamous features. Cancer 1977;39:2497-502.

29. Landon G, Ordoñez NG. Clear cell variant of medullary carcinoma of the thyroid. Hum Pathol 1985;16:844-7.

30. Giri D, Gultekin SH, Ward RF, Hurley JR, Hoda SA. Clear-cell follicular adenoma of ectopic thyroid in the submandibular region. Endocr Pathol 1998;9:347-51.

31. Wenig BM, Adair CF, Heffess CS. Primary mucoepidermoid carcinoma of the thyroid gland: a report of six cases and a review of the literature of a follicular epithelial-derived tumor. Hum Pathol 1995;26:1099-108.

32. Franssila KO, Harach HR, Wasenius VM. Mucoepidermoid carcinoma of the thyroid. Histopathology 1984;8:847-60.

33. Katoh R, Sugai T, Ono S, et al. Mucoepidermoid carcinoma of the thyroid gland. Cancer 1990;65:2020-7.

34. Mizukami Y, Matsubara F, Hashimoto T, et al. Primary mucoepidermoid carcinoma in the thyroid gland. A case report including an ultrastructural and biochemical study. Cancer 1984;53:1741-5.

35. Rhatigan RM, Roque JL, Bucher RL. Mucoepidermoid carcinoma of the thyroid gland. Cancer 1977;39:210-4.

36. Baloch ZW, Solomon AC, LiVolsi VA. Primary mucoepidermoid carcinoma and sclerosing mucoepidermoid carcinoma with eosinophilia of the thyroid gland: a report of nine cases. Mod Pathol 2000;13:802-7.

37. Ando M, Nakanishi Y, Asai M, Maeshima A, Matsuno Y. Mucoepidermoid carcinoma of the thyroid gland showing marked ciliation suggestive of its pathogenesis. Pathol Int 2008;58:741-4.

38. Beckner ME, Shultz JJ, Richardson T. Solid and cystic ultimobranchial body remnants in the thyroid. Arch Pathol Lab Med 1990;114:1049-52.

39. Rocha AS, Soares P, Machado JC, et al. Mucoepidermoid carcinoma of the thyroid: a tumour histotype characterised by P-cadherin neoexpression and marked abnormalities of E-cadherin/catenins complex. Virchows Arch 2002;440:498-504.

40. Harach HR. Thyroid follicles with acid mucins in man: a second kind of follicles? Cell Tissue Res 1985;242:211-5.

41. Harach HR, Day ES, de Strizic NA. Mucoepidermoid carcinoma of the thyroid. Report of a case with immunohistochemical studies. Medicina (B Aires) 1986;46:213-6.

42. Minagawa A, Iitaka M, Suzuki M, et al. A case of primary mucoepidermoid carcinoma of the thyroid: molecular evidence of its origin. Clin Endocrinol (Oxf) 2002;57:551-6.

43. Bondeson L, Bondeson AG, Thompson NW. Papillary carcinoma of the thyroid with mucoepidermoid features. Am J Clin Pathol 1991;95:175-9.

44. Trovisco V, Vieira de Castro I, Soares P, et al. BRAF mutations are associated with some histological types of papillary thyroid carcinoma. J Pathol 2004;202:247-51.

45. Miranda RN, Myint MA, Gnepp DR. Composite follicular variant of papillary carcinoma and mucoepidermoid carcinoma of the thyroid. Report of a case and review of the literature. Am J Surg Pathol 1995;19:1209-15.

46. Cameselle-Teijeiro J, Febles-Pérez C, Sobrinho-Simões M. Papillary and mucoepidermoid carcinoma of the thyroid with anaplastic transformation: a case report with histologic and immunohistochemical findings that support a provocative histogenetic hypothesis. Pathol Res Pract 1995;191:1214-21.

47. Bhaijee F, Pepper DJ, Pitman KT, Bell D. New developments in the molecular pathogenesis of head and neck tumors: a review of tumor-specific fusion oncogenes in mucoepidermoid carcinoma, adenoid cystic carcinoma, and NUT midline carcinoma. Ann Diagn Pathol 2011;15:69-77.

48. Chan JK, Albores-Saavedra J, Battifora H, Carcangiu ML, Rosai J. Sclerosing mucoepidermoid carcinoma of the thyroid with eosinophilia. A distinctive low-grade malignancy arising from the metaplastic follicles of Hashimoto's thyroiditis. Am J Surg Pathol 1991;15:438-48.

49. Albores-Saavedra J, Gu X, Luna MA. Clear cells and thyroid transcription factor I reactivity in sclerosing mucoepidermoid carcinoma of the thyroid gland. Ann Diagn Pathol 2003;7:348-53.

50. Hunt JL, LiVolsi VA, Barnes EL. p63 expression in sclerosing mucoepidermoid carcinomas with eosinophilia arising in the thyroid. Mod Pathol 2004;17:526-9.

51. Solomon AC, Baloch ZW, Salhany KE, Mandel S, Weber RS, LiVolsi VA. Thyroid sclerosing mucoepidermoid carcinoma with eosinophilia: mimic of Hodgkin disease in nodal metastases. Arch Pathol Lab Med 2000;124:446-9.

52. Sim SJ, Ro JY, Ordoñez NG, Cleary KR, Ayala AG. Sclerosing mucoepidermoid carcinoma with eosinophilia of the thyroid: report of two patients, one with distant metastasis, and review of the literature. Hum Pathol 1997;28:1091-6.

53. Lowe D, Jorizzo J, Hutt MS. Tumor-associated eosinophilia: a review. J Clin Pathol 1981;34:1343-8.

54. Nicolaides AR, Rhys Evans P, Fisher C. Adeno-squamous carcinoma of the thyroid gland. J Laryngol Otol 1989;103:978-9.

55. Eom TI, Koo BY, Kim BS, et al. Coexistence of primary squamous cell carcinoma of thyroid with classic papillary thyroid carcinoma. Pathol Int 2008;58:797-800.

56. Lam KY, Lo CY, Liu MC. Primary squamous cell carcinoma of the thyroid gland: an entity with aggressive clinical behaviour and distinctive cytokeratin expression profiles. Histopathology 2001;39:279-86.

57. Mahoney JP, Saffos RO, Rhatigan RM. Follicular adenoacanthoma of the thyroid gland. Histopathology 1980;4:547-57.

58. Syed MI, Stewart M, Syed S, et al. Squamous cell carcinoma of the thyroid gland: primary or secondary disease? J Laryngol Otol 2011;125:3-9.

59. Ryska A, Ludvíková M, Rydlová M, Cáp J, Zalud R. Massive squamous metaplasia of the thyroid gland—report of three cases. Pathol Res Pract 2006;202:99-106.

60. Vollenweider I, Hedinger C. Solid cell nests (SCN) in Hashimoto's thyroiditis. Virchows Arch A Pathol Anat Histopathol 1988;412:357-63.

61. Harach HR. Histological markers of solid nests of the thyroid. With some emphasis on their expression in thyroid ultimobranchial-related tumors. Acta Anat (Basel) 1985;124:111-6.

62. Harach HR. Solid cell nests of the thyroid. J Pathol 1988;155:191-200.

63. Louis DN, Vickery AL Jr, Rosai J, Wang CA. Multiple branchial cleft-like cysts in Hashimoto's thyroiditis. Am J Surg Pathol 1989;13:45-9.

64. Mlynek ML, Richter HJ, Leder LD. Mucin in carcinomas of the thyroid. Cancer 1985;56:2647-50.

65. Gherardi G. Signet ring cell 'mucinous' thyroid adenoma: a follicle cell tumour with abnormal accumulation of thyroglobulin and a peculiar histochemical profile. Histopathology 1987;11:317-26.

66. Rigaud C, Bogomoletz WV. "Mucin secreting" and "mucinous" primary thyroid carcinomas: pitfalls in mucin histochemistry applied to thyroid tumours. J Clin Pathol 1987;40:890-5.

67. Mendelsohn G. Signet-cell simulating microfollicular adenoma of the thyroid. Am J Surg Pathol 1984;8:705-8.

68. Brisigotti M, Lorenzini P, Alessi A, Fabbretti G, Baldoni C. Mucin-producing adenoma of the thyroid gland. Tumori 1986;72:211-4.

69. Yoshida J, Tanimura A, Yamashita H, Matsuo K. Signet ring cell adenoma of the thyroid with mucin predominance. Thyroid 1999;9:401-4.

70. Cruz MC, Marques LP, Sambade CC, Sobrinho-Simões MA. Primary mucinous carcinoma of the thyroid. Surg Pathol 1991;4:266-73.

71. Deligdisch L, Subhani Z, Gordon RE. Primary mucinous carcinoma of the thyroid gland: report of a case and ultrastructural study. Cancer 1980;45:2564-7.

72. Diaz-Perez R, Quiroz H, Nishiyama RH. Primary mucinous adenocarcinoma of thyroid gland. Cancer 1976;38:1323-5.

73. Harada T, Shimaoka K, Hiratsuka M, Hirokawa M, Tsukayama C. Mucin-producing carcinoma of the thyroid gland—a case report and review of the literature. Jpn J Clin Oncol 1984;14:417-24.

74. Sobrinho-Simões MA, Nesland JM, Johannessen JV. A mucin-producing tumor in the thyroid gland. Ultrastruct Pathol 1985;9:277-81.

75. Cretney A, Mow C. Mucinous variant of follicular carcinoma of the thyroid gland. Pathology 2006;38:184-6.

76. Harach HR. Thyroid follicles with acid mucins in man: a second kind of follicles? Cell Tissue Res 1985;242:211-5.

77. Harach HR. Thyroglobulin in human thyroid follicles with acid mucin. J Pathol 1991;164:261-3.

78. Chan JK, Tse CC. Mucin production in metastatic papillary carcinoma of the thyroid. Hum Pathol 1988;19:195-200.

79. Morari EC, Silva JR, Guilhen AC, et al. Muc-1 expression may help characterize thyroid nodules but does not predict patients' outcome. Endocr Pathol 2010;21:242-9.

80. Abrosimov A, Saenko V, Meirmanov S, et al. The cytoplasmic expression of MUC1 in papillary thyroid carcinoma of different histological variants and its correlation with cyclin D1 overexpression. Endocr Pathol 2007;18:68-75.

81. Baek SK, Woo JS, Kwon SY, Lee SH, Chae YS, Jung KY. Prognostic significance of the MUC1 and MUC4 expressions in thyroid papillary carcinoma. Laryngoscope 2007;117:911-6.

82. Alves P, Soares P, Fonseca E, Sobrinho-Simões M. Papillary thyroid carcinoma overexpresses fully and underglycosylated mucins together with native and sialylated simple mucin antigens and histo-blood group antigens. Endocr Pathol 1999;10:315-24.

83. Alves P, Soares P, Rossi S, Fonseca E, Sobrinho-Simões M. Clinicopathologic and prognostic significance of the expression of mucins, simple mucin antigens and histo-blood group antigens in papillary thyroid carcinoma. Endocr Pathol 1999;10:305-13.

84. Uccella S, La Rosa S, Finzi G, Erba S, Sessa F. Mixed mucus-secreting and oncocytic carcinoma of the thyroid: pathologic, histochemical, immunohistochemical, and ultrastructural study of a case. Arch Pathol Lab Med 2000;124:1547-52.

85. Kondo T, Kato K, Nakazawa T, Miyata K, Murata S, Katoh R. Mucinous carcinoma (poorly differentiated carcinoma with extensive extracellular mucin deposition) of the thyroid: a case report with immunohistochemical studies. Hum Pathol 2005;36:698-701.

86. Mizukami Y, Nakajima H, Annen Y, Michigishi T, Nonomura A, Nakamura S. Mucin-producing poorly differentiated adenocarcinoma of the thyroid. A case report. Pathol Res Pract 1993;189:608-12; discussion 612-5.

87. Carcangiu ML, Steeper T, Zampi G, Rosai J. Anaplastic thyroid carcinoma. A study of 70 cases. Am J Clin Pathol 1985;83:135-58.

88. Fernandes BJ, Bedard YC, Rosen I. Mucus-producing medullary cell carcinoma of the thyroid gland. Am J Clin Pathol 1982;78:536-40.

89. Zaatari GS, Saigo PE, Huvos AG. Mucin production in medullary carcinoma of the thyroid. Arch Pathol Lab Med 1983;107:70-4.

90. Golouh R, Us-Krasovecf M, Auersperg M, Jancar J, Bondi A, Eusebi V. Amphicrine-composite calcitonin and mucin-producing carcinoma of the thyroid. Ultrastruct Pathol 1985;8:197-206.

91. D'Antonio A, Addesso M, De Dominicis G, Boscaino A, Liguori G, Nappi O. Mucinous carcinoma of thyroid gland. Report of a primary and a metastatic mucinous tumour from ovarian adenocarcinoma with immunohistochemical study and review of literature. Virchows Arch 2007;451:847-51.

92. Kuma S, Hirokawa M, Miyauchi A, Kakudo K. Oncocytic thyroid carcinoma with extensive myxoid stroma. Histopathology 2003;42:514-6.

93. Murakami S, Sakata H, Okubo K, Tsuji Y, Kayano H. Thyroid adenoma with extensive extracellular mucin deposition: report of a case. Surg Today 2007;37:226-9.

239

12 MEDULLARY THYROID CARCINOMA AND C-CELL HYPERPLASIA

MEDULLARY THYROID CARCINOMA

Definition. *Medullary thyroid carcinoma* is a malignant tumor of the thyroid gland composed of cells showing evidence of C-cell differentiation (1,2). These tumors are also referred to as *C-cell carcinoma, solid carcinoma with amyloid stroma*, and *neuroendocrine carcinoma of the thyroid gland*.

General Features. A report of an amyloid-containing thyroid tumor first appeared in the literature in 1910 (3). Brandenburg (4) reported a second case in 1954 and suggested that the amyloid was produced by the tumor cells. The major features of this tumor type, which include a solid nonfollicular growth pattern, stromal amyloid deposits, and a high incidence of lymph node metastasis, were defined in 1959 by Hazard et al. (5) who suggested the term medullary (solid) thyroid carcinoma. Interestingly, R.C. Horn (6), 8 years earlier, had described a type of thyroid carcinoma characterized by sharply defined round or ovoid compact cell groups in a background of hyalinized connective tissue and noted that it was of intermediate malignancy. In retrospect, at least some of the cases reported by Horn represented medullary thyroid carcinomas.

In 1961, Sipple (7) reported a case of thyroid carcinoma associated with pheochromocytoma and an apparent parathyroid adenoma. In a detailed literature review, Sipple noted an increased incidence of thyroid cancer in patients with pheochromocytoma, with a risk 14 times greater than in the general population. Williams et al. (8) subsequently reported that the thyroid tumors associated with pheochromocytomas were medullary thyroid carcinomas. In the same year, Williams proposed that medullary thyroid carcinoma was derived from parafollicular cells, based on comparative studies in dogs and rats (9). Bussolati and Pearse (10) demonstrated the parafollicular cell origin of calcitonin, which had been discovered by Copp et al. (11)

more than a decade earlier. Subsequent studies confirmed the presence of calcitonin in tumor extracts and in the plasma of affected individuals (12,13).

Medullary thyroid carcinoma comprises up to 10 percent of all thyroid malignancies (2,14). These tumors occur sporadically or in heritable forms with an autosomal dominant pattern of inheritance. Sporadic tumors account for approximately 75 percent of all cases and occur with equal frequency in different parts of the world (15). The prevalence of this tumor type in unselected autopsy series is less than 0.7 percent (16–25). As might be anticipated, the prevalence in surgical series of patients with nodular thyroid disease in whom abnormal calcitonin levels were identified during screening studies is considerably higher than in autopsy series (26–34). In rare instances, the sporadic tumors occur in association with Hashimoto disease, but this occurrence is probably fortuitous (35). Some data suggest that chronic hypercalcemia may be associated with an increased incidence of these tumors (36).

In contrast to their rarity in humans, medullary carcinomas occur commonly in many rat strains, and their prevalence increases with the age of the animal (37). Vitamin D3 administration increases the frequency of the tumors in rats, whereas animals on a vitamin D-restricted diet have a lower incidence of C-cell tumors, when compared to controls on a normal diet (38,39). Medullary thyroid carcinomas also occur commonly in bulls, where they are classified as ultimobranchial neoplasms (40).

The incidence of medullary carcinoma is not increased in humans treated by irradiation to the head and neck. Data in experimental animals, however, suggest that rats treated with low doses of ^{131}I have an increased incidence of these tumors. Interestingly, high levels of calcium in drinking water do not potentiate the effects of radiation on C-cells in these studies (38,39).

Table 12-1

FAMILIAL MEDULLARY THYROID CARCINOMA SYNDROMES

	MEN 2A[a]	MEN 2B	FMTC[b]
OMIM[c]	171400	162300	155240
Syndrome	Sipple syndrome	Williams-Pollock syndrome; Gorlin-Vickers syndrome; Wagenmann-Froboese syndrome	
Relative frequency	55-90%	5-10%	5-35%
Commonly involved codons	634, 609, 611. 618, 620, 630, 631	918, 883	768, 790, 791, 804, 649, 891, 609, 611, 618, 620, 630, 631
Mean age (years) at clinical presentation of thyroid tumors	25-35	10-20	45-55
Medullary thyroid carcinoma	>90%	>90%	>90%
Pheochromocytoma	30-50%	50%	–
Hyperparathyroidism	15-30%	–	–

[a]MEN = multiple endocrine neoplasia; FMTC = familial medullary thyroid carcinoma.
[b]FMTC most likely represents a phenotypic variant of MEN 2A with low penetrance of pheochromocytoma and hyperparathyroidism.
[c]Online Mendelian Inheritance in Man number.

Medullary thyroid carcinomas are highly penetrant in patients with the multiple endocrine neoplasia (MEN) 2 syndromes. It has been estimated that more than 90 percent of carriers of the affected gene will develop these tumors (41). MEN 2A-associated tumors account for up to 90 percent of all heritable medullary thyroid carcinomas in some series. Affected patients also have pheochromocytomas in approximately 30 to 50 percent of the cases and parathyroid abnormalities in 15 to 30 percent (Table 12-1) (7,11,14,41–43).

Occasional kindreds manifest thyroid tumors exclusively, and these cases are classified as *familial medullary thyroid carcinoma* (FMTC) (Table 12-1) (44,45). The definition of FMTC and its separation from MEN 2A is controversial (46). According to guidelines from the American Thyroid Association, the most rigid definition for FMTC is multigenerational transmission of medullary thyroid carcinoma in which no family member has pheochromocytoma or hyperparathyroidism. A less rigid definition is the presence of four affected family members without other features of MEN 2A. Because of the subsequent development of pheochromocytoma and hyperparathyroidism in some families previously classified as FMTC, this disorder is now thought to represent a phenotypic variant of MEN 2A

with low penetrance of pheochromocytoma and hyperparathyroidism (Table 12-1) (47).

Some kindreds with MEN 2A or FMTC also have cutaneous lichen amyloidosis, which typically appears as pruritic plaques over the upper back (48,49). It has been suggested that the presence of this disorder should prompt molecular studies to rule out MEN 2A. In several of the patients reported by Verga et al. (49), pruritus had been present since infancy. According to this study, pruritus played a pivotal role in the development of the cutaneous lichen amyloidosis, with the amyloid deposits developing as a result of repeated scratching. Hirschsprung disease has been associated with MEN 2A in a few families and also occurs in occasional patients with FMTC (50).

MEN 2B is the most phenotypically distinctive type of the MEN 2 syndromes and also has the most aggressive clinical course (41,51–53). It accounts for approximately 5 to 10 percent of all MEN 2 cases. Pheochromocytomas occur in up to 50 percent of affected patients, but hyperparathyroidism, in contrast to MEN 2A, is absent (Table 12-1). Additionally, patients with MEN 2B may have musculoskeletal abnormalities (marfanoid habitus, pes cavus, pectus excavatum); neuromas of the lips, tongue, and conjunctiva; medullated corneal nerves; urinary

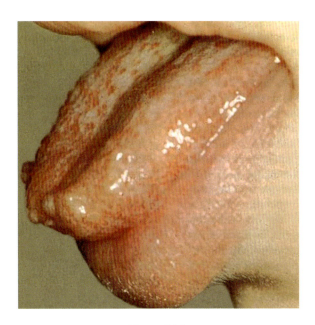

Figure 12-1

MULTIPLE ENDOCRINE NEOPLASIA 2B

Multiple mucosal neuromas are present in the tongue and lips of a patient with multiple endocrine neoplasia (MEN) 2B.

ganglioneuromatosis and malformations; and intestinal ganglioneuromatosis (fig. 12-1). The latter features need not be present in MEN 2B, and their presence is not pathognomonic of this disorder (41).

Molecular Pathogenesis. All of the MEN 2 syndromes develop as a consequence of germline mutations of the *RET* gene on chromosome 10q11.2 (54,55). The *RET* proto-oncogene encompasses 21 exons and encodes a receptor tyrosine kinase with three isoforms that are generated by alternative splicing of the 3^1 region (56). RET receptors have an extracellular domain (including ligand binding, cadherin-like, and cysteine-rich subdomains) that is involved in the recognition and binding of RET ligands and coreceptors, a transmembrane domain, and an intracellular segment with the two tyrosine kinase domains (TK1, TK2) required for autophosphorylation of the tyrosine residues within the TK domain of each RET molecule (57). RET is expressed in a variety of neural crest derivatives (C-cells, adrenal medulla, extra-adrenal paraganglia, sympathetic and enteric ganglia), parathyroid gland, and urogenital tract (58). Mice homozygous for a targeted *RET* mutation develop to term but

demonstrate both renal agenesis or dysgenesis and absence of enteric neurons, but do not have evidence of neoplastic disorders (59).

The ligands for RET are members of the glial cell line–derived neurotrophic factor (GDNF) family and include GDNF, neuturin, artemin, and persphin. The receptors for the GDNF family are membrane-bound adaptor molecules and RET, which form a trimeric receptor system that includes glycosyl-phosphatidyl (anchored coreceptor alpha 1-4 as a ligand binding component and RET as an activation signaling component) (60). Activation of the RET receptor leads to activation of downstream signaling pathways, including RAS/ERK, ERK5, p38, MAPK, PLC gamma, PI3-kinase, JNK, STAT, and SRC (61).

Activating germline mutations of *RET*, resulting in aberrant activation of RET receptors, have been identified in MEN 2A, MEN 2B, and FMTC (41,62–68). The mutations are of the missense type and affect primarily exons 10 and 11, with less frequent mutations affecting exons 13, 14, 15, and 16. Most mutations in patients with MEN 2A and FMTC affect the cysteine-rich extracellular domain of the receptor protein. Codon 634 mutations are present in approximately 80 percent of MEN 2A patients while mutations in codons 609, 618, and 620 account for more than 60 percent of cases of FMTC and those patients with the Hirschsprung phenotype. In patients with MEN 2A, the codon 634 mutations have a strong genotype-phenotype correlation with the development of pheochromocytoma and hyperparathyroidism (69). The most common mutation of codon 634 is *TGC-CGC* (Cys-Arg)

Mutations affecting the tyrosine kinase domain (codon 918) are present in the germline of a high proportion of patients with MEN 2B and in a subset of tumors in patients with sporadic medullary thyroid carcinoma (65–67). This mutation results in the replacement of methionine with threonine. Codon 883 mutations, which result in the substitution of phenylalanine for alanine, occur in a small subset of patients with MEN 2B (70).

MEN 2-associated mutations have high transforming activities for NIH 3T3 cells, suggesting that the underlying tumorigenic mechanism results from dominant oncogenic conversion rather than loss of tumor suppressor function (71). Moreover, targeting of MEN 2A mutant

RET to C-cells in transgenic mice results in the development of C-cell hyperplasia or medullary thyroid carcinoma in 100 percent of the animals, in addition to mammary and parotid gland carcinomas in 50 percent (72). Mutations of the *GDNF* gene, on the other hand, have not been implicated in the development of MEN 2 syndromes (73).

The mechanisms of gain of function mutations of the *RET* proto-oncogene depend on the affected codon. For example, mutations of codons 609, 611, 618, 620, 630, and 634 constitutively activate the tyrosine kinase receptor by ligand-independent dimerization and cross phosphorylation in the absence of its ligands and coreceptors (71). Patients with FMTC may have the same mutations as those present in MEN 2A or mutations of codons 768, 790, 791, 804, 844, and 891 (55). The latter mutations may interfere with ATP binding of the tyrosine kinase receptor. The codon 918 mutation results in alterations of the substrate recognition pocket of the catalytic core. This change may then lead to aberrant downstream signals resulting in the MEN 2B phenotype (70,74).

Inactivating germline *RET* mutations have been implicated in approximately 50 percent of familial and 15 percent of Hirschsprung disease-related cases (75). The cosegregation of Hirschsprung disease and MEN 2A is rare but has been documented in some patients with codon 609, 611, and 620 mutations. The codon 620 mutations account for 12 percent of the genetic variants associated with MEN 2A but are responsible for up to 50 percent of combined Hirschsprung disease-related MEN 2A cases (76). The codon 620 mutation has been referred to as the Janus mutation since it results in both gain of function leading to neoplasia (thyroid gland, adrenal gland) and in loss of function in the same individual (76). A few patients with FMTC have also been reported to have Hirschsprung disease. Cutaneous lichen amyloidosis is closely linked to mutations in codon 634 (49).

Somatic mutations of codon 918 have been reported in up to 80 percent of cases of sporadic medullary thyroid carcinoma (54,55,66). This mutation, which is identical to the 918 germline mutation in MEN 2B, results in the substitution of threonine for methionine. Rarely, other codons are mutated in these tumors.

The codon 918 mutation arises as an event in tumor progression within a single tumor or in a metastatic clone (54,62). The 918 mutation in sporadic tumors is nonhomogeneous and occurs in subsets of most tumors and among subsets of metastases. In the study reported by Eng et al. (54), one of two medullary carcinomas occurring in patients with MEN 2A carried a somatic codon 918 mutation in addition to a MEN 2A-associated germline mutation. While some studies (77–79) have reported that the 918 mutation is associated with a poor clinical outcome, other studies (80) have failed to confirm this claim. Moura et al. (81) have studied a series of sporadic medullary thyroid carcinomas (65 percent *RET* positive; 35 percent *RET* negative) with respect to other mutational events. Somatic *H-RAS* and *K-RAS* mutations were found in 56 and 12 percent of *RET*-negative cases, respectively (81). These findings suggest that *RAS* and *RET* represent alternative genetic events in sporadic medullary thyroid carcinoma (81). Similar results have been reported by other groups (82). An additional family of genes, designated Sprouty (Spry), has also been implicated in the development of medullary thyroid carcinoma. The studies of Macia et al. (83) have demonstrated that the Spry1 promoter is frequently methylated in these tumors, and that its expression is reduced, consistent with a tumor suppressor function.

Both medullary thyroid carcinoma and C-cell hyperplasia occur in transgenic mice with the cysteine-634-arginine or methionine-918-threonine mutations expressed under the control of the calcitonin gene promoter (84,85). Similar tumors have been reported in transgenic mice with the cysteine-634 mutation fused to the Moloney virus long terminal repeat (72). Transgenic mice constructed with the dopamine β-hydroxylase promoter to direct the expression of methionine-918-threonine develop tumors identical to human ganglioneuromas in the sympathetic nervous system and adrenal medulla (86).

Clinical Features. Sporadic medullary thyroid carcinoma is primarily a tumor of middle-aged adults, with a female to male ratio of 1.3:1.0 (2,8,14,15,87). Generally, most patients with sporadic tumors present with a painless thyroid nodule that is typically cold on scintigraphic scan. In the series reported by Kebebew et al. (88), nearly 75 percent of patients presented with a thyroid mass while 15 percent had local symptoms of dysphagia, dyspnea, or hoarseness. Cervical lymph node metastases may be evident at presentation, and in some cases, distant metastases are also present.

Affected patients present with a variety of signs and symptoms in addition to the thyroid mass. Patients with metastatic disease, for example, may have severe diarrhea or flushing, symptoms related to the high circulating levels of calcitonin. The tumors may produce a wide array of peptides, amines, and prostaglandins that also have been implicated in the development of diarrhea and flushing (89). Some tumors produce adrenocorticotrophic hormone (ACTH) and pro-opiomelanocortins, which are responsible for the development of Cushing syndrome (90). This syndrome occurs in approximately 0.6 percent of patients with medullary thyroid carcinoma and survival following its recognition is poor (91). Although very high levels of calcitonin may be present in patients with advanced medullary thyroid carcinoma, hypocalcemia is virtually nonexistent.

Patients with MEN 2A generally present with clinical evidence of thyroid tumors between the ages of 25 and 35 years, with a female to male ratio of 1.3:1.0 (15,41,92,93). The age of presentation has become progressively younger with the development of calcitonin screening studies in the 1970s (13,94) and molecular diagnostic testing for *RET* mutations in the 1990s (41,55,62,63,95,96). In approximately 10 percent of patients, pheochromocytomas become evident before the appearance of the thyroid tumors. The pheochromocytomas are commonly bilateral and multicentric, and are preceded by phases of adrenal medullary hyperplasia (97,98). Malignant pheochromocytomas are present in less than 4 percent of patients with MEN 2A, a frequency of malignancy that does not differ significantly from that observed in patients with nonsyndromic pheochromocytomas. Rare examples of composite pheochromocytomas have been reported in association with MEN 2A. Hyperparathyroidism occurs in up to 30 percent of affected patients. The resected parathyroid glands typically show evidence of chief cell hyperplasia, which is indistinguishable from that observed in patients with other forms of familial or sporadic hyperplasia.

The age of onset of thyroid tumors in patients with MEN 2B is considerably younger than that observed in patients with MEN 2A or FMTC (41,52,97,99,100). Prior to the advent of genetic and biochemical screening studies, the age of onset of thyroid tumors was between 10 to 20 years. More recent studies have demonstrated that medullary carcinomas can occur in MEN 2B patients of less than 1 year of age. Moreover, the tumors tend to be more aggressive than those occurring in MEN 2A patients (51,52,97,101). More than 50 percent of MEN 2B patients have de novo mutations, primarily affecting codon 918.

The age of onset of thyroid tumors in FMTC is 45 to 55 years of age, comparable to that observed in patients with sporadic medullary carcinoma (45). By definition, these patients lack evidence of adrenal medullary or parathyroid disease.

Laboratory Diagnosis. The laboratory diagnosis of medullary thyroid carcinoma has undergone a remarkable evolution over the past 30 years. Prior to the development of the radioimmunoassay for calcitonin, most patients with medullary thyroid carcinoma presented with thyroid masses, with or without regional nodal involvement (13,102). Current studies indicate that most medullary thyroid carcinomas secrete calcitonin into the serum. In an analysis of more than 800 cases, the prevalence rate of nonsecretory tumors was 0.83 percent (103). The extent of serum calcitonin elevation correlates strongly with tumor burden in most patients with advanced disease. Evaluation of serum calcitonin has also been recommended for patients with nodular thyroid disease, according to the guidelines proposed by the European Thyroid Cancer Task Force (104). It should be remembered, however, that moderate elevations of calcitonin may occur in patients with renal failure, paraneoplastic production by nonthyroidal neuroendocrine tumors, hypergastrinemia, hypercalcemia, Hashimoto thyroiditis, and interference from heterophil antibodies (104).

The observation that calcitonin secretion could be stimulated by the administration of secretagogues, such as calcium gluconate or pentagastrin, formed the basis of highly successful large scale screening studies in the 1970s

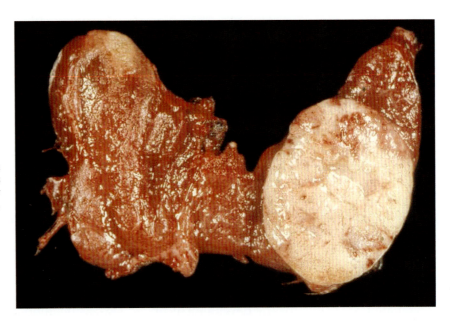

Figure 12-2

SPORADIC MEDULLARY THYROID CARCINOMA

The tumor is confined to a single thyroid lobe and appears sharply circumscribed. (Courtesy of Dr. X. Matias-Guiu, Lleida, Spain.)

and 1980s for the early detection of tumors in patients with MEN 2, MEN 2B, and FMTC (13,92,105,106).

Genetic studies in the mid 1990s were successful in establishing the molecular basis of the heritable forms of medullary carcinoma. These findings facilitated the development of molecular diagnostic testing procedures for the identification of carriers of the mutant gene. Current recommendations from the American Thyroid Association indicate that all patients with these tumors should be tested for *RET* mutations, including patients with apparent sporadic tumors (46,107). Peripheral blood leukocytes can be tested for mutations by the polymerase chain reaction (PCR) for the most commonly involved *RET* exons including 10, 11, 13–16, and possibly exon 8. Approximately 98 percent of carriers are correctly identified by this type of analysis, which is available in a number of commercial and university-based laboratories.

When a mutation is found, all first-degree relatives must be screened in order to identify carriers. If the PCR analysis is negative, the remaining exons can be sequenced. If this extended mutational analysis is negative in the index case, haplotype or genetic linkage analysis can be considered. If all of these tests are negative, the family should be informed of the low probability of heritable medullary carcinoma. Provocative testing of calcitonin may be performed if the family is not reassured of the low probability of hereditary disease on the basis of genetic testing.

Gross Findings. Medullary carcinomas vary in size from those that are barely visible to those that replace an entire lobe of the thyroid gland (1,2,5,8). The tumors are sharply circumscribed but are usually nonencapsulated (fig. 12-2). In rare instances, however, they may be surrounded by a fibrous capsule. On cross section, they are tan to pink, with a moderately firm consistency; others are firm and fibrotic, with areas of granular yellow discoloration that represent focal calcifications.

The smaller tumors generally occur at the junction of the upper and middle thirds of the lobes in which C-cells normally predominate. When the tumors become very large, they may replace one entire lobe and extend into the contralateral lobe, perithyroidal soft tissues, and trachea (fig. 12-3). While sporadic tumors most commonly present as unilateral lesions, the heritable tumors usually involve both lobes of the gland and are typically multicentric (figs. 12-4, 12-5) (2,41).

Microscopic Findings. Medullary thyroid carcinomas exhibit a wide variety of histologic patterns that mimic the entire spectrum of primary thyroid tumors, including follicular, papillary, and undifferentiated carcinomas (2,5,8,108–110). In fact, some degree of follicle formation is found in a high proportion of cases (111). The prototypic medullary carcinoma

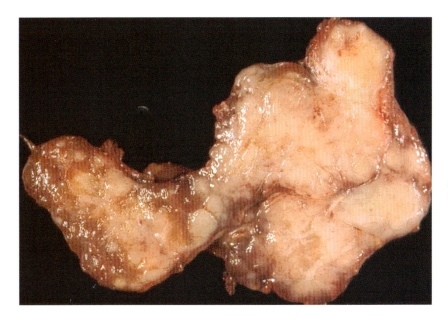

Figure 12-3

SPORADIC MEDULLARY THYROID CARCINOMA

The tumor has replaced both lobes. (Courtesy of Dr. X. Matias-Guiu, Lleida, Spain.)

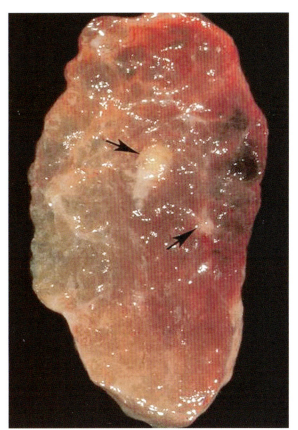

Figure 12-4

MEN 2A-ASSOCIATED MEDULLARY THYROID CARCINOMA

Multiple small foci of tumor are present within this thyroid lobe (arrows).

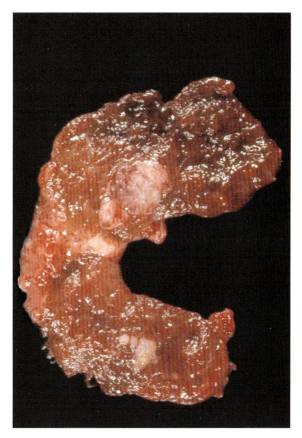

Figure 12-5

MEN 2A-ASSOCIATED MEDULLARY THYROID CARCINOMA

Tumor foci are present in both thyroid lobes. (Courtesy of Dr. X. Matias-Guiu, Lleida, Spain.)

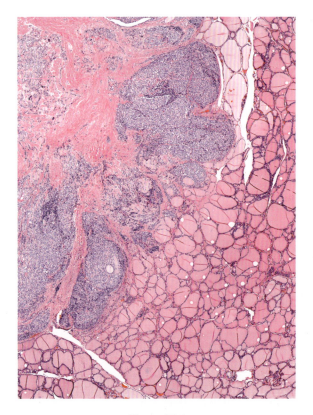

Figure 12-6

MEDULLARY THYROID CARCINOMA

Although this tumor appeared to be sharply circumscribed on gross examination, microscopic examination shows extension into the adjacent thyroid parenchyma.

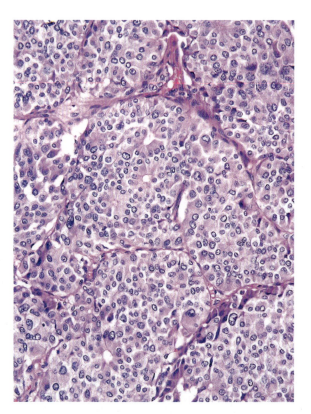

Figure 12-7

MEDULLARY THYROID CARCINOMA

This tumor has a predominant lobular growth pattern.

has a lobular, trabecular, insular, or sheet-like growth pattern (figs. 12-6–12-10). While most of the tumors appear grossly circumscribed, microscopic examination almost always shows extension of the tumor into the adjacent normal thyroid gland (fig. 12-6).

Individual tumor cells may be round, polygonal, or spindle shaped, with frequent admixtures of these cell types (figs. 12-11–12-14). In the round and polygonal cells, the nuclei have coarsely clumped or speckled chromatin and generally inconspicuous nucleoli. Occasional nuclear pseudoinclusions, similar to those seen in papillary thyroid carcinoma, may be present. Binucleate cells are common and giant cells with multiple nuclei may be evident (112). Spindle cells have elongated nuclei with a chromatin distribution similar to that seen in the polygonal and round cells (fig. 12-14). Most medullary carcinomas exhibit low to moderate

degrees of nuclear pleomorphism and mitotic activity is generally low (113). Occasional cases, however, may exhibit more marked degrees of pleomorphism and mitotic activity.

The cytoplasm varies from eosinophilic to basophilic, and is finely granular in well-fixed preparations (2,5,8). In some cases, however, the cytoplasm appears clear. Occasional mucin-positive cytoplasmic vacuoles are present (114–116). Zaatari et al. (117) found mucicarmine-positive deposits in up to 40 percent of cases, with intracellular deposits in 8 percent.

Foci of necrosis and hemorrhage are uncommon in small tumors, but more frequent in larger ones. Lymphatic and vascular invasion may be seen at the advancing front of the tumor (fig. 12-15) and, in advanced cases, lymphatic invasion may be present in the contralateral lobe.

Stromal amyloid deposits occur in up to 90 percent of cases (figs. 12-16, 12-17), including

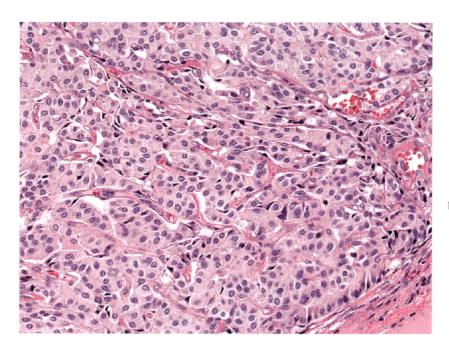

Figure 12-8

**MEDULLARY
THYROID CARCINOMA**

This tumor has nesting and trabecular growth patterns.

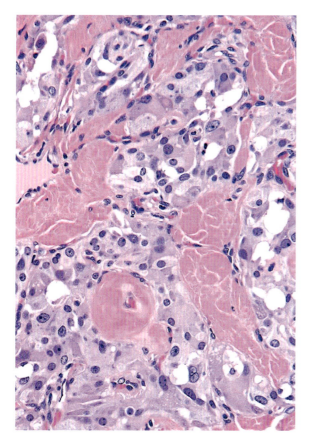

Figure 12-9

MEDULLARY THYROID CARCINOMA

Dense fibrous tissue is present between groups of tumor cells.

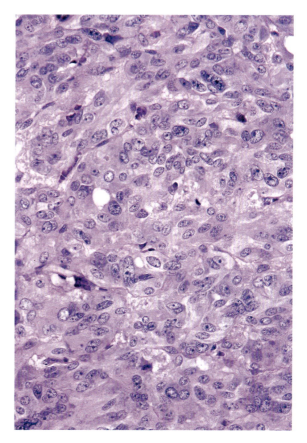

Figure 12-10

MEDULLARY THYROID CARCINOMA

This tumor has a solid growth pattern.

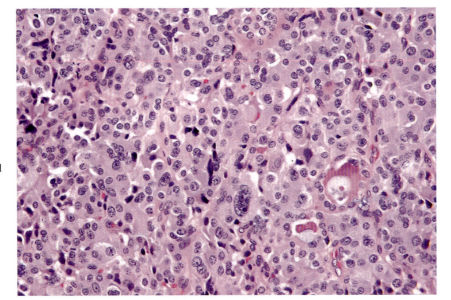

Figure 12-11

MEDULLARY THYROID CARCINOMA

Occasional cells have enlarged hyperchromatic nuclei.

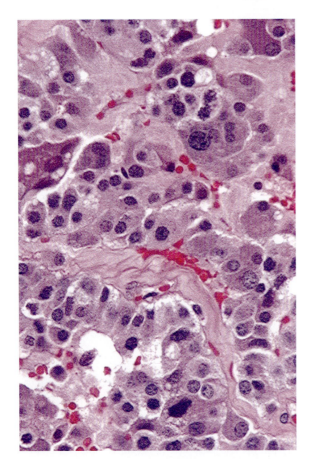

Figure 12-12

MEDULLARY THYROID CARCINOMA

The tumor cells have a distinct plasmacytoid appearance.

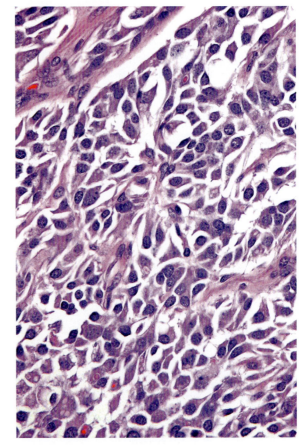

Figure 12-13

MEDULLARY THYROID CARCINOMA

The tumor cells have mixed epithelioid and spindle cell features.

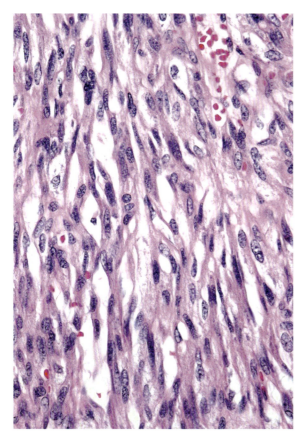

Figure 12-14

MEDULLARY THYROID CARCINOMA

This tumor is composed of spindle-shaped cells.

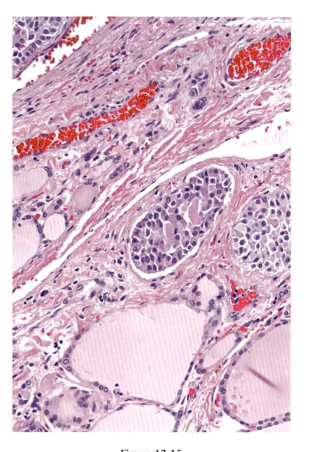

Figure 12-15

MEDULLARY THYROID CARCINOMA

Foci of lymphovascular invasion are present at the interface of the tumor with the adjacent thyroid gland.

micromedullary carcinomas (2,5,8,118,119). The amyloid deposits are Congo red positive, with typical green birefringence in polarized light (fig. 12-18), while crystal violet stains the amyloid deposits metachromatically. The amyloid deposits have a fibrillar ultrastructure that is identical to that seen in other forms of amyloidosis (fig. 12-19). Antibodies to calcitonin generally demonstrate positive staining within the amyloid. Although earlier studies suggested that the amyloid in these tumors was derived from the calcitonin precursor (120), more recent studies utilizing mass spectrometric analysis indicate that full length calcitonin is the sole constituent of amyloid in medullary carcinoma (121). In some instances, the amyloid may elicit a foreign body giant cell reaction (fig. 12-20). Calcification of the amyloid may occur (fig. 12-21) and occasional tumors contain psammoma bodies. A few medullary

carcinomas consist almost exclusively of amyloid, and it may be difficult to distinguish them from amyloid goiters (fig. 12-17) (122).

Histochemical and Immunohistochemical Findings. With the advent of immunohistochemistry, histochemical stains are of limited value for the diagnosis of medullary thyroid carcinoma in current daily practice. However, they are reviewed at this point primarily for historical purposes. Medullary carcinomas are typically argyrophilic, as demonstrated with the Grimelius method and other argyrophil staining methods (123,124). In most cases, the tumor cells show moderate to weak positivity, although occasional cells stain strongly. The most intensely positive cells often have a dendritic morphology. The Masson Fontana stain is usually negative, although occasional cases contain scattered argentaffin- positive cells. The

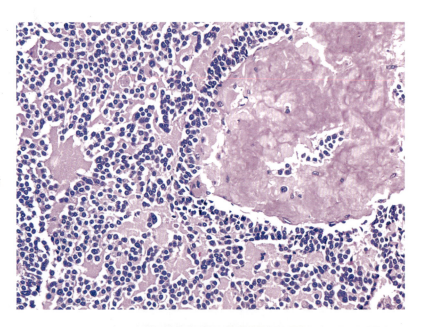

Figure 12-16

MEDULLARY THYROID CARCINOMA

This tumor contains deposits of amyloid.

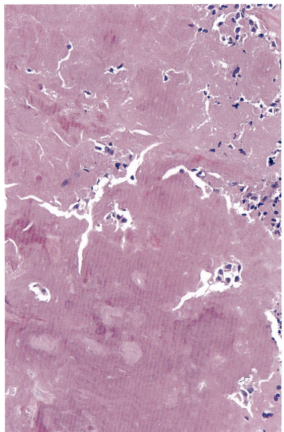

Figure 12-17

MEDULLARY THYROID CARCINOMA

This tumor is replaced almost completely by amyloid. (Figures 12-17 and 12-18 are from the same case.)

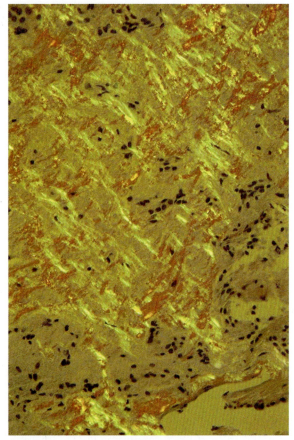

Figure 12-18

MEDULLARY THYROID CARCINOMA

This Congo red stain examined under polarized light shows green birefringence.

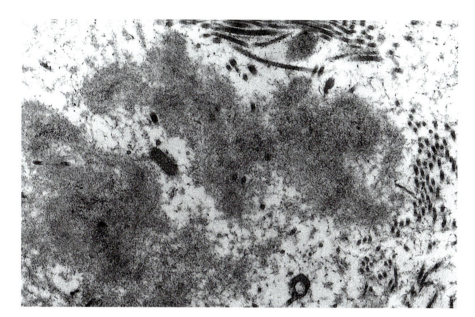

Figure 12-19

MEDULLARY THYROID CARCINOMA

This electron micrograph demonstrates fibrillar amyloid deposits together with densely stained collagen fibrils.

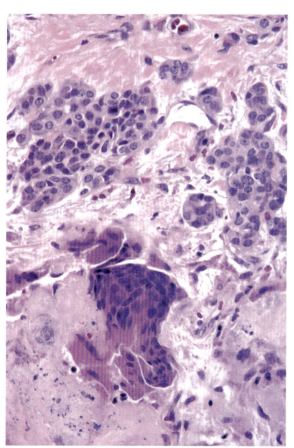

Figure 12-20

MEDULLARY THYROID CARCINOMA

A foreign body giant cell is present within the amyloid of this tumor.

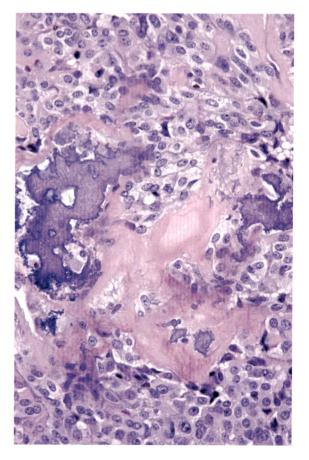

Figure 12-21

MEDULLARY THYROID CARCINOMA

The amyloid in this case is focally calcified.

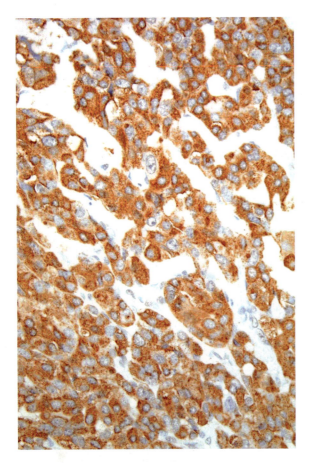

Figure 12-22

MEDULLARY THYROID CARCINOMA

Immunoperoxidase stain for calcitonin.

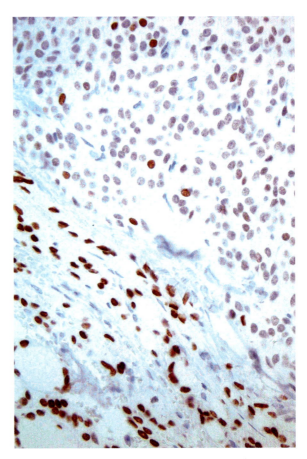

Figure 12-23

MEDULLARY THYROID CARCINOMA

Normal thyroid follicular cells (lower left) stain strongly for thyroid transcription factor (TTF)-1, while the tumor cell nuclei (upper right) are weakly reactive.

tumor cells exhibit metachromasia following treatment with hydrochloric acid and toluidine or coriphosphine O (masked metachromasia).

Calcitonin is present in 80 to 90 percent of medullary carcinomas (fig. 12-22) (125,126). Many cases show extensive calcitonin staining throughout the tumor, while others show only focal and weak reactivity. The calcitonin gene-related peptide is also commonly present within the tumors (127). Some tumors that are negative for calcitonin and the calcitonin gene-related peptide may give positive signals for calcitonin messenger RNA using in situ hybridization (128). Other tumors that are negative for calcitonin and calcitonin mRNA may be positive for the calcitonin gene-related peptide (129).

Medullary thyroid carcinomas are positive for thyroid transcription factor (TTF)-1, a property that they share with normal thyroid and tumors of follicular cell origin, although less intensely than the latter (fig. 12-23) (130). Stains for thyroglobulin are typically negative in these tumors, although entrapped normal thyroid follicles may stain positively (figs. 12-24, 12-25). Medullary carcinomas are positive for low molecular weight cytokeratins and exhibit a CK7-positive/CK20-negative phenotype (125). Vimentin is variably present within the tumor cells, and some tumors contain subpopulations of neurofilament-positive cells.

The tumors are positive for a wide spectrum of generic neuroendocrine markers including neuron-specific enolase (131), chromogranin (132), and synaptophysin (fig. 12-26) (133) (also see chapter 1). Since neuron-specific enolase may also be expressed in tumors of follicular cell

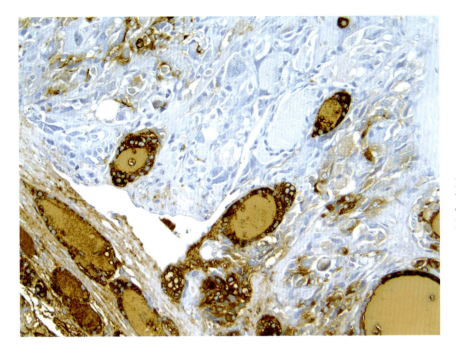

Figure 12-24

**MEDULLARY
THYROID CARCINOMA**

Normal thyroid follicles (lower left) stain for thyroglobulin, while the tumor (upper right) contains scattered thyroglobulin-positive follicles.

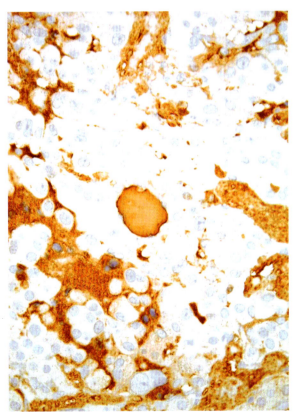

Figure 12-25

MEDULLARY THYROID CARCINOMA

Colloid and interstitial deposits are positive for thyroglobulin, while the tumor cells are negative.

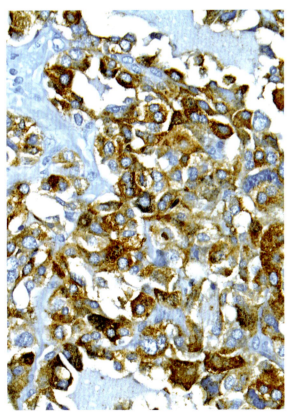

Figure 12-26

MEDULLARY THYROID CARCINOMA

Immunoperoxidase stain for chromogranin.

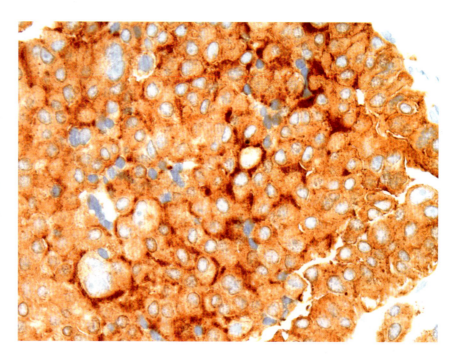

Figure 12-27

**MEDULLARY
THYROID CARCINOMA**

Immunoreactivity for carcino-embryonic antigen (CEA) with a monoclonal CEA antibody is present predominantly within the plasma membranes of the tumor cells.

origin, it is not a useful differential diagnostic marker. Chromogranin is a more specific marker for medullary carcinoma and may be more sensitive than calcitonin for the identification of this tumor type. Histaminase is also present in a high proportion of cases but is not specific for medullary thyroid carcinoma (134–136).

Many other peptides have been found within these tumors, and their presence has been confirmed by radioimmunoassays of tumor extracts. Both somatostatin (124,137–140) and gastrin-releasing peptide (141–143) are present in subpopulations of normal C-cells, and both of these peptides are commonly expressed in medullary carcinomas (144). Generally, somatostatin immunoreactivity is present in single cells or in small cell groups, which most often comprise less than 5 percent of the tumor cell population (138). The somatostatin-positive cells often have a dendritic morphology, with branching cell processes extending between adjacent tumor cells. Somatostatin receptors are also present within these tumors (145). Other peptides that may be present include ACTH (90), other pro-opiomelanocortins, neurotensin, substance P, vasoactive intestinal peptide, chorionic gonadotropin, and prolactin-stimulating factor (146–148). In rare instances, the tumors contain cells immunoreactive for glucagon, gastrin, and insulin (124,149). The tumors may also contain

catecholamines and serotonin (149). Similar to the distribution of certain peptide hormones in these tumors, serotonin immunoreactivity is often present in cells with a dendritic morphology.

Galectin-3 is present in approximately 90 percent of sporadic and heritable medullary thyroid carcinomas, while foci of C-cell hyperplasia are reportedly negative for this marker (150). Carcinoembryonic antigen (CEA) levels are typically high in the plasma of patients with medullary carcinoma. Correlative immuno-histochemical studies have demonstrated that nearly 100 percent of these tumors exhibit CEA positivity (fig. 12-27) (151–155). Several groups have demonstrated that certain medullary carcinomas lose the ability to synthesize and secrete calcitonin (156,157). Such cases, however, often maintain their capacity for CEA synthesis. In fact, calcitonin-negative areas in medullary carcinoma are frequently positive for CEA (152). The finding of decreasing levels of calcitonin in the presence of increasing levels of CEA generally predicts an aggressive clinical course (158).

Ultrastructural Findings. A characteristic feature of medullary carcinoma is the presence of membrane-bound secretory granules that represent sites of storage of calcitonin and other peptides (123,159–161). Type I granules have an average diameter of 280 nm, with moderately dense, finely granular contents that are

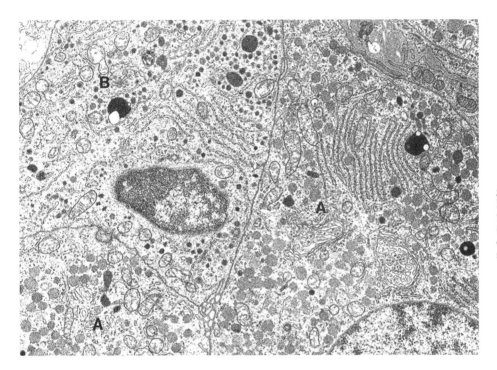

Figure 12-28

MEDULLARY THYROID CARCINOMA

In this electron micrograph, the tumor cells have a predominance of type I secretory granules (A). One cell has a predominance of type II secretory granules (B).

Figure 12-29

MEDULLARY THYROID CARCINOMA

This electron micrograph demonstrates sparsely granulated spindle-shaped tumor cells.

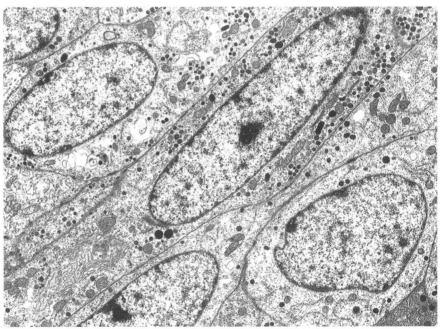

closely applied to the limiting membranes of the granules. Type II granules have an average diameter of 130 nm, with more electron-dense contents that are separated from the membranes by a narrow electron-lucent space (figs. 12-28, 12-29) (123). Generally, neoplastic C-cells have smaller numbers of granules than hyperplastic or normal C-cells.

Cytologic Findings. See chapter 20.

Differential Diagnosis. Medullary carcinomas may mimic the entire spectrum of benign and malignant thyroid tumors (110,162). True papillary variants are rare while pseudo-papillary changes that result from artifactual separation of tumor cells are more common. Papillary carcinomas of follicular cell origin have enlarged and irregularly shaped nuclei with an overlapping, ground-glass appearance, grooves, and pseudoinclusions. The nuclei of medullary carcinoma cells, on the other hand, are round with punctate chromatin. Nuclear pseudoinclusions may be present in medullary carcinoma, but they are considerably less common than in papillary carcinoma. Psammoma bodies are rarely present in medullary carcinoma. Medullary carcinomas are positive for calcitonin, chromogranin, and synaptophysin while papillary carcinomas are positive for thyroglobulin. Occasional papillary carcinomas contain abundant stromal collagen with foci of hyalinization that mimic amyloid. The often solid pattern of the sclerosing variants of papillary carcinoma, together with the prominent stroma, may be confused with medullary carcinoma; however, the sclerosing variants are negative for amyloid, lack calcitonin, and are positive for thyroglobulin.

Since medullary carcinomas may contain follicles they must be distinguished from follicular cell neoplasms. The latter tumors are positive for thyroglobulin but lack calcitonin, chromogranin, and synaptophysin immunoreactivity. Medullary carcinomas may also have oncocytic or clear cell features similar to those occurring in follicular cell tumors. Entrapped normal follicles are frequent in medullary carcinomas, particularly at their peripheries. True mixed follicular and C-cell tumors due occur, but are exceptionally rare. TTF-1 is present within follicular- and C-cell–derived tumors although the intensity of staining is usually less in the latter.

Medullary carcinomas must also be distinguished from poorly differentiated carcinomas that have insular, trabecular, or solid growth patterns. The stroma of insular carcinomas is negative for amyloid while the tumor cells are variably positive for thyroglobulin and TTF-1. Since medullary carcinomas often exhibit a solid growth pattern, some have been classified in the past as undifferentiated (anaplastic) carcinomas. Medullary carcinomas, however, lack the anaplasia, mitotic activity, and necrosis that characterize undifferentiated carcinomas. Medullary carcinomas of spindle and giant cell types may be distinguished from undifferentiated carcinomas by calcitonin immunoreactivity in the former group.

Studies by Nieuwenhuijzen-Kruseman et al. (163) have suggested that certain undifferentiated thyroid carcinomas may, in fact, represent medullary carcinomas. In a series of 14 anaplastic carcinomas, 9 exhibited both argyrophilia and calcitonin immunoreactivity. Martinelli et al. (164) described a case of anaplastic thyroid carcinoma that, in addition to argyrophilia and calcitonin immunoreactivity, also had mucinous and squamous differentiation. Anaplastic transformation of medullary carcinoma has also been reported by Zeman et al. (165). Others, however, have not been able to confirm the presence of calcitonin in undifferentiated carcinoma (166).

The distinction of small cell medullary carcinoma from malignant lymphoma and plasmacytoma may be difficult, particularly in small biopsy or cytologic samples. The demonstration of CD45 and additional markers of T- and B-cell differentiation supports the diagnosis of lymphoma while the presence of immunoglobulins and CD138 establishes the diagnosis of plasmacytoma.

Small cell carcinoma of the lung and other sites may metastasize to the thyroid gland and mimic medullary carcinoma of small cell type. Since TTF-1 is expressed both in lung and thyroid tumors, the presence of this marker is not a useful discriminant. Moreover, calcitonin and generic neuroendocrine markers may be present in both tumor types. Other neuroendocrine tumors that may metastasize to the thyroid gland and mimic medullary thyroid carcinoma include carcinoid and atypical carcinoid tumors. The diagnosis of metastatic neuroendocrine tumors to the thyroid gland is favored in the presence of multiple tumor foci, a predominant interstitial growth pattern, folliculotropism, and rosette formations with lumens and cuticular borders (167). In these instances, careful clinical and radiologic examination may be helpful in identifying a pulmonary or extrapulmonary primary.

Since mucin may be present in medullary carcinomas, these tumors must also be distinguished from mucinous carcinomas that have metastasized to the thyroid gland. The demonstration of calcitonin in a mucinous tumor within the thyroid gland establishes its C-cell origin.

The hyalinizing trabecular tumor is typically encapsulated, as are some variants of medullary carcinoma (168). A trabecular pattern is present in both tumor types and both may exhibit areas of hyalinization resembling amyloid. The stroma of medullary carcinoma, however, is positive for amyloid whereas the stroma of hyalinizing trabecular tumors stains only for collagen. While medullary carcinomas stain for calcitonin and CEA, these markers are negative in hyalinizing trabecular tumors. Occasional hyalinizing trabecular tumors, however, may be positive for chromogranin.

Medullary carcinomas may also be difficult to distinguish from paragangliomas. The latter tumors are positive for chromogranin and synaptophysin but are negative for calcitonin. In paragangliomas, a population of S-100–positive sustentacular cells is typically present at the periphery of the cell nest.

Occasional intrathyroidal parathyroid adenomas are difficult to distinguish from medullary carcinomas. Parathyroid tumors are positive for parathyroid hormone and chromogranin, while stains for calcitonin are negative.

Spread and Metastases. Medullary thyroid carcinomas most commonly metastasize to the central compartment and lateral cervical lymph nodes. In most patients with palpable thyroid tumors, lymph node metastases occur in the central compartment in 50 to 75 percent, in the ipsilateral jugulocarotid chain in 50 to 60 percent, and the contralateral jugulocarotid chain in 25 to 50 percent of patients with sporadic medullary thyroid carcinomas (169,170). Hematogenous metastases occur most commonly in lung, liver, and bone. Metastases to a variety of other sites, including the adrenal gland (171,172), pituitary gland (173), and breast (174) have also been reported.

Treatment and Prognosis. Medullary thyroid carcinoma of both sporadic and heritable types is treated optimally by total thyroidectomy. According to the recommendations of the American Thyroid Association, patients with suspected or known tumors, without evidence of local invasion or cervical nodal metastases, should be treated by total thyroidectomy with central lymph node dissection (level 6). A minority view considers ipsilateral cervical node dissection (levels 2 to 5) as an option (46). In patients with clinical evidence of ipsilateral cervical nodal disease, total thyroidectomy with central and modified cervical dissection is recommended. Preoperative ultrasound of cervical nodes is of value in determining whether a contralateral dissection is indicated (170).

Treatment for advanced disease includes surgery, radiation, chemoembolization, standard chemotherapy, and more recently developed, targeted chemotherapies (175). In particular, targeted therapies that inhibit RET and other tyrosine kinases have shown promise in the treatment of locally advanced and metastatic tumor (176–179).

According to the 2009 Management Guidelines from the American Thyroid Association, the specific type of mutation is important in the timing of prophylactic thyroidectomy for patients with MEN 2 (46). The risk stratification includes four groups, designated A-D, as summarized in Table 12-2, together with recommendations for timing of thyroidectomy.

Postoperative calcitonin levels usually stabilize within 72 hours after thyroidectomy. Postoperative surveillance is required for the monitoring of persistent, recurrent, or metastatic disease. The development of new calcitonin elevation, or the development of clinically evident disease, should prompt a metastatic work-up (170).

Both calcitonin and CEA serum doubling times have been used as prognostic indices in patients with medullary carcinoma (180,181). In one study (166), when the calcitonin doubling time was less than 6 months, 5- and 10-year survival rates were 25 and 8 percent, respectively, while doubling times between 6 months and 2 years were associated with 5- and 10-year survival rates of 92 and 37 percent, respectively. In contrast, patients with calcitonin doubling times of greater than 2 years were all alive at the end of the study. Some studies have suggested that CEA doubling time has a higher predictive value than calcitonin doubling time (181). These results suggest that calcitonin and CEA doubling times may be superior to initial clinical staging as a prognostic predictor.

Based on a review of nine series, the 5-year survival rates of patients with medullary carcinoma range from 65 to 89 percent while 10-year survivals range from 47 to 86 percent (88,182–187). Numerous histologic and immunohistochemical parameters, including cellular composition (spindle cell versus round cell), pleomorphism, extent of amyloid deposition,

Table 12-2

TIMING OF PROPHYLACTIC THYROIDECTOMY IN PATIENTS WITH MEN 2[a]

| | Risk Level | | | |
	A	B	C	D
Codon	768, 790, 791, 804, 649, 891	609, 611, 618, 620, 630, 631	634	918, 883
MEN 2 subtypes	FMTC[b]	FMTC/MEN 2A	MEN 2A	MEN 2B
MTC[c] age of onset[d]	Adult	5 years	<5 years	<1 year
Timing of thyroidectomy	Age 5–10 or when calcitonin levels increase	5 years	<5 years	First months of life

[a]MEN 2 = multiple endocrine neoplasia type 2.
[b]FMTC = familial medullary thyroid carcinoma.
[c]MTC = medullary thyroid carcinoma.
[d]Based on the earliest age of presence of MTC in screened populations.

immunohistochemical features, and extent of calcitonin staining, have been examined as potential prognostic parameters and none has proven to be significant in multivariate analyses. Instead, vascular invasion has been reported as an adverse predictor of disease-free status (188,189). Stromal desmoplasia has also been suggested as an important parameter to predict metastatic potential (190). Studies assessing tumor proliferative activity have demonstrated that metastasizing medullary thyroid carcinomas had higher Ki-67 indices than those that remained localized to the thyroid gland (191). Subsequent studies have shown that sporadic tumors with somatic *RET* mutations and Ki-67 indices in excess of 50 cells/mm^2 had a more aggressive course than mutation-negative tumors with low Ki-67 indices (192). As with other thyroid tumors, patient age (greater than 50 years) and stage are the most important prognostic factors. In the study reported by Kebebew et al. (88), age and stage were the only two independent prognostic factors in patients with these tumors. Male sex approached statistical significance in univariate analyses and most likely represents a minor risk factor. While patients with cervical lymph node metastases are more likely to have recurrent or persistent disease, this parameter is not associated with a significantly higher mortality rate.

In Kebebew's series of 104 patients with sporadic and heritable medullary carcinomas (88), 49.4 percent were cured, 12.3 percent had recurrent tumor, and 38.3 percent had persistent tumor. The mean follow-up time was 8.6 years,

with 10.7 percent and 13.5 percent cause-specific mortality rates at 5 and 10 years, respectively. In this series, 32 percent of the patients with heritable tumors were diagnosed by genetic or biochemical screening studies. These patients had a lower incidence of cervical node metastases and 94.7 percent were cured at last follow-up, as compared with patients with sporadic tumors. Patients presenting with the systemic symptoms of diarrhea, bone pain, and flushing had widespread metastatic disease and one third of these patients died within 5 years.

In a multicenter French study of 170 young patients with *RET* germline mutations, Rohmer et al. (193) concluded that disease-free survival was best predicted by TNM staging and a preoperative basal calcitonin level of less than 30 pg/mL. All patients had total thyroidectomies before a mean age of 11 years, together with central node dissection in two thirds of the cases. Ninety percent of patients treated after 1992 were disease free as compared to 62.1 percent treated before 1993. The combined disease-free rate was 87 percent for the two groups. Combining both groups, normal C-cell distribution, C-cell hyperplasia, or micromedullary carcinoma (defined as smaller than 1 cm) were found in 88 percent of cases while 12 percent had tumors 1 cm or larger; 60 percent of the patients were N0, 9 percent were N1, and 30.7 percent were NX. The authors concluded that the TNM status was more important than genotype for predicting outcome and that cure was achieved in all patients with basal calcitonin levels under 30 pg/mL.

MEDULLARY CARCINOMA VARIANTS

Papillary Variant

Rarely, medullary carcinomas exhibit a true papillary pattern in which the component cells are aligned along fibrovascular stalks (194). In the cases described by Kakudo et al. (195), the tumors also exhibited solid foci characteristic of medullary carcinoma. The presence of a pseudopapillary pattern is considerably more common (fig. 12-30). The latter change results from artifactual separation of groups of tumor cells away from points of vascular supply. As a result, groups of tumor cells appear to be attached to stromal elements of the tumor, with intervening "empty" spaces.

Follicular (Tubular) Variant

Medullary carcinomas may be composed wholly or in part of follicular structures that resemble follicular cell neoplasms (118,194,196–199). The tumor cells form follicles lined by cells that resemble those seen in the more solid areas of the tumor (fig. 12-31). The lumens of the follicles appear empty or contain an eosinophilic colloid-like substance. Although the origin of this material is unknown, it most likely represents calcitonin and other secreted proteins, as suggested by the fact that immunostains for calcitonin reveal variable degrees of reactivity within these areas while stains for thyroglobulin are negative.

Small Cell Variant

The small cell variant is characterized by the presence of cells with round to ovoid hyperchromatic nuclei and scant cytoplasm (fig. 12-32) (200,201). The cells most closely resemble those of the intermediate variant of small cell carcinoma, and some resemble neuroblastoma. The presence of calcitonin, calcitonin-gene related peptide, or other peptides (somatostatin, gastrin-releasing peptide) is characteristic of the C-cell differentiation in these tumors.

The small cell variant exhibits a compact, trabecular, or diffuse growth pattern. The tumor cells may be negative for calcitonin, but stains for CEA are usually strongly positive. Mitotic activity may be high and foci of necrosis present. This variant occurs in a pure form or is admixed with more typical foci of tumor.

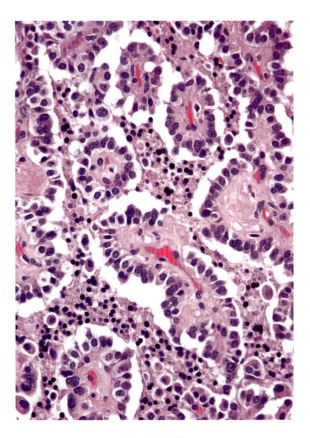

Figure 12-30

MEDULLARY THYROID CARCINOMA WITH PSEUDOPAPILLARY FEATURES

This tumor shows extensive pseudopapillary changes.

Eusebi et al. (202) have reported two cases of small cell thyroid carcinoma that were classified as apparent primary thyroid oat cell carcinomas (fig. 12-33). Both tumors were positive for chromogranin and synaptophysin but were negative for thyroglobulin and calcitonin by immunohistochemistry. Both tumors were also negative for calcitonin messenger RNA by in situ hybridization studies. On the basis of these studies, Eusebi et al. concluded that such cases should be separated from small cell medullary carcinomas and should be classified as primary small (oat) cell carcinomas of the thyroid gland. It has been suggested that some small cell thyroid tumors may be related to the Ewing tumor family on the basis of *EWSR1-FLI1* rearrangements (203).

Giant Cell Variant

Isolated tumor giant cells, characterized by multiple nuclei and abundant eosinophilic

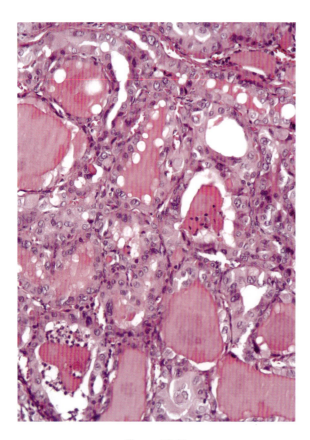

Figure 12-31

**MEDULLARY THYROID
CARCINOMA: FOLLICULAR VARIANT**

This tumor has a predominant follicular pattern of growth.

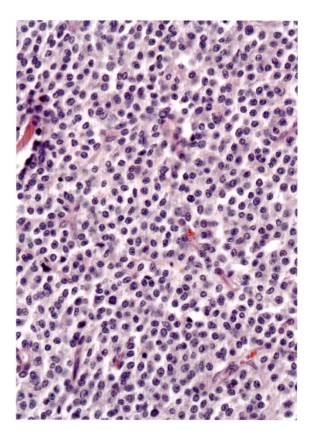

Figure 12-32

**MEDULLARY THYROID CARCINOMA:
SMALL CELL VARIANT**

This tumor is composed of small cells.

cytoplasm, are found in occasional medullary carcinomas. Some tumors contain a predominance of these cells (fig. 12-34) (112,201). Typically, the giant cell areas are admixed with foci of more typical medullary carcinoma. The tumor giant cells are positive for calcitonin.

Clear Cell Variant

Medullary carcinomas may be composed wholly or in part of cells with optically clear cytoplasm (fig. 12-35). Landon and Ordonez (204) described a medullary carcinoma composed predominantly of large polygonal cells with clear cytoplasm. In other areas, the tumor was composed of spindle-shaped cells with eosinophilic cytoplasm. The clear cells were negative for mucins and did not contain appreciable amounts of glycogen. The tumor stained positively for calcitonin and contained dense-core secretory granules ultrastructurally.

Melanotic Variant

Melanin pigment has been described in a variety of peptide- and amine-producing tumors, including medullary thyroid carcinoma (fig. 12-36). Marcus et al. (205) described a case of nonfamilial medullary thyroid carcinoma that contained collections of dendritic argentaffin-positive cells. The dendritic cells were negative for calcitonin while the remaining cells within the tumor were positive. Ultrastructurally, the argentaffin-positive cells contained typical melanosomes. Beerman et al. (206) demonstrated both melanosomes and calcitonin-containing secretory granules within the same tumor cells. These tumors may also be positive for HMB-45 (207).

Oncocytic Variant

Rare examples of medullary carcinoma with oncocytic features have been reported (fig. 12-

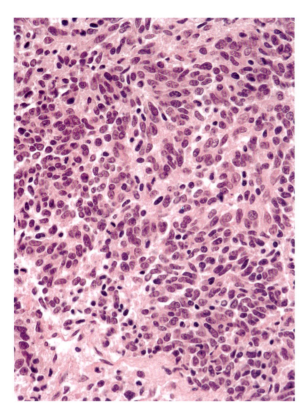

Figure 12-33

**SMALL CELL NEUROENDOCRINE
CARCINOMA OF THYROID GLAND**

This tumor is composed of small cells with high nuclear:
cytoplasmic ratios. (Courtesy of Dr. V. Eusebi, Bologna, Italy.)

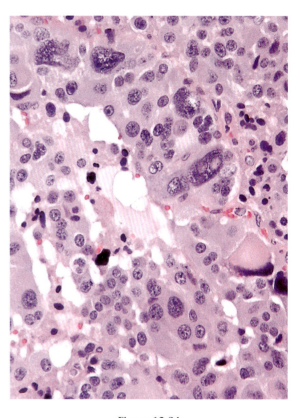

Figure 12-34

**MEDULLARY THYROID CARCINOMA:
GIANT CELL VARIANT**

This tumor is composed of multifocal collections of
pleomorphic giant cells with nuclear pseudoinclusions.

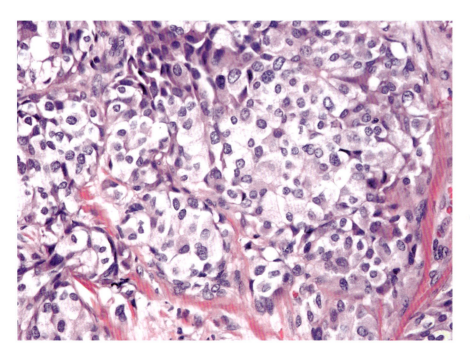

Figure 12-35

**MEDULLARY
THYROID CARCINOMA:
CLEAR CELL VARIANT**

This tumor is composed of
cells with clear cytoplasm.

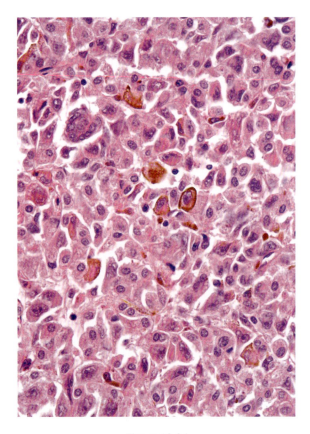

Figure 12-36

MEDULLARY THYROID CARCINOMA: MELANOTIC VARIANT

This tumor contains scattered melanin-positive cells.

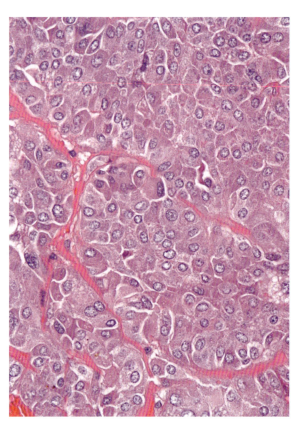

Figure 12-37

MEDULLARY THYROID CARCINOMA: ONCOCYTIC VARIANT

This tumor is composed of large cells with granular eosinophilic cytoplasm (oncocytes).

37) (208,209). In the case reported by Dominguez-Malagon et al. (208), 60 to 70 percent of the tumor cells were of the oncocytic type while the remainder had features of conventional medullary carcinoma. The tumor cells had a trabecular arrangement and were separated by an amyloid-free fibrous stroma. The tumor cells contained numerous mitochondria and a few membrane-bound secretory granules. There was strong positivity for calcitonin, chromogranin, and CEA but thyroglobulin was negative.

Squamous Cell Variant

Foci of squamous metaplasia are exceptionally seen in medullary carcinoma. The case reported by Dominguez-Malagon et al. (208) was calcitonin negative but showed diffuse positivity for neuron-specific enolase and chromogranin and focal positivity for CEA. Focal deposits of stromal amyloid were also present in this case.

Amphicrine Cell Variant

Golough et al. (210) described a case of medullary carcinoma in which approximately 30 percent of the tumor cells had a signet ring morphology (fig. 12-38). Combined Alcian blue and Grimelius stains revealed that approximately 5 percent of the tumor cells were both alcianophilic and argyrophilic. Ultrastructurally, the tumor cells contained both mucin deposits and membrane-bound secretory granules.

Paraganglioma-Like Variant

Occasional medullary carcinomas are encapsulated and arranged in a broad trabecular pattern with an amyloid-negative hyalinized stroma, resembling hyalinizing trabecular adenoma (paraganglioma-like thyroid adenoma) (fig. 12-39) (211,212). Huss and Mendelsohn (213) reported two such cases that were calcitonin positive and

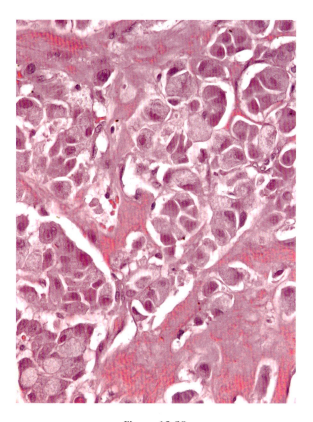

Figure 12-38

MEDULLARY THYROID CARCINOMA: AMPHICRINE CELL VARIANT

The vacuolated tumor cells contain both mucin and calcitonin (amphicrine type). (Courtesy of Dr. V. Eusebi, Bologna, Italy.)

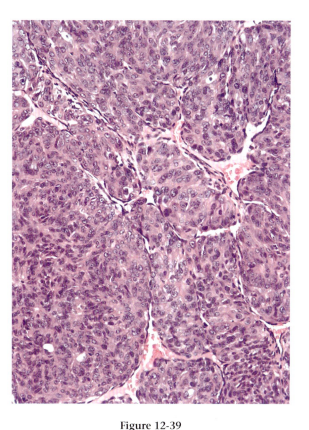

Figure 12-39

MEDULLARY THYROID CARCINOMA: PARAGANGLIOMA-LIKE VARIANT

This tumor has a paraganglioma-like pattern.

classified as medullary thyroid carcinomas. Some of these cases also contain scattered S-100–positive sustentacular-type cells (214,215).

Angiosarcoma-Like Variant

Occasional medullary carcinomas have pseudosarcomatous features. These may be mistaken for angiosarcomas (216).

Encapsulated Variant

Almost all neoplasms composed of C-cells are carcinomas, although occasional examples of tumors interpreted as C-cell adenomas are reported (217). In 1988, Kodama et al. (218) described two cases of C-cell adenoma, each of which measured 4 cm in diameter. The tumors were composed of cells that were fusiform to cuboidal, with small elliptical nuclei. Neither tumor contained amyloid or foci of calcification.

In contrast to most medullary carcinomas, stains for CEA were negative and there was no evidence of increased CEA levels in the serum. Calcitonin levels were markedly elevated and the tumor cells stained strongly for this peptide. The term "C-cell adenoma" has been suggested for completely encapsulated C-cell tumors (219); however, until more is known about the biology of these tumors, it is best to regard them as *encapsulated medullary carcinomas*.

Medullary Microcarcinoma

The term *medullary microcarcinoma* is used to describe sporadic or heritable tumors measuring less than 1 cm in diameter (figs. 12-40, 12-41) (220–222). These tumors may exhibit nesting, trabecular, or diffuse growth patterns. Occasional microcarcinomas have a microfollicular growth pattern resembling small follicular adenoma or adenomatous foci. Most of the reported cases have been incidental findings in

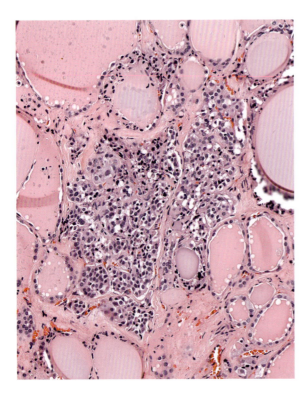
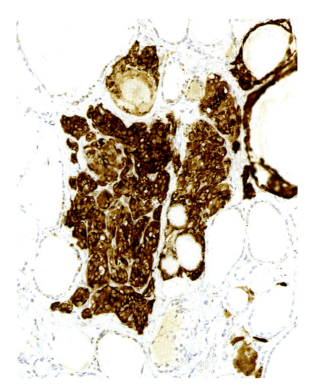

Figure 12-40

MEDULLARY THYROID MICROCARCINOMA

Left: This tumor was discovered incidentally in a patient with multinodular goiter. The central portion of the lesion shows early fibrosis.

Right: The cells are positive for calcitonin. There was a mild degree of C-cell hyperplasia immediately adjacent to the lesion, but the contralateral lobe had a normal C-cell distribution. *RET* mutation analysis was negative.

thyroid glands removed for other reasons or in patients with nodular thyroid disease who have been screened for calcitonin abnormalities.

The prognosis of patients with medullary microcarcinoma is generally excellent; however, occasional microcarcinomas (particularly those that are symptomatic or associated with significant preoperative hypercalcitoninemia or postoperative hypercalcitoninemia) give rise to nodal and distant metastases (220). One study has suggested that the term "medullary microcarcinoma" should be applied to those tumors measuring less than 0.5 cm since none of the patients with tumors of this size had evidence of nodal disease or hypercalcitoninemia (223).

Heritable Forms of Medullary Carcinoma

The histopathologic features of the tumors in patients with heritable medullary carcinoma are virtually indistinguishable from those occurring sporadically, except for their bilaterality, multi-

focality, and association with C-cell hyperplasia (figs. 12-42, 12-43) (2,8,14,15,41,110). Correlative light and electron microscopic studies have demonstrated that foci of early medullary thyroid carcinoma are characterized by the extension of C-cells through the basement membranes of C-cell–filled follicles (123,224). This observation has been confirmed by immunostains for type IV collagen (225).

Invasion is associated with areas of early fibrosis between the infiltrating C-cells as they extend into the thyroid interstitium (fig. 12-44). Further progression is characterized by increasing degrees of fibrosis between the tumor cell nests (fig. 12-45).

MIXED MEDULLARY AND FOLLICULAR CELL CARCINOMA

Definition. *Mixed medullary and follicular cell carcinoma* is a tumor showing the morphologic features of medullary carcinoma with

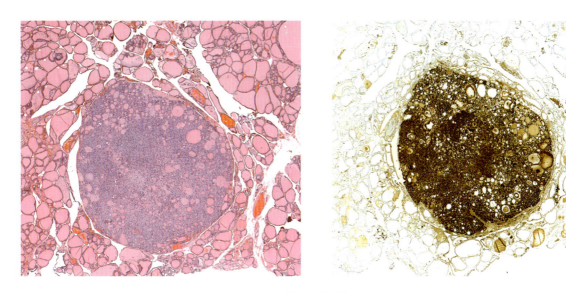

Figure 12-41

MEDULLARY THYROID MICROCARCINOMA

Left: This tumor was discovered incidentally in a patient with multinodular goiter. There is entrapment of normal follicles, predominantly at the periphery of the tumor.

Right: The tumor cells are positive for calcitonin. There is no evidence of associated C-cell hyperplasia.

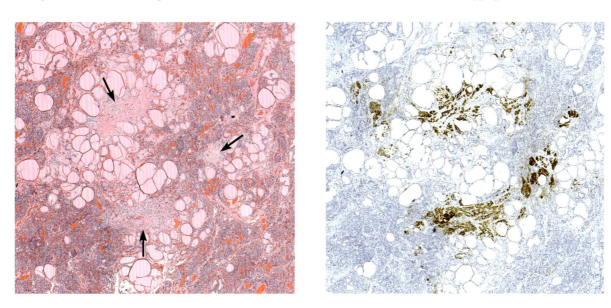

Figure 12-42

MEN 2A-ASSOCIATED MEDULLARY THYROID CARCINOMA

Left: There are multiple foci of tumor in this lobe (arrows). The contralateral lobe also contained multiple tumor deposits.
Right: The foci are positive for calcitonin.

immunoreactive calcitonin and the morphologic features of follicular or papillary carcinomas with immunoreactive thyroglobulin (1,226,227). These tumors have been referred to by a variety of terms, including *mixed follicular* (or *papillary*) and *C-cell carcinoma, biphasic carcinoma, differentiated carcinoma (intermediate type), composite/compound carcinoma,* and *stem cell carcinoma* (227). The tumors may occur sporadically or in heritable forms.

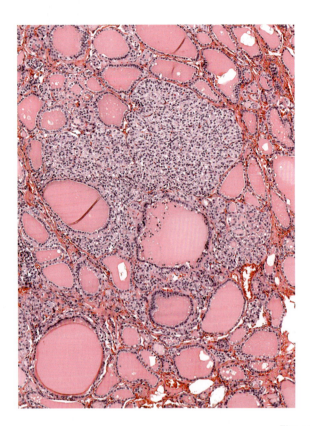 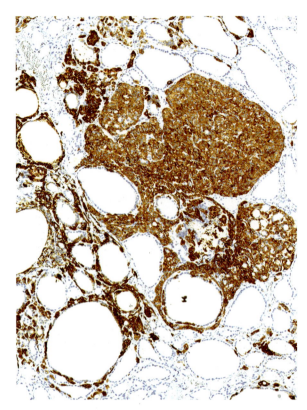

Figure 12-43

MEN 2A-ASSOCIATED MEDULLARY THYROID CARCINOMA

Left: The tumor cells have incorporated adjacent normal follicles. Multiple foci of tumor were present in both lobes.
Right: The tumor cells contain less immunoreactive calcitonin than the adjacent hyperplastic C-cells.

General Features. C-cell and follicular cell neoplasms, including papillary thyroid carcinomas, may occur as anatomically distinct synchronous lesions (fig. 12-46) or as intimately admixed tumors (228–237). True mixed medullary and follicular cell carcinomas are rare, accounting for 0.15 percent of all thyroid tumors (227). It has been suggested that the existence of mixed tumors may explain the occasional cases of medullary thyroid carcinoma that have the capacity for radioactive iodine uptake (226).

There is considerable controversy with respect to the histogenesis of these tumors. Some authors have favored an origin from a common stem cell capable of differentiating into both follicular cell and C-cell lineages. This hypothesis is supported by the demonstration of calcitonin and thyroglobulin in the same cells both in primary tumors and nodal metastases (230). In addition, in situ hybridization studies have demonstrated calcitonin and thyroglobulin messenger RNAs in a small subset of single tumor cells (229).

An alternative hypothesis suggests that the two components are not derived from a single progenitor cell since they demonstrate different patterns of mutations, allelic losses, and clonal composition. Molecular studies have indicated that the follicular components in some mixed tumors are often oligoclonal or polyclonal and more frequently exhibit hyperplastic rather than neoplastic features (238). These observations suggest that at least a subset of mixed tumors is composed of medullary carcinoma containing hyperplastic follicles. According to the "hostage hypothesis," entrapped non-neoplastic follicles are stimulated by trophic factors leading to hyperplastic follicular foci (238). Subsequent acquired genetic defects in follicular cells lead to neoplastic transformation and the development of papillary or follicular neoplasms.

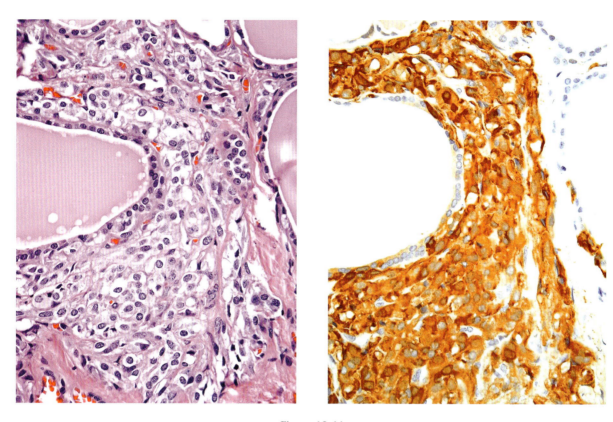

Figure 12-44

MEN 2A-ASSOCIATED MEDULLARY THYROID CARCINOMA

Left: The tumor cells have extended beyond the follicle into the adjacent thyroid interstitium. There is a mild degree of fibrosis around the infiltrating C-cells.

Right: The tumor cells are positive for calcitonin.

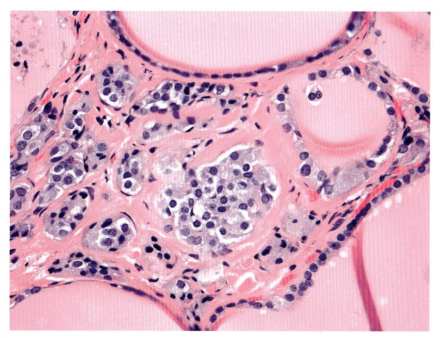

Figure 12-45

MEN 2A-ASSOCIATED MEDULLARY THYROID CARCINOMA

Groups of infiltrating tumor cells are surrounded by a fibrous stroma.

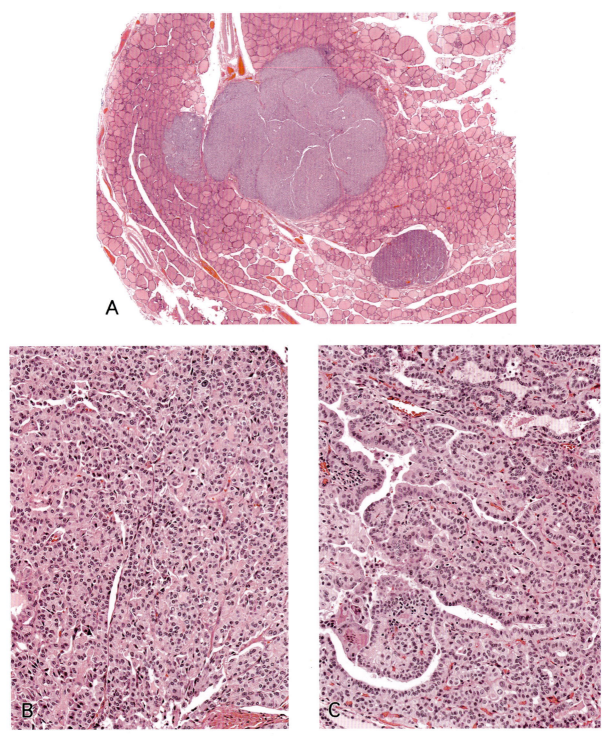

Figure 12-46

MEN 2A-ASSOCIATED MEDULLARY THYROID CARCINOMA AND SYNCHRONOUS PAPILLARY THYROID CARCINOMA

A: The larger lobulated mass is a medullary thyroid carcinoma. The smaller nodule at the lower right is a papillary thyroid carcinoma.

B: The medullary carcinoma has a predominant solid growth pattern. The calcitonin stain was positive.

C: The papillary carcinoma component has well-defined papillary features and was negative for calcitonin.

Some kindreds with *RET* point mutations have both papillary and medullary carcinomas. According to one study, the frequency of occult papillary carcinoma in patients with medullary carcinoma was higher than that occurring in patients undergoing thyroidectomies for goiters or nodules (14.8 percent versus 6.8 percent) (fig. 12-46) (239). Whether this difference is due to more extensive sampling of the medullary carcinoma cases, however, is unknown. Certain *RET* mutations exhibit constitutive kinase activity and are mitogenic for thyroid follicular cells, although at a lower level than *RET/PTC1* mutations (240). These studies suggest that *RET* point mutations behave as conditional oncogenes for follicular cells. The fact that the transforming activities are modest in follicular cells may explain the uncommon association of medullary and follicular carcinomas.

RET51 cDNA has been used to construct transgenic mice with the most frequent MEN 2A mutation (Cys-634-Arg), expressed under the control of the human calcitonin promoter. The animals developed medullary carcinomas and follicular cell tumors resembling papillary carcinoma depending on the founder line examined (241). Interestingly, one founder line developed compound medullary/papillary carcinoma.

Clinical Features. The mean age in 36 reported cases was 48 years, with a male to female ratio of 1.3:1.0 (227). Most patients present with a thyroid mass that is cold on scintigraphic scan and solid on ultrasonographic examination.

Gross and Microscopic Findings. Most tumors present as solid, white, nonencapsulated masses measuring 3 to 4 cm in diameter. They appear microscopically as medullary carcinomas that are admixed with follicular-derived elements in varying proportions (figs. 12-47–12-50). The diagnosis depends on the demonstration of thyroglobulin-positive follicles deep within the tumor. The cells lining the follicles often have enlarged and occasionally hyperchromatic nuclei which are larger than those of the non-neoplastic follicular cells in the adjacent normal thyroid gland.

In those cases of mixed medullary and papillary carcinoma, the nuclei of the papillary carcinoma component are enlarged, with clearing, groove formation, and pseudoinclusions. The follicular and papillary components are

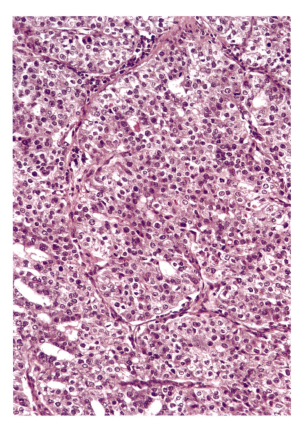

Figure 12-47

MIXED MEDULLARY AND FOLLICULAR CARCINOMA OF DIFFERENTIATED (INTERMEDIATE) TYPE

The solid areas resemble medullary thyroid carcinoma and are characterized by the presence of polyhedral cells arranged in compact lobules. (Courtesy of Dr. O. Ljungberg, Malmo, Sweden.)

positive for thyroglobulin while the medullary components are positive for neuroendocrine markers and calcitonin.

Mixed oncocytic, poorly differentiated, and undifferentiated carcinomas have also been reported to occur in association with medullary carcinomas (227). Both medullary- and follicular-derived components have been recognized in lymph node metastases.

Differential Diagnosis. Mixed medullary and follicular cell neoplasms must be distinguished from medullary thyroid carcinomas with entrapped follicles, as discussed earlier. In general, entrapped follicles are most often present at the peripheries of the tumors, although they may be present in more central regions. In addition, extracellular deposits of thyroglobulin released

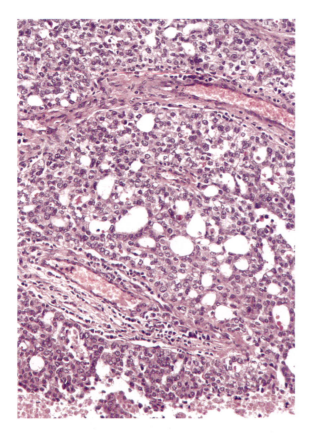

Figure 12-48

MIXED MEDULLARY AND FOLLICULAR CARCINOMA OF DIFFERENTIATED (INTERMEDIATE) TYPE

The tumor cells form follicular structures that are lined by cells with features similar to those noted in the solid areas. (Courtesy of Dr. O. Ljungberg, Malmo, Sweden.)

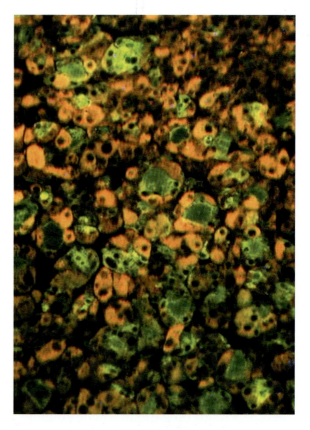

Figure 12-49

MIXED MEDULLARY AND FOLLICULAR CARCINOMA OF DIFFERENTIATIATED (INTERMEDIATE) TYPE

Thyroglobulin stains with a fluorescein-labeled antibody (green), while calcitonin stains with a rhodamine-labeled antibody (orange). (Courtesy of Dr. O. Ljungberg, Malmo, Sweden.)

from disrupted follicular cells may diffuse around and into the neoplastic C-cells. Mixed tumors must also be distinguished from the follicular (tubular) variant of medullary thyroid carcinoma. The cells surrounding the follicular structures in the latter entity are positive for calcitonin and negative for thryoglobulin. Similarly, the papillary variant of medullary thyroid carcinoma is positive for calcitonin and negative for thyroglobulin.

Treatment and Prognosis. Patients are treated by total thyroidectomy with central lymph node dissection. Those tumors with a follicular/papillary component may respond to radioactive iodine. Most patients develop nodal metastases, and distant metastases occur in approximately 25 percent of cases, with involvement of lung, liver, or bone.

C-CELL HYPERPLASIA

Definition. *C-cell hyperplasia* is a multifocal proliferative condition characterized by an increased mass of C-cells within the follicles of the thyroid gland.

General Features. C-cell hyperplasia is an uncommon entity that has been studied most extensively in patients with heritable medullary thyroid carcinoma syndromes. This disorder was identified initially by provocative tests of calcitonin reserve and more recently by molecular testing procedures for mutations in the *RET* proto-oncogene. In patients with the various MEN 2 syndromes, C-cell hyperplasia is a preneoplastic condition that precedes the development of the multifocal medullary carcinomas that characterize these conditions

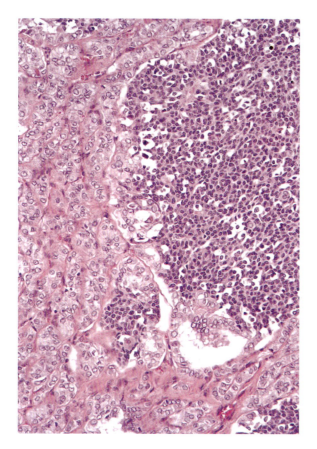

Figure 12-50

MIXED MEDULLARY AND FOLLICULAR CARCINOMA

In this case, several nests of medullary carcinoma are present within a solid trabecular, poorly differentiated carcinoma. (Courtesy of Dr. M. Papotti, Turin, Italy.)

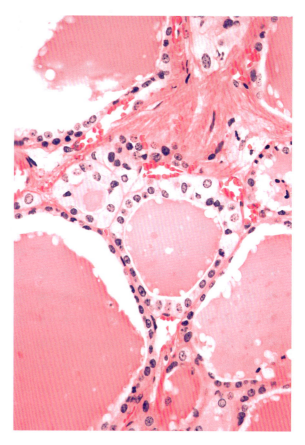

Figure 12-51

MEN 2A-ASSOCIATED DIFFUSE C-CELL HYPERPLASIA

The number of C-cells is increased, as compared to normal. They have clear cytoplasm and mild variation in nuclear size.

(13,92,94,106,242–248). MEN 2-associated C-cell hyperplasia is also referred to as *primary (neoplastic) C-cell hyperplasia* (figs. 12-51–12-57) (249). In contrast, patients with nonheritable forms of C-cell hyperplasia (*secondary* or *physiologic C-cell hyperplasia*), including cases of microdissected C-cell hyperplasia adjacent to sporadic medullary carcinomas, lack evidence of *RET* point mutations, despite the presence of codon 918 mutations in the tumors (250).

Secondary C-cell hyperplasia is associated with a variety of conditions, including aging populations (251), Hashimoto thyroiditis (252,253), goitrous hypothyroidism (254), and hypercalcemic and hypergastrinemic states (figs. 12-58–12-60) (255,256). It is found adjacent to follicular cell neoplasms and adenomatous nodules (257) and metastases to the thyroid gland (*peritumoral*

C-cell hyperplasia) (258). C-cell hyperplasia also occurs in patients with the PTEN hamartoma syndrome (259,260).

In many rat strains, C-cell hyperplasia occurs in an age-dependent manner and is frequently associated with multifocal medullary carcinomas, particularly after the age of 2 years (37,261). Many of the affected animals also have evidence of pheochromocytoma, pituitary adenoma, and pancreatic endocrine neoplasms. Similar changes have also been described in the bull (262). Experimental studies have shown that the chronic administration of calcitonin secretagogues may lead to the development of C-cell hyperplasia in some species (263).

Clinical Features. The clinical features of patients with MEN 2-associated C-cell hyperplasia have been discussed in the section on medullary

273

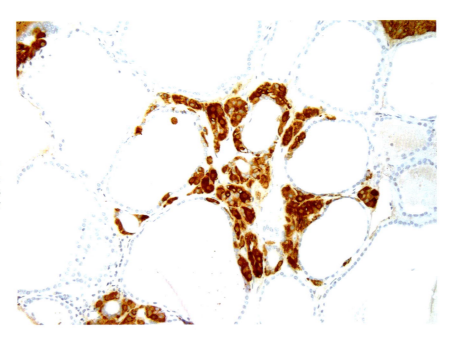

Figure 12-52

MEN 2A-ASSOCIATED DIFFUSE C-CELL HYPERPLASIA

The C-cell proliferation surrounds individual follicles (immunoperoxidase stain for calcitonin).

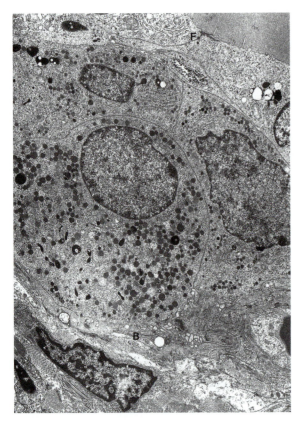

Figure 12-53

MEN 2A-ASSOCIATED DIFFUSE C-CELL HYPERPLASIA

C-cells proliferate between follicular cells (F) and the follicular basal lamina (B).

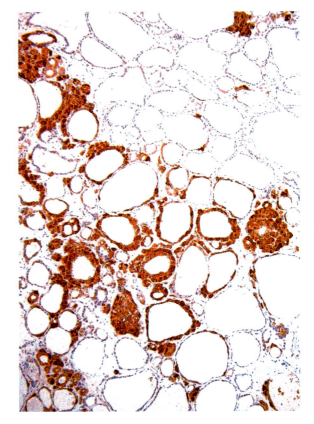

Figure 12-54

MEN 2A-ASSOCIATED DIFFUSE AND NODULAR C-CELL HYPERPLASIA

Some of the follicles are replaced by nodular aggregates of C-cells (immunoperoxidase stain for calcitonin).

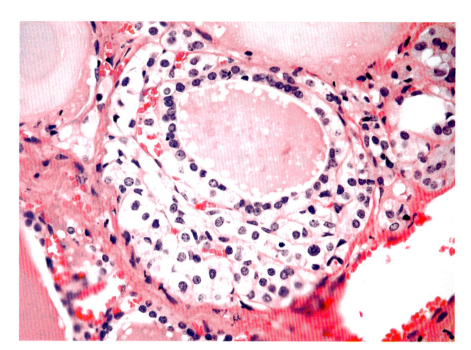

Figure 12-55

MEN 2A-ASSOCIATED NODULAR C-CELL HYPERPLASIA

C-cells completely surround a follicle. The overlying C-cells are atrophic.

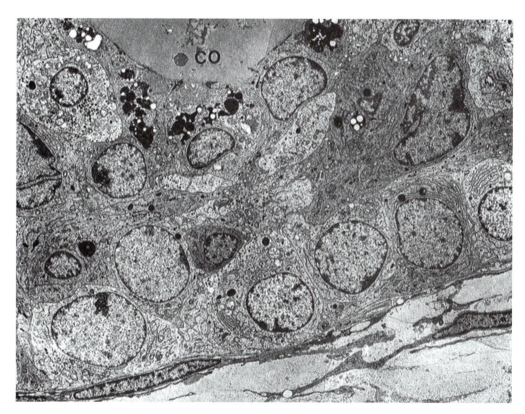

Figure 12-56

MEN 2A-ASSOCIATED NODULAR C-CELL HYPERPLASIA

In this electron micrograph, a small amount of colloid (CO) is present in the center of the follicle. The C-cells are separated from the interstitium by the follicular basal lamina. (Fig. 3 from DeLellis RA, Nunnemacher G, Wolfe HJ. C-cell hyperplasia. An ultrastructural analysis. Lab Invest 1977;36:240.)

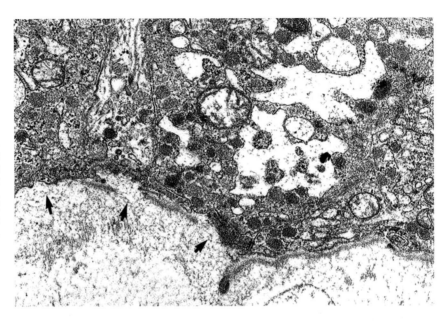

Figure 12-57

MEN 2A-ASSOCIATED NODULAR C-CELL HYPERPLASIA

In this electron micrograph, the basal lamina shows multiple gaps (arrows). There was evidence of stromal invasion in other areas. (Fig. 19 from DeLellis RA, Wolfe HJ. The pathobiology of the human calcitonin (C) cell: a review. Pathol Annu 1981;16(Pt. 2):42.)

carcinoma. Secondary C-cell hyperplasia is usually discovered as an incidental finding.

Gross Findings. Thyroid glands from patients with MEN 2-associated C-cell hyperplasia show no gross abnormalities (41,224,264). In those patients with positive molecular testing results, each lobe of the thyroid gland should be blocked in its entirety. C-cell hyperplasia is most likely to be found in sections corresponding to the middle third of the lateral lobes. Secondary C-cell hyperplasia is usually an incidental microscopic finding in thyroid glands removed for other causes.

Microscopic Findings. According to current criteria, C-cell hyperplasia is defined by the presence of at least 50 C-cells per low-power microscopic field (100X) (254). The component cells have round to ovoid, centrally placed nuclei with fairly coarse chromatin and inconspicuous nucleoli. The cytoplasm varies from amphophilic to clear (figs. 12-51–12-53). Diffuse C-cell hyperplasia is characterized by bilateral and multifocal increased numbers of C-cells within follicles, while focal hyperplasia is characterized by the partial replacement of the follicular space by C-cells, often in an eccentric pattern (224). With further progression, the follicles are filled with expansile foci of proliferating C-cells (nodular C-cell hyperplasia).

Ultrastructurally, the proliferating C-cells are separated from the thyroid interstitium by the follicular basal lamina in diffuse, focal, and nodular C-cell hyperplasia (figs. 12-54–12-56)

(123,224,243). Basal lamina defects are particularly common in nodular C-cell hyperplasia (fig.12-57). The latter changes may represent an early phase of the transition to invasive carcinoma.

The C-cells in heritable medullary thyroid carcinoma syndromes often, but not invariably, exhibit some degree of dysplasia (figs. 12-51–12-55) The term "neoplastic" hyperplasia has been proposed by Perry et al. (249) to define MEN 2-associated (primary) C-cell hyperplasia that reflects the atypia of the proliferating C-cells. Interestingly, in 1978 Carney et al. (52) proposed that C-cell hyperplasia associated with MEN 2 syndromes is a preinvasive carcinoma or carcinoma in situ. Further evidence for the neoplastic nature of C-cell hyperplasia has come from molecular studies of microdissected foci of thyroid glands from patients with MEN 2A (265). These studies have shown that foci of C-cell hyperplasia are monoclonal, with inactivation of the same allele in both thyroid lobes. Moreover, the foci have different secondary alterations involving the tumor suppressor genes p53, *RB1*, *WT1*, and *NF1*. These findings, together with the downregulation of apoptosis, are consistent with an intraepithelial neoplastic process and suggest that early clonal expansions precede the migration of C-cell precursors into the thyroid lobes in MEN 2A (265). Despite these observations, most investigators continue to use the term C-cell hyperplasia for the preinvasive stages of C-cell proliferation.

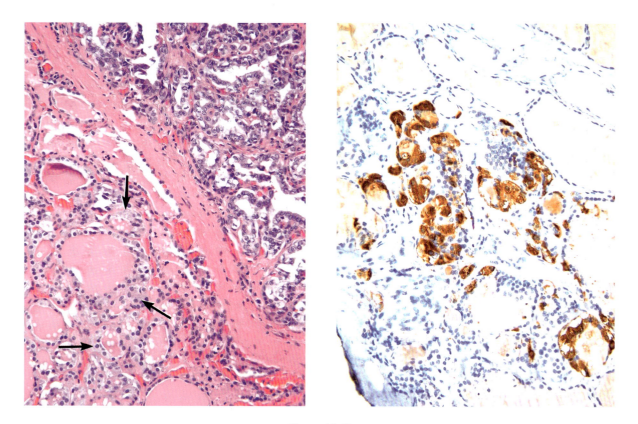

Figure 12-58

SECONDARY (PHYSIOLOGIC) C-CELL HYPERPLASIA ADJACENT TO PAPILLARY THYROID CARCINOMA

Left: The papillary thyroid carcinoma is present in the upper right portion of this field. The adjacent normal thyroid is at the left. Groups of hyperplastic C-cells are present in the normal thyroid tissue (arrows).

Right: Immunoperoxidase stain for calcitonin in the adjacent normal thyroid demonstrates C-cell hyperplasia.

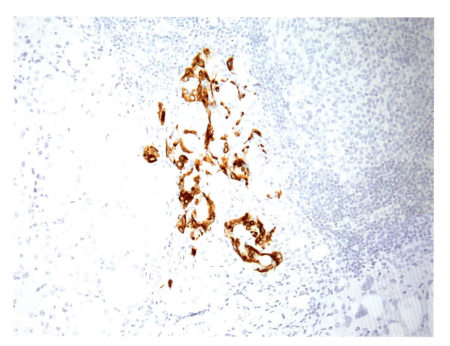

Figure 12-59

SECONDARY (PHYSIOLOGIC) C-CELL HYPERPLASIA IN HASHIMOTO THYROIDITIS

Immunoperoxidase stain for calcitonin shows an area of C-cell hyperplasia adjacent to a lymphoid follicle (upper right).

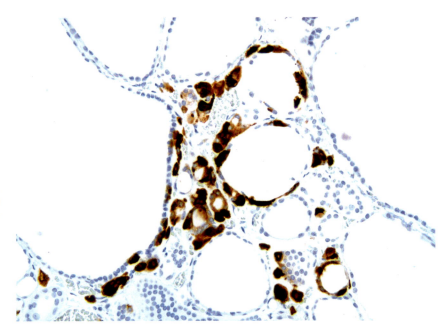

Figure 12-60

SECONDARY (PHYSIOLOGIC) C-CELL HYPERPLASIA ASSOCIATED WITH HYPERCALCEMIA

The number of C-cells is increased, as compared to normal (immunoperoxidase stain for calcitonin).

The view that C-cell hyperplasia is a precursor and marker of MEN 2-associated medullary thyroid carcinoma has been challenged by several studies (266,267). In a series of 30 patients with nodular (adenomatous) thyroid disease and abnormal pentagastrin-stimulated calcitonin levels, Kaserer et al. (266) reported 19 patients (female to male: 14 to 5) with medullary thyroid carcinoma and 11 males but no females with C-cell hyperplasia only, as defined by greater than 50 C-cells per low-power field. Six of 16 patients with apparent sporadic medullary thyroid carcinomas had concomitant C-cell hyperplasia, 3 of whom had newly diagnosed MEN 2, as proven by genetic studies. On the basis of these observations, Kaserer concluded that C-cell hyperplasia was an unreliable marker for heritable medullary thyroid carcinoma and that it had a preneoplastic potential in the absence of *RET* germline mutations.

Possible explanations for these observations are the following: 1) the observed C-cell hyperplasia in sporadic tumor cases represents the upper limit of normal C-cell distribution; 2) the C-cell hyperplasia is analogous to secondary (physiologic) C-cell hyperplasia found adjacent to papillary and follicular tumors; or 3) some sporadic medullary thyroid carcinomas may, in fact, develop against a background of C-cell hyperplasia. Mears and Diaz-Cano (268) have re-analyzed the data in the Kaserer study (267) and

concluded that multifocal and bilateral invasive medullary carcinomas associated with expansile intraepithelial neoplasia (C-cell hyperplasia) represent familial disease in 98 percent of cases. The probability of sporadic disease associated with nodular and neoplastic C-cell hyperplasia was calculated as 1.87 percent. It is likely, therefore, that a small subset of sporadic medullary thyroid carcinomas are preceded by C-cell hyperplasia that is morphologically indistinguishable from MEN 2-associated ("neoplastic") C-cell hyperplasia. Accordingly, molecular studies should be performed to rule out *RET* germline mutations in equivocal cases.

Differential Diagnosis. The distinction between the upper limit of normal C-cell distribution and secondary (physiologic) hyperplasia may be very difficult (figs. 12-58–12-60). This is due, in part, to the wide variations in C-cell distribution in normal individuals and the variations in C-cell density in different portions of the thyroid lobes (269,270). For example, C-cell density is particularly high in the vicinity of solid cell nests. Perry et al. (249) have suggested that "neoplastic" C-cell hyperplasia is recognizable in routinely stained sections on the basis of mild to moderate nuclear atypia. They further suggest that physiologic (secondary) C-cell hyperplasia requires immunostains for calcitonin for its identification, because of the lack of nuclear atypia. It should be recognized, however, that normal C-cells, particularly in the area of the ultimobranchial bodies, may exhibit considerable nuclear enlargement and hyperchromasia. Similar changes may also be evident in some cases of secondary (physiologic) C-cell hyperplasia (fig. 12-58).

Foci of nodular C-cell hyperplasia are occasionally difficult to distinguish from a variety of other changes, including squamous metaplasia (271,272), solid cell nests (271), intrathyroidal thymic or parathyroid nests, palpation thyroiditis (multifocal granulomatous thyroiditis)

(273), and tangential cuts of normal follicles. The latter are composed of polyhedral cells with well-defined cell borders and centrally placed nuclei, which are identical to those of the adjacent follicular cells. Most of the other entities are discussed in other portions of this Fascicle.

Treatment and Prognosis. Patients with MEN 2-associated C-cell hyperplasia are treated by total thyroidectomy with central compartment lymph node dissection (46,88). In the absence of coexisting medullary thyroid carcinoma, the cure rate is almost 100 percent.

REFERENCES

1. Hedinger CH, Williams ED, Sobin LH. Histological typing of thyroid tumors. WHO International Classification of Tumors, 2nd ed. Berlin: Springer-Verlag; 1988.
2. Matias-Guiu X, DeLellis RA, Moley JF, et al. Medullary thyroid carcinoma. In: DeLellis RA, Lloyd RV, Heitz PU, Eng C, eds. Pathology and genetics of tumours of endocrine organs (WHO Classification of Tumours). Lyon: IARC Press; 2004;86-91.
3. Stoffel E. Lokales amyloid der Schildrüse. Anat Physiol Klin Med 1910;201:245-51.
4. Brandenburg W. [Metastasizing amyloid goiter.] Zentrabl Allg Path 1954;91:422-8. [German]
5. Hazard JB, Hawk WA, Crile G Jr. Medullary (solid) carcinoma of the thyroid; a clinicopathologic entity. J Clin Endocrinol Metab 1959;19:152-61.
6. Horn RC. Carcinoma of the thyroid. Description of a distinctive morphological variant and report of seven cases. Cancer 1951;4:697-707.
7. Sipple JH. The association of pheochromocytoma with carcinoma of the thyroid gland. Am J Med 1961;31:163-6.
8. Williams ED, Brown CL, Doniach I. Pathological and clinical findings in a series of 67 cases of medullary carcinoma of the thyroid. J Clin Pathol 1966;19:103-13.
9. Williams ED. Histogenesis of medullary carcinoma of the thyroid. J Clin Pathol 1966;19:114-8.
10. Bussolati G, Pearse AG. Immunofluorescent localization of calcitonin in the C cells of the pig and dog thyroid. J Clin Endocrinol 1967;37:205-9.
11. Copp DH, Cameron EC, Cheney BA, Davidson AG, Henze KG. Evidence of calcitonin—a new hormone from the parathyroid that lowers serum calcium. Endocrinology 1962;70:638-49.
12. Tashjian AH Jr, Melvin EW. Medullary carcinoma of the thyroid gland. Studies of thyrocalcitonin in plasma and tumor extracts. N Engl J Med 1968;279:279-83.
13. Melvin KE, Miller HH, Tashjian AH Jr. Early diagnosis of medullary carcinoma of the thyroid by means of calcitonin assay. N Engl J Med 1971;285:1115-20.
14. Sizemore GW. Medullary carcinoma of the thyroid gland. Semin Oncol 1987;14:306-14.
15. Lips CJ, Vasen HF, Lamers CB. Multiple endocrine neoplasia syndromes. Crit Rev Oncol Hematol 1988;2:117-84.
16. Autelitano F, Spagnoli LG, Santeusano G, Villaschi S, Autelitano M. [Occult carcinoma of the thyroid gland: an epidemiological study of autopsy material.] Ann Ital Chir 1990;61:141-6. [Italian]
17. Bondeson L, Ljungberg O. Occult thyroid carcinoma at autopsy in Malmo, Sweden. Cancer 1981;47:319-23.
18. Chong PY. Thyroid carcinomas in Singapore autopsies. Pathology 1994;26:20-2.
19. Furmanchuk AW, Roussak N, Ruchti C. Occult thyroid carcinomas in the region of Minsk, Belarus. An autopsy study of 215 patients. Histopathology 1993;23:319-25.
20. Komorowski RA, Hanson GA. Occult thyroid pathology in the young adult: an autopsy study of 138 patients without clinical thyroid disease. Hum Pathol 1988;19:689-96.

21. Lang W, Borrusch H, Bauer L. Occult carcinomas of the thyroid. Evaluation of 1,020 sequential autopsies. Am J Clin Pathol 1988;90:72-6.

22. Martinez-Tello FJ, Martinez-Cabruja R, Fernandez-Martin J, Lasso-Oria C, Ballestin-Carcavilla C. Occult carcinoma of the thyroid. A systematic autopsy study from Spain of two series performed with two different methods. Cancer 1993;15:4022-9.

23. Neuhold N, Kaiser H, Kaserer K. Latent carcinoma of the thyroid in Austria: a systematic autopsy study. Endocr Pathol 2001;12:23-31.

24. Nielsen B, Zetterlund B. Malignant thyroid tumours at autopsy in a Swedish goitrous population. Cancer 1985;55:1041-3.

25. Thorvaldsson SE, Tulinius H, Bjornsson J, Bjarnason O. Latent thyroid carcinoma in Iceland at autopsy. Pathol Res Pract 1992;12:23-31.

26. Elisei R, Bottici V, Luchetti F, et al. Impact of routine measurement of serum calcitonin on the diagnosis and outcome of medullary thyroid cancer: experience in 10,864 patients with nodular thyroid disorders. J Clin Endocrinol Metab 2004;89:163-8.

27. Hahm JR, Lee MS, Min YK, et al. Routine measurement of serum calcitonin is useful for early detection of medullary thyroid carcinoma in patients with nodular thyroid diseases. Thyroid 2001;11:78-80.

28. Karanikas G, Moameni A, Poetzl C, et al. Frequency and relevance of elevated calcitonin levels in patients with neoplastic and non-neoplastic thyroid disease and in healthy subjects. J Clin Endocrinol Metab 2004;89:515-9.

29. Scheuba C, Kaserer K, Moritz A, et al. Sporadic hypercalcitoninemia: clinical and therapeutic consequences. Endocr Related Cancer 2009; 16:243-53.

30. Niccoli P, Wion-Barbot N, Caron P, et al. Interest of routine measurement of serum calcitonin: study in a large series of thyroidectomized patients. The French Medullary Study Group. J Clin Endocrinol Metab 1992;82:338-41.

31. Ozgen AG, Hamulu F, Bayraktar F, et al. Evaluation of routine basal serum calcitonin measurement for early diagnosis of medullary thyroid carcinoma in seven hundred seventy-three patients with nodular goiter. Thyroid 1999;9:579-82.

32. Pacini F, Fontanelli M, Fugazzola L, et al. Routine measurement of serum calcitonin in nodular thyroid diseases allows the preoperative diagnosis of unsuspected medullary thyroid carcinoma. J Clin Endocrinol Metab 1994;78:826-9.

33. Rieu M, Lame MC, Richard A, et al. Prevalence of sporadic medullary thyroid carcinoma: the importance of routine measurement of serum calcitonin in the diagnostic evaluation of thyroid nodules. Clin Endocrinol 1995;42:453-60.

34. Vierhapper H, Raber W, Bieglmayer C, Kaserer K, Weinhäusl A, Niederle B. Routine measurement of plasma calcitonin in nodular thyroid diseases. J Clin Endocrinol Metab 1997;82:1589-93.

35. Weiss LM, Weinberg DS, Warhol MJ. Medullary carcinoma arising in a thyroid with Hashimoto's disease. Am J Clin Pathol 1983;80:534-8.

36. LiVolsi VA, Feind CR. Incidental medullary thyroid carcinoma in sporadic hyperparathyroidism. An expansion of the concept of C-cell hyperplasia. Am J Clin Pathol 1979;71:595-9.

37. DeLellis RA, Nunnemacher G, Bitman WR, et al. C-cell hyperplasia and medullary thyroid carcinoma in the rat. An immunohistochemical and ultrastructural analysis. Lab Invest 1979;40:140-54.

38. Thurston V, Williams ED. Experimental induction of C cell tumours in thyroid by increased dietary content of vitamin D3. Acta Endocrinol (Copenh) 1982;100:41-5.

39. Triggs SM, Williams ED. Experimental carcinogenesis in the rat thyroid follicular and C cells. A comparison of the effect of variation in dietary calcium and of radiation. Acta Endocrinol (Copehn) 1977;85:84-92.

40. Black HE, Capen CC, Young DM. Ultimobranchial thyroid neoplasms in bulls. A syndrome resembling medullary thyroid carcinoma in man. Cancer 1973;32:865-78.

41. Gimm O, Morrison CD, Suster S, Komminoth P, Mulligan L, Sweet KM. Multiple endocrine neoplasia type 2. In: DeLellis RA, Lloyd RV, Heitz PU, Eng C, eds. Pathology and genetics of tumours of endocrine organs (WHO Classification of Tumours). 2004;211-17.

42. Saadi AA. Management and prevention of familial medullary carcinoma of the thyroid. Prog Clin Biol Res 1979;34:343-50.

43. Schimke RN, Hartmann WH. Familial amyloid producing medullary thyroid carcinoma and pheochromocytoma. A distinct genetic entity. Ann Intern Med 1965;63:1027-39.

44. Sobol H, Narod SA, Schuffenecher I, Amos C, Ezekowitz RA, Lenoir GM. Hereditary medullary thyroid carcinoma: genetic analysis of three related syndromes. Henry Ford Hosp Med J 1989;37:109-11.

45. Farndon JR, Leight GS, Dilley WG, et al. Familial medullary thyroid carcinoma without associated endocrinopathies: a distinct clinical entity. Br J Surg 1986;73:278-81.

46. American Thyroid Association Guidelines Task Force, Kloos R, Eng C, et al. Medullary thyroid cancer: management guidelines of the American Thyroid Association. Thyroid 2009;19:565-612.

47. Moers AM, Landsvater RM, Schaap C, et al. Familial medullary thyroid carcinoma; not a distinct clinical entity? Genotype-phenotype correlation in a large family. Am J Med 1996;101:635-41.

48. Gagel RF, Levy ML, Donovan DT, Alford BR, Wheeler T, Tschen JA. Multiple endocrine neoplasia type 2a associated with cutaneous lichen amyloidosis. Am Intern Med 1989;111:802-6.

49. Verga U, Fugazzola L, Cambiaghi S, et al. Frequent association between MEN 2A and cutaneous lichen amyloidosis. Clin Endocrinol (Oxf) 2005;59:156-61.

50. Verdy M, Weber AM, Roy CC, Morin CL, Cadotte M, Brochu P. Hirschsprung's disease in a family with multiple endocrine neoplasia type 2. J Pediatr Gastroenterol Nutr 1982;1:603-7.

51. Carney JA, Hayles AB. Alimentary tract manifestations of multiple endocrine neoplasia, type 2b. Mayo Clin Proc 1977;52:543-8.

52. Carney JA, Sizemore GW, Hayles AB. Multiple endocrine neoplasia, type 2b. Pathobiol Annu 1978:8:105-53.

53. Gorlin RJ, Sedano HO, Vickers RA, Cercenka J. Multiple mucosal neuromas, pheochromocytoma and medullary carcinoma of the thyroid—a syndrome. Cancer 1968;22:293-9.

54. Eng C, Mulligan LM, Healey CS, et al. Heterogeneous mutation of the RET proto-oncogene in subpopulations of medullary thyroid carcinomas. Cancer Res 1996;56:2167-70.

55. Eng C. RET proto-oncogene in the development of human cancer. J Clin Oncol 1999:17:380-3.

56. Takahashi M, Buma Y, Iwamoto T, Inaguma Y, Ikeda H, Hiai Hl. Cloning and expression of the ret proto-oncogene encoding a tyrosine kinase with two potential transmembrane domains. Oncogene 1988;3:571-8.

57. Ichihara M, Murakumo Y, Takahashi M. RET and neuroendocrine tumors. Cancer Lett 2004:204:197-211.

58. Pachnis V, Mankoo B, Costantini F. Expression of the c-ret proto-oncogene during mouse embryogenesis. Development 1993;119:1005-17.

59. Schuchardt A, Dagati V, Larsson-Bloomberg L, Costantini F, Pachnis V. Defects in the kidney and enteric nervous system of mice lacking the tyrosine kinase receptor Ret. Nature 1994;367:380-3.

60. Treanor JJ, Goodman L, de Sauvage F, et al. Characterization of the multicomponent receptor for GDNF. Nature 1996;381:80-3.

61. Lai AZ, Gujral TS, Mulligan LM. RET signaling in endocrine tumors: delving deeper into molecular mechanisms. Endocr Pathol 2007;18:57-67.

62. Mulligan LM, Kwok JB, Healey CS, et al. Germline mutations of the RET proto-oncogene in multiple endocrine neoplasia type 2A. Nature 1993;363:458-60.

63. Donis-Keller H, Dou S, Chi D, et al. Mutations in the RET proto-oncogene are associated with MEN 2A and FMTC. Hum Mol Genet 1993;2:851-6.

64. Mulligan LM, Eng C, Healey CS, et al. Specific mutations of the RET proto-oncogene are related to disease phenotype in MEN 2A and FMTC. Nat Genet 1994;6:70-4.

65. Hofstra RM, Landsvater RM, Ceccherini I, et al. A mutation the RET proto-oncogene associated with multiple endocrine neoplasia type 2B and sporadic medullary thyroid carcinoma. Nature 1994;367:375-6.

66. Eng C, Smith DP, Mulligan LM, et al. Point mutation within the tyrosine kinase domain of the RET proto-oncogene in multiple endocrine neoplasia type 2B and related sporadic tumours. Hum Mol Genet 1994;3:237-41.

67. Carlson KM, Dou S, Chi D, et al. Single missense mutation in the tyrosine kinase catalytic domain of the RET proto-oncogene in associated with multiple endocrine neoplasia type 2B. Proc Natl Acad Sci USA 1994;91:1579-83.

68. Hoff AO, Cote GJ, Gagel RF. Multiple endocrine neoplasia. Annu Rev Physiol 2000;62:377-411.

69. Eng C, Clayton D, Schuffenecker I, et al. The relationships between specific RET proto-oncogene mutations and disease phenotype in multiple endocrine neoplasia type 2. International RET mutation consortium analysis. JAMA 1996;276:1575-9.

70. Gimm O, Marsh DJ, Andrew SD, et al. Germline dinucleotide mutation in codon 883 of the RET proto-oncogene in multiple endocrine neoplasia type 2B without codon 918 mutation. J Clin Endocrinol Metab 1997;81:3902-4.

71. Santoro M, Carlomagno F, Romano A, et al. Activation of RET as a dominant transforming gene by germline mutations of MEN2A and MEN2B. Science 1995;267:381-3.

72. Kawai K, Iwashita T, Murakami H, et al. Tissue specific carcinogenesis in transgenic mice expressing the RET protooncogene with a multiple endocrine neoplasia type 2A mutation. Cancer Res 2000;60:5254-60.

73. Marsh DJ, Zheng Z, Arnold A, et al. Mutation analysis of glial cell line derived neutropic factor, a ligand for an RET/coreceptor complex in multiple endocrine neoplasia type 2 and sporadic neuroendocrine tumors. J Clin Endocrinol Metab 1997;82:3025-8.

74. Songyang S, Carraway KL 3rd, Eck MJ, et al. Catalytic specificity of protein-tyrosine kinases is critical for selective signalling. Nature 1995;373:536-9.

75. Amiel J, Sproat-Emison E, Garcia-Barcelo M, et al. Hirschsprung disease, associated with syndromes and genetics: a review. J Med Genetics 2008;45:1-14.

76. Arighi E, Popsueva A, Degl'Innocenti D, et al. Biological effects of the dual phenotypic Janus mutation of RET cosegregating with both multiple endocrine neoplasia type 2 and Hirschsprung's disease. Mol Endocrinol 2004;18:1004-17.

77. Zedenius J, Wallin G, Hamberger G, Nordenskjöld M, Weber G, Larsson C. Somatic and MEN 2A de novo mutations identified in the RET proto-oncogene by screening of sporadic MTCs. Hum Mol Genet 1994;3:1259-62.

78. Romei C, Elisei R, Pinchera A, et al. Somatic mutations of the ret protooncogene in sporadic medullary thyroid carcinoma are not restricted to exon 16 and are associated with tumor recurrence. J Clin Endocrinol Metab 1996;81:1619-22.

79. Elisei R, Cosci B, Romei C, et al. Prognostic significance of RET oncogene mutations in sporadic thyroid carcinoma: a 10 year follow-up study. J Clin Endocrinol Metab 2008;93:682-7.

80. Marsh DJ, Learoyd DL, Andrew SD, et al. Somatic mutations in the RET proto-oncogene in sporadic medullary thyroid carcinoma. Clin Endocrinol (Oxf.) 1996;44:249-57.

81. Moura MM, Cavaco BM, Pinto AE, Leite V. High prevalence of RAS mutations in RET-negative sporadic medullary thyroid carcinomas. J Clin Endocrinol Metab 2011;96:E863-8.

82. Agrawal N, Jiao Y, Sausen M, et al. Exomic sequencing of medullary thyroid cancer reveals dominant and mutually exclusive oncogenic mutations in RET and RAS. J Clin Endocrinol Metab 2013;98:E364-9.

83. Macia A, Gallel P, Vaquero M, et al. Sprouty1 is a candidate tumor-suppressor gene in medullary thyroid carcinoma. Oncogene 2012;31:3961-72.

84. Reynolds L, Jones K, Winton DJ, et al. C-cell and thyroid epithelial tumours and altered follicular development in transgenic mice expressing the long isoform of MEN 2A RET. Oncogene 2001;20:3986-94.

85. Acton DS, Velthuyzen D, Lips CJ, Höppener JW. Multiple endocrine neoplasia type 2B mutation in human RET oncogene induces medullary thyroid carcinoma in transgenic mice. Oncogene 2000;19:3121-5.

86. Sweetser DA, Froelick GJ, Matsumoto AM, et al. Ganglioneuroma and renal abnormalities are induced by activated RET (MEN2B) in transgenic mice. Oncogene 1999;18:877-86.

87. Chong GC, Beahrs OH, Sizemore GW, Woolner LH. Medullary carcinoma of the thyroid gland. Cancer 1975;35:695-704.

88. Kebebew E, Ituarte PH, Siperstein AE, Duh QY, Clark OH. Medullary thyroid carcinoma: clinical characteristics, treatment, prognostic factors, and a comparison of staging systems. Cancer 2000;88:1139-48.

89. Williams ED, Karim SM, Sandler M. Prostaglandin secretion by medullary carcinoma of the thyroid. A possible cause of the associated diarrhea. Lancet 1968;1:22-3.

90. Williams ED, Morales AM, Horn RC. Thyroid carcinoma and Cushing's syndrome. A report of two cases with review of the common features of the "non endocrine" tumours associated with Cushing's syndrome. J Clin Pathol 1968;21:129-35.

91. Barbosa SL, Rodien P, Leboulleux S, et al. Ectopic adrenocorticotropic hormone-syndrome in medullary carcinoma of the thyroid: a retrospective analysis and review of the literature. Thyroid 2005;15:618-23.

92. Gagel RF, Tashjian AH Jr, Cummings T, et al. The clinical outcome of prospective screening for multiple endocrine neoplasia type 2a. An 18-year experience. N Engl J Med 1988;318:478-84.

93. Kakudo K, Carney JA, Sizemore GW. Medullary carcinoma of the thyroid. Biologic behavior of the sporadic and familial neoplasm. Cancer 1985;55:2818-21.

94. Wolfe HJ, Melvin KE, Cervi-Skinner SJ, et al. C-cell hyperplasia preceding medullary thyroid carcinoma. N Engl Med 1973;289:437-41.

95. Grauer A, Raue F, Gagel RF. Changing concepts in the management of hereditary and sporadic medullary thyroid carcinoma. Endocrinol Metab Clin North Am 1990;19:613-35.

96. Mathew CG, Chin KS, Easton DF, et al. A linked genetic marker for multiple endocrine neoplasia type 2A on chromosome 10. Nature 1987;328:527-8.

97. Carney JA, Sizemore GW. Tyce GM. Bilateral adrenal medullary hyperplasia in multiple endocrine neoplasia, type 2: the precursor of bilateral pheochromocytoma. Mayo Clin Proc 1975;50:3-10.

98. DeLellis RA, Wolfe HJ, Gagel RF, et al. Adrenal medullary hyperplasia. A morphometric analysis in patients with familial medullary thyroid carcinoma. Am J Pathol 1976;83:177-96.

99. Schminke RN, Hartmann WH, Prout TE, Rimoin DL. Syndrome of bilateral pheochromocytoma, medullary thyroid carcinoma and multiple neuromas. A possible regulatory defect in the differentiation of chromaffin tissue. N Engl J Med 1968;279:1-17.

100. Brauckhoff M, Machens A, Lorenz K, Bjøro T, Varhaug JE, Dralle H. Surgical curability of medullary thyroid cancer in multiple endocrine neoplasia 2B: a changing perspective. Ann Surg 2014;259:800-6.

101. Norton JA, Froome LC, Farrell RE, Wells SA Jr. Multiple endocrine neoplasia type IIb: the most aggressive form of medullary thyroid carcinoma. Surg Clin North Am 1979;59:109-18.

102. Wells SA Jr, Baylin SB, Leight GS, Dale JK, Dilley WG, Farndon JR. The importance of early diagnosis in patients with hereditary medullary thyroid carcinoma. Ann Surg 1982;195:595-9.

103. Frank-Raue K, Machens A, Leidig-Bruckner G, et al. Prevalence and clinical spectrum of nonsecretory medullary thyroid carcinoma in a series of 839 patients with sporadic medullary thyroid carcinoma. Thyroid 2013;23:294-300.

104. Pacini F, Schlumberger M, Dralle H, et al. European consensus for the management of patients with differentiated thyroid carcinoma of the follicular epithelium. Eur J Endocrinol 2006;154:787-803.

105. Goltzman D, Potts JT Jr, Ridgway RC, Maloof F. Calcitonin as a tumor marker. Use of the radioimmunoassay for calcitonin in the postoperative evaluation of patients with medullary thyroid carcinoma. N Engl J Med 1974;290:1035-9.

106. Saad MF, Ordonez NG, Rashid RK, et al. Medullary carcinoma of the thyroid. A study of the clinical features and prognostic factors in 161 patients. Medicine (Baltimore) 1984;63:319-42.

107. Ball DW. American Thyroid Association Guidelines for management of medullary thyroid cancer: an adult endocrinology perspective. Thyroid 2009;19:547-50.

108. Hazard JB. The C cells (parafollicular cells) of the thyroid gland and medullary thyroid carcinoma. A review. Am J Pathol 1977:88:213-50.

109. Lertprasertsuke N, Kakudo K, Nakamura A, et al. C cell carcinoma of the thyroid. Follicular variant. Acta Pathol Jpn 1989;39:393-9.

110. Rosai J, Carcangiu ML, DeLellis RA. Tumors of the thyroid gland. Atlas of Tumor Pathology, 3rd Series, Fascicle 5. Washington DC: American Registry of Pathology; 1992.

111. Sobrinho-Simões M, Sambade C, Nesland JM, Holm R, Damjanov I. Lectin histochemistry and ultrastructure of medullary carcinoma of the thyroid gland. Arch Pathol Lab Med 1990;114:369-75.

112. Kakudo, K, Miyauchi A, Ogihara T, et al. Medullary carcinoma of the thyroid. Giant cell type. Arch Pathol Lab Med 1978;102:445-7.

113. Lee TK, Myers RT, Marshall RB, Bond MG, Kardon B. The significance of mitotic rate: a retrospective study of 127 thyroid carcinomas. Hum Pathol 1985;16:1042-6.

114. Aldabagh SM, Trujillo YP, Taxy JB. Occult medullary thyroid carcinoma. Unusual histological variant presenting with metastatic disease. Am J Clin Pathol 1986;845:247-50.

115. Fernandes BJ, Bedard YC, Rosen I. Mucus-producing medullary cell carcinoma of the thyroid gland. Am J Clin Pathol 1982;78:536-40.

116. Martin-Lacave I, Gonzalez-Campora R, Moreno Fernandez A, Sanchez Gallego F, Mantero C, Galera-Davidson H. Mucosubstances in medullary carcinoma of the thyroid. Histopathology 1988;13:55-6.

117. Zaatari GS, Saigo PE, Huvos AG. Mucin production in medullary carcinoma of the thyroid. Arch Pathol Lab Med 1983;107:70-4.

118. Etit D, Faquin WC, Gaz R, Randolph G, DeLellis RA, Pilch BZ. Histopathologic and clinical features of medullary microcarcinoma and C-cell hyperplasia in prophylactic thyroidectomies for medullary carcinoma: a study of 42 cases. Arch Pathol Lab Med 2008;132:1767-73.

119. Westermark P, Johnson KH. The polypeptide hormone-derived amyloid forms: nonspecific alterations or signs of abnormal peptide processing? APMS 1988;96:475-83.

120. Sletten K, Westermark P, Natvig JB. Characterization of amyloid fibril proteins from medullary carcinoma of the thyroid. J Exp Med 1976;143:993-8.

121. Khurana R, Agarwal A, Bajpai VK, et al. Unraveling the amyloid associated with human medullary thyroid carcinoma. Endocrinology 2004;145:5465-70.

122. James PD. Amyloid goitre. J Clin Pathol 1972;25:683-6.

123. DeLellis RA, Wolfe HJ. The pathobiology of the human calcitonin (C)-cell: a review. Pathol Annu 1981:16(Pt 2):25-52.

124. Sikri KL, Vardell IM, Hamid QA, et al. Medullary carcinoma of the thyroid. An immunocytochemical and histochemical study of 25 cases using eight separate markers. Cancer 1985;56:2481-91.

125. Shin SJ, Treaba DO, DeLellis RA. Immunohistology of endocrine tumors. In: Dabbs DJ, ed. Diagnostic immunohistology: theranostic and genomic applications, 4th ed. Philadelphia: Saunders Elsevier; 2014:205-60.

126. Stanta G, Carcangiu ML, Rosai J. The biochemical and immunohistochemical profile of thyroid neoplasia. Pathol Annu 1988;23:129-57.

127. Steenbergh PH, Höppener JW, Zandberg J, Van de Ven WJ, Jansz HS, Lips CJ. Calcitonin gene related peptide coding sequence is conserved in the human genome and is expressed in medullary thyroid carcinoma. J Clin Endocrinol Metab 1984;59:358-60.

128. Lloyd RV. Use of molecular probes in the study of endocrine diseases. Hum Pathol 1987;18:1199-211.

129. Nakazawa T, Cameselle-Teijeiro J, Vinagre C, et al. C-cell-derived calcitonin-free neuroendocrine carcinoma of the thyroid: the diagnostic inportance of CGRP immunoreactivity. Int J Surg Pathol 2014 [Epub ahead of print].

130. Kaufmann O, Dietel M. Expression of thyroid transcription factor-1 in pulmonary and extrapulmonary small cell carcinomas and other neuroendocrine carcinomas of various primary sites. Histopathology 2000;36:415-20.

131. Schröder S, Böcker W, Baisch H, et al. Prognostic factors in medullary thyroid carcinoma. Survival in relation to age, sex, stage, histology, immunocytochemistry, and DNA content. Cancer 1988;61:806-16.

132. Schmid KW, Fischer-Colbrie R, Hagn C, Jasani B, Williams ED, Winkler H. Chromogranin A and B and secretogranin II in medullary carcinomas of the thyroid. Am J Surg Pathol 1987;11:551-6.

133. Gould VE, Wiedenmann B, Lee I, et al. Synaptophysin expression in neuroendocrine neoplasms as determined by immunocytochemistry. Am J Pathol 1987:126:243-57.

134. Baylin SB, Beaven MA, Engleman K, Sjoerdsma A. Elevated histaminase activity in medullary carcinoma of the thyroid gland. N Engl J Med 1972;283:1239-44.

135. Lippman SM, Medelsohn G, Trump DL, Wells SA Jr, Baylin SB. The prognostic and biological significance of cellular heterogeneity in medullary thyroid carcinoma: a study of calcitonin, L-dopa decarboxylase, and histaminase. J Clin Endocrinol Metab 1982;54:233-40.

136. Mendelsohn G, Eggleston JC, Weisburger WR, Gann DS, Baylin SB. Calcitonin and histaminase in C-cell hyperplasia and medullary thyroid carcinoma. A light microscopic and immunohistochemical study. Am J Pathol 1978;92:35-52.

137. Capella C, Bordi C, Monga G, et al. Multiple endocrine cell types in thyroid medullary carcinoma. Evidence for calcitonin, somatostatin, ACTH, 5HT and small granule cells. Virchows Arch A Pathol Anat Histol 1978;377:111-28.

138. Scopsi L, Ferrari C, Pilotti S, et al. Immunocytochemical localization and identification of prosomatostatin gene products in medullary carcinoma of human thyroid gland. Hum Pathol 1990;21:820-30.

139. Sundler F, Alumets J, Håkanson R, Björklund L, Ljungberg O. Somatostatin-immunoreactive cells in medullary carcinoma of the thyroid gland. Am J Pathol 1977;88:381-6.

140. Yamada Y, Ito S, Matsubara Y, Kobayashi S. Immunohistochemical demonstration of somatostatin-containing cells in the human, dog, and rat thyroids. Tohoku J Exp Med 1977;122:87-92.

141. Matsubayashi S, Yanaihara C, Ohkubo M, et al. Gastrin-releasing peptide immunoreactivity in medullary thyroid carcinoma. Cancer 1984;53:2472-7.

142. Sunday ME, Wolfe HJ, Roos BA, Chin WW, Spindel ER. Gastrin-releasing peptide gene expression in developing hyperplastic and neoplastic human thyroid C-cells. Endocrinology 1988;122:1551-8.

143. Yamaguchi K, Abe K, Adachi I, et al. Concomitant production of immunoreactive gastrin-releasing peptide and calcitonin in medullary carcinoma of the thyroid. Metabolism 1984;33:724-7.

144. Franc B, Chayvialle JA, Modigliani E, et al. Plasma and tumor levels of somatostatin (SRIF) and somatostatin immunohistochemistry in medullary thyroid carcinoma: apparently discrepant preliminary results. Henry Ford Hosp Med J 1987;35:147-8.

145. Reubi JC, Chayvialle JA, Franc B, Cohen R, Calmettes C, Modigliani E. Somatostatin receptors and somatostatin content in medullary thyroid carcinomas. Lab Invest 1991;64:567-73.

146. Birkenhäger JC, Upton GV, Seldenrath HJ, Krieger DT, Tashjian AH Jr. Medullary thyroid carcinoma: ectopic production of peptides with ACTH-like, corticotrophin releasing factor-like and prolactin production-stimulating activities. Acta Endocrinol (Copenh) 1976;83:280-92.

147. Ohashi M, Yanase T, Fujio N, Ibayashi H, Kinjo M, Matsuo H. Alpha neoendorphin-like immunoreactivity in medullary carcinoma of the thyroid. Cancer 1987;59:277-80.

148. Roth KA, Bensch KG, Hoffman AR. Characterization of opioid peptides in human thyroid medullary carcinoma. Cancer 1987;59:850-6.

149. Uribe M, Fenoglio-Preiser CM, Grimes M, Feind C. Medullary carcinoma of the thyroid gland. Clinical, pathological, and immunohistochemical features with review of the literature. Am J Surg Pathol 1985;9:577-94.

150. Faggiano A, Talbot M, Lacroix L, et al. Differential expression of galectin-3 in medullary thyroid carcinoma and C-cell hyperplasia. Clin Endocrinol 2002;57:813-9.

151. Burtin P, Calmettes C, Fondaneche MC. CEA and non-specific cross-reacting antigen (NCA) in medullary carcinomas of the thyroid. Int J Cancer 1979;23:741-5.

152. DeLellis RA, Rule AH, Spiler I, Nathanson L, Tashjian AH Jr, Wolfe HJ. Calcitonin and carcinoembryonic antigen as tumor markers in medullary thyroid carcinoma. Am J Clin Pathol 1978;70:587-94.

153. DeLellis RA, Wolfe HJ, Rule AH. Carcinoembryonic antigen as a tissue marker in medullary thyroid carcinoma. New Engl J Med 1978;299:1082.

154. Ishikawa N, Hamada S. Association of medullary carcinoma of the thyroid and carcinoembryonic antigen. Br J Cancer 1976;34:111-5.

155. Schröder S, Kloppel G. Carcinoembryonic antigen and nonspecific cross-reacting antigen in thyroid cancer. An immunocytochemical study using polyclonal and monoclonal antibodies. Am J Surg Pathol 1987;11:100-8.

156. Saad MF, Ordòñez NG, Guido JJ, Samaan NA. The prognostic value of calcitonin immunostaining in medullary carcinoma of the thyroid. J Clin Endocrinol Metab 1984;59:850-6.

157. Trump DL, Mendelsohn G, Baylin SB. Discordance between plasma calcitonin and tumor-cell mass in medullary thyroid carcinoma. N Engl J Med 1979;301:253-5.

158. Mendelsohn G, Wells SA, Baylin SB. Relationship of tissue carcinoembryonic antigen and calcitonin to tumor virulence in medullary thyroid carcinoma. An immunohistochemical study in early, localized and virulent disseminated stages of disease. Cancer 1984;54:657-62.

159. Braunstein H, Stephens CL, Gibson RL. Secretory granules in medullary carcinoma of the thyroid. Electron microscopic demonstration. Arch Pathol 1968;85:306-13.

160. Dämmrich J, Ormanns W, Schäffer R. Electron microscopic demonstration of calcitonin in human medullary carcinoma of the thyroid by the immunogold staining method. Histochemistry 1984;81:369-72.

161. Huang SN, Goltzman D. Electron and immuno-electron microscopic study of thyroidal medullary carcinoma. Cancer 1978;41:2226-35.

162. Normann T, Johannessen JV, Gautvik KM, Olsen BR, Brennhovd IO. Medullary carcinoma of the thyroid. Diagnostic problems. Cancer 1976;38:366-77.

163. Nieuwenhuizjen Kruseman AC, Bosman FT, van Bergen Henegouw JC, Cramier-Knijnenburg G, Brutel de la Riviera G. Medullary differentiation of anaplastic thyroid carcinoma. Am J Clin Pathol 1982;77:541-7.

164. Martinelli G, Bazzocchi F, Govoni E, Santini D. Anaplastic type of medullary thyroid carcinoma. An ultrastructural and immunohistochemical study. Virchows Arch A Pathol Anat Histopathol 1983;400:61-7.

165. Zeman V, Němec J, Platil A, Zamrazil V, Pohunková D, Neradilová M. Anaplastic transformation of medullary thyroid cancer. Neoplasma 1978;25:249-55.

166. Carcangiu ML. Steeper T, Zampi G, Rosai J. Anaplastic thyroid carcinoma. A study of 70 cases. Am J Clin Pathol 1985;83:135-58.

167. Matias-Guiu X, LaGuette J, Puras-Gil AM, Rosai J. Metastatic neuroendocrine tumors to the thyroid gland mimicking medullary carcinoma: a pathologic and immunohistochemical study of six cases. Am J Surg Pathol 1997;21:754-62.

168. Carney JA, Ryan J, Goellner JR. Hyalinizing trabecular adenoma of the thyroid gland. Am J Surg Pathol 1987;11:583-91.

169. Scollo C, Baudin E, Travagli JP, et al. Rationale for central and bilateral lymph node dissection in sporadic and hereditary medullary thyroid cancer. J Clin Endocrinol Metab 2003;88:2070-5.

170. Moo-Young TA, Traugott AL, Moley JF. Sporadic and familial medullary thyroid carcinoma: state of the art. Surg Clin North Am 2009;89:1193-1204.

171. Lack EE. Tumors of the adrenal glands and extraadrenal paraganglia. AFIP Atlas of Tumor Pathology, 4th Series, Fascicle 8. Washington DC: American Registry of Pathology; 2007:262.

172. Sand M, Uecker S, Bechara FG, et al. Simultaneous ectopic adrenocorticotropic hormone syndrome and adrenal metastasis of a medullary thyroid carcinoma causing paraneoplastic Cushing's syndrome. Int Semin Surg Oncol 2007;4:15.

173. Conway A, Wiernik A, Rawaal A, Lam C, Mesa H. Occult primary medullary thyroid carcinoma presenting with pituitary and parotid metastases: case report and review of the literature. Endocr Pathol 2012;23:115-22.

174. Ricciato MP, Lombardi CP, Raffaelli M, De Rosa A, Corsello SM. Metastatic breast involvement from medullary thyroid carcinomas: a clue to consider the need of early diagnosis and adequate surgical strategy. Thyroid 2010;20:831-2.

175. Griebeler ML, Gharib H, Thompson GB. Medullary thyroid carcinoma. Endocr Pract 2013; 19:703-11.

176. Giunti S, Antonelli A, Amorosi A, Santarpia L. Cellular signaling pathway alterations and potential targeted therapies for medullary thyroid carcinoma. Int J Endocrinol 2013;2013:803171.

177. Ton GN, Banaszynski ME, Kolesar JM. Vandetanib: a novel targeted therapy for the treatment of metastatic or locally advanced medullary thyroid cancer. Am J Health Syst Pharm 2013;70:849-55.

178. Bible KC, Suman VJ, Molina JR, et al. A Multicenter phase 2 trial of pazopanib in metastatic and progressive medullary thyroid carcinoma: MC057H. J Clin Endocrinol Metab 2014;99:1687-93.

179. Metzger R, Milas M. Inherited cancer syndromes and the thyroid. Cur Opin Oncol 2014;26:51-6.

180. Barbet J, Campion L, Kraeber-Bodere F, Chatel JF, GTE Study Group. Prognostic impact of serum calcitonin and carcinoembryonic antigen doubling-times in patients with medullary thyroid carcinoma. J Clin Endocrinol Metab 2005;90:6077-84.

181. Meijer JA, le Cessie S, van der Hout WB, et al. Calcitonin and carcinoembryonic antigen doubling times as prognostic factors in medullary thyroid carcinoma: a structured meta-analysis. Clin Endocrinol (Oxf) 2010;72:534-42.

182. Bergholm U, Adami HO, Bergstrom R, et al. Clinical characteristics in sporadic and familial medullary thyroid carcinoma. A nationwide study of 249 patients in Sweden from 1959 through 1981. Cancer 1989;63:1196-204.

183. Raue F, Kotzerke J, Reinwein D, et al. Prognostic factors in medullary thyroid carcinoma: evaluation of 741 patients from the German Medullary Thyroid Carcinoma Register. Clin Invest 1993;71:7-12.

184. Modigliani E, Cohen R, Campos JM, et al. Prognostic factors for survival and for biochemical cure in medullary thyroid carcinoma: results in 899 patients. The GETC Study Group. Groupe d'Etude des Tumeurs a calcitonine. Clin Endocrinol 1998;48:265-73.

185. Brierley JD, Tsang R, Simpson WJ, Gospodarowicz M, Sutcliffe S, Panzarella T. Medullary thyroid cancer: analysis of survival and prognostic factors and the role of radiation therapy in local control. Thyroid 1996;6:305-10.

186. Dottorini ME, Assi A, Sironi M, Sangalli G, Spreafico G, Colombo L. Multivariate analysis of patients with medullary thyroid carcinoma: prognostic significance and impact on treatment of clinical and pathological variables. Cancer 1996;77:1556-65.

187. Scopsi L, Sampietro G, Boracchi P, et al. Multivariate analysis of prognostic factors in sporadic medullary thyroid carcinoma. A retrospective study of 109 consecutive patients. Cancer 1996;78:2173-83.

188. Rios A, Rodriguez JM, Acosta JM, et al. Prognostic value of histological and immunochemical characteristics for predicting the recurrence of medullary thyroid carcinoma. Ann Surg Oncol 2010;17:2444-51.

189. Abraham DT, Low TH, Messina M, et al. Medullary thyroid carcinoma: long-term outcomes of surgical treatment. Ann Surg Oncol 2011;18:219-25.

190. Koperek O, Scheuba C, Cherenko M, et al. Desmoplasia in medullary thyroid carcinoma: a reliable indicator of metastatic potential. Histopathology 2008;52:623-30.

191. Tisell LE, Oden A, Muth A, et al. The Ki67 index a prognostic marker in medullary thyroid carcinoma. Br J Cancer 2003;89:2093-7.

192. Mian C, Pennelli G, Barollo S, et al. Combined RET and Ki-67 assessment in sporadic medullary thyroid carcinoma: a useful tool for patient risk stratification. Eur J Endocrinol 2011;164:971-6.

193. Rohmer V, Vidal-Trecan G, Bourdelot A, et al. Prognostic factors of disease free survival after thyroidectomy in 170 young patients with a RET germline mutation: a multicenter study of the Group Francais d'Etude des Tumeurs Endocrines. J Clin Endocrinol Metab 2011;96:509-18.

194. Sambade C, Baldague-Faria A, Cardoso-Oliveira M, Sobrinho-Simões M. Follicular and papillary variants of medullary thyroid carcinoma. Pathol Res Pract 1988;184:98-107.

195. Kakudo K, Miyauchi A, Takai S, et al. C cell carcinoma of the thyroid—papillary type. Acta Pathol Jpn 1979;29:653-9.

196. Papotti M, Sambataro D, Pecchioni C, Bussolati G. The pathology of medullary carcinoma of the thyroid: review of the literature and personal experience on 62 cases. Endocr Pathol 1996;7:1-2.

197. Harach HR, Williams ED. Glandular (tubular and follicular) variants of medullary carcinoma of the thyroid. Histopathology 1983;7:83-97.

198. Lertprasertsuke N, Kakudo K, Nakamura A, et al. C-cell carcinoma of the thyroid. Follicular variant. Acta Pathol Jpn 1989;39:393-9.

199. Valenta LJ, Michel-Bechet M, Mattson JC, Singer FR. Microfollicular thyroid carcinoma with amyloid rich stroma, resembling medullary carcinoma of the thyroid (MCT). Cancer 1977;39:1573-86.

200. Albores-Saavedra J, LiVolsi VA, Williams ED. Medullary carcinoma. Semin Diagn Pathol 1985;2:137-46.

201. Mendelsohn G, Baylin SB, Bigner SH, Wells SA, Eggleston JC. Anaplastic variants of medullary thyroid carcinoma: a light microscopic and immunohistochemical study. Am J Surg Pathol 1980;4:333-41.

202. Eusebi V, Damiani S, Riva C, Lloyd RV, Capella C. Calcitonin free oat-cell carcinoma of the thyroid gland. Virchows Arch A Pathol Anat Histopathol 1990;417:267-71.

203. Eloy C, Oliveira M, Vieira J, Teixeira MR, Cruz J, Sobrinho-Simões M. Carcinoma of the thyroid with ewing family tumor elements and favorable prognosis: report of a second case. Int J Surg Pathol 2014;22:260-5.

204. Landon G, Ordòñez NG. Clear cell variant of medullary carcinoma of the thyroid. Hum Pathol 1985;16:844-7.

205. Marcus JN, Dise CA, LiVolsi VA. Melanin production in a medullary thyroid carcinoma. Cancer 1982;49:2518-26.

206. Beerman H, Rigaud C, Bogomeletz WV, Hollander H, Veldhuizen H. Melanin production in black medullary thyroid carcinoma (MTC). Histopathology 1990;16:227-34.

207. Singh K, Sharma MC, Jain D, Kumar R. Melanotic medullary carcinoma of the thyroid—report of a case with brief review of literature. Diagn Pathol 2008;3:2.

208. Dominguez-Malagon H, Delgado-Chavez R, Torres-Najera M, Gould E, Albores-Saavedra J. Oxyphil and squamous variants of medullary thyroid carcinoma. Cancer 1989;63:1183-8.

209. Harach HR, Bergholm U. Medullary (C cell) carcinoma of the thyroid with features of follicular oxyphilic cell tumors. Histopathology 1988;13:645-56.

210. Golouh R, Us-Krasovec M, Auersperg M, Jancar J, Bondi A, Eusebi V. Amphicrine—composite calcitonin and mucin producing—carcinoma of the thyroid. Ultrastruct Pathol 1985;8:197-206.

211. Carney JA, Ryan J, Goellner JR. Hyalinizing trabecular adenoma of the thyroid gland. Am J Surg Pathol 1987;11:583-91.

212. Bronner M, LiVolsi VA, Jennings T. PLAT: Paraganglioma-like adenomas of the thyroid. Surg Pathol 1988;1:383-9.

213. Huss LJ, Mendelsohn G. Medullary carcinoma of the thyroid gland: an encapsulated variant resembling the hyalinizing trabecular (paraganglioma-like) adenoma of thyroid. Mod Pathol 1990;3:581-5.

214. Magro G, Grasso S. Sustentacular cells in sporadic paraganglioma-like medullary thyroid carcinoma: report of a case with diagnostic and histogenetic considerations. Pathol Res Pract 2000;196:55-9.

215. Bockhorn M, Sheu SY, Frilling A, Molmenti E, Schmid KW, Broelsch CE. Paraganglioma-like medullary thyroid carcinoma: a rare entity. Thyroid 2005;15:1363-7.
216. Laforga JB, Aranda FI. Pseudosarcomatous features in medullary thyroid carcinoma, spindle-cell variant. Report of a case studied by FNA and immunohistochemistry. Diagn Cytopathol 2007;35:424-8.
217. Beskid M, Lorenc R, Rosciszewska A. C-cell thyroid adenoma in man. J Pathol 1971;103:1-4.
218. Kodama T, Okamoto T, Fujimoto Y, et al. C cell adenoma of the thyroid: a rare but distinct clinical entity. Surgery 1988;104:997-1003.
219. Mendelsohn G, Oertel JE. Encapsulated medullary thyroid carcinomas: differentiation from "atypical" adenomas by calcitonin immunohistochemistry. Lab Invest 1981;44:43A.
220. Guyetant S, Dupre F, Bigorgne JC, et al. Medullary thyroid microcarcinoma: a clinicopathologic retrospective study of 38 patients with no prior familial disease. Hum Pathol 1999;30:957-63.
221. Albores-Saavedra JA, Kruegan JE. C-cell hyperplasia and medullary thyroid microcarcinoma. Endocr Pathol 2001;12:365-77.
222. Mizukami Y, Kurumaya H, Nonomura A, et al. Sporadic medullary microcarcinoma of the thyroid. Histopathology 1992;21:375-7.
223. Pillarisetty VG, Katz SC, Ghossein RA Tuttle RM, Shaha AR. Micromedullary thyroid cancer: how micro is truly micro? Ann Surg Oncol 2009;16:2875-81.
224. DeLellis RA, Nunnemacher G, Wolfe HJ. C-cell hyperplasia. An ultrastructural analysis. Lab Invest 1977;36:237-48.
225. McDermott MB, Swanson PE, Wick MR. Immunostains for collagen type IV discriminate between C-cell hyperplasia and microscopic medullary carcinoma in multiple endocrine neoplasia type 2A. Hum Pathol 1995;26:1308-12.
226. Hellman DE, Kartchner M, Van Antwerp JD, Salmon SE, Patton DD, O'Mara R. Radioiodine in the treatment of medullary carcinoma of the thyroid. J Clin Endocrinol Metab 1979:48:451-8.
227. Papotti M, Bussolati G, Komminoth P, Matias-Guiu X, Volante M. Mixed medullary and follicular cell carcinoma. In: DeLellis RA, Lloyd RV, Heitz PU, Eng C, eds. Pathology and genetics of tumours of endocrine organs (WHO Classification of Tumours). 2004:92-3.
228. Hales M, Rosenau W, Okerlund MD, Galante M. Carcinoma of the thyroid with a mixed medullary and follicular pattern: morphological, immunohistochemical, and clinical laboratory studies. Cancer 1982;50:1352-9.
229. Papotti M, Negro F, Carney JA, Bussolati G, Lloyd RV. Mixed medullary-follicular carcinoma of the thyroid. A morphological, immunohistochemical and in situ hybridization analysis of 11 cases. Virchows Arch 1997;430:397-405
230. Holm R, Sobrinho-Simões M, Nesland JM, Johannessen JV. Concurrent production of calcitonin and thyroglobulin by the same neoplastic cells. Ultrastruct Pathol 1986;10:241-8.
231. LiVolsi VA. Mixed thyroid carcinoma: a real entity? Lab Invest 1987;57:237-9.
232. Ljungberg O, Bondeson L, Bondeson AG. Differentiated thyroid carcinoma, intermediate type: a new tumor entity with features of follicular and parafollicular carcinoma. Hum Pathol 1984;15:218-28.
233. Ljungberg O, Ericsson UB, Bondesson L, Thorell J. A compound follicular-parafollicular cell carcinoma of the thyroid: a new tumor entity? Cancer 1983;52;1053-61.
234. Pfaltz M, Hedinger CE, Mühlethaler JP. Mixed medullary and follicular carcinoma of the thyroid. Virchows Arch A Pathol Anat Histopathol 1983;400:53-9.
235. Sobrinho-Simões M, Nesland J, Johannessen JV. Farewell to the dual histogenesis of thyroid tumors? Ultrastruct Pathol 1985;8:iii-v.
236. Albores-Saavedra J, Gorraez de la Mora T, de la Torre-Rendon F, Gould E. Mixed medullary papillary carcinoma of the thyroid: a previously unrecognized variant of thyroid carcinoma. Hum Pathol 1990;21:1151-5.
237. Sadow PM, Hunt JL. Mixed medullary-follicular derived carcinomas of the thyroid gland. Adv Anat Pathol 2010;17:282-5.
238. Volante M, Papotti M, Roth J, et al. Mixed medullary-follicular thyroid carcinoma. Molecular evidence for a dual origin of tumor components. Am J Pathol 1999;155:1499-509.
239. Vantyghem MC, Pigny P, Leteurtre E, et al. Thyroid carcinomas involving follicular and parafollicular C cells: seventeen cases with characterization of RET oncogenic activation. Thyroid 2004;14:842-7.
240. Melillo RM, Cirafici AM, DeFalco V, et al. The oncogenic activity of RET point mutants for follicular thyroid cells may account for the occurrence of papillary thyroid carcinoma in patients affected by familial medullary thyroid carcinoma. Am J Pathol 2004;165:511-21.
241. Reynolds L, Jones K, Winton DJ, et al. C-cell and thyroid epithelial tumours and altered follicular development in transgenic mice expressing the long isoform of MEN 2A RET. Oncogene 2001;20:3986-94.
242. Wells SA Jr, Ontjes DA, Cooper CW, et al. The early diagnosis of medullary carcinoma of the thyroid gland in patients with multiple endocrine neoplasia type II. Ann Surg 1975;182:362-70.
243. Asaadi AA. Ultrastructure in C cell hyperplasia in asymptomatic patients with hypercalcitoninemia and a family history of medullary thyroid carcinoma. Hum Pathol 1981;12:617-22.

244. Schürch W, Babäi F, Boivin Y, Verdy M. Light-electron microscopic and cytochemical studies on the morphogenesis of familial medullary thyroid carcinoma. Virchows Arch A Pathol Anat Histol 1977;376:29-46.

245. Frilling A, Dralle H, Eng C, Raue F, Broelsch CE. Presymptomatic DNA screening in families with multiple endocrine neoplasia type 2 and familial medullary thyroid carcinoma. Surgery 1995;118:1099-103.

246. Moline J, Eng C. Multiple endocrine neoplasia type 2: an overview. Genet Med 2011;13:755-64.

247. Wells SA Jr, Pacini F, Robinson BG, Santoro M. Multiple endocrine neoplasia type 2 and familial medullary thyroid carcinoma: an update. J Clin Endocrinol Metab 2013;98:3149-64.

248. Krampitz GW, Norton JA. RET gene mutations (genotype and phenotype) of multiple endocrine neoplasia type 2 and familial medullary thyroid carcinoma. Cancer 2014;120:1920-31.

249. Perry A, Molberg K, Albores-Saavedra J. Physiologic versus neoplastic C-cell hyperplasia of the thyroid: separation of distinct histologic and biologic entities. Cancer 1996;77:750-6.

250. Saggiorato E, Rapa I, Garino F, et al. Absence of RET gene point mutations in sporadic thyroid C-cell hyperplasia. J Mol Diagn 2007;9:214-9.

251. O'Toole K, Fenoglio-Preiser C, Pushparaj N. Endocrine changes associated with the human aging process: III. Effect of age on the number of calcitonin immunoreactive cells in the thyroid gland. Hum Pathol 1985:16:991-1000.

252. Biddinger PW, Brennan MF, Rosen PP. Symptomatic C-cell hyperplasia associated with chronic lymphocytic thyroiditis. Am J Surg Pathol 1991;15:599-604.

253. Libbey NP, Nowakowski KJ, Tucci JR. C-cell hyperplasia of the thyroid in a patient with goitrous hypothyroidism and Hashimoto's thyroiditis. Am J Surg Pathol 1989;13:71-7.

254. Albores-Saavedra J. C-cell hyperplasia. Am J Surg Pathol 1989;13:987-9.

255. LiVolsi VA, Feind CR, LoGerfo P, Tashjian AH Jr. Demonstration by immunoperoxidase staining of hyperplasia of parafollicular cells in the thyroid gland in hyperparathyroidism. J Clin Endocrinol Metab 1973;37:550-9.

256. Wolfe HJ, DeLellis RA, Scott RT, Tasjhjian AH Jr. C-cell hyperplasia in chronic hypercalcemia in man. [Abstract]. Am J Pathol 1975;78:20A.

257. Albores-Saavedra J, Monforte H, Nadji M, Morales AR. C-cell hyperplasia in thyroid tissue adjacent to follicular cell tumors. Hum Pathol 1988;19:795-9.

258. Scopsi L, Di Palma S, Ferrari C, Holst JJ, Rehfeld JF, Rilke F. C-cell hyperplasia accompanying thyroid diseases other than medullary thyroid carcinoma: an immunocytochemical study by means of antibodies to calcitonin and somatostatin. Mod Pathol 1991;4:297-304.

259. Zambrano E, Holm I, Glickman J, et al. Abnormal distribution and hyperplasia of thyroid C-cells in PTEN-associated tumor syndromes. Endocr Pathol 2004;15:55-64.

260. Laury AR, Bongiovanni M, Tille JC, Kozakewich H, Nosé V. Thyroid pathology in PTEN-hamartoma tumor syndrome: characteristic findings of a distinct entity. Thyroid 2011;21:135-44.

261. Boorman GA, Hollander CF. Animal model of human disease: medullary carcinoma of the thyroid in the rat. Am J Pathol 1976;83:237-40.

262. Capen CC, Black HE. Animal model of human disease. Medullary thyroid carcinoma, multiple endocrine neoplasia, Sipple's syndrome. Animal model: ultimobranchial thyroid neoplasm in the bull. Am J Pathol 1974;74:377-80.

263. Capen CC, Young DM. Fine structural alterations in thyroid parafollicular cells of cows in response to experimental hypercalcemia induced by vitamin D. Am J Pathol 1969;57:365-82.

264. Wolfe HJ, DeLellis RA. Familial medullary thyroid carcinoma and C cell hyperplasia. Clin Endocrinol Metab 1981;10:351-65.

265. Diaz-Cano S, DeMiguel M, Blanes A, Tashjian R, Wolfe HJ. Germline RET 634 mutation positive MEN 2A-related C-cell hyperplasias have genetic features consistent with intraepithelial neoplasia. J Clin Endocrinol Metab 2001;86:3948-51.

266. Kaserer K, Scheuba C, Neuhold N, et al. C-cell hyperplasia and medullary thyroid carcinoma in patients routinely screened for serum calcitonin. Am J Surg Pathol 1998;22:722-8.

267. Kaserer K, Scheuba C, Neuhold N, et al. Sporadic versus familial medullary thyroid microcarcinoma: a histopathologic study of 50 consecutive patients. Am J Surg Pathol 2001;25:1245-51.

268. Mears L, Diaz-Cano SJ. Difference between familial and sporadic medullary thyroid carcinomas. Am J Surg Pathol 2003;27:266-7.

269. Guyetant S, Rousselet MC, Durigon M, et al. Sex-related C cell hyperplasia in the normal human thyroid: a quantitative autopsy study. J Clin Endocrinol Metab 1997;82:42-7.

270. Lips CJ, Leo JR, Berends MJ, et al. Thyroid C-cell hyperplasia and micronodules in close relatives of MEN-2A patients: pitfalls in early diagnosis and revaluation of criteria for surgery. Henry Ford Hosp Med J 1987;35:133-8.

271. Yamaoka Y. Solid cell nest (SCN) of human thyroid gland. Acta Pathol Jpn 1973;23:493-506.

272. Vollenweider I, Hedinger C. Solid cell nests (SCN) in Hashimoto's thyroiditis. Virchows Arch A Pathol Anat Histopathol 1988;412:357-63.

273. Carney JA, Moore SB, Northcutt RC, Woolner LB, Stillwell GK. Palpation thyroiditis (multifocal granulomatous folliculitis). Am J Clin Pathol 1975;64:639-47.

13 SARCOMAS OF THE THYROID GLAND

GENERAL CONSIDERATIONS

Sarcomas are malignant tumors with a mesenchymal phenotype. They presumably arise from one of the stromal components of the thyroid gland.

A sarcoma of the thyroid gland should be a straightforward subject, both conceptually and in practice, using the following reasoning: 1) the thyroid gland, like any other organ, has a mesenchymal (stromal) component; 2) this component, like that of any other site, can undergo malignant transformation; 3) the result should be a sarcoma not significantly different from those arising from analogous mesenchymal cell types in the somatic soft tissues or in other organs, and therefore diagnosable by using similar criteria. Unfortunately, this seemingly logical reasoning cannot be rigidly applied to sarcomas of the thyroid gland because undifferentiated (anaplastic) carcinomas may resemble various sarcomas to such a degree as to render the differential diagnosis difficult or even impossible. The thyroid gland is not the only organ in the body in which this situation arises; nevertheless, it seems to be here, more than at any other site, that the vexing antinomy between observed differentiation and assumed histogenesis is more sorely tested (1). This is discussed at length in chapter 9. The important point is that most malignant thyroid tumors with a sarcomatoid appearance are undifferentiated carcinomas, in the sense that they exhibit telltale signs of epithelial differentiation by either morphologic or immunohistochemical criteria. Therefore, such tumors should be regarded as undifferentiated thyroid carcinomas "in the absence of indisputable proof to the contrary," as recommended by the World Health Organization (WHO) Committee for the Histologic Typing of Thyroid Tumors (2).

The WHO committee also states that the diagnosis of thyroid sarcoma should only be made in tumors lacking all evidence of epithelial differentiation and showing definite evidence of specific sarcomatous differentiation. This definition may be too restrictive. There is no reason, for instance, why a fibrosarcoma (a tumor that does not show a specific pattern of sarcomatous differentiation) could not occur in the thyroid gland. In view of the above considerations, however, the WHO proposal seems logical and has been adopted in the 2004 edition of the WHO section on Tumors of the Thyroid Gland, which does not have a general chapter on sarcomas, but acknowledges the existence of specific rare types of thyroid sarcomas.

The age of the patient at the time of diagnosis is another diagnostic factor. Since undifferentiated thyroid carcinomas are exceptionally rare before the age of 50 years, the possibility of any given sarcoma-like thyroid tumor actually being a true sarcoma increases proportionally as the patient's age decreases. Another diagnostic possibility is a sarcoma of the soft tissues of the neck that has invaded the thyroid gland secondarily, even if this phenomenon is just as unusual as a true primary thyroid sarcoma.

Many isolated case reports of thyroid sarcoma are on record, and the range of specific diagnoses used for them is wide. It includes *fibrosarcoma* (3,4), *liposarcoma* (5–7), *leiomyosarcoma* (8,9), *osteosarcoma* (10), *chondrosarcoma* (11), *malignant peripheral nerve sheath tumor* (12,13), *Ewing sarcoma/primitive neuroectodermal tumor (PNET)* (14), *follicular dendritic cell sarcoma* (15), and *malignant (diffuse) hemangiopericytoma* (16). One of the reported cases of thyroid leiomyosarcoma developed in a child with congenital immunodeficiency which was Epstein-Barr virus related (figs. 13-1–13-3) (17). Another case was detected 4 years after a hysterectomy for uterine leiomyosarcoma (18); in this situation, it becomes impossible to determine whether the thyroid tumor is a metastasis from the uterine tumor or a second primary, although the former scenario seems more likely.

Figure 13-1

THYROID LEIOMYOSARCOMA

This tumor was strongly immuno-reactive for smooth muscle actin and negative for keratin and thyroid transcription factor (TTF)-1.

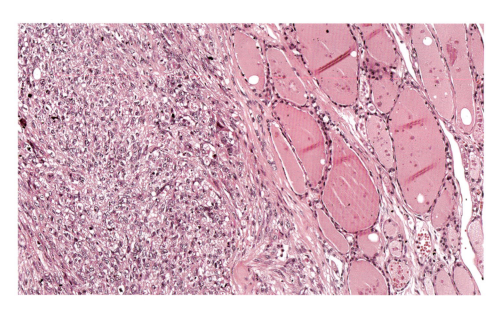

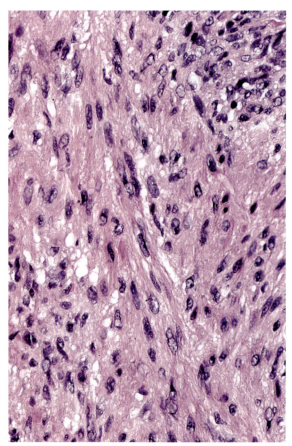

Figure 13-2

THYROID LEIOMYOSARCOMA

The pattern of growth is fascicular. The cytoplasm of the tumor cells has a fibrillary acidophilic quality.

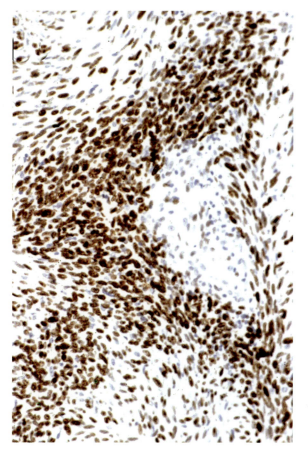

Figure 13-3

THYROID LEIOMYOSARCOMA

The tumor cells are positive for Epstein-Barr virus encoded RNA (EBER). The patient had a congenital immuno-deficiency.

Few of these reported thyroidal "sarcomas" qualify as such if the WHO criteria are strictly applied. Fortunately, the issue is of no great practical significance, since their natural history and response to therapy do not differ significantly from those of undifferentiated carcinomas. The outstanding exception is angiosarcoma, a highly controversial entity that deserves to be discussed separately because of its distinct epidemiologic, morphologic, immunohistochemical, and ultrastructural peculiarities.

ANGIOSARCOMA

Definition. *Angiosarcoma* is a malignant tumor exhibiting endothelial cell differentiation. Theoretically, any malignant tumor of the blood vessels could be called an angiosarcoma. In practice, however, the term is reserved for those tumors exhibiting endothelial (rather than pericytic, glomic, or vascular smooth muscle) differentiation. In common parlance, angiosarcoma is used synonymously with *malignant hemangioendothelioma,* the latter being a more specific and accurate, but less popular, designation.

General Features. One of the most striking features of thyroid angiosarcoma is that most of the reported cases are from mountainous areas, especially the Alpine regions of central Europe, which in the past were said to comprise as much as 16 percent of all thyroid malignancies (19). The identification of this tumor type and the heated defense about its authenticity came primarily from Swiss authors (20,21). Historically, most American pathologists have been skeptical about the existence of this entity, favoring the alternative hypothesis that most, if not all, of the reported cases are in reality undifferentiated carcinomas with an angiosarcomatoid appearance (22). Some European pathologists have adopted a similar point of view (23).

In recent years, evidence has accumulated that a thyroid malignancy exhibiting phenotypical features of endothelial cell differentiation in the absence of epithelial markers does exist. Its predilection for mountainous regions had been linked to the iodine deficiency that existed in those areas and the nodular hyperplasia (goiter) that was its natural consequence. Indeed, thyroid angiosarcoma develops in most instances against this background. It has been hypothesized that the marked vascularization

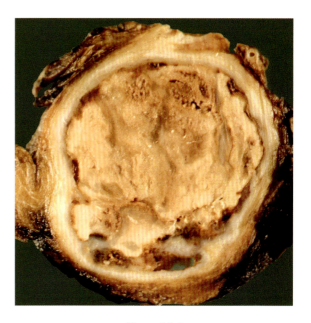

Figure 13-4

THYROID ANGIOSARCOMA
This tumor is almost completely necrotic.

that takes place in hyperplastic glands (and which caused formidable technical difficulties at surgery in years past) is the milieu on which angiosarcoma arises. Thyroid angiosarcoma is not limited to these regions, however, or to goitrous glands (24–28). Judging from the widely divergent conclusions reached about these issues by the various authors, the controversy is far from subsiding (29–31).

Clinical Features. Most patients are elderly individuals with a history of longstanding goiter who have noticed sudden enlargement, sometimes painful, of the thyroid gland. In Egloff's series (32), the average age at the time of diagnosis was 62 years. In some instances, signs due to metastatic spread, such as chest pain and hemothorax resulting from pleuropulmonary metastases, are already evident at presentation.

Gross Findings. The tumor is typically large, with extensive areas of necrosis and hemorrhage (figs. 13-4, 13-5). The latter may result in blood-filled cystic cavities resembling hematomas. Although almost always invasive, the cut surface may appear nodular and well-circumscribed (33).

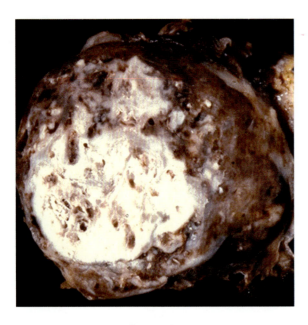

Figure 13-5

THYROID EPITHELIOID ANGIOSARCOMA

This tumor is characteristically necrotic and hemorrhagic. (Courtesy of Dr. V. Eusebi, Bologna, Italy.)

Microscopic Findings. Like angiosarcomas elsewhere, the distinguishing feature of this tumor when it involves the thyroid gland is the presence of freely anastomosing vascular channels lined by atypical endothelial cells (fig. 13-6). This may be associated with a papillary configuration resulting from a predominantly intraluminal pattern of growth (19,32), or may represent only a focal finding in what is otherwise a poorly differentiated neoplasm with a predominantly solid pattern of growth.

The shape of the tumor cells ranges from spindled to epithelioid (34). Multinucleated and other bizarre cellular forms are unusual. The tumor cells lining the vascular spaces are plumper than those located between them. Some of the epithelioid cells may exhibit intracytoplasmic vacuoles, sometimes containing intact or fragmented red blood cells. These formations are thought to represent attempts at vascular lumen formation.

The nuclei of the epithelioid endothelial cells are often large and vesicular, with regular outlines, and endowed with a prominent amphophilic or eosinophilic nucleolus connected by chromatin strands to the nuclear membrane, a useful diagnostic clue (fig. 13-7). The eosino-

philic cytoplasm is abundant in the epithelioid endothelial cells but less so in the spindle forms. Mitoses, both typical and atypical, are invariably found, often in large numbers.

The pattern of growth is nearly always highly invasive. Thyroid follicles are first displaced and then destroyed by the growth of the tumor. On occasion, the sarcoma grows within the wall of sizable intrathyroidal arteries, between the two elastic laminae. A constant feature is the presence of extensive fresh and old hemorrhage, the latter represented by conglomerates of hemosiderin-laden macrophages. Tumor necrosis is usually widespread.

Immunohistochemical Findings. In addition to the expected strong and relatively nonspecific reactivity for vimentin, the cells of angiosarcoma stain in greater or lesser degree for all the endothelial cell markers. Factor VIII-related antigen (fig. 13-8) (35–40), although a highly specific marker, is very labile and prone to diffusion into the surrounding tissues. Thus, spurious factor VIII-related antigen positivity may result from nonspecific uptake of antigen-rich serum and platelets by the tumor cells. Ulex europaeus I receptor is also expressed by epithelial cells in individuals with blood group O (fig. 13-9). CD34, in addition to endothelial cells, also stains a large variety of mesenchymal cells and their tumors. CD31 exhibits a much greater degree of specificity for endothelial cells than CD34, and is sometimes positive in CD34-negative vascular tumors (fig. 13-10). FLI-1, originally isolated from the tumor cells of Ewing sarcoma/PNET, also intensely decorates the nuclei of normal and neoplastic endothelial cells. Epithelioid angiosarcomas are often immunoreactive for keratin, a feature (shared with their counterparts in bone and other sites) that adds another twist to the controversy concerning the differential diagnosis between thyroid angiosarcoma and undifferentiated carcinoma (fig. 13-11) (24,41,42).

The recently described ERG transcription factor, an endothelial marker belonging to the ETS family of transcription factors, is expressed in nearly all benign and malignant vascular tumors. Alas, it is also detectable in the cells of prostatic carcinoma and occasional other tumors (43). In the better-differentiated areas of the tumor, the formation of vascular channels

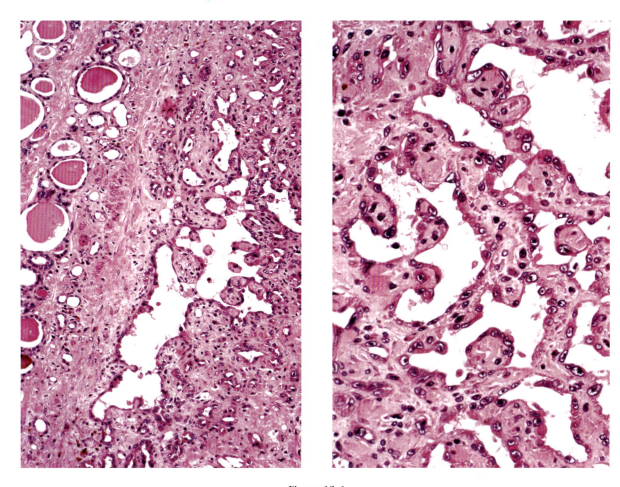

Figure 13-6

THYROID ANGIOSARCOMA

Left: The tumor is composed of anastomosing vascular channels.
Right: High-power view of the anastomosing vascular channels.

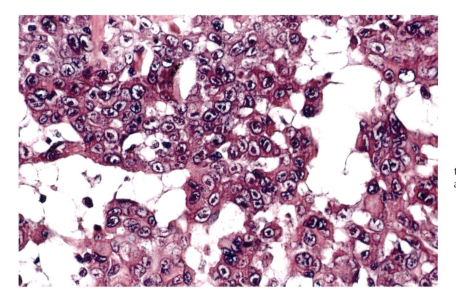

Figure 13-7

**THYROID
ANGIOSARCOMA**

The tumor cells have an epithelioid appearance. The nucleoli are prominent.

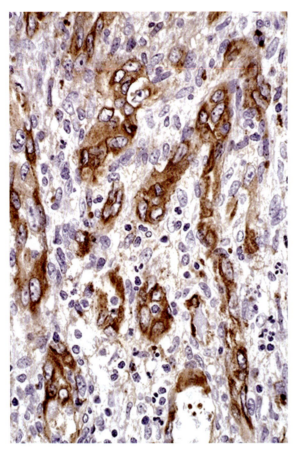

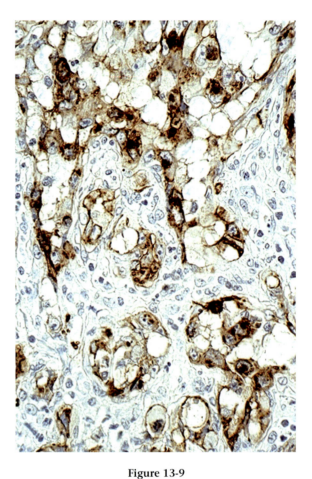

Figure 13-8

THYROID ANGIOSARCOMA

These plump epithelioid endothelial cells are strongly positive for factor VIII-related antigen.

Figure 13-9

THYROID ANGIOSARCOMA

There is strong immunoreactivity of the neoplastic elements for Ulex europaeus I lectin.

Figure 13-10

THYROID ANGIOSARCOMA

Intense positivity of the tumor cells for CD31.

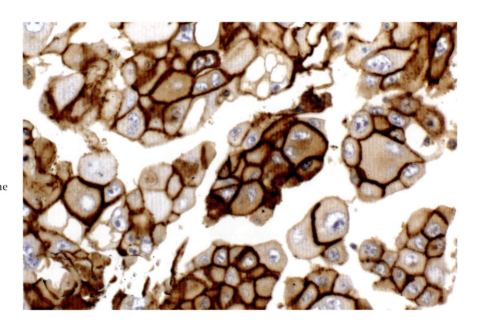

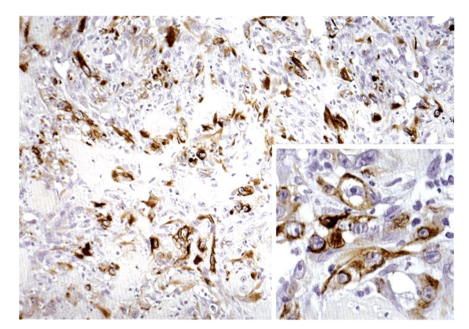

Figure 13-11

THYROID ANGIOSARCOMA

The tumor cells are strongly immunoreactive for keratin. Inset: High-power view.

Figure 13-12

THYROID ANGIOSARCOMA

An immunostain for type IV collagen shows the presence of the basal lamina component around groups of tumor cells, thus highlighting the formation of primitive vascular tubules.

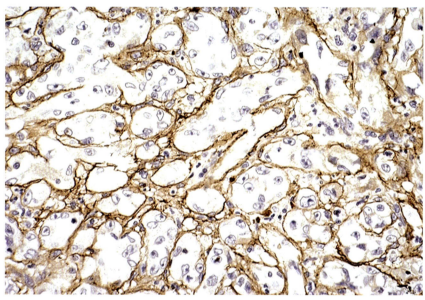

is accompanied by the deposition of basement membrane, a feature that can be evidenced by the demonstration of type IV collagen or laminin (fig. 13-12) (44).

Of all the above markers, CD31, FLI-1, and ERG are regarded at present as the most useful for the immunohistochemical detection of endothelial cell differentiation in tumors, including those arising in the thyroid gland.

Ultrastructural Findings. The better-differentiated tumor cells exhibit basal lamina formation, primitive cell junctions, numerous pinocytotic vesicles, and a variable number of cytoplasmic filaments. The latter are more abundant in the epithelioid cell types. In some tumor cells, intracytoplasmic vacuoles are seen, bordered by a membrane featuring pinocytotic vesicles. These formations are analogous to those present in neoformed normal vessels and are interpreted as an early sign of vascular lumen formation (44).

The Weibel-Palade bodies are a specific ultrastructural feature of endothelial cells. They are rod-shaped, membrane-bound cytoplasmic organelles that contain a variable number of tubules of approximately 15-nm diameter and which are the storage site for factor VIII-related protein (45). These structures are commonly present in the better-differentiated tumors but not necessarily in the poorly differentiated ones. Their absence, therefore, does not rule out a diagnosis of angiosarcoma (24,33).

Molecular Genetic Findings. The expression of vascular endothelial growth factor (VEGF) is increased in angiosarcoma of the thyroid gland. Nuclear accumulation of p53, associated with MDM2 immunoreactivity, in the absence of the *TP53* gene mutation, has been shown in some tumors (46). The extent of p53 immunoreactivity in angiosarcoma, however, appears lower than that reported for undifferentiated thyroid carcinoma (28).

Differential Diagnosis. In addition to the comments above, the differentiation of thyroid angiosarcoma and undifferentiated (anaplastic) carcinoma is discussed in connection with the latter (see chapter 9). A low-grade/borderline form of vascular tumor, known as epithelioid hemangioendothelioma, has been reported in the thyroid gland (47).

Treatment and Prognosis. Thyroid angiosarcoma is an exceedingly malignant tumor. It grows rapidly, infiltrates beyond the gland, and metastasizes distantly, particularly to lung and lymph nodes. Swiss authors have emphasized the high frequency of subpleural hemorrhagic tumor nodules, often associated with massive hemothorax (19). Response to radiation therapy or chemotherapy is poor, and the mortality rate is at least as high as that for undifferentiated carcinoma.

REFERENCES

1. Hedinger CE. Sarcomas of the thyroid gland. In: Hedinger CE, ed. Thyroid cancer. Berlin: Springer-Verlag; 1969:47-52.
2. Hedinger CE. Histological typing of thyroid tumours. New York: Springer-Verlag, 1988.
3. Chesky VE, Hellwig CA, Welch JW. Fibrosarcoma of the thyroid gland. Surg Gynecol Obstet 1960;111:767-70.
4. Shin WY, Aftalion B, Hotchkiss E, Schenkman R, Berkman J. Ultrastructure of a primary fibrosarcoma of the human thyroid gland. Cancer 1979;44:584-91.
5. Andrion A, Gaglio A, Dogliani N, Bosco E, Mazzucco G. Liposarcoma of the thyroid gland. Fine-needle aspiration cytology, immunohistology, and ultrastructure. Am J Clin Pathol 1991;95:675-9.
6. Mitra A, Fisher C, Rhys-Evans P, Harmer C. Liposarcoma of the thyroid. Sarcoma 2004;8:91-6.
7. Huang GW, Li YX, Hu ZL. Primary myxoid liposarcoma of the thyroid gland. J Clin Pathol 2009;62:1037-8.
8. Kawahara E, Nakanishi I, Terahata S, Ikegaki S. Leiomyosarcoma of the thyroid gland. A case report with a comparative study of five cases of anaplastic carcinoma. Cancer 1988;62:2558-63.
9. Thompson LD, Wenig BM, Adair CF, Shmookler BM, Heffess CS. Primary smooth muscle tumors of the thyroid gland. Cancer 1997;79:579-87.
10. Ohbu M, Kameya T, Wada C, et al. Primary osteogenic sarcoma of the thyroid gland: a case report. Surg Pathol 1989;2:67-72.
11. Tseleni-Balafouta S, Arvanitis D, Kakaviatos N, Paraskevakou H. Primary myxoid chondrosarcoma of the thyroid gland. Arch Pathol Lab Med 1988;112:94-6.
12. Thompson LD, Wenig BM, Adair CF, Heffess CS. Peripheral nerve sheath tumors of the thyroid gland: a series of four cases and a review of the literature. Endocr Pathol 1996;7:309-18.
13. Pallares J, Pérez-Ruiz L, Ros S, et al. Malignant peripheral nerve sheath tumor of the thyroid: A clinicopathological and ultrastructural study of one case. Endocr Pathol 2004;15:167-74.
14. Adapa P, Chung TW, Popek EJ, Hunter JV. Extraosseous Ewing sarcoma of the thyroid gland. Pediatr Radiol 2009;39:1365-8.
15. Yu L, Yang SJ. Primary follicular dendritic cell sarcoma of the thyroid gland coexisting with Hashimoto's thyroiditis. Int J Surg Pathol 2011;19:502-5.
16. Proks C. Generalized hemangiopericytoma of the thyroid gland (report of a case). Neoplasma 1961;8:219-24.
17. Tulbah A, Al-Dayel F, Fawaz I, Rosai J. Epstein-Barr virus-associated leiomyosarcoma of the thyroid in a child with congenital immunodeficiency: a case report. Am J Surg Pathol 1999;23:473-6.

18. Piana S, Valli R, Foscolo AM. Thyroid leiomyosarcoma: primary or metastasis? That's the question! Endocr Pathol 2011;22:226-8.

19. Egloff B. The hemangioendothelioma. In: Hedinger CE, ed. Thyroid cancer. Berlin: Springer-Verlag; 1969:52-9. (UICC monograph series; Vol 12.)

20. Hedinger CE. Geographic pathology of thyroid diseases. Pathol Res Pract 1981;171:285-92.

21. Hedinger E. Zur Lehre der Struma sarcomatosa. I. Die Blutgefässendotheliome der Struma. Frankfurt Z Pathol 1909;3:487-540.

22. Klinck GH. Hemangioendothelioma and sarcoma of the thyroid. In: Hedinger CE, ed. Thyroid cancer. Berlin: Springer-Verlag; 1969:60-3. (UICC monograph series; Vol 12.)

23. Krisch K, Holzner JH, Kokoschka R, Jakesz R, Niederle B, Roka R. Hemangioendothelioma of the thyroid gland—true endothelioma or anaplastic carcinoma? Pathol Res Pract 1980;170:230-42.

24. Eusebi V, Carcangiu ML, Dina R, Rosai J. Keratin-positive epithelioid angiosarcoma of thyroid. A report of four cases. Am J Surg Pathol 1990;14:737-47.

25. Tanda F, Massarelli G, Bosincu L, Cossu U. Angiosarcoma of the thyroid: a light, electron microscopic and histoimmunological study. Hum Pathol 1988;19:742-5.

26. Beer TW. Malignant thyroid haemangioendothelioma in a non-endemic goitrous region, with immunohistochemical evidence of a vascular origin. Histopathology 1992;20:539-41.

27. Maiorana A, Collina G, Cesinaro AM, Fano RA, Eusebi V. Epithelioid angiosarcoma of the thyroid. Clinicopathological analysis of seven cases from non-Alpine areas. Virchows Arch 1996;429:131-7.

28. Ryska A, Ludvikova M, Szepe P, Boor A. Epithelioid haemangiosarcoma of the thyroid gland. Report of six cases from a non-Alpine region. Histopathology 2004;44:40-6.

29. Mills SE, Stallings RG, Austin MB. Angiomatoid carcinoma of the thyroid gland. Anaplastic carcinoma with follicular and medullary features mimicking angiosarcoma. Am J Clin Pathol 1986;86:674-8.

30. Tötsch M, Dobler G, Feichtinger H, Sandbichler P, Ladurner D, Schmid KW. Malignant hemangioendothelioma of the thyroid. Its immunohistochemical discrimination from undifferentiated thyroid carcinoma. Am J Surg Pathol 1990;14:69-74.

31. Ritter JH, Mills SE, Nappi O, Wick MR. Angiosarcoma-like neoplasms of epithelial organs: true endothelial tumors or variants of carcinoma? Semin Diagn Pathol 1995;12:270-82.

32. Egloff B. The hemangioendothelioma of the thyroid. Virchows Arch A Pathol Anat Histopathol 1983;400:119-42.

33. Chan YF, Ma L, Boey JH, Yeung HY. Angiosarcoma of the thyroid. An immunohistochemical and ultrastructural study of a case in a Chinese patient. Cancer 1986;57:2381-8.

34. Lamovec J, Zidar A, Zidanik B. Epithelioid angiosarcoma of the thyroid gland. Report of two cases. Arch Pathol Lab Med 1994;118:642-6.

35. Guarda LA, Ordóñez NG, Smith JL Jr, Hanssen G. Immunoperoxidase localization of factor VIII in angiosarcomas. Arch Pathol Lab Med 1982;106:515-6.

36. Mukai K, Rosai J, Burgdorf WH. Localization of factor VIII-related antigen in vascular endothelial cells using an immunoperoxidase method. Am J Surg Pathol 1980;4:273-6.

37. Pfaltz M, Hedinger C, Saremaslani P, Egloff B. Malignant hemangioendothelioma of the thyroid and factor VIII-related antigen. Virchows Arch A Pathol Anat Histopathol 1983;401:177-84.

38. Ruchti C, Gerber HA, Schaffner T. Factor VIII-related antigen in malignant hemangioendothelioma of the thyroid: additional evidence for the endothelial origin of this tumor. Am J Clin Pathol 1984;82:474-80.

39. Schäffer R, Ormanns W. [Immunohistochemical detection of factor VIII antigen in malignant hemangioendotheliomas of the thyroid. A contribution to histogenesis.] Schweiz Med Wochenschr 1983;113:601-5. [German]

40. Vollenweider I, Hedinger C, Saremaslani P, Pfaltz M. Malignant hemangioendothelioma of the thyroid. Immunohistochemical evidence of heterogeneity. Pathol Res Pract 1989;184:376-81.

41. Gray MH, Rosenberg AE, Dickersin GR, Bhan AK. Cytokeratin expression in epithelioid vascular neoplasms. Hum Pathol 1990;21:212-7.

42. van Haelst UJ, Pruszczynski M, ten Cate LN, Mravunac M. Ultrastructural and immunohistochemical study of epithelioid hemangioendothelioma of bone: coexpression of epithelial and endothelial markers. Ultrastruct Pathol 1990;14:141-9.

43. Miettinen M, Wang ZF, Paetau A, et al. ERG transcription factor as an immunohistochemical marker for vascular endothelial tumors and prostatic carcinoma. Am J Surg Pathol 2011;35:432-41.

44. Rosai J, Sumner HW, Kostianovsky M, Pérez-Mesa C. Angiosarcoma of the skin. A clinicopathologic and fine structural study. Hum Pathol 1976;7:83-109.

45. Carstens PH. The Weibel-Palade body in the diagnosis of endothelial tumors. Ultrastruct Pathol 1981;2:315-25.

46. Zietz C, Rossle M, Haas C, et al. MDM-2 oncoprotein overexpression, p53 gene mutation and VEGF up-regulation in angiosarcomas. Am J Pathol 1998;153:1425-33.

47. Siddiqui MT, Evans HL, Ro JY, Ayala AG. Epithelioid haemangioendothelioma of the thyroid gland: a case report and review of literature. Histopathology 1998;32:473-6.

14 MALIGNANT LYMPHOMA OF THE THYROID GLAND AND RELATED LESIONS

MALIGNANT LYMPHOMA

Definition. *Primary malignant lymphoma* is a malignant tumor composed of lymphoid cells or their progeny involving the thyroid gland. The term is usually reserved for those cases in which the thyroid gland is the predominant, often exclusive and presumably primary, site of involvement. This process should be clearly separated from secondary involvement of the thyroid gland by a systemic lymphoma or leukemia, which in autopsy studies has been found to occur in approximately 10 percent of the cases (1). Primary thyroid lymphoma constitutes approximately 8 percent of all thyroid malignancies (2).

Predisposing Factors. In over 80 percent of the cases of thyroid lymphoma, the residual non-neoplastic gland exhibits features of autoimmune thyroiditis of either Hashimoto or lymphocytic type. The frequency of this association is clearly significant and much higher than that found between thyroiditis and thyroid carcinoma (3). The existence of a causal relationship between the two disorders is now widely accepted (4–6). Although it is possible that in some cases the presence of lymphoma in the thyroid gland may induce the thyroiditis, it seems more likely that, in most instances, it is the thyroiditis that predisposes the patient to the development of the lymphoma.

The situation is analogous to that seen at several other sites, in which prolonged antigenic stimulation has been shown to elicit the development of a lymphoid malignancy. A typical example is the salivary gland lymphoma arising in patients with Sjögren syndrome. There are some epidemiologic data supporting this interpretation. A comparison between populations of Iceland and northeast Scotland has shown that the presence of thyroiditis, prevalence of thyroid antibodies, and thyroid lymphoma were all considerably more common in the Scotland group (7). To put the above facts in perspective,

however, it should be pointed out that only an exceedingly small percentage of patients with thyroiditis develop a malignant lymphoma of the thyroid gland.

Another possible etiopathogenetic factor for the development of thyroid lymphoma is exposure of the gland to radiation. A few suggestive cases have been reported in which the exposure was external radiation to the neck or thymic area (8). There is no convincing evidence that administration of [131-I]P255I results in an increased incidence of this type of malignancy.

Clinical Features. Most cases of primary thyroid lymphoma are seen in middle-aged or elderly patients. The most common age at presentation is in the sixties. The ratio of women to men ranges from 2:1 to 8:1 in the various series (9). The common clinical presentation is thyroid enlargement, which is often firm or hard and may be fixed.

The duration of the symptoms is usually short. Hoarseness, dysphagia, and/or dyspnea occur in about 25 percent, and cord paresis in about 17 percent of the patients. As expected, these symptoms are more common in tumors exhibiting extrathyroidal extension (10,11).

Most patients are euthyroid, and the tumor presents as one or more cold nodules on thyroid scan (12). Of 50 cases collected during a 9-year period from the population-based Danish Lymphoma Registry, 76 percent of patients had localized disease (stages I-II) and 24 percent had disseminated lymphoma (stages III-IV) (9).

Gross Findings. The gross features depend on the microscopic type of lymphoma. In most instances the tumor presents as a solid mass with a homogeneous, bulging white surface featuring the "fish-flesh" appearance classically associated with lymphoma in general (figs. 14-1, 14-2). The interface between the tumor and adjacent gland is usually ill defined, and encapsulation is absent. Large or peripherally located lesions tend to invade the thyroid capsule and extend

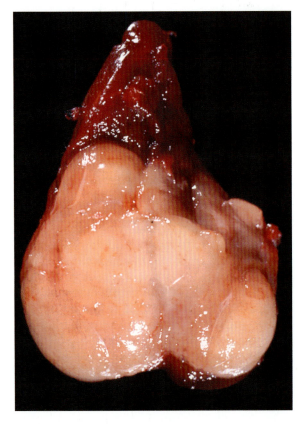

Figure 14-1

MALIGNANT LYMPHOMA

The cut surface is homogeneous, bulging, and tan colored, without appreciable necrosis or hemorrhage.

into the surrounding soft tissue. Necrosis and hemorrhage are uncommon, in contrast with their almost universal presence in undifferentiated (anaplastic) carcinoma.

Microscopic Findings. The overwhelming majority of primary thyroid lymphomas are of non-Hodgkin type and have a B-cell phenotype (13). Anscombe and Wright (14) postulated that nearly all primary thyroid lymphomas belong to the mucosa-associated lymphoid tissue (MALT) family of neoplasms, i.e., that they are of marginal zone B-cell derivation. They base their proposal, originally advanced by Isaacson, Wright, and coworkers (15–17), on the presence of lymphoid packing of the follicles (which they regard as a form of lymphoepithelial lesion), frequent plasmacytoid differentiation, tendency of the tumor to remain localized for long periods, and predilection for other sites of MALT (e.g., the gastrointestinal tract) when relapse occurs.

Following this all-embracing scheme, Derringer et al. (18) divided their primary thyroid lymphomas into: (low-grade) marginal zone B-cell lymphomas (MZBCL) (30 cases); diffuse large B-cell lymphomas (DLBCL) (41 cases); and DLBCL with MZBCL (also known as high-grade MZBCL) (36 cases). The pattern of growth of these tumors is usually diffuse but it may be follicular (see below). As with extranodal MZBCL

Figure 14-2

MALIGNANT LYMPHOMA

The typical "fish-flesh" appearance of this tumor is clearly appreciated on the cut surface of this gross specimen.

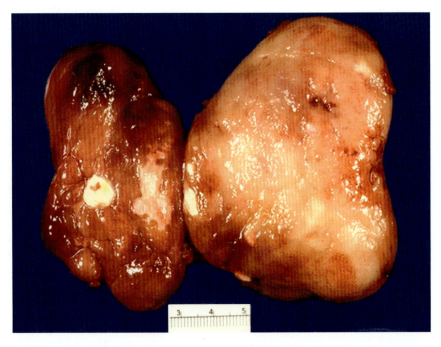

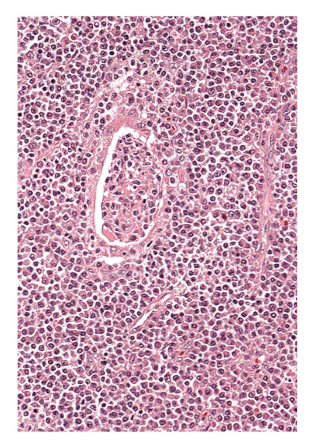

Figure 14-3

MARGINAL ZONE B-CELL LYMPHOMA

The packing of follicles by the tumor cells is an important diagnostic clue.

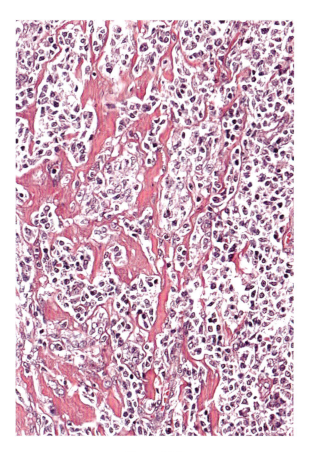

Figure 14-4

LARGE CELL LYMPHOMA

The nesting pattern induced by the fibrous bands is similar to that often seen in mediastinal lymphomas.

at other sites, it is the presence of a destructive infiltrate replacing the normal parenchyma that morphologically distinguishes the lymphoma from a reactive process. In the thyroid gland, this distinction may be difficult considering that some cases of Hashimoto thyroiditis have very florid lymphoid hyperplasia. Entrapment and invasion of thyroid follicles is the rule with lymphomas of the thyroid gland, and it is usually extensive.

Some of the tumor cells are present between the follicular cells, and others accumulate within the follicular lumens, producing lymphoepithelial lesions (fig. 14-3). Compagno and Oertel (19) remarked on the high frequency and diagnostic importance of this "follicular packing" by the malignant lymphoid cells, even if the change is also seen (although generally to a lesser degree) in thyroiditis and Graves disease (20). The close

intermingling of neoplastic and follicular cells, and the common presence of abnormalities in the latter, either as a reaction to the lymphoma or (when oncocytic) as an expression of the preexisting thyroiditis, are the main reasons why thyroid lymphomas are misdiagnosed as undifferentiated small cell carcinomas (2).

Another potential source of confusion is the fact that some lymphomas (particularly those composed of large cells) are associated with the formation of fibrous bands that compartmentalize the tumor cells into well-defined solid nests, a feature analogous to that seen with higher frequency in large cell lymphomas of thymus, retroperitoneum, and other locations (fig. 14-4) (21,22). A feature of diagnostic importance is the spreading of tumor cells along the wall of blood vessels, some of which lie beneath the intima, narrowing but not obliterating the lumen (3,23).

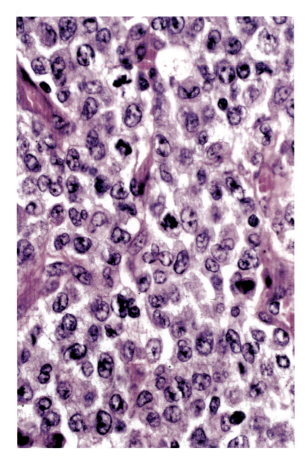

Figure 14-5

LARGE CELL LYMPHOMA

High-power view shows large vesicular nuclei (some bilobed), prominent nucleoli, and a fair amount of cytoplasm.

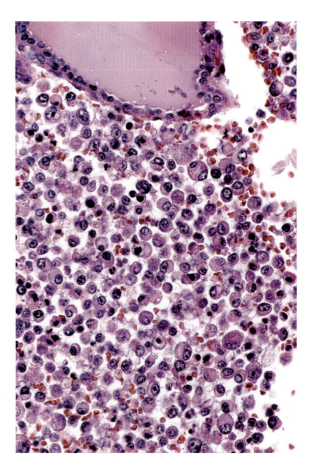

Figure 14-6

LYMPHOPLASMACYTOID LYMPHOMA

Most of the tumor cells have a distinct plasmacytoid appearance.

Microscopically, the conventional (low-grade) form of MZBCL consists of predominantly small lymphoid cells with variable proportions of centrocyte-like cells, plasma cells, lymphoplasmacytoid lymphocytes, monocytoid B-cells, and interspersed large transformed lymphocytes. DLBCLs are composed of large lymphoid cells with centroblastic-like, immunoblastic, monocytoid B-cell, or immunoblastic/plasmacytoid features (figs. 14-5–14-7) (24). DLBCL with MZBCL exhibits an admixture of the two components, the former usually representing over 50 percent of the entire tumor area (25). Only when the large-sized blast cells (centroblastic-like, immunoblastic) form solid, proliferating sheets, can DLBCL be confidently diagnosed within a conventional (low-grade) MZBCL. Although DLBCL with MZBCL is also known as high-grade MZBCL, the use of this term is no longer recommended by most hematopathologists. Cases with a large cell component should be diagnosed as DLBCL, noting that they arise in association with conventional MZBCL. A high percentage of MZBCLs and a smaller number of DLBCLs exhibit focal or extensive plasmacytoid features; these tumors should not be equated with plasmacytomas. Exceptionally, MZBCLs show focal signet ring features and thus simulate metastatic adenocarcinoma (26).

Most thyroid lymphomas with follicular growth are examples of MZBCL with reactive follicles, often colonized or distorted by the neoplastic cells; nevertheless, bona fide follicular lymphomas of the thyroid gland do exist. Bacon et al. (27) described 22 such cases, which they divided into a classic ("adult") group carrying a

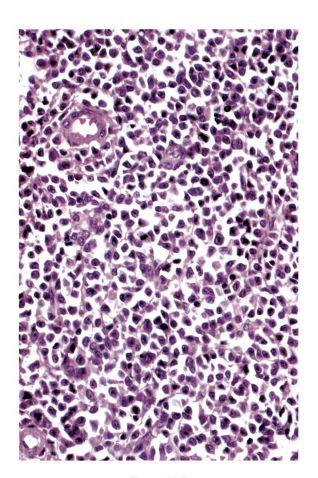

Figure 14-7

MARGINAL ZONE B-CELL LYMPHOMA

Diffuse infiltration of the thyroid gland by small round lymphoid cells.

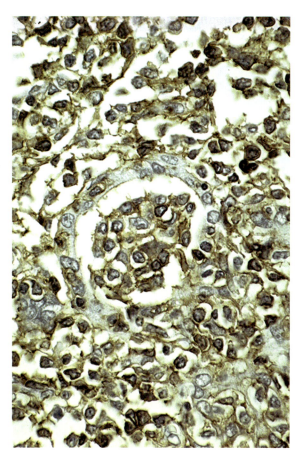

Figure 14-8

LARGE CELL LYMPHOMA

The tumor cells in this field are positive for CD45, including those located within an entrapped follicle. The epithelial follicular cells are negative.

t(14;18)/*IGH-BCL2* or expression of BCL-2, and a second group lacking this molecular genetic alteration. Isolated examples of Burkitt lymphoma are also on record (28).

Immunohistochemical Findings. The tumor cells are consistently positive for CD45 (fig. 14-8). In keeping with the B-cell derivation of nearly all cases, they also exhibit immunoreactivity for pan-B-cell markers, such as CD20. CD10 is negative, and CD5 is rarely coexpressed with pan-B-cell markers. As in other MZBCLs, staining for CD21 and CD35 shows a distorted meshwork of follicular dendritic cells, corresponding to the reactive follicles colonized by the neoplastic lymphocytes. Immunoglobulin light chain restriction is easily demonstrable on fresh suspended cells or frozen sections, and less consistently in formalin-fixed, paraffin-embedded

material (29). The reader is referred to the specialized hematopathology textbooks for a detailed description of the other lymphoid markers that these tumors may exhibit. Only exceptionally do primary thyroid lymphomas exhibit T-cell markers, but a handful of such cases are on record, including a few examples of anaplastic large cell lymphoma (28,30–32).

Stains for keratin or thyroglobulin are useful in delineating the entrapped follicles and in highlighting the close intermingling of neoplastic lymphoid cells (which are negative for these two markers) and the entrapped, atrophic, or hyperplastic follicular cells (which are highly reactive for both) (fig. 14-9A–C). Diffusion of thyroglobulin from the entrapped follicles may create difficulties of interpretation, however (fig. 14-9D).

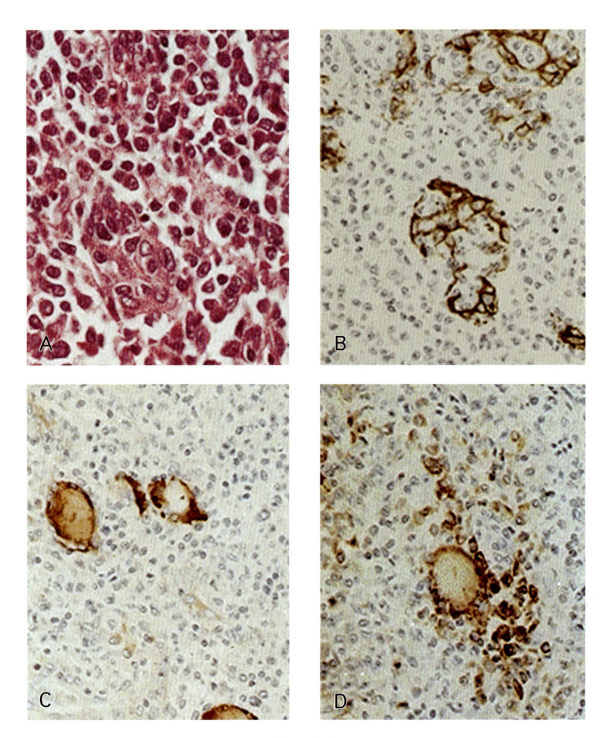

Figure 14-9

LARGE CELL LYMPHOMA

A: The hematoxylin and eosin (H&E)-stained section shows entrapment and infiltration of thyroid follicles by tumor cells.

B: Immunostaining for keratin illustrates the entrapment and distortion of epithelial follicular cells by lymphoma.

C: Immunostaining for thyroglobulin shows several entrapped follicles.

D: Another area of the same tumor stained for thyroglobulin shows that the latter has diffused out from an entrapped follicle and been absorbed nonspecifically by the adjacent malignant lymphoma cells. These cells have thus acquired an apparent positivity for this marker.

Ultrastructural Findings. The electron microscopic features are similar to those seen in malignant lymphomas elsewhere. The most important determination to be made at the electron microscopic level is documentation of the absence of epithelial markers, such as desmosomes, in the malignant cells (being careful not to misinterpret the entrapped follicular cells as neoplastic elements).

Molecular Genetic Findings. Sequence analysis of immunoglobulin genes supports the concept that lymphomas of the thyroid gland may develop from Hashimoto thyroiditis (33). The demonstration of light and heavy immunoglobulin chain genes is very useful in cases where MZBCL needs to be distinguished from thyroiditis (usually Hashimoto type) with florid lymphoid hyperplasia (34). Nevertheless, in some cases of Hashimoto thyroiditis the results of molecular studies for immunoglobulin gene clonality are not always easy to interpret due to the presence of clonal bands associated with a polyclonal smear pattern after gel electrophoresis of polymerase chain reaction products (35).

MZBCL is associated with balanced chromosomal translocations that deregulate the expression of several genes: *MALT1* (at 18q21), *BCL10* (at 18q21), *FOXP1* (at 3p14.1). The prevalence of these alterations depends on the primary site of the lymphoma, i.e., gastric versus salivary gland. A common rearrangement in thyroid lymphoma is the t(3;14)(p14.1;q32), which juxtaposes *IGH* to *FOXP1* (36,37).

Cytologic Findings. See chapter 20.

Spread and Metastases. Malignant lymphoma of the thyroid gland invades locally until eventually most or all of the gland is replaced by tumor. At that stage, direct extension into the surrounding soft tissues is the rule. Regional lymph nodes may also be affected. When this is the case, the involvement may be only focal, as if the tumor had metastasized from the thyroid gland. This phenomenon is analogous to that sometimes seen with lymphomas of other organs (e.g., stomach) in relation to their respective regional nodes. When post-treatment relapse occurs, it often involves the gastrointestinal tract, sometimes exclusively (3,14).

Treatment and Prognosis. Although some authors have questioned the need for a thyroidectomy in primary thyroid lymphoma (11,38), in most institutions the therapeutic policy is to remove the affected gland (12). This seems a sensible approach, similar to that generally advocated for lymphomas of other extranodal sites. The excision should be followed by high-dose irradiation to the field, including the regional lymph nodes. Whether chemotherapy is indicated in patients with localized disease remains controversial, but there is an increasing tendency to use it (13,39,40). In cases with extrathyroid involvement, it seems reasonable to avoid surgical resection and proceed directly to radiation therapy, which is usually combined with chemotherapy. The latter is mandatory in patients with stage III-IV disease.

In older series, the most important prognostic factor in malignant lymphoma of the thyroid gland was the presence or absence of extrathyroid extension, i.e., the stage of the disease (41). This feature still retains prognostic validity, although the differences are not as striking in more recent series (10,12).

The tumor type is also prognostically important, in that MZBCLs confer a better prognosis than DLBCLs (18). In a small series of patients with stage I-II disease treated at Stanford University with high-dose regional irradiation after excision, there was an 83.3 percent survival rate at 3 years and a 75 percent relapse-free survival rate at 2 years (39). There was not a single instance of local recurrence. In a series from Japan composed of 79 cases, the overall 5-year survival rate was 74 percent (42), and in a series from the Mayo Clinic composed of 103 cases, the corresponding figure for patients seen through 1979 was 50 percent (12).

OTHER LYMPHOID TUMORS AND TUMOR-LIKE CONDITIONS

Hodgkin Lymphoma

It is exceptional for *Hodgkin lymphoma* to involve primarily the thyroid gland. As in many other extranodal sites, most cases so diagnosed in the past would be classified otherwise today. Nevertheless, indisputable cases of Hodgkin lymphoma of the thyroid are on record. Most of the cases are of the nodular sclerosis subtype of the classic form, and some show concomitant involvement of the regional lymph nodes (figs. 14-10–14-12) (43,44). Involvement of the

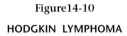

Figure14-10

HODGKIN LYMPHOMA

The nodularity seen in the cut surface of this specimen is a clue to the diagnosis of the nodular sclerosis variant of classic Hodgkin lymphoma.

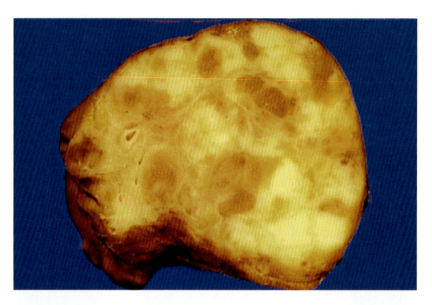

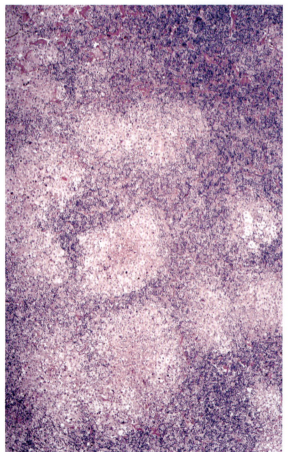

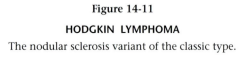

Figure 14-11

HODGKIN LYMPHOMA

The nodular sclerosis variant of the classic type.

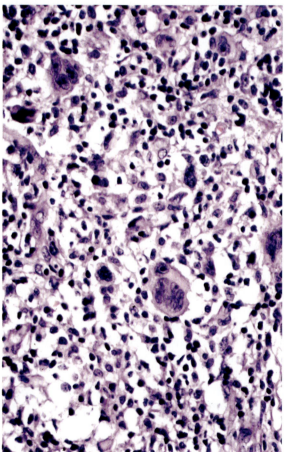

Figure 14-12

HODGKIN LYMPHOMA

High-power view shows numerous Reed-Sternberg cells in a polymorphic lymphoid background.

thyroid gland by systemic Hodgkin lymphoma is also rare; it was seen in only 2 percent of the cases in the series of Shimaoka et al. (45).

Plasmacytoma

Involvement of the thyroid gland by a malignant proliferation of plasma cells can be seen as an expression of widespread myeloma or as the only manifestation of the disease (46). When the latter is the case, the term *plasmacytoma* is used (47). The disease, even if localized, may be accompanied by detectable immunoglobulin abnormalities in the serum (48,49).

Plasmacytoma should be distinguished from malignant lymphomas exhibiting plasmacytoid features (a phenomenon that can be seen both in MZBCL and DLBCL), not always an easy task (50). In "true" plasmacytoma, all of the tumor cells have the appearance of plasma cells exhibiting various degrees of immaturity or atypia, whereas in the lymphomas, the plasmacytoid elements alternate with cells of lymphoid type. Immunoglobulin light chain restriction is present immunohistochemically (51). Plasmacytoma may be associated with amyloid deposits and a foreign body reaction, features that may simulate the appearance of medullary carcinoma.

Primary plasmacytoma of the thyroid, like malignant lymphoma, is often accompanied by evidence of autoimmune thyroiditis in the residual portion of the gland (47,52). The differential diagnosis includes plasma cell granuloma (see below).

Plasma Cell Granuloma and Related Lesions

Plasma cell granuloma is the term used for a tumor-like condition of inflammatory nature and unknown etiology in which plasma cells predominate. As in other organs in which this process occurs (e.g., lung and oral cavity), it is distinguished from plasmacytoma by the mature appearance of all the plasma cells, the presence of Russell bodies (sometimes in large numbers), the admixture with other inflammatory cells, the conspicuous fibrosis, and, most important, the demonstration of light chain polyclonality on immunohistochemical or flow cytometric evaluation (53,54).

The cases reported as *pseudolymphoma* of the thyroid gland (51) may be the expression of a pathogenetically similar phenomenon; however, the definition and existence of this process remain controversial. As in other organs, it is doubtful that it represents a distinct entity. Similar comments apply to the cases reported as *inflammatory pseudotumor* of the thyroid, in which spindle cells of alleged myofibroblastic nature predominate over the plasma cells (55).

REFERENCES

1. Shimaoka K, Sokal JE, Pickren JW. Metastatic neoplasms in the thyroid gland. Pathological and clinical findings. Cancer 1962;15:557-65.
2. Heimann R, Vannineuse A, De Sloover C, Dor P. Malignant lymphomas and undifferentiated small cell carcinoma of the thyroid: a clinicopathological review in the light of the Kiel classification for malignant lymphomas. Histopathology 1978;2:201-13.
3. Williams ED. Malignant lymphoma of the thyroid. Clin Endocrinol Metab 1981:10:379-89.
4. Holm LE, Blomgren H, Löwhagen T. Cancer risks in patients with chronic lymphocytic thyroiditis. N Engl J Med 1985;312:601-4.
5. Kato I, Tajima K, Suchi T, et al. Chronic thyroiditis as a risk factor of B-cell lymphoma in the thyroid gland. Jpn J Cancer Res 1985;76:1085-90.
6. Santana V, Rose NR. Neoplastic lymphoproliferation in autoimmune disease: an updated review. Clin Immunol Immunopathol 1992;63:205-13.
7. Williams ED, Doniach I, Bjarnason O, Michie W. Thyroid cancer in an iodide rich area. A histopathological study. Cancer 1977;39:215-22.
8. Bisbee AC, Thoeny RH. Malignant lymphoma of the thyroid following irradiation. Cancer 1975;35:1296-9.
9. Pedersen RK, Pedersen NT. Primary non-Hodgkin's lymphoma of the thyroid gland: a population based study. Histopathology 1996;28:25-32.
10. Burke JS, Butler JJ, Fuller LM. Malignant lymphomas of the thyroid: a clinical pathologic study of 35 patients including ultrastructural observations. Cancer 1977;39:1587-602.

11. Rasbach DA, Mondschein MS, Harris NL, Kaufman DS, Wang CA. Malignant lymphoma of the thyroid gland: a clinical and pathologic study of twenty cases. Surgery 1985;98:1166-70.

12. Devine RM, Edis AJ, Banks PM. Primary lymphoma of the thyroid: a review of the Mayo Clinic experience through 1978. World J Surg 1981;5:33-8.

13. Ha CS, Shadle KM, Medeiros LJ, et al. Localized non-Hodgkin lymphoma involving the thyroid gland. Cancer 2001;91:629-35.

14. Anscombe AM, Wright DH. Primary malignant lymphoma of the thyroid—a tumour of mucosa-associated lymphoid tissue: review of seventy-six cases. Histopathology 1985;9:81-97.

15. Hyjek E, Isaacson PG. Primary B cell lymphoma of the thyroid and its relationship to Hashimoto thyroiditis. Hum Pathol 1988;19:1315-26.

16. Isaacson P, Wright DH. Extranodal malignant lymphoma arising from mucosa-associated lymphoid tissue. Cancer 1984;53:2515-24.

17. Isaacson PG, Androulakis-Papachristou A, Diss TC, Pan L, Wright DH. Follicular colonization in thyroid lymphoma. Am J Pathol 1992;141:43-52.

18. Derringer GA, Thompson LD, Frommelt RA, Bijwaard KE, Heffess CS, Abbondanzo SL. Malignant lymphoma of the thyroid gland: a clinicopathologic study of 108 cases. Am J Surg Pathol 2000;24:623-39.

19. Compagno J, Oertel JE. Malignant lymphoma and other lymphoproliferative disorders of the thyroid gland. A clinicopathologic study of 245 cases. Am J Clin Pathol 1980;74:1-11.

20. Matias-Guiu X, Esquius J. Lymphoepithelial lesion in the thyroid. A non-specific histological finding. Pathol Res Pract 1991;187:296-300.

21. Perrone T, Frizzera G, Rosai J. Mediastinal diffuse large-cell lymphoma with sclerosis. A clinicopathologic study of 60 cases. Am J Surg Pathol 1986;10:176-91.

22. Rosas-Uribe A, Rappaport H. Malignant lymphoma, histiocytic type with sclerosis (sclerosing reticulum cell sarcoma). Cancer 1972;29:946-53.

23. Oertel JE, Heffess CS. Lymphoma of the thyroid and related disorders. Semin Oncol 1987;14:333-42.

24. Mizukami Y, Michigishi T, Nonomura A, et al. Primary lymphoma of the thyroid: a clinical, histological and immunohistochemical study of 20 cases. Histopathology 1990;17:201-9.

25. Skacel M, Ross CW, Hsi ED. A reassessment of primary thyroid lymphoma: high-grade MALT-type lymphoma as a distinct subtype of diffuse large B-cell lymphoma. Histopathology 2000;37:10-8.

26. Allevato PA, Kini SR, Rebuck JW, Miller JM, Hamburger JI. Signet ring cell lymphoma of the thyroid: a case report. Hum Pathol 1985;16:1066-8.

27. Bacon CM, Diss TC, Ye H, et al. Follicular lymphoma of the thyroid gland. Am J Surg Pathol 2009;33:22-34.

28. Thieblemont C, Mayer A, Dumontet C, et al. Primary thyroid lymphoma is a heterogeneous disease. J Clin Endocrinol Metab 2002;87:105-11.

29. Aozasa K, Ueda T, Katagiri S, Matsuzuka F, Kuma K, Yonezawa T. Immunologic and immunohistologic analysis of 27 cases with thyroid lymphomas. Cancer 1987;60:969-73.

30. Mizukami Y, Matsubara F, Hashimoto T, et al. Primary T-cell lymphoma of the thyroid. Acta Pathol Jpn 1987;37:1987-95.

31. Motoi N, Ozawa Y. Malignant T-cell lymphoma of the thyroid gland associated with Hashimoto's thyroiditis. Pathol Int 2005;55:425-30.

32. Abdul-Rahman ZH, Gogas HJ, Tooze JA, et al. T-cell lymphoma in Hashimoto's thyroiditis. Histopathology 1996;29:455-9.

33. Moshynska OV, Saxena A. Clonal relationship between Hashimoto thyroiditis and thyroid lymphoma. J Clin Pathol 2008;61:438-44.

34. Takano T, Miyauchi A, Matsuzuka F, et al. Detection of monoclonality of the immunoglobulin heavy chain gene in thyroid malignant lymphoma by vectorette polymerase chain reaction. J Clin Endocrinol Metab 2005;90:720-3.

35. Saxena A, Alport EC, Moshynska O, Kanthan R, Boctor MA. Clonal B cell populations in a minority of patients with Hashimoto's thyroiditis. J Clin Pathol 2004;57:1258-63.

36. Campo E, Chott A, Kinney MC, et al. Update on extranodal lymphomas. Conclusions of the Workshop held by the EAHP and the SH in Thessaloniki, Greece. Histopathology 2006;48:481-504.

37. Streubel B, Vinatzer U, Lamprecht A, Raderer M, Chott A. T(3;14)(p14.1;q32) involving IGH and FOXP1 is a novel recurrent chromosomal aberration in MALT lymphoma. Leukemia 2005;19:652-8.

38. Ansell SM, Grant CS, Habermann TM. Primary thyroid lymphoma. Semin Oncol 1999;26:316-23.

39. Chak LY, Hoppe RT, Burke JS, Kaplan HS. Non-Hodgkin's lymphoma presenting as thyroid enlargement. Cancer 1981;48:2712-6.

40. Watanabe N, Noh JY, Narimatsu H, et al. Clinicopathological features of 171 cases of primary thyroid lymphoma: a long-term study involving 24533 patients with Hashimoto's disease. Br J Haematol 2011;153:236-43.

41. Woolner LB, McConahey WM, Beahrs OH, Black BM. Primary malignant lymphoma of the thyroid. Review of forty-six cases. Am J Surg 1966;111:502-23.

42. Aozasa K, Inoue A, Tajima K, Miyauchi A, Matsuzuka F, Kuma K. Malignant lymphomas of the thyroid gland. Analysis of 79 patients with emphasis on histologic prognostic factors. Cancer 1986;58:100-4.

43. Feigin GA, Buss DH, Paschal B, Woodruff RD, Myers RT. Hodgkin's disease manifested as a thyroid nodule. Hum Pathol 1982;13:774-6.

44. Wang SA, Rahemtullah A, Faquin WC, Roepke J, Harris NL, Hasserjian RP. Hodgkin's lymphoma of the thyroid: a clinicopathologic study of five cases and review of the literature. Mod Pathol 2005;18:1577-84.

45. Shimaoka K, Sokal JE, Pickren JW. Metastatic neoplasms in the thyroid gland. Pathological and clinical findings. Cancer 1962;15:557-65.

46. Shimaoka K, Gailani S, Tsukada Y, Barcos M. Plasma cell neoplasm involving the thyroid. Cancer 1978;41:1140-6.

47. Aozasa K, Inoue A, Yoshimura H, Miyauchi A, Matsuzuka F, Kuma K. Plasmacytoma of the thyroid gland. Cancer 1986;58:105-10.

48. Ottó S, Péter I, Végh S, Juhos E, Besznyák I. Gamma-chain heavy-chain disease with primary thyroid plasmacytoma. Arch Pathol Lab Med 1986;110:893-6.

49. Rubin J, Johnson JT, Killeen R, Barnes L. Extramedullary plasmacytoma of the thyroid associated with a serum monoclonal gammopathy. Arch Otolaryngol Head Neck Surg 1990;116:855-9.

50. Aihara H, Tsutsumi Y, Ishikawa H. Extramedullary plasmacytoma of the thyroid, associated with follicular colonization and stromal deposition of polytypic immunoglobulins and major histocompatibility antigens. Possible categorization in MALT lymphoma. Acta Pathol Jpn 1992;42:672-83.

51. Aozasa K. Ueda T, Katagiri S, Matsuzuka F, Kuma K, Yonezawa T. Immunologic and immunohistologic analysis of 27 cases with thyroid lymphomas. Cancer 1987;60:969-73.

52. Cremonini A, Ponzoni M, Beretta E, et al. Plasma cell granuloma of the thyroid gland: a challenging diagnostic problem. Int J Surg Pathol 2012;20:500-6.

53. Holck S. Plasma cell granuloma of the thyroid. Cancer 1981;48:830-2.

54. Yapp R, Linder J, Schenken JR, Karrer FW. Plasma cell granuloma of the thyroid. Hum Pathol 1985;16:848-50

55. Kojima M, Suzuki M, Shimizu K, Masawa N. Inflammatory pseudotumor of the thyroid gland showing prominent myofibroblastic proliferation. A case report. Endocr Pathol 2009;20:186-90.

PARATHYROID TUMORS

Parathyroid tumors are discussed in another section of this Fascicle, but they are briefly mentioned here since some aspects of these neoplasms impact upon the thyroid gland. Intrathyroidal parathyroid neoplasms can look like primary thyroid tumors to the surgeon and may present interpretative problems for the pathologist at the microscopic level. True *intrathyroidal parathyroid glands* are rare (about 0.2 percent) compared with the high frequency of these glands abutting the thyroid gland (1). These intrathyroidal or perithyroidal parathyroid glands may be affected by adenoma, primary or secondary chief cell hyperplasia, and carcinoma (2). The formation of follicles with intraluminal colloid-like material may closely simulate the microscopic appearance of a follicular thyroid neoplasm. The occurrence of parathyroid tumor cells with clear or oncocytic cytoplasm can lead to confusion with clear cell or oncocytic thyroid neoplasms, respectively.

The light microscopic features that favor a parathyroid over a thyroid origin are a more intricate vascular pattern, prominence of the endothelial cells, more pronounced nesting pattern, smaller size of the individual cells, and thinner tumor trabeculae (3). Cytoplasmic glycogen, as evidenced by periodic acid–Schiff (PAS) staining, is generally more abundant in parathyroid than in thyroid clear cells. For the cases in which the distinction cannot be made on morphologic grounds, immunohistochemical stains for thyroglobulin (negative), FLI-1 (negative), parathyroid hormone (positive), and synaptophysin (positive) should settle the issue. Furthermore, parathyroid tumors, unlike differentiated tumors of thyroid follicular or C-cell derivation, do not express thyroid transcription factor (TTF)-1 (4).

PARAGANGLIOMA

A handful of cases of primary *paraganglioma* of the thyroid gland have been reported (5–10), one of which behaved aggressively (9). Most appear authentic based on the description and photographic documentation; in particular, the cases seen in association with unilateral or bilateral paragangliomas of the carotid body seem incontrovertible (7,11). Microscopically, they are encapsulated and composed of nests ("Zellballen") of chromogranin-positive tumor cells surrounded by S-100 protein–positive sustentacular cells (figs. 15-1–15-3) (12). The sources for these tumors are

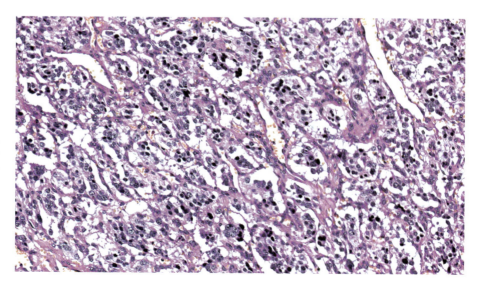

Figure 15-1

PARAGANGLIOMA

The nesting ("Zellballen") pattern of this tumor involving the thyroid gland is characteristic.

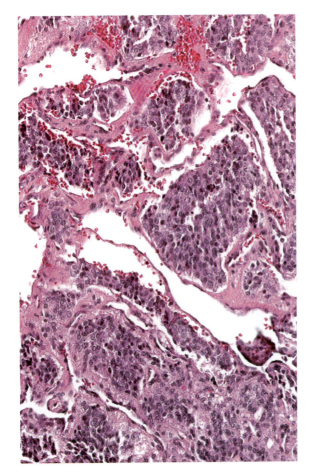

Figure 15-2

PARAGANGLIOMA

The "Zellballen" are large, with irregular contours.

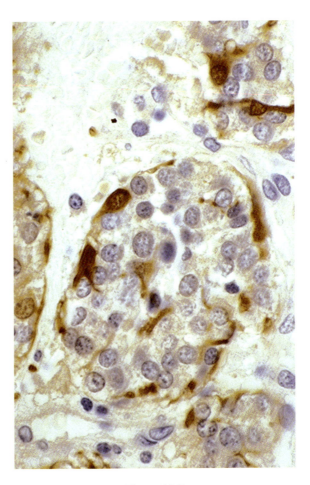

Figure 15-3

PARAGANGLIOMA

The cells positive for S-100 protein, usually located at the periphery of the "Zellballen," are thought to represent sustentacular cells.

small paraganglia located in or immediately beneath the thyroid capsule (13).

Before accepting a diagnosis of primary thyroid paraganglioma, it is important to consider the following three alternatives. First, paraganglioma of the carotid body or other cervical paraganglia may grow in close proximity to or even extend into the thyroid gland. The distinction is entirely dependent on the surgical and gross findings, since their microscopic, ultrastructural, and immunohistochemical features are identical. Also, paragangliomas may develop at any site as components of several tumor syndromes, including the pheochromocytoma-paraganglioma syndrome, caused by inactivating germline mutations in the Krebs cycle succinate dehydrogenase B (*SDHB*), C (*SDHC*), or D (*SDHD*)

genes that are present in 10 to 30 percent of apparently sporadic tumors. Immunohistochemistry for SDHB is effective in identifying syndromic cases that are typically SDHD negative (14). Second, hyalinizing trabecular adenoma of thyroid gland has a nesting pattern that may result in a paraganglioma-like appearance, to the point that the term paraganglioma-like adenoma of the thyroid (PLAT) was originally proposed for it (15). The presence of trabeculae and occasional follicles, immunoreactivity for thyroglobulin, and overall negativity for chromogranin and other neuroendocrine markers should establish the distinction with ease.

Finally, medullary thyroid carcinoma with a nesting (paraganglioma-like) pattern of growth

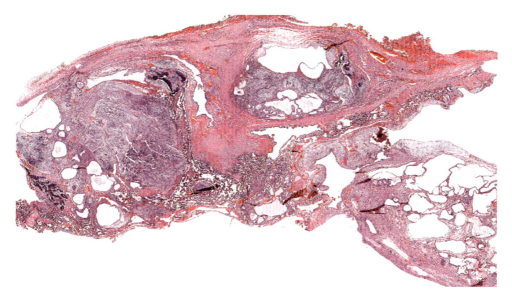

Figure 15-4

CERVICAL TERATOMA

The tumor was entirely composed of mature elements.

may be difficult to distinguish from paraganglioma because of the numerous features that these two neuroendocrine tumors share. The most important criterion in favor of medullary thyroid carcinoma is the immunohistochemical demonstration of calcitonin or calcitonin gene-related peptide. Features supportive of paraganglioma are the immunohistochemical demonstration of opioid peptides and the detection by either electron microscopy or immunohistochemistry (S-100 protein staining) of sustentacular cells at the periphery of the tumor nests (fig. 15-3) (16). Unfortunately, none of these features can be regarded as absolute, since calcitonin may be undetectable for technical or other reasons in medullary thyroid carcinomas while occasionally present in paragangliomas, opioid peptides have been found in some thyroid medullary carcinomas, and sustentacular cells have been described in neuroendocrine neoplasms other than paragangliomas (such as carcinoid tumors).

TERATOMA

The neck is not an unusual site for the occurrence of *teratomas* in neonates and infants (17,18). They are usually located in the midneck and can reach huge dimensions (19–22). In some instances, emergency surgery is needed because of symptoms resulting from compression of the upper respiratory tract (23).

At the gross level, most of these tumors have a multiloculated cystic appearance, which may be combined with smaller solid areas. Microscopically, the usual haphazard admixture of tissues derived from all three germ layers (including neural tissue, with a predominance of neuroglial elements) is identified (figs. 15-4–15-6). Nearly all of the reported cases in neonates and infants have been mature microscopically and have followed a benign clinical course. The latter is also true for most of the teratomas exhibiting some degree of histologic immaturity (18).

Many cervical teratomas partially involve the thyroid gland. Intimate intermingling of teratomatous elements with thyroid follicles and the presence of a pseudocapsule are the criteria used to favor a thyroid origin for them. Otherwise, they do not differ from the cervical teratomas that are anatomically separate from the thyroid gland.

Teratomas of the thyroid gland developing in adults differ from the above; most have the microscopic features of malignancy and an aggressive clinical course (19,24–30). It is our impression, however, that some of these cases do not qualify as true germ cell neoplasms. Some of the published examples (31,32) and some practically identical cases that we have personally observed may actually be malignant primitive neuroepithelial tumors. The cartilage and other mesenchymal tissues present in them may be explained by the fact that much of the mesenchyme of the neck is of neural crest derivation. Other reported cases of malignant teratoma of the thyroid gland (28,33) have been reinterpreted

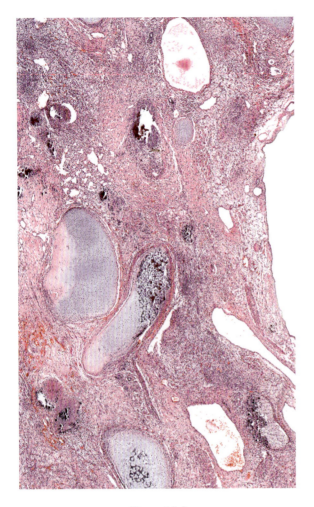

Figure 15-5

CERVICAL TERATOMA

Cartilaginous nodules are seen, some of which are undergoing ossification.

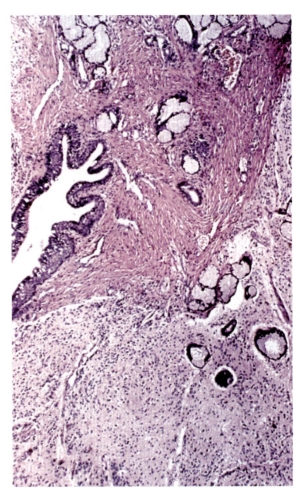

Figure 15-6

CERVICAL TERATOMA

There is a disorderly admixture of mature and immature tissue types.

by us as neoplasms showing thymic or related branchial pouch differentiation (see below).

Exceptionally, other germ cell neoplasms, such as yolk sac tumor, can involve the thyroid gland (34).

SOLITARY FIBROUS TUMOR

Solitary fibrous tumor can involve primarily the thyroid gland (35–37). The behavior is generally benign, but aggressive cases have been documented (35,38,39). The microscopic appearance is similar to that of solitary fibrous tumors elsewhere.

Typical features include a hemangiopericytomatous pattern of growth, alternation of hypercellular and hypocellular areas, deposition of keloid-like collagen, and immunoreactivity for CD34, CD99, and BCL-2 (figs. 15-7, 15-8) (35,38,39). It is likely that cases reported in the past as hemangiopericytoma of thyroid gland belong to this category.

OTHER BENIGN SOFT TISSUE–TYPE TUMORS

Isolated cases of *hemangioma* (40–42), *lymphangioma* (43), *hemangiopericytoma* (but see previous paragraph) (44,45), *angiolipoma* (46,47), *diffuse lipomatosis (thyrolipomatosis)* (48), *schwannoma* (49–51), *granular cell tumor* (52–54), and *leiomyoma* (49) of the thyroid gland have been reported.

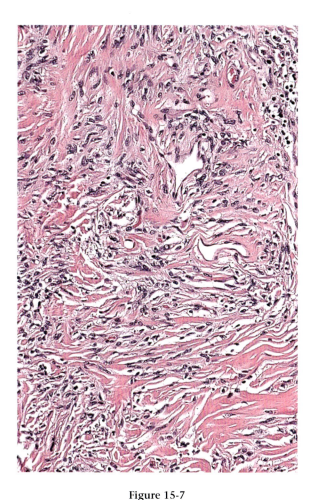

Figure 15-7

SOLITARY FIBROUS TUMOR

The hemangiopericytoma-like pattern is a common feature of this tumor.

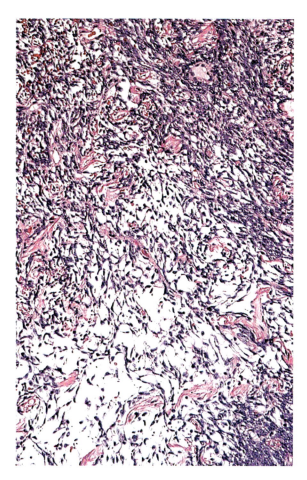

Figure 15-8

SOLITARY FIBROUS TUMOR

Typical alternation of hypercellular and hypocellular areas is seen.

TUMORS WITH THYMIC OR RELATED BRANCHIAL POUCH DIFFERENTIATION

There is a family of cervical tumors that have features consistent with an origin from branchial pouch derivatives and which exhibit differentiation toward thymic tissue (fig. 15-9). Although not of thyroid origin, a brief mention of these lesions is appropriate, not only because they can be found adjacent to or even within the thyroid gland but also because the microscopic appearance of some of them resembles some forms of primary thyroid carcinoma.

Ectopic Cervical Thymoma

Ectopic cervical thymoma is the easiest lesion from the group to recognize because its mi-

croscopic appearance mirrors that of its most common counterpart in the mediastinum. The usual location is the anterolateral neck, generally deep to the sternomastoid muscle. It can be subjacent to or inside the lower pole of the thyroid gland. When this is the case, the clinical diagnosis of a primary thyroid nodule is usually made. Residual ectopic thymic tissue is often found at the periphery. As in the mediastinum, the tumor can be encapsulated or invasive, the former greatly predominating.

Microscopically, most of the reported cases belong to the type AB thymoma of the World Health Organization (WHO) classification (fig. 15-9). As such, they are an admixture of type A- and type B-like thymomas, as similarly named

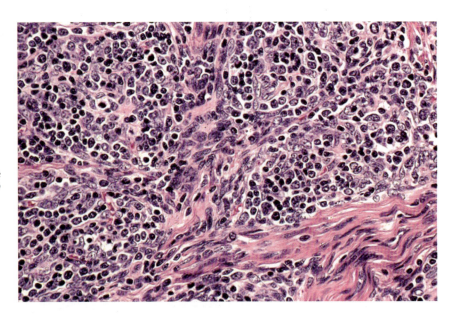

Figure 15-9

ECTOPIC CERVICAL THYMOMA

This thymoma, located in the neck, is of AB type in the WHO classification.

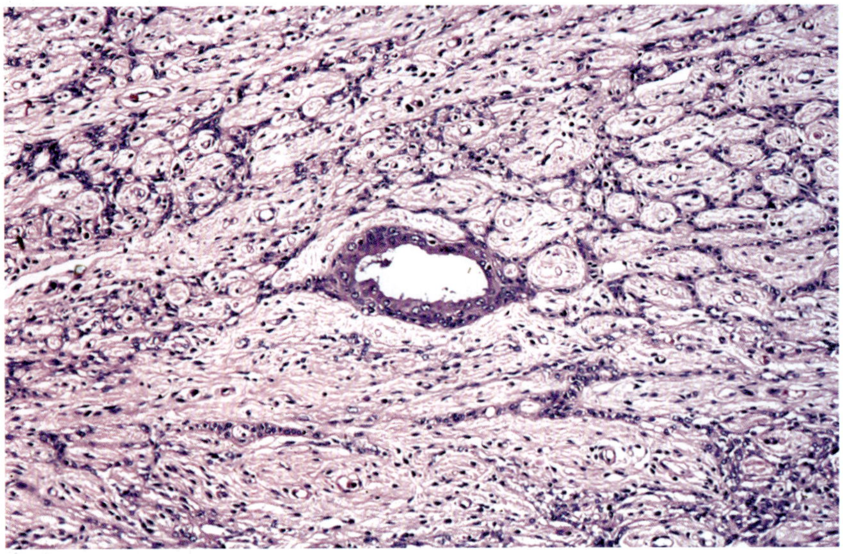

Figure 15-10

ECTOPIC HAMARTOMATOUS THYMOMA

Most of the tumor is composed of mesenchymal-like spindle cells, but the central cystic structure lined by squamous epithelium points to the correct diagnosis.

tumors are in their usual orthotopic mediastinal location (55–59). Curiously, ectopic cervical thymomas show a great predilection for females.

Ectopic Hamartomatous Thymoma

Ectopic hamartomatous thymoma is not likely to be confused with a primary thyroid neoplasm on the basis of either location or microscopic appearance. It is mentioned here only for the sake of completeness.

The typical location is the supraclavicular or suprasternal region. Microscopically, a proliferation of bland-looking spindle cells simulating mesenchymal or schwannian elements is seen admixed with solid or cystic epithelial islands and mature adipose tissue (figs. 15-10–15-13). The spindle cells have an epithelial phenotype ultrastructurally (desmosomes and tonofibrils) and immunohistochemically (keratin positivity). In contrast to ectopic cervical thymoma, ectopic hamartomatous thymoma predominates in men. The behavior of the published cases has invariably been benign (56,60,61).

Spindle Epithelial Tumor with Thymus-Like Differentiation

We have proposed the acronym SETTLE (*spindle epithelial tumor with thymus-like differentiation*)

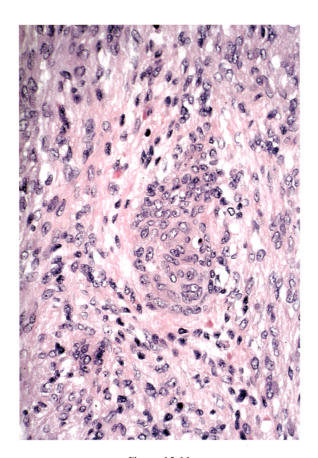

Figure 15-11

ECTOPIC HAMARTOMATOUS THYMOMA

An obvious epithelial nest is surrounded by mesenchymal-like cells.

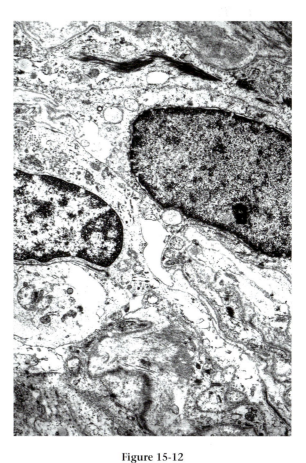

Figure 15-12

ECTOPIC HAMARTOMATOUS THYMOMA

Ultrastructurally, the tonofilaments and desmosomes attest on top of the figure to the epithelial nature of the tumor.

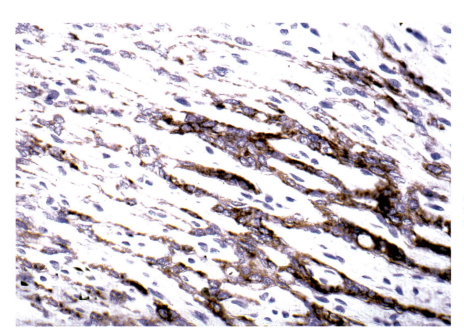

Figure 15-13

ECTOPIC HAMARTOMATOUS THYMOMA

The keratin immunostain shows the transition between the two components of the tumor

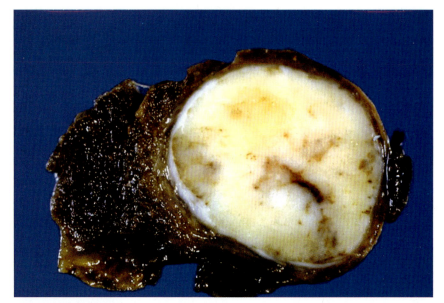

Figure 15-14

SPINDLE EPITHELIAL TUMOR WITH THYMUS-LIKE DIFFERENTIATION

The gross appearance is nondescript and similar to that of a thyroid follicular neoplasm.

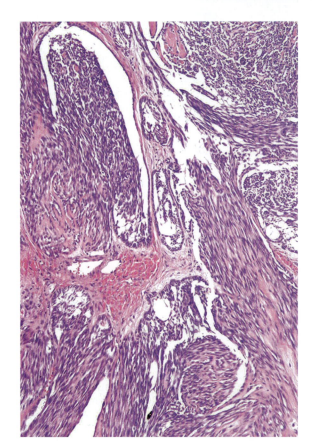

Figure 15-15

SPINDLE EPITHELIAL TUMOR WITH THYMUS-LIKE DIFFERENTIATION

Low-power view shows the nesting and fascicular arrangement of the tumor cells.

(56) for a tumor that was previously reported as *thyroid spindle cell tumor with mucous cysts* (62) and *malignant teratoma of the thyroid* (33,63). It occurs predominantly in children and young adults (mean age, 15 years) and typically presents as a thyroid nodule.

At the gross level, the lesion can be encapsulated, partially circumscribed, or infiltrative (fig. 15-14). The cut surface is firm, grayish white to tan, and vaguely whorled; small cysts may be visible. Residual thyroid tissue is often identified at the periphery.

Microscopically, the tumor is highly cellular and traversed by sclerotic bands that result in the formation of incompletely demarcated nodules (fig. 15-15). The diagnostic feature is the admixture of fairly monotonous spindle cells and plumper cells showing obvious epithelial differentiation (fig. 15-16). Interstitial accumulation of mucin is a constant feature, and vascular invasion may be present.

The spindle cells show ultrastructural and immunohistochemical features of epithelial cells, similar to those of ectopic hamartomatous thymoma (fig. 15-17). The cells with a clear-cut epithelial appearance at the light microscopic level may appear ultrastructurally as complex narrow tubules, small papillae, trabecular islands, and solid sheets, all blending imperceptibly with the predominant spindle cell component. In addition, in many cases there are branching cystic

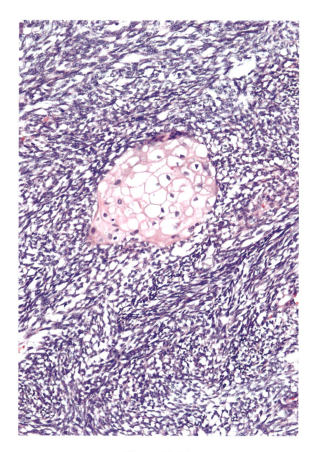

Figure 15-16

**SPINDLE EPITHELIAL TUMOR
WITH THYMUS-LIKE DIFFERENTIATION**

An island of squamous epithelium is surrounded by a predominant spindle cell component. The biphasic appearance of this tumor and the hypercellular but monotonous quality of the spindle cell component may lead to a mistaken diagnosis of synovial sarcoma.

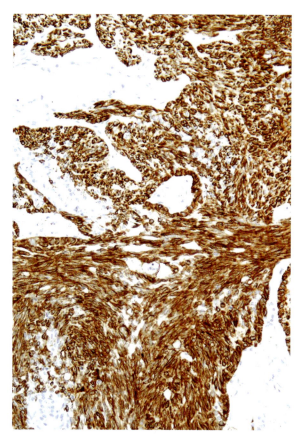

Figure 15-17

**SPINDLE EPITHELIAL TUMOR
WITH THYMUS-LIKE DIFFERENTIATION**

Strong immunoreactivity for keratin is present throughout.

glands lined by mucinous or respiratory-type epithelium with basally located nuclei (fig. 15-18). SETTLE lacks the gene fusion (*SS18/SSX1* or *SS18/SSX2*) associated with synovial sarcoma, a tumor that it closely resembles morphologically (64).

SETTLE is characterized by the occasional development of late distant metastases to lung, mediastinum, or kidney (as late as 25 years after resection of the original tumor).

Carcinoma Showing Thymus-Like Differentiation

Carcinoma showing thymus-like differentiation, which we have designated as CASTLE (56) and which was first described by Miyauchi et al. (66)

as *intrathyroidal epithelial thymoma*, occurs in adults (mean age, 48.5 years) and presents as a thyroid mass (56,65–68). It involves predominantly one of the lower lobes of the thyroid gland and often extends to the juxtathyroid soft tissue. It is hard and lobulated, and its cut surface is gray to pinkish gray (fig. 15-19).

Microscopically, the tumor is divided into irregularly shaped lobules and cords by fibrous septa infiltrated by lymphocytes and plasma cells (fig. 15-20). The tumor cells have large vesicular nuclei, prominent nucleoli, fairly abundant cytoplasm, and indistinct cell borders (fig. 15-21). The overall appearance is similar to that of thymic carcinoma, of which it may represent its ectopic counterpart. Mitotic activity is scanty. Foci of definite squamous differentiation

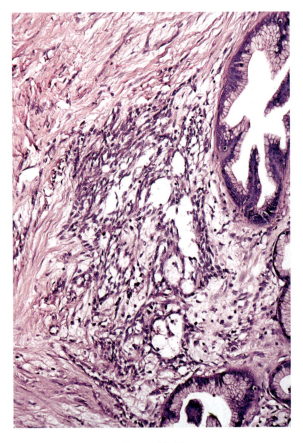

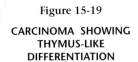

Figure 15-18

**SPINDLE EPITHELIAL TUMOR
WITH THYMUS-LIKE DIFFERENTIATION**

Mucus-secreting glands are admixed with a cellular spindle cell component exhibiting irregular microcystic formations.

may be present, and there may be perivascular spaces containing lymphocytes.

Immunohistochemically, the tumor cells are reactive for cytokeratin and CD5, and negative for thyroglobulin and calcitonin. Neuroendocrine differentiation may be present, as in its mediastinal counterpart (69). Ultrastructurally, the cells of CASTLE exhibit elongated cell processes, tonofilaments, and numerous desmosomes. The natural history is generally characterized by a slow evolution and a tendency for late local recurrence (as long as 15 years after the initial diagnosis) (68).

The differential diagnosis includes primary undifferentiated or squamous cell thyroid carcinoma and metastatic carcinoma (particularly from upper aerodigestive tract, lung, and mediastinum). Features favoring the diagnosis of CASTLE include a lobulated pattern of expansile growth, lymphocytic infiltration, perivascular spaces, low mitotic count, paucity of neutrophils, and immunoreactivity for CD5 (56).

Salivary Gland-Type Tumors

Cases of *pleomorphic adenoma* of the thyroid gland with features analogous in all regards to those of the homonymous salivary gland tumor (including the presence of myoepithelial cells and cartilage) have been reported (70,71). Occasional papillary thyroid carcinomas can mimic the growth pattern of *adenoid cystic carcinoma* (72).

Figure 15-19

**CARCINOMA SHOWING
THYMUS-LIKE
DIFFERENTIATION**

Grossly, the tumor is solid, lobulated, and yellowish. It involves both the peripheral thyroid gland and the perithyroidal tissues.

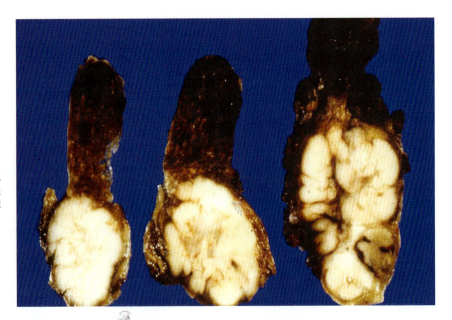

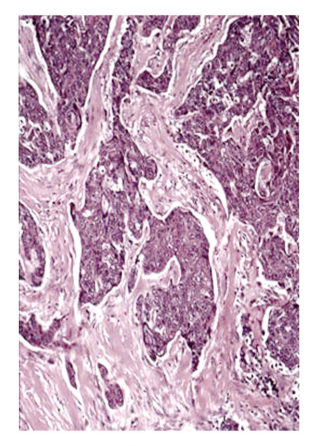

Figure 15-20

**CARCINOMA SHOWING
THYMUS-LIKE DIFFERENTIATION**

The epithelial tumor nests separated from each other by wide collagenous bands are similar to those seen in conventional thymic carcinoma of mediastinum, of which this tumor represents an ectopic counterpart.

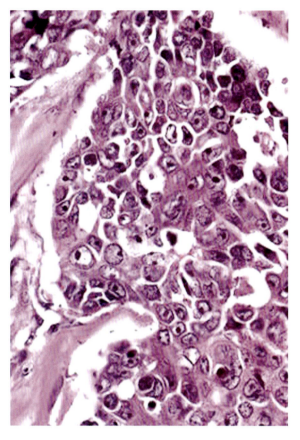

Figure 15-21

**CARCINOMA SHOWING
THYMUS-LIKE DIFFERENTIATION**

High-power view of the tumor shows an evident squamous appearance.

REFERENCES

1. Akerström G, Malmaeus J, Bergström R. Surgical anatomy of human parathyroid glands. Surgery 1984;95:14-21.
2. Sawady J, Mendelsohn F, Sirota RL, Taxy JB. The intrathyroidal hyperfunctioning parathyroid gland. Mod Pathol 1989;2:652-7.
3. LiVolsi VA. Surgical pathology of the thyroid. In: Major problems in pathology; Vol 22 (series). Philadelphia: WB Saunders; 1990.
4. Mantovani G, Corbetta S, Romoli R, Alberti L, Beck-Peccoz P, Spada A. Absence of thyroid transcription factor-1 expression in human parathyroid and pituitary glands. Mol Cell Endocrinol 2001;182:13-7.

5. Banner B, Morecki R, Eviatar A. Chemodectoma in the mid-thyroid region. J Otolaryngol 1979;8:271-3.
6. Buss DH, Marshall RB, Baird FG, Myers RT. Paraganglioma of the thyroid gland. Am J Surg Pathol 1980;4:589-93.
7. Haegert DG, Wang NS, Ferrer PA, Seemayer TA, Thelmo W. Non-chromaffin paragangliomatosis manifesting as a cold thyroid nodule. Am J Clin Pathol 1974;61:561-70.
8. Kay S, Montague JW, Dodd RW. Nonchromaffin paraganglioma (chemodectoma) of thyroid region. Cancer 1975;36:582-5.

9. Mitsudo SM, Grajower MD, Balbi H, Silver C. Malignant paraganglioma of the thyroid gland. Arch Pathol Lab Med 1987;111:378-80.

10. González Poggioli N, López Amado M, Pimentel MT. Paraganglioma of the thyroid gland: a rare entity. Endocr Pathol 2009;20:62-5.

11. Hughes JH, El-Mofty S, Sessions D, Liapis H. Primary intrathyroidal paraganglioma with metachronous carotid body tumor: report of a case and review of the literature. Pathol Res Pract 1997;193:791-6.

12. LaGuette J, Matias-Guiu X, Rosai J. Thyroid paraganglioma: a clinicopathologic and immunohistochemical study of three cases. Am J Surg Pathol 1997;21:748-53.

13. Zak F, Lawson W. Glomic (paraganglionic) tissue in the larynx and capsule of the thyroid gland. Mt Sinai J Med 1972;39:82-90

14. van Nederveen FH, Gaal J, Favier J, et al. An immunohistochemical procedure to detect patients with paraganglioma and phaeochromocytoma with germline SDHB, SDHC, or SDHD gene mutations: a retrospective and prospective analysis. Lancet Oncol 2009;10:764-71.

15. Libbey NP, Hemstreet MK, Butmarc JR, Tibbetts LM, Tucci JR. Paraganglioma-like adenomas of the thyroid (PLAT): incidental lesions with unusual features in a patient with nodular goiter. Endocr Pathol 1997;8:143-51.

16. Schroder HD, Johannsen L. Demonstration of S-100 protein in sustentacular cells of pheochromocytomas and paragangliomas. Histopathology 1986;10:1023-33.

17. Bale GF. Teratoma of the neck in the region of the thyroid gland; a review of the literature and report of 4 cases. Am J Pathol 1950;26:565-79.

18. Riedlinger WF, Lack EE, Robson CD, Rahbar R, Nosé V. Primary thyroid teratomas in children: a report of 11 cases with a proposal of criteria for their diagnosis. Am J Surg Pathol 2005;29:700-6.

19. Newsted T Jr, Shirkey HC. Teratoma of the thyroid region: report of a case with seven-year follow-up. Am J Dis Child 1964;107:88-95.

20. Silberman R, Mendelson IR. Teratoma of the neck: report of two cases and review of the literature. Arch Dis Child 1960;35:159-70.

21. Stone HH, Henderson WD, Guidio FA. Teratomas of the neck. Am J Dis Child 1967;113:222-4.

22. Weitzner S. Benign teratoma of the neck in an infant. Am J Dis Child 1964;107:84-5.

23. Fisher JE, Cooney DR, Voorhess ML, Jewett TC Jr. Teratoma of thyroid gland in infancy: review of the literature and two case reports. J Surg Oncol 1982;21:135-40.

24. Buckley NJ, Burch WM, Leight GS. Malignant teratoma of the thyroid gland in an adult: a case report and a review of the literature. Surgery 1986;100:932-7.

25. Buckwalter JA, Layton JM. Malignant teratoma in the thyroid gland of an adult. Ann Surg 1954;139:218-23.

26. Hajdu SI, Hajdu EO. Malignant teratoma of the neck. Arch Pathol 1967;83:567-70.

27. Kier R, Silverman PM, Korobkin M, Wain S, Leight G, Burch W Jr. Malignant teratoma of the thyroid in an adult: CT appearance. J Comput Assisted Tomogr 1985;9:174-6.

28. Murao T, Nakanishi M, Toda K, Konishi H. Malignant teratoma of the thyroid gland in an adolescent female. Acta Pathol Jpn 1979;29:109-17.

29. O'Higgins N, Taylor S. Malignant teratoma in the adult thyroid gland. Br J Clin Pract 1975;29:237-8.

30. Bowker CM, Whittaker RS. Malignant teratoma of the thyroid: case report and literature review of thyroid teratoma in adults. Histopathology 1992;21:81-3.

31. Kimler SC, Muth WF. Primary malignant teratoma of the thyroid: case report and literature review of cervical teratomas in adults. Cancer 1978;42:311-7.

32. Craver RD, Lipscomb JT, Suskind D, Velez MC. Malignant teratoma of the thyroid with primitive neuroepithelial and mesenchymal sarcomatous components. Ann Diagn Pathol 2001;5:285-92.

33. Kingsley DP, Elton A, Bennett MH. Malignant teratoma of the thyroid. Case report and review of the literature. Br J Cancer 1968;22:7-11.

34. Furtado LV, Leventaki V, Layfield LJ, Lowichik A, Muntz HR, Pysher TJ. Yolk sac tumor of the thyroid gland: a case report. Pediatr Dev Pathol 2011;14:475-9.

35. Rodriguez I, Ayala E, Caballero C, et al. Solitary fibrous tumor of the thyroid gland: report of seven cases. Am J Surg Pathol 2001;25:1424-8.

36. Tanahashi J, Kashima K, Daa T, et al. Solitary fibrous tumor of the thyroid gland: report of two cases and review of the literature. Pathol Int 2006;56:471-7.

37. Verdi D, Pennelli G, Pelizzo MR, Toniato A. Solitary fibrous tumor of the thyroid gland: a report of two cases with an analysis of their clinical and pathological features. Endocr Pathol 2011;22:165-9.

38. Cameselle-Teijeiro J, Varela-Durán J, Fonseca E, Villanueva JP, Sobrinho-Simões M. Solitary fibrous tumor of the thyroid. Am J Clin Pathol 1994;101:535-8.

39. Kie JH, Kim JY, Park YN, Lee MK, Yang WI, Park JS. Solitary fibrous tumour of the thyroid. Histopathology 1997;30:365-8.

40. Pickleman JR, Lee JF, Straus FH 2nd, Paloyan E. Thyroid hemangioma. Am J Surg 1975;129:331-6.

41. Clarke MR, Boppana S. Hemangioma of the thyroid gland in an adolescent with chronic lymphocytic thyroiditis and adenomatous hyperplasia. Endocr Pathol 1998;9:185-9

42. Huang SA, Tu HM, Harney JW, et al. Severe hypothyroidism caused by type 3 iodothyronine deiodinase in infantile hemangiomas. N Engl J Med 2000;343:185-9.

43. Gardner DF, Frable WJ. Primary lymphangioma of the thyroid gland. Arch Pathol Lab Med 1989;113:1084-5.

44. Hansen T, Gaumann A, Ghalibafian M, Höferlin A, Heintz A, Kirkpatrick CJ. Haemangiopericytoma of the thyroid gland in combination with Hashimoto's disease. Virchows Arch 2004;445:315-9.

45. Ostrowski ML, Cartwright J Jr, Maldonado JE, Mody D, LiVolsi VA. Hemangiopericytoma of the thyroid, an unusual spindle cell lesion. Int J Surg Pathol 1995;4:311-8.

46. Palazzo JP, Coté SA. Primary angiolipoma of the thyroid gland: a case report. Int J Surg Pathol 2005;13:305-7.

47. Dimosthenous K, Righi A, Puccetti M, Lorenzini P. Angiolipoma of the thyroid gland. Int J Surg Pathol 2009;17:65-7.

48. Ge Y, Luna MA, Cowan DF, Truong LD, Ayala AG. Thyrolipoma and thyrolipomatosis: 5 case reports and historical review of the literature. Ann Diagn Pathol 2009;13:384-9.

49. Andrion A, Bellis D, Delsedime L, Bussolati G, Mazzucco G. Leiomyoma and neurilemoma: report of two unusual non-epithelial tumours of the thyroid gland. Virchows Arch A Pathol Anat Histopathol 1988;413:367-72.

50. Delaney WE, Fry KE. Neurilemoma of the thyroid gland. Ann Surg 1964;160:1014-6.

51. Thompson LD, Wenig BM, Adair CF, Heffess CS. Peripheral nerve sheath tumors of the thyroid gland: a series of four cases and a review of the literature. Endocr Pathol 1996;7:309-8.

52. Baloch ZW, Martin S, LiVolsi VA. Granular cell tumor of the thyroid: a case report. Int J Surg Pathol 2005;13:291-4.

53. Bowry M, Almeida B, Jeannon JP. Granular cell tumor of the thyroid gland: a case report and review of the literature. Endocr Pathol 2011;22:1-5.

54. Milias S, Hytiroglou P, Kourtis D, Papadimitriou CS. Granular cell tumour of the thyroid gland. Histopathology 2004;44:190-1.

55. Bothra R, Dahiya SL, Treisman E, Goodman P. Cervical thymoma. Int Surg 1975;60:301-2.

56. Chan JK, Rosai J. Tumors of the neck showing thymic or related branchial pouch differentiation: a unifying concept. Hum Pathol 1991;22:349-67.

57. Martin JM, Randhawa G, Temple WJ. Cervical thymoma. Arch Pathol Lab Med 1986;110:354-7.

58. Ridenhour CE, Henzel JH, DeWeese MS, Kerr SE. Thymoma arising from undescended cervical thymus. Surgery 1970;67:614-9.

59. Yamashita H, Murakami N, Noguchi S, et al. Cervical thymoma and incidence of cervical thymus. Acta Pathol Jpn 1983;33:189-94.

60. Fetsch JF, Weiss SW. Ectopic hamartomatous thymoma: clinicopathologic, immunohistochemical, and histogenetic considerations in four new cases. Hum Pathol 1990;21:662-8.

61. Rosai J, Limas C, Husband EM. Ectopic hamartomatous thymoma. A distinctive benign lesion of the lower neck. Am J Surg Pathol 1984;8:501-13.

62. Harach HR, Saravia Day E, Franssila KO. Thyroid spindle cell tumor with mucous cysts. An intrathyroid thymoma? Am J Surg Pathol 1985;9:525-30.

63. Murao T, Nakanishi M, Toda K, Konishi H. Malignant teratoma of the thyroid gland in an adolescent female. Acta Pathol Jpn 1979;29:109-17.

64. Folpe AL, Lloyd RV, Bacchi CE, Rosai J. Spindle epithelial tumor with thymus-like differentiation: a morphologic, immunohistochemical, and molecular genetic study of 11 cases. Am J Surg Pathol 2009;33:1179-86.

65. Miyauchi A, Kuma K, Matsuzuka F, et al. Intrathyroidal epithelial thymoma: an entity distinct from squamous cell carcinoma of the thyroid. World J Surg 1985;9:128-35.

66. Damiani S, Filotico M, Eusebi V. Carcinoma of the thyroid showing thymoma-like features. Virchows Arch A Pathol Anat Histopathol 1991;418:463-6.

67. Kakudo K, Mori I, Tamaoki N, Watanabe K. Carcinoma of possible thymic origin presenting as a thyroid mass: a new subgroup of squamous cell carcinoma of the thyroid. J Surg Oncol 1988;138:187-92.

68. Miyauchi A, Ishikawa H, Maeda M. [Intrathyroidal epithelial thymoma: a report of 6 cases with immunohistochemical and ultrastructural studies.] Endocr Surg 1989;6:289-95. [Japanese]

69. Yamazaki M, Fujii S, Daiko H, Hayashi R, Ochiai A. Carcinoma showing thymus-like differentiation (CASTLE) with neuroendocrine differentiation. Pathol Int 2008;58:775-9.

70. Lange MJ. Pleomorphic adenoma of the thyroid containing salivary gland cells with pseudocartilage and myoepithelial cells. Int Surg 1974;59:178-9.

71. Levy GH, Marti JL, Cai G, et al. Pleomorphic adenoma arising in an incidental midline isthmic thyroid nodule: a case report and review of the literature. Hum Pathol 2012;43:134-7.

72. Baloch ZW, Segal JP, LiVolsi VA. Unique growth pattern in papillary carcinoma of the thyroid gland mimicking adenoid cystic carcinoma. Endocr Pathol 2011;22:200-5.

16 SECONDARY TUMORS OF THE THYROID GLAND

The thyroid gland may be directly invaded by carcinomas of the pharynx, larynx, trachea, esophagus, and parathyroid gland, as well as by metastatic tumors in adjacent cervical lymph nodes originated from these and other sites. Postcricoid and subglottic laryngeal tumors have a particular tendency to extend into the thyroid gland via the thyroidal cartilages (1). Most of these tumors are of squamous cell type, and the fact that the thyroid gland involvement is a secondary event is usually obvious by the clinical and radiographic features. Because of the rarity of primary squamous cell carcinoma of the thyroid, the possibility of a metastasis should be considered whenever this tumor type is found in a thyroid biopsy, particularly if the tumor is well to moderately well differentiated. Also, parathyroid tumors, unlike differentiated tumors of thyroid follicular and C-cell derivation, do not express thyroid transcription factor (TTF)-1 (2).

Blood-borne metastases to the thyroid gland are common at autopsy in patients with widespread malignancy, particularly melanoma and carcinomas of kidney, lung, breast, gastrointestinal tract, head and neck region, and uterus (figs. 16-1–16-3) (3). In one large series, metastases to the thyroid gland were found in 9.5 percent of 1,980 patients who died of malignancy in other organs (4). These metastases, however, were the cause of clinically detectable thyroid enlargement or functional disturbances of this organ in only 25 percent or less of the cases. In other series, the incidence of metastatic thyroid involvement has been lower, ranging from 0.5 to 4.0 percent (3,5).

Occasional cancers metastatic to the thyroid gland are accompanied by hyperthyroidism, presumably as a result of the destruction of the follicles by tumor and the massive release of thyroid hormones (6). Sometimes the metastases lodge within a primary thyroid tumor, as an expression of the odd phenomenon known as tumor-to-tumor metastasis. It has been suggested that follicular adenomas are more

likely to be the recipients of metastatic tumors than non-neoplastic thyroid tissue (fig. 16-4). Renal cell carcinoma, lung carcinoma, breast carcinoma, adenocarcinoma of large bowel, and melanoma are the most common "donor" tumors (7–9).

On gross examination, secondary deposits in the thyroid gland are frequently multiple. Microscopically, they show a predominantly interstitial pattern of infiltration: the follicles are surrounded and deformed by the tumor but rarely infiltrated. Occasionally, however,

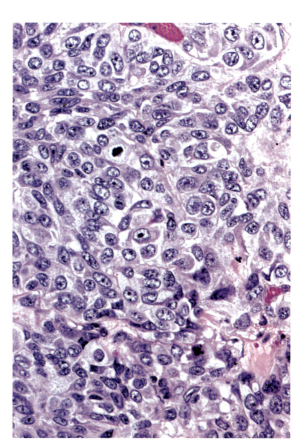

Figure 16-1

MALIGNANT MELANOMA METASTATIC TO THYROID
Note the large nuclei and the prominent nucleoli.

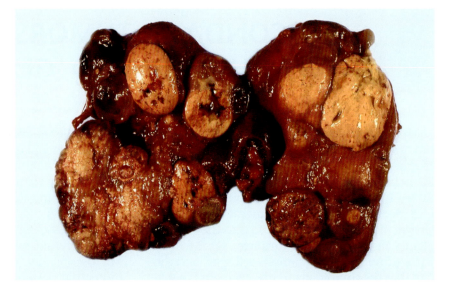

Figure 16-2

RENAL CELL CARCINOMA METASTATIC TO THYROID

Multiple nodules are present throughout the gland.

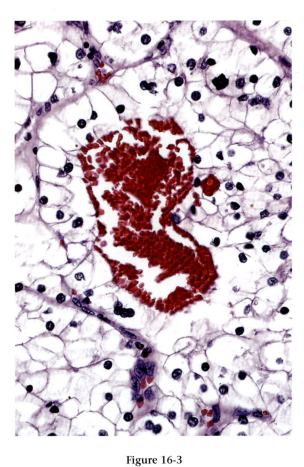

Figure 16-3

CLEAR CELL RENAL CELL CARCINOMA METASTATIC TO THYROID

The "bloody gland" in the center is an important clue to the diagnosis.

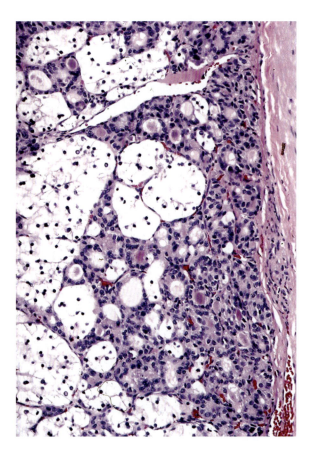

Figure 16-4

CLEAR CELL RENAL CELL CARCINOMA METASTATIC TO A THYROID FOLLICULAR ADENOMA

The rest of the thyroid gland was uninvolved. Follicular adenomas seem to be more likely "recipients" of metastases than the normal thyroid gland.

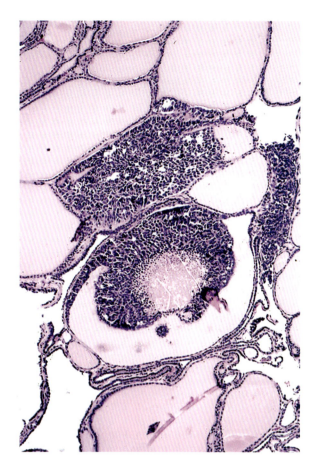

Figure 16-5

**ATYPICAL CARCINOID TUMOR OF
LUNG METASTATIC TO THYROID**

There is "folliculotropism" of the tumor cells.

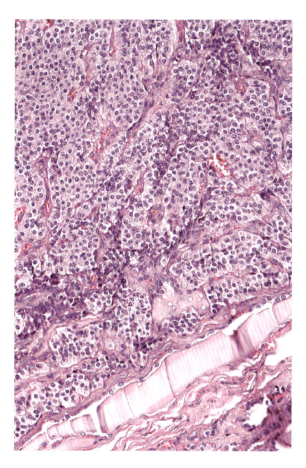

Figure 16-6

**CARCINOID TUMOR OF LUNG
METASTATIC TO THYROID**

The main entity in the differential diagnosis is medullary carcinoma.

there is extensive permeation of the follicles, and the pattern simulates a primary neoplasm. A peculiar manifestation of this phenomenon is the "folliculotropism" sometimes exhibited by carcinoid tumors of lung when metastasizing to the thyroid gland (fig. 16-5) (10).

The most significant type of thyroid metastasis clinically is the one that presents as a thyroid mass while the original source remains occult, thus simulating a primary tumor or thyroiditis (6,11). The most common of these are renal cell carcinoma (by far), large bowel adenocarcinoma, and melanoma (12–15). Carcinoid tumors also metastasize to the thyroid gland and simulate a medullary carcinoma of that organ (fig. 16-6) (10).

Metastatic renal cell carcinoma deserves special mention (16). It may present as a thy-

roid mass while the primary renal tumor is totally silent or as long as 16 or 22 years after nephrectomy (17–19). The metastasis may be limited to the thyroid gland or also involve other sites, particularly the pancreas (20). The thyroid nodule may be solitary or multiple, and the microscopic appearance is usually that of the clear cell type of renal cell carcinoma. The obvious entities in the differential diagnosis are the primary thyroid neoplasms exhibiting clear cell changes (see chapter 11).

Features favoring a diagnosis of metastatic renal cell carcinoma are multiplicity of tumor nodules, marked vascularization provided by sinusoidal vessels, "follicles" (in reality, glandular lumens) packed with red blood cells ("bloody

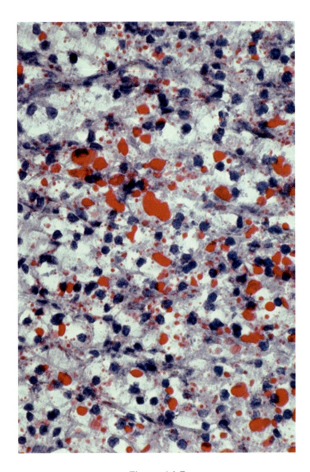

Figure 16-7

RENAL CELL CARCINOMA METASTATIC TO THYROID

There is strong oil red O positivity, indicative of neutral fat in the cytoplasm.

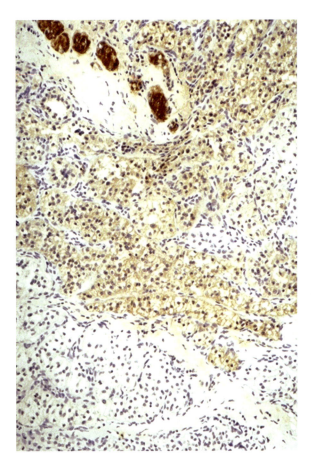

Figure 16-8

RENAL CELL CARCINOMA METASTATIC TO THYROID

Some of the thyroglobulin from the entrapped follicles located in the upper left has diffused out and been nonspecifically absorbed by the adjacent tumor cells, which have thus acquired a spurious positivity for this marker.

glands"), and a prominent water-clear appearance of the cytoplasm with little, if any, granularity. The latter feature is particularly important because the cells of a thyroid primary follicular clear cell tumor usually maintain a certain degree of cytoplasmic granularity, which becomes more noticeable in periodic acid–Schiff (PAS)-stained slides (see figs. 16-3, 16-4) (17).

The PAS stain is otherwise of only limited use in this differential diagnosis. The absence of glycogen is against a diagnosis of metastatic renal cell carcinoma, but its presence, even in large amounts, does not rule out the alternative possibility of a primary thyroid tumor. Similar considerations apply to lipid stains (fig. 16-7). The most useful ancillary methods in this situation are immunohistochemical stains for thyroglobulin, TTF-1, and the renal cell carcinoma marker carbonic anhydrase IX (CAIX) (21). The latter, a recently described marker, is consistently positive in renal cell carcinoma and negative in primary thyroid neoplasms (21).

Thyroglobulin is negative in metastatic tumors and usually positive (at least focally) in primary neoplasms. Alas, the interpretation requires caution for two reasons. First, the amount of this marker in primary clear cell tumors of the thyroid gland may be scanty, most of the space in the cytoplasm having been occupied by vacuoles (17). Second, entrapment of normal follicles by the tumor followed by thyroglobulin diffusion and absorption by the metastatic cells

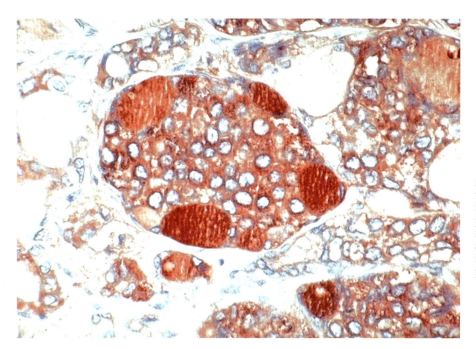

may occur and be misinterpreted as a positive result (fig. 16-8) (17). A similar phenomenon occurs with metastatic tumors from other sites (fig. 16-9). The TTF-1 stain is very useful in these circumstances, with the proviso that lung adenocarcinomas (and, occasionally, tumors from other organs, like extrapulmonary small cell neuroendocrine carcinoma) also stain for this marker. A specific situation in which immunostaining for thyroglobulin or for TTF-1 has very limited use is in the differentiation of primary undifferentiated (anaplastic) thyroid carcinoma and metastatic undifferentiated carcinoma from another site (such as lung, pancreas, or kidney), for the simple reason that it is likely be negative in both situations. When faced with this scenario, a metastatic tumor should be favored over a primary undifferentiated carcinoma if the tumor nodule is small, stuck between normal follicles, and multiple (as opposed of a large tumor mass with extrathyroid extension).

Just as important as secondary tumors that can simulate primary thyroid neoplasms, is the reciprocal situation. Primary thyroid tumors for which the danger of misinterpretation as secondary neoplasms is particularly high include those with clear cell, mucinous (including signet ring), and squamous changes; columnar cell carcinoma; and the family of tumors showing thymic or related branchial pouch differentiation (see chapter 15) (22). Also, the occasional renal cell carcinoma containing thyroid-like macrofollicular areas may closely simulate dilated thyroid follicles (23).

REFERENCES

1. Harrison DF. Thyroid gland in the management of laryngopharyngeal cancer. Arch Otolaryngol 1973;97:301-2.

2. Mantovani G, Corbetta S, Romoli R, Alberti L, Beck-Peccoz P, Spada A. Absence of thyroid transcription factor-1 expression in human parathyroid and pituitary glands. Mol Cell Endocrinol 2001;182:13-7.

3. Nakhjavani MK, Gharib H, Goellner JR, van Heerden JA. Metastasis to the thyroid gland. A report of 43 cases. Cancer 1997;79:574-8.

4. Shimaoka K, Sokal JE, Pickren JW. Metastatic neoplasms in the thyroid gland. Pathological and clinical findings. Cancer 1962;15:557-65.

5. Lam KY, Lo CY. Metastatic tumors of the thyroid gland: a study of 79 cases in Chinese patients. Arch Pathol Lab Med 1998;122:37-41.

6. Ivy HK. Cancer metastatic to the thyroid: a diagnostic problem. Mayo Clin Proc 1984;59:856-9.

7. Mizukami Y, Saito K, Nonomura A, et al. Lung carcinoma metastatic to microfollicular adenoma of the thyroid. A case report. Acta Pathol Jpn 1990;40:602-8.

8. Ro JY, Guerrieri C, el-Naggar AK, Ordóñez NG, Sorge JG, Ayala AG. Carcinomas metastatic to follicular adenomas of the thyroid gland. Report of two cases. Arch Pathol Lab Med 1994;118:551-6.

9. Baloch ZW, LiVolsi VA. Tumor-to-tumor metastasis to follicular variant of papillary carcinoma of thyroid. Arch Pathol Lab Med 1999;123:703-6.

10. Matias-Guiu X, LaGuette J, Puras-Gil AM, Rosai J. Metastatic neuroendocrine tumors to the thyroid gland mimicking medullary carcinoma: a pathologic and immunohistochemical study of six cases. Am J Surg Pathol 1997;21:754-62.

11. Elliott RH Jr, Frantz VK. Metastatic carcinoma masquerading as primary thyroid cancer: a report of authors' 14 cases. Ann Surg 1960;151:551-61.

12. Tibaldi JM, Shapiro LE, Mahadevia PS. Thyroiditis mimicked by metastatic carcinoma to the thyroid. Mayo Clin Proc 1986;61:399-400.

13. Czech JM, Lichtor TR, Carney JA, van Heerden JA. Neoplasms metastatic to the thyroid gland. Surg Gynecol Obstet 1982;155:503-5.

14. McCabe DP, Farrar WB, Petkov TM, Finkelmeier W, O'Dwyer P, James A. Clinical and pathologic correlations in disease metastatic to the thyroid gland. Am J Surg 1985;150:519-23.

15. Wychulis AR, Beahrs OH, Woolner LB. Metastases of carcinoma to the thyroid gland. Ann Surg 1964;160:169-77.

16. Heffess CS, Wenig BM, Thompson LD. Metastatic renal cell carcinoma to the thyroid gland: a clinicopathologic study of 36 cases. Cancer 2002;95:1869-78.

17. Carcangiu ML, Sibley RK, Rosai J. Clear cell change in primary thyroid tumors. A study of 38 cases. Am J Surg Pathol 1985;9:705-22.

18. Green LK, Ro JY, Mackay B, Ayala AG, Luna MA. Renal cell carcinoma metastatic to the thyroid. Cancer 1989;63:1810-5.

19. Sindoni A, Rizzo M, Tuccari G, et al. Thyroid metastases from clear cell renal carcinoma 18 years after nephrectomy. Ann Endocrinol (Paris) 2010;71:127-30.

20. Iesalnieks I, Winter H, Bareck E, et al. Thyroid metastases of renal cell carcinoma: clinical course in 45 patients undergoing surgery. Assessment of factors affecting patients' survival. Thyroid 2008;18:615-24.

21. Cimino-Mathews A, Sharma R, Netto GJ. Diagnostic use of PAX8, CAIX, TTF-1, and TGB in metastatic renal cell carcinoma of the thyroid. Am J Surg Pathol 2011;35:757-61.

22. Rigaud C, Bogomoletz WV, Delisle MJ, Diebold MD, Caulet T. [Metastatic cancers of the thyroid gland. Diagnostic difficulties.] Bull Cancer (Paris) 1987;74:117-27. [French]

23. Fadare O, Lam S, Rubin C, Renshaw IL, Nerby CL. Papillary renal cell carcinoma with diffuse clear cells and thyroid-like macrofollicular areas. Ann Diagn Pathol 2010;14:284-91.

17 TUMOR-LIKE CONDITIONS OF THE THYROID GLAND

Listed in this section is a heterogeneous group of non-neoplastic thyroid disorders that can simulate a neoplastic process at the gross or microscopic level. Aspects of some of these conditions have already been discussed in other chapters.

NODULAR HYPERPLASIA

General Features. *Nodular hyperplasia* (*nodular* or *multinodular goiter, adenomatoid* or *adenomatous goiter, adenomatous hyperplasia*) is a common thyroid disease. The form known as *endemic goiter* is the result of low iodine content of the water and soil; it can be largely prevented by adding iodine to common salt (1–3) or by intramuscular injections of iodized oil (R. Cooke, personal communication, 2004). The deficiency in thyroid hormone production induced by the iodine deficiency leads to an increase in thyroid-stimulating hormone (TSH) secretion, which results initially in a hyperplastic gland with tall follicular epithelial cells and small amounts of colloid (*parenchymatous goiter*), and later in follicular atrophy with abundant storage of colloid (*colloid goiter*). As expected, many transitional forms exist within this continuous spectrum (see chapter 1).

The form known as *sporadic nodular goiter* is by far the most common in the United States. Some cases are associated with lymphocytic or Hashimoto thyroiditis and are viewed as the nodular forms of these immune-mediated inflammatory diseases. The incidence in the general adult population is 3 to 5 percent clinically and about 50 percent at autopsy (4,5).

The pathogenesis of thyroid nodular hyperplasia remains poorly understood (6). It may represent a multifactorial and multistep process, which includes a genetic predisposition, an initially diffuse hyperplasia of the gland (which may be due to iodine deficiency, nutritional goitrogens, and autoimmunity, all of which may lead to a series of mutational events in the follicular cells. Tongue-in-cheek, we would like to add the type of goiter that Michelangelo Buonarroti claimed to have developed from the prolonged strain to the neck suffered while painting the Sistine Chapel, being that he was standing on a scaffold, with his head and neck greatly overextended (fig. 17-1). Just as odd is the fact that he likened his goiter to that developing in cats due to "the bad water in Lombardy" (7).

Amusing anecdotes aside, it is possible that some of the above-listed events are "activating," and through their interaction with various

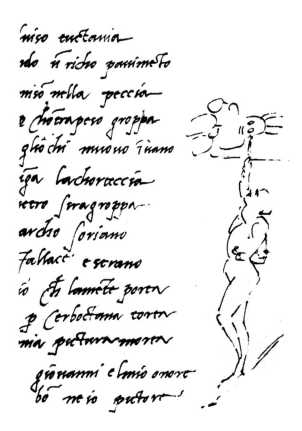

Figure 17-1

MICHELANGELO'S GOITER

Michelangelo's caricature of himself painting the Sistine Chapel ceiling while standing on a scaffold. Note the large protrusion in the anterior neck ("goiter") resulting from the overextension of the head. The adjacent sonnet is also by him.

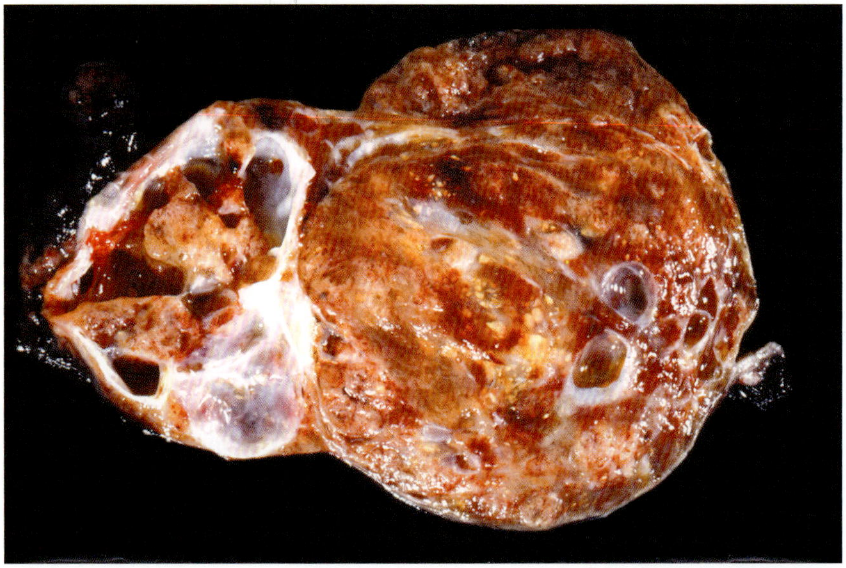

Figure 17-2

NODULAR HYPERPLASIA

This large multinodular lesion with extensive secondary changes was located in the mediastinum.

growth factors lead to the formation of "clones," which become the niduses for the formation of clinically apparent nodules (8). Many nodules (particularly the "dominant" nodules that develop in the background of nodular hyperplasia) are monoclonal when evaluated using X-chromosome inactivation patterns (8). These studies have limitations due to the significant size of the embryonal X-chromosome inactivation area that in the thyroid gland is about 0.5-1.0 cm² (9), but results consistent with a monoclonal cell population are identical to those obtained in many follicular adenomas.

Other features make the distinction between some hyperplastic nodules and true thyroid neoplasms difficult. Chromosomal alterations that are simple but detectable by both conventional karyotyping and ploidy analysis, particularly trisomy 7 but also translocations involving 17q13, are found in some hyperplastic nodules (10,11). They are present in 5 to 10 percent of common hyperplastic nodules, but in a higher proportion of those with adenomatous features (11). TSH receptor (TSHr)-activating mutations, identical to those found in hyperfunctioning "toxic" adenomas, have been described in hyperfunctioning, scintigraphically "hot" areas of multinodular goiters and even in microscopic, autoradiographically hot foci of about 30 percent of euthyroid goiters (8,12). Even activating *RAS* mutations of the type found in follicular adenomas and carcinomas occur in a few hy-

perplastic nodules (13). The monoclonal origin, the occurrence of chromosomal abnormalities, and the presence of oncogenic mutations in at least some hyperplastic nodules (usually those with adenomatous features) argue in favor of a neoplastic nature of nodules in goiters. Although these considerations are not an issue for routine histologic diagnosis, they are important for understanding the development of thyroid nodular hyperplasia. They reflect the difficulty in drawing a line between hyperplasia and neoplasia, a situation common to many endocrine proliferative conditions.

Clinical Features. Most patients are euthyroid and present with a multinodular gland that may become very large, cause tracheal and esophageal obstruction, and produce considerable disfigurement. In cases accompanied by a firm, larger, "dominant" nodule, the clinical distinction from a true neoplasm may be impossible. Hemorrhage within a nodule can cause sudden enlargement and pain. Cases associated with thyroid hyperfunction are referred to as *toxic nodular hyperplasia*. Some cases of thyroid nodular hyperplasia are located substernally and resemble superior mediastinal tumors.

Gross Findings. The thyroid gland is enlarged and its shape is distorted; one lobe may be larger than the other (figs. 17-2–17-4). Glands weighing over 2,000 g have been recorded. The thyroid capsule may be stretched but is intact. On cross section, multiple nodules are seen,

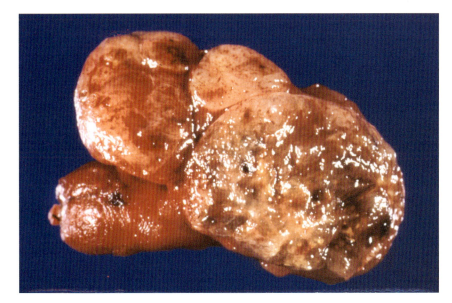

Figure 17-3

NODULAR HYPERPLASIA

The entire gland is involved by ill-defined nodules, many of which show cystic and hemorrhagic secondary changes.

Figure 17-4

NODULAR HYPERPLASIA

Variously sized nodules are present in this cut-surface view, some incompletely encapsulated. There is secondary hemorrhage, necrosis, and cystic degeneration.

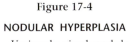

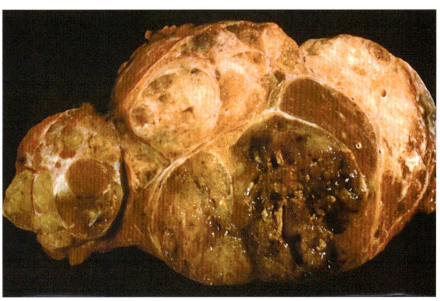

some partially encapsulated. Secondary changes, in the form of hemorrhage, calcification, and cystic degeneration, are common, especially in the larger nodules (figs. 17-5, 17-6).

Microscopic Findings. Microscopically, there is a wide range of appearances. Some nodules are composed of markedly dilated follicles lined by flattened epithelium, others are extremely cellular, and still others are composed predominantly or exclusively of oncocytes or, rarely, cells with clear cytoplasm. Some of the dilated follicles have a conglomerate of small active follicles at one pole, representing hyperplastic forms of "Sanderson polsters" (see chapter 1). Rupture of follicles may lead to a granulomatous reaction to the colloid, with the appearance of histiocytes and foreign body-type multinucleated giant cells. Areas of fresh and old hemorrhage, coarse fibrous trabeculation, and foci of calcification (of nonpsammomatous type) are common.

Occasionally, osseous metaplasia is seen. Greatly thickened vessels with calcified media may be present at the periphery of the gland. A variable number of mononuclear inflammatory cells are present in the stroma in many of

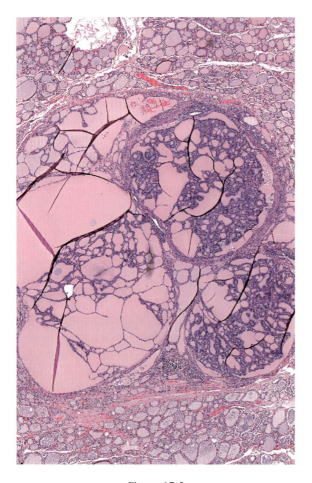

Figure 17-5

NODULAR HYPERPLASIA

The cluster of hyperplastic nodules shows focal cystic change and lacks encapsulation.

the cases, indicating the coexistence of chronic thyroiditis. Autolytic changes occur more rapidly in hyperplastic than in normal glands. In rare cases, the stroma undergoes focal adipose metaplasia. True psammoma bodies may be seen in nodular hyperplasia, but they are rare (14). Their presence should suggest a papillary carcinoma nearby.

Differential Diagnosis. Nodular hyperplasia can simulate a malignant tumor via several mechanisms, including hypercellularity of some of the nodules, focal presence of vesicular nuclei, occurrence of papillary formations, and development of parasitic nodules (15). The papillae that are seen in nodular hyperplasia tend to be located within cystically dilated follicles, with their tips pointing toward the center of that follicle (i.e., they have a so-called centripetal orientation). Similar to the papillae of diffuse hyperplasia, those present in nodular hyperplasia are characteristically lined by columnar or tall cuboidal epithelial cells with basophilic cytoplasm and basally located, perfectly round nuclei with smooth contours (figs. 17-7, 17-8). The apical surface of the benign papillae of nodular hyperplasia stains slightly or not at all with Alcian blue or epithelial membrane antigen (EMA), whereas the surface of the papillae of papillary carcinoma usually reacts strongly with both markers (16).

The criteria for distinguishing nodular hyperplasia from follicular adenoma are discussed in chapter 5, and the controversial issue of a possible relationship between nodular hyperplasia

Figure 17-6

NODULAR HYPERPLASIA

One of the hyperplastic nodules is very cellular, whereas another has undergone complete cystic degeneration, with pseudocapsular formation and focal calcification.

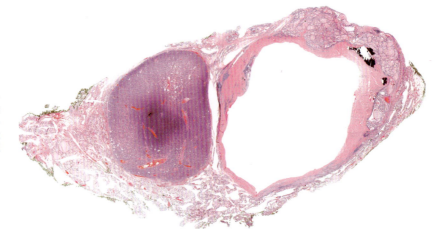

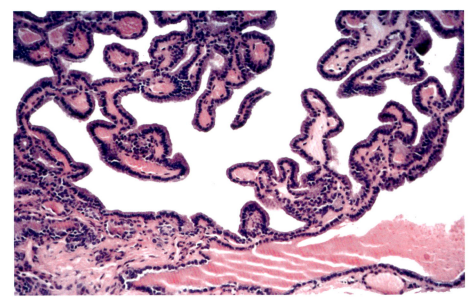

Figure 17-7

BENIGN PAPILLAE IN NODULAR HYPERPLASIA

This hyperplastic nodule is highly papillary, closely resembling papillary carcinoma on low-power examination.

Figure 17-8

BENIGN PAPILLAE IN NODULAR HYPERPLASIA

Features favoring the benign nature of these papillae are the basal location of the nuclei, their round regular contours, the lack of nuclear clearing, the pale quality of the cytoplasm, and the tall shape of the cells. The latter feature should not lead to an overdiagnosis of papillary carcinoma (including its tall cell variant).

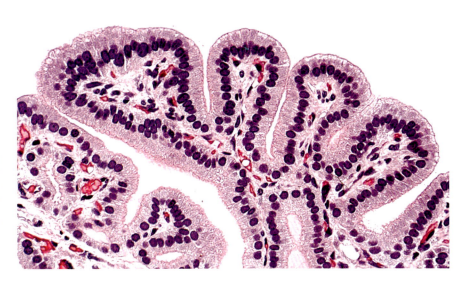

and thyroid carcinoma is discussed in chapter 6. Based on some of the considerations discussed above, molecular diagnostic methods may not be much better than conventional histology in distinguishing hyperplastic thyroid nodules from true neoplasms. Exceptionally, foci of extramedullary hematopoiesis are found in nodular hyperplastic thyroid glands, foreshadowing the clinical evidence of agnogenic myeloid metaplasia (17,18).

DIFFUSE HYPERPLASIA

General Features. *Graves disease* is one of the two major forms of autoimmune thyroid disease (19,20). The diffusely hyperplastic gland of this disorder simulates malignancy in three ways: 1) through the presence of well-developed papillary formations, some of which are endowed with a central fibrovascular core; 2) through the presence of large vesicular nuclei in the follicular epithelium; and 3) through the occasional extension of the hyperplastic process outside the confines of the thyroid gland. The nuclear clearing is not nearly as well developed as that seen in papillary thyroid carcinoma and is even less pronounced than that sometimes associated with Hashimoto thyroiditis. The benign nature of the papillary formations is recognized by their widespread occurrence throughout the gland, the lack of a fibrous stromal response, and the papillae

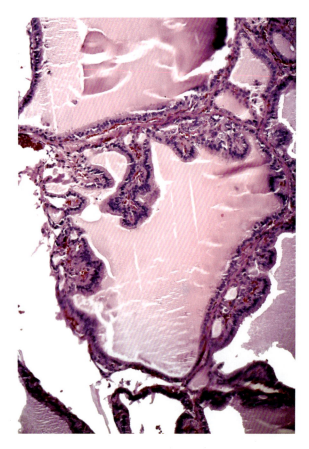

Figure 17-9

BENIGN PAPILLAE IN DIFFUSE HYPERPLASIA

The "centripetal" orientation of these short papillae toward the center of a cystically dilated follicle is an important clue to their benign nature.

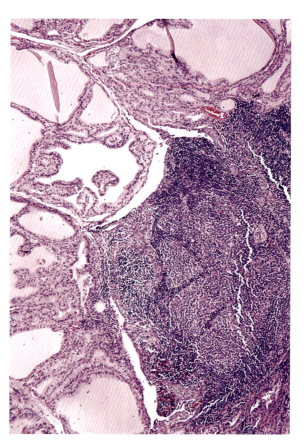

Figure 17-10

DIFFUSE HYPERPLASIA

Hyperplastic thyroid follicles, some featuring short papillary formations, are adjacent to a large lymphoid nodule with prominent germinal centers.

that are usually lined by columnar follicular cells characterized by perfectly round, basally located, normochromatic or hyperchromatic nuclei and abundant basophilic cytoplasm (figs. 17-9–17-12). Immunohistochemically, p27kip1 is significantly higher in the papillae of diffuse hyperplasia than in those of papillary carcinoma, but this stain should rarely be needed (21). Therapy of Graves disease with ^{131}I can lead to the development of nodularity, cyst formation, marked oncocytic changes, and pronounced nuclear atypia (22).

In some cases of Graves disease, hyperplastic follicular cells are present in the adjacent perithyroid soft tissue. This potentially misleading feature may not represent spread from the thyroid gland itself but rather the expression of concomitant hyperplasia of preexisting nor-

mal thyroid follicles embedded in the skeletal muscle of the neck and anatomically separate from the thyroid gland, a microscopic finding often seen in normal individuals (see chapter 1) (23). Whatever the mechanism, infiltration of skeletal muscle fibers by this highly cellular thyroid tissue may result in a mistaken diagnosis of malignancy. If the patient's hyperthyroid status is known and it is realized that the morphologic changes in the extrathyroid tissue are those of diffuse hyperplasia (and therefore not different from those present inside the gland) this error should be avoidable.

DYSHORMONOGENETIC GOITER

General Features. The term *dyshormonogenetic goiter* is applied to a group of genetically determined thyroid hyperplasias resulting from

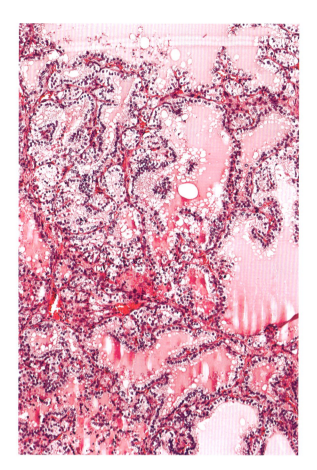

Figure 17-11

DIFFUSE HYPERPLASIA

The proliferating follicles have a complex arrangement with innumerable small pseudopapillae.

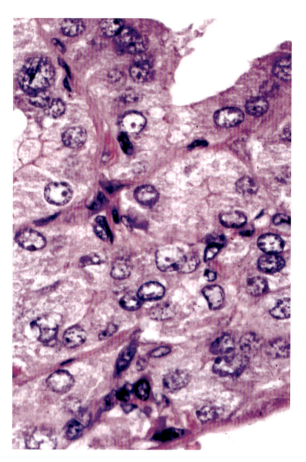

Figure 17-12

DIFFUSE HYPERPLASIA

The clear appearance of most nuclei may lead to a mistaken diagnosis of papillary carcinoma. However, the nuclear clearing is only partial, most of the nucleoli are centrally located, the cellular contours are regular, and the abundant cytoplasm has a pale granular (nononcocytic) quality.

defective thyroglobulin synthesis (mostly related to thyroglobulin gene mutations [24]) or, less commonly, from defects in thyroid hormone synthesis (25). Known types of the former include unresponsiveness to TSH, defects in iodine transport or organification, defective iodotyrosine coupling, and deiodinase defects (26,27). A form due a mutation of the pendrin gene and associated with sensorineural deafness is known as *Pendred syndrome* (28) In all of these conditions, the absence of feedback to the pituitary gland leads to the continuous hypersecretion of TSH and a markedly hyperactive thyroid gland.

Clinical and Microscopic Findings. Most of the cases are seen in patients younger than 24 years, and the typical presentation is in the form of goiter accompanied by hypothyroidism. The gland is invariably enlarged and multinodular, weighing up to 600 g in one large series (figs. 17-13, 17-14) (29). The hypercellularity can be extreme and is often accompanied by bizarre (large, hyperchromatic, or misshapen) nuclear forms (figs. 17-15, 17-16). The pattern of growth may be solid, microfollicular, with papillary formations, or with insular features (30). Fibrosis, a common finding, may simulate capsular invasion. Encapsulated nodules may develop, and the capsule may appear focally violated by the hyperplastic process (31–33). Clues to the diagnosis include young age of presentation, familial incidence (in the absence of iodine deficiency), a bewildering heterogeneity of architectural and cytologic

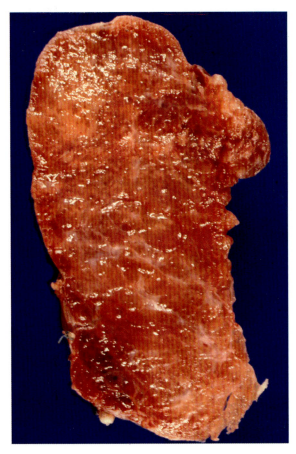

Figure 17-13

DYSHORMONOGENETIC GOITER

The cut surface shows fine nodularity and a reddish color due to the increased vascularization.

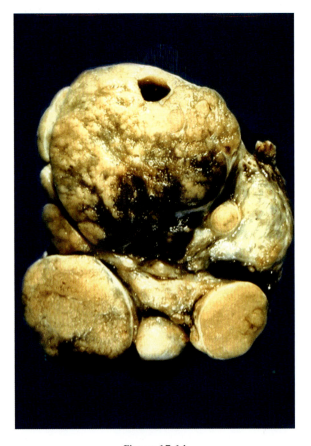

Figure 17-14

DYSHORMONOGENETIC GOITER

The cut surface of a thyroid gland from a patient with dyshormonogenetic goiter shows marked hyperplastic changes associated with secondary hemorrhage and fibrosis.

Figure 17-15

DYSHORMONOGENETIC GOITER

The low-power appearance is not substantially different from that of the usual (sporadic) from of nodular hyperplasia.

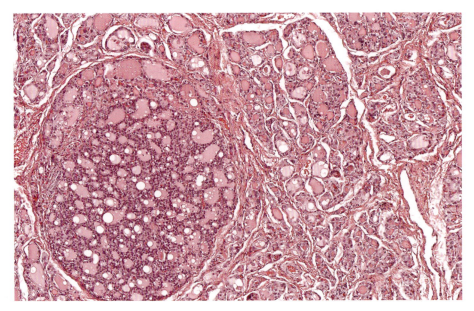

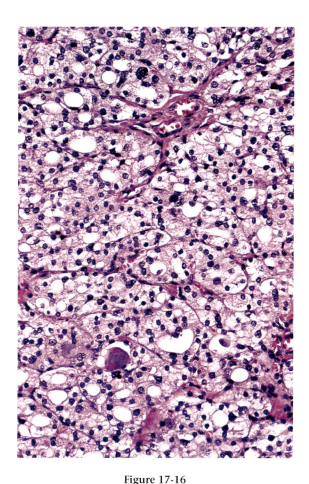

Figure 17-16

DYSHORMONOGENETIC GOITER

The follicular cells of this hypercellular gland have clear cytoplasm and hyperchromatic nuclei, some of large size.

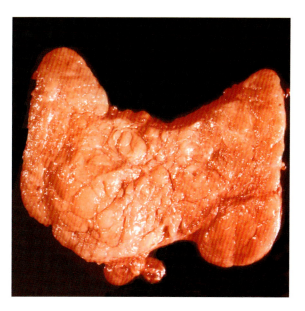

Figure 17-17

HASHIMOTO THYROIDITIS

"Meaty" hyperplastic gland with a multinodular appearance due to the concomitant nodular hyperplasia (nodular Hashimoto thyroiditis).

features, scarcity of intraluminal colloid, and the fact that most of the bizarre nuclear forms are found in the thyroid tissue located between the hyperplastic nodules rather than in the nodules themselves (29). Some correlation exists between the specific type of genetic aberration and the pathologic features present (34).

It should be apparent from the above that to make a diagnosis of malignancy when such a background is present is a difficult task, to the point that some observers believe that it can only be made if metastases have occurred. We regard this position as unreasonably restrictive and believe that the diagnosis of malignancy is justified if the conventional cytoarchitectural features of the entity are present, independent of the presence of dyshormonogenetic goiter-related changes (35,36). Well-documented

cases associated with distant metastases are on record (37).

The differential diagnosis of dyshormonogenetic goiter also includes iatrogenic goiter resulting from the administration of antithyroidal agents (29). Other genetically determined conditions in which the thyroid gland is often involved are discussed in chapter 19.

THYROIDITIS

Hashimoto Thyroiditis

General Features. *Hashimoto thyroiditis* is the prototype of autoimmune thyroid disease, which begins with the activation of thyroid antigen-specific helper T cells (38,39). According to one theory, this activation usually results from a viral infection, but conclusive evidence for a viral etiology is lacking (40). There is instead strong epidemiologic evidence in favor of a genetic component in the pathogenesis of this disease (41).

Clinical and Microscopic Findings. Hashimoto thyroiditis usually presents as a bilateral diffuse enlargement of the gland (figs. 17-17, 17-18). The two key morphologic features are oncocytic change of the follicular epithelium

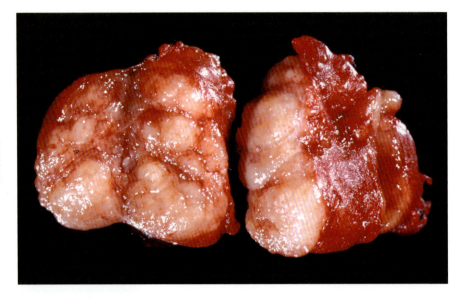

Figure 17-18

HASHIMOTO THYROIDITIS

The cut surface shows vague nodularity, signaling the early changes of nodular hyperplasia in a background of Hashimoto thyroiditis.

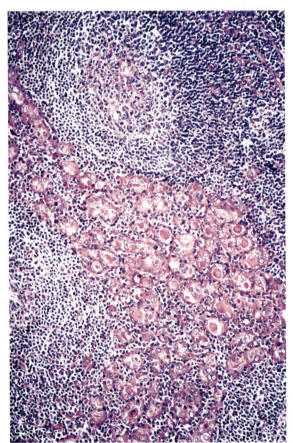

Figure 17-19

HASHIMOTO THYROIDITIS

Clusters of follicular cells with oncocytic features are admixed with a heavy lymphoid infiltrate containing germinal centers.

and a variously intense lymphoid infiltrate, predominantly composed of T cells and associated with B cell–containing germinal centers lacking evidence of clonality (fig. 17-19) (42).

Hashimoto thyroiditis can simulate a thyroid neoplasm in several ways. The nuclei of scattered oncocytic follicular cells may show marked enlargement, hyperchromasia, and abnormal shapes, features that they share with oncocytes of other organs and which should not be necessarily taken as a sign of malignancy or even of neoplastic transformation. Conversely, the nuclei of these cells may be vesicular and overlapping, their appearance thus approaching that of the ground-glass nuclei of papillary carcinoma (figs. 17-20, 17-21).

When Hashimoto thyroiditis is associated with diffuse hyperplasia (*"hashitoxicosis"*) or nodular hyperplasia (*nodular Hashimoto thyroiditis*), papillary formations may be seen. The criteria for distinguishing them from the papillae of papillary carcinoma are similar to those used when inflammatory changes are absent (see below).

Sharply outlined follicular-patterned nodules of varying cellularity may develop within the inflamed gland, requiring differentiation from follicular and oncocytic neoplasms (fig. 17-22). "Parasitic nodules" (i.e., thyroid nodules anatomically separate from the thyroid gland) developing in patients with Hashimoto thyroiditis may share the same morphologic abnormalities (including the nuclear alterations described

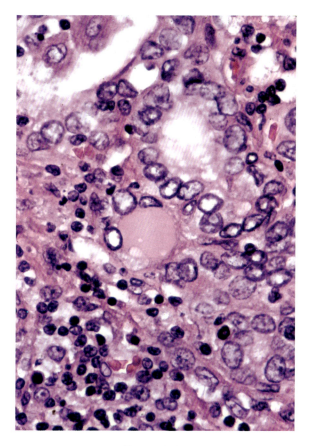

Figure 17-20

HASHIMOTO THYROIDITIS

The overlapping, partially clear nuclei in this case of Hashimoto thyroiditis simulate papillary carcinoma, a difficult differential diagnosis.

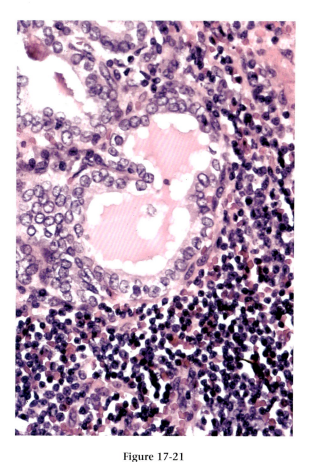

Figure 17-21

HASHIMOTO THYROIDITIS

The nuclei are partially clear, but the changes are subtle and present throughout the gland without mass formation. They are not, therefore, sufficient to establish a diagnosis of papillary carcinoma.

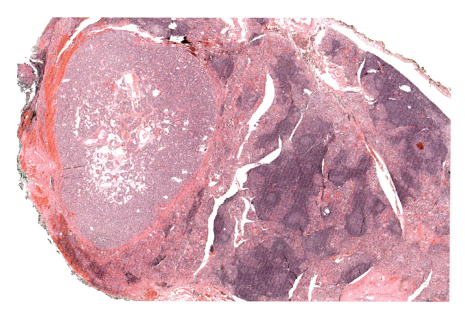

Figure 17-22

HASHIMOTO THYROIDITIS AND NODULAR HYPERPLASIA

This combined pattern is sometimes referred to as nodular Hashimoto thyroiditis.

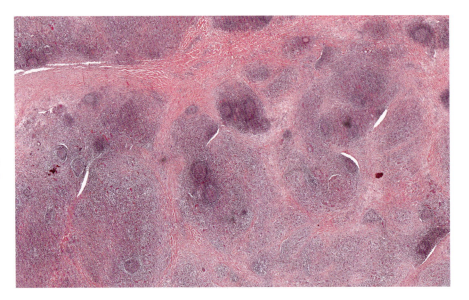

Figure 17-23

FIBROUS VARIANT OF HASHIMOTO THYROIDITIS

The prominent nodular configuration results from extensive fibrosis.

above), thus mimicking a lymph node involved by thyroid carcinoma (see chapter 18).

Prominent solid nests with a squamoid appearance that exhibit a mild degree of nuclear atypia may be seen in Hashimoto thyroiditis (particularly in the fibrous variant) (figs. 17-23–17-25) (43). Some represent metaplastic thyroid follicles, while others are hyperplastic solid cell nests (44). They should be distinguished from primary and metastatic squamous cell carcinomas and from the sclerosing mucoepidermoid carcinoma with eosinophilia that probably arises from these nests (see chapter 15) (45). Ductular structures thought to be a manifestation of phylogenic regression also have been described (46).

Large intrathyroidal squamous-lined cystic formations that closely resemble branchial cleft cysts may be seen in Hashimoto thyroiditis (fig. 17-26) (47). Although the association between the two processes seems established, similar lymphoepithelial cysts can also be seen in otherwise normal glands (48).

Several lines of evidence, including molecular data, point to a pathogenetic link between Hashimoto thyroiditis and thyroid carcinoma. Although this relationship is not straightforward, the follicular cells in Hashimoto thyroiditis can acquire chromosomal alterations when they proliferate to form discrete nodules (49), show loss of heterozygosity at tumor suppressor gene loci (50), and harbor oncogenic *RET/PTC* rearrangements, albeit at a very low frequency (51).

The cytologic features of Hashimoto thyroiditis are described in chapter 20 and the possible relationship between Hashimoto thyroiditis and thyroid carcinoma is discussed in chapter 7.

Subacute Granulomatous (DeQuervain) Thyroiditis

Subacute granulomatous (DeQuervain) thyroiditis can simulate a malignancy clinically and grossly when it has a focal rather than diffuse character due to the ill-defined nature of its margins (fig. 17-27). Microscopic examination resolves the issue with the recognition of the presence of folliculocentric giant cell-containing granulomas, often surrounding and phagocytosing clumps of colloid material. Immunohistochemically, there is strong reactivity for CA17-9, particularly in the late stage of the disease (52).

Fibrosing (Riedel) Thyroiditis

Fibrosing (Riedel) thyroiditis is notorious because of its carcinoma-like appearance at the time of surgery. This appearance results from the extension of the fibrosing process outside the thyroid gland into the surrounding soft tissue. The diagnosis is usually obvious microscopically because of the heavy deposition of collagen (some of it having a keloid-like quality), prominent lymphoplasmacytic infiltrate (which is polyclonal), phlebitis, and a fairly unremarkable appearance of the intervening follicles (figs. 17-28, 17-29) (53,54). Fibrosing thyroiditis should be distinguished from the

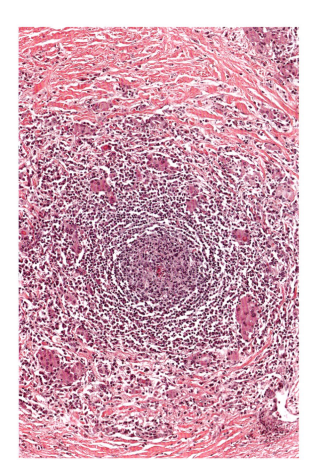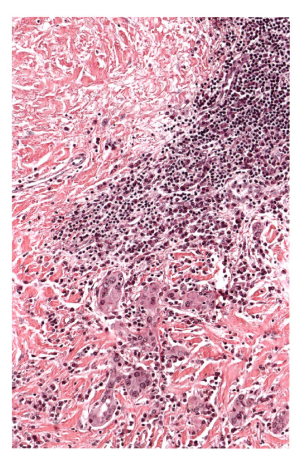

Figure 17-24

FIBROUS VARIANT OF HASHIMOTO THYROIDITIS

Left: A large lymphoid follicle with a prominent germinal center is surrounded by a fibrotic shell containing atrophic thyroid follicles with oncocytic features.

Right: A high-power view shows that the residual thyroid follicles are scanty and atrophic.

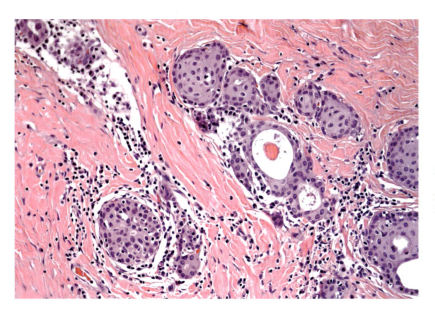

Figure 17-25

SQUAMOUS NESTS IN FIBROUS HASHIMOTO THYROIDITIS

Most of these structures are follicles with squamous metaplasia (some with a residual lumen). The main differential diagnosis is with solid cell nests.

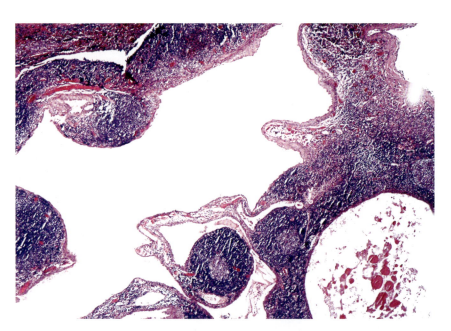

Figure 17-26

BRANCHIAL CLEFT CYST-LIKE FORMATION INSIDE A THYROID AFFECTED BY HASHIMOTO THYROIDITIS

Lesions with a similar pathogenesis can be seen in the salivary glands and thymus.

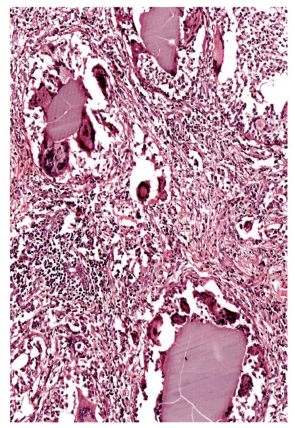

Figure 17-27

GRANULOMATOUS THYROIDITIS

The folliculocentric inflammatory infiltrate is rich in foreign body-type multinucleated giant cells. The follicular lining has been largely destroyed.

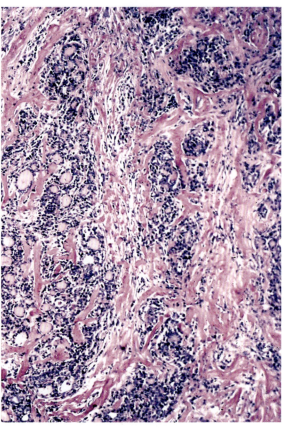

Figure 17-28

FIBROSING (RIEDEL) THYROIDITIS

Extensive fibrosis is accompanied by parenchymal atrophy and a lymphocytic infiltrate. The collagen has a sharply outlined, keloid-like quality.

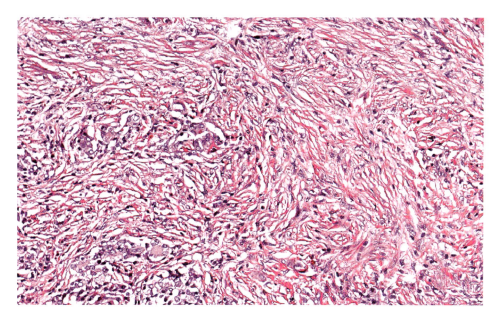

Figure 17-29

FIBROSING (RIEDEL) THYROIDITIS

Extensive fibrosis with almost complete atrophy of the thyroid follicles.

spindle cell type of undifferentiated (anaplastic) carcinoma, which exhibits obvious cytologic atypia, high mitotic rate, and necrosis; from the desmoplastic reaction that may accompany papillary carcinoma, which in some instances may be extremely florid and acquire a nodular fasciitis-like quality (55); and from large cell malignant lymphoma with sclerosis.

The etiology is unknown, but the prevailing view is that it is one of the manifestations of the group of sclerosing inflammatory diseases generically known as inflammatory fibrosclerosis, which also includes retroperitoneal fibrosis (Ormond disease), sclerosing mesenteritis, and sclerosing cholangitis (56). A high level of the rare IgG4 immunoglobulin is a feature of this disease group, including Riedel thyroiditis (57), and can be identified by immunohistochemistry in the plasma cells on histologic sections from lesional tissue (58). Although clearly a different disease from Hashimoto thyroiditis (including the fibrous variant of the latter), it may coexist with it (59,60). Furthermore, it has been noted that in the IgG4-related disease the fibrosis tends to be predominantly interfollicular rather than interlobular or scar type (61).

Multifocal Fibrosing (Sclerosing) Thyroiditis

Multifocal fibrosing (sclerosing) thyroiditis is a term we have proposed for a thyroid disorder characterized by multiple (sometimes innumerable), microscopic stellate-shaped foci composed of cellular fibroblastic tissue. These foci may entrap a few thyroid follicles and are often surrounded by hypercellular follicles radiating from the center. At low magnification, the individual lesions are reminiscent of the type of papillary carcinoma traditionally known as occult sclerosing carcinoma and currently designated papillary microcarcinoma or papillary microtumor (see chapter 7), from which it is distinguished by the absence of the cytoarchitectural features of papillary carcinoma (figs. 17-30–17-32) (62). Furthermore, although a given thyroid gland may harbor two or more papillary microcarcinomas, we are not aware of them ever presenting in the widespread fashion that characterizes this entity. The fact that occasionally a bonafide papillary microcarcinoma is present at the edge of one of these lesions complicates matters.

The etiology and pathogenesis of this process are not known, but the appearance is suggestive of the following sequence: idiopathic multifocal injury, follicular loss, replacement by scar-like tissue, reactive hyperplasia of the adjacent follicles, and, in some cases, development of a papillary microcarcinoma. Parenthetically, such a sequence would be pathogenetically similar to the one that has been thought to operate in radial scar of the breast. The alternative hypothesis, recently backed by a molecular finding (absence of *BRAF* mutations) is that multifocal fibrosing thyroiditis is an "incidental bystander" in the process and a reflection of the background thyroiditis (63).

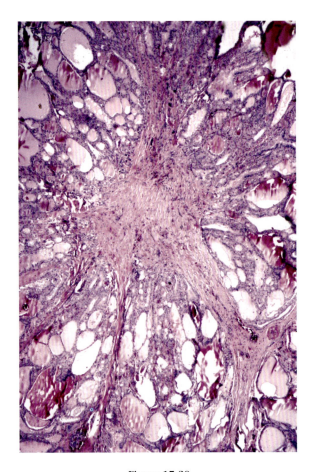

Figure 17-30

MULTIFOCAL FIBROSING THYROIDITIS

The radial scar appearance of the lesion is reminiscent of that seen in the breast lesion carrying the same designation.

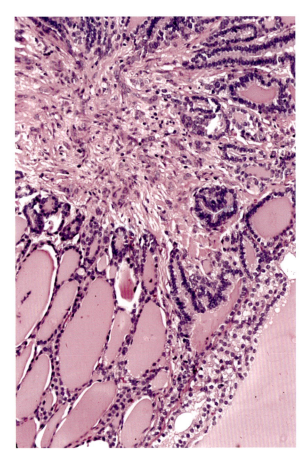

Figure 17-31

MULTIFOCAL FIBROSING THYROIDITIS

A ring of hyperplastic elongated thyroid follicles surrounds the central area of scarring. The nuclear features of papillary carcinoma were absent.

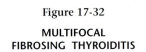

Figure 17-32

MULTIFOCAL FIBROSING THYROIDITIS

Scar tissue entraps atrophic follicles in the central portion of the lesion. The cytologic features of papillary carcinoma were lacking.

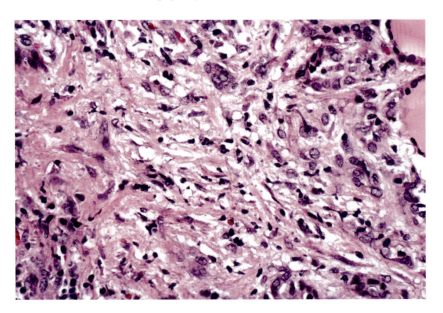

Malakoplakia

Malakoplakia has been described as exceptionally involving the thyroid gland and mimicking a malignant neoplasm clinically (64). The disease is recognized by the presence of an inflammatory infiltrate rich in histiocytes, some of which contain Michaelis-Gutmann bodies. The disease, which may be associated with Hashimoto thyroiditis, is thought to be due to an acquired defect of macrophage bactericidal digestion (65).

Other Forms of Thyroiditis

Other inflammatory/reactive conditions that may involve the thyroid gland include *palpation thyroiditis* (*multifocal granulomatous folliculitis*) (fig. 17-33) (66), *postpartum thyroiditis* and the possible related *spontaneous silent thyroiditis* (67,68), *postoperative necrotizing granuloma* (69), *sarcoidosis* (70), and *Wegener granulomatosis* (71). The latter two can simulate a thyroid tumor clinically. Inflammatory thyroid lesions of various types are frequent in patients infected with human immunodeficiency virus (HIV), especially those with active disease (72).

MISCELLANEOUS LESIONS

Langerhans Cell Histiocytosis

Langerhans cell histiocytosis (*Langerhans cell granulomatosis, histiocytosis X, eosinophilic granuloma*) involves the thyroid gland only exceptionally, sometimes in isolation and more often as part of a multisystem disease (73–75). The process can simulate a malignancy clinically (76). There may be dual involvement of the thyroid and parathyroid glands (77). Some cases are associated with Hashimoto thyroiditis and Graves disease (78). The most intriguing association is with papillary carcinoma, which can manifest in several ways (79): 1) with the thyroid gland involved by both processes; 2) with a cervical lymph node containing both metastatic papillary carcinoma and Langerhans cell histiocytosis; and 3) with Langerhans cell histiocytosis present in cervical lymph nodes draining a papillary carcinoma (80–83).

The microscopic features of Langerhans cell histiocytosis of the thyroid gland are similar to those seen in other sites. The diagnosis is made by the identification of Langerhans cells against the appropriate background, which usually in-

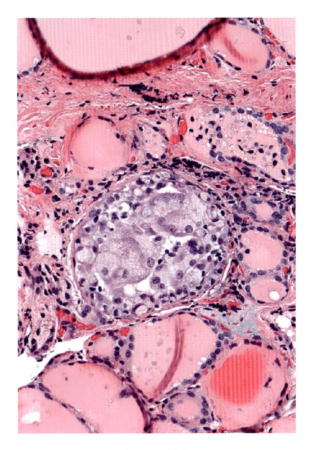

Figure 17-33

SO-CALLED PALPATION THYROIDITIS

A single follicle shows degeneration of the lining epithelium and packing of the lumen by multinucleated giant cells and lymphocytes.

cludes a variable number of eosinophils (figs. 17-34, 17-35) (84).

Rosai-Dorfman Disease

Several cases of thyroid involvement by *Rosai-Dorfman disease* (*sinus histiocytosis with massive lymphadenopathy*) have been reported, almost always in females. Some probably represent secondary extension from adjacent lymph nodes (85). In others, the thyroid gland is the site of primary involvement. Clinically, Rosai-Dorfman disease may simulate subacute thyroiditis and anaplastic carcinoma (86,87). The remainder of the gland is often affected by lymphocytic or Hashimoto thyroiditis (88). Also, involvement of anterior cervical-midline lymph nodes by Rosai-Dorfman disease may clinically simulate a thyroid mass (89).

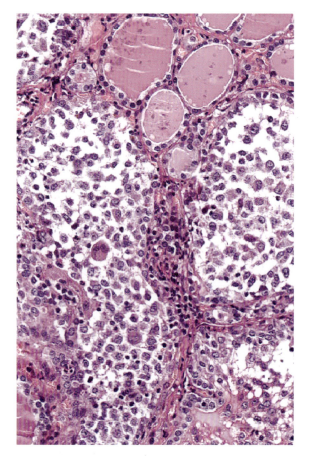

Figure 17-34

LANGERHANS CELL HISTIOCYTOSIS

Intrathyroidal highly cellular nodules are largely composed of Langerhans cells, some multinucleated.

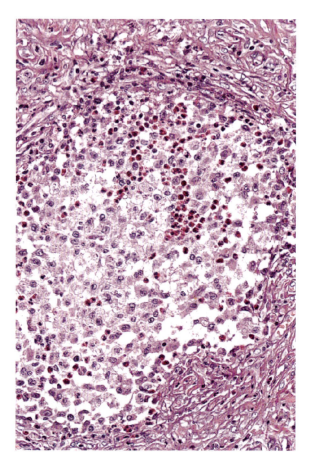

Figure 17-35

LANGERHANS CELL HISTIOCYTOSIS

Alternating clusters of Langerhans cells and eosinophils in a nodule surrounded by fibrous tissue.

RADIATION CHANGES

Exposure of the thyroid gland to external radiation, whether accidental or therapeutic, results in a variety of morphologic alterations. Low-dose radiation (less than 1,500 rads), which has been used in the past for a variety of benign conditions, has a marked potential for inducing thyroid alterations on a long-term basis. The most common abnormalities are nodular hyperplasia (which reached an incidence of 16.5 percent in one series [90]) and follicular adenoma (91). Similar changes occur after high-dose irradiation, such as that administered for Hodgkin lymphoma (92). In both instances, the hyperplastic nodules may be extremely hypercellular and exhibit marked cytologic atypia, characterized by nuclear enlargement, vesicular changes with nucleolar prominence, nuclear crowding,

and hyperchromasia (fig. 17-36). This atypia is distributed in a random fashion within the various nodules. The combination of radiation-induced nuclear atypia and papillary hyperplastic changes can result in a very disturbing microscopic picture. Other abnormalities often seen in these glands include fibrosis, hyalinization, and chronic inflammation.

A dramatic example of the consequences of accidental external radiation is the accident at the Chernobyl nuclear power station in April 1986, as a result of which a large segment of the population of the Republic of Belarus was exposed to high doses of radiation. Radioiodines, mainly ^{131}I, were abundant in the fallout and resulted in a variety of neoplastic and nonneoplastic diseases of the thyroid gland, which are still being monitored and categorized. The

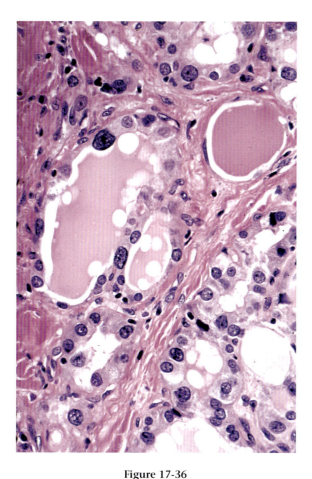

Figure 17-36

**THYROID FOLLICLES WITH
RADIATION-INDUCED CHANGES**

There is marked nuclear pleomorphism and hyperchromasia, but the follicular architecture is preserved.

tumors (mainly papillary carcinoma) are discussed in chapter 7. The non-neoplastic conditions included nodular goiter, diffuse hyperplasia, lymphocytic thyroiditis, perifollicular fibrosis, follicular atrophy, and cellular atypia (93).

RET/PTC gene rearrangements (often *RET/ PTC3*) are present in many radiation-associated papillary carcinomas that develop after therapeutic radiation to the neck or after the Chernobyl accident. These rearrangements are sometimes detected in postradiation cases diagnosed histologically as follicular adenomas or hyperplastic nodules. Other oncogenic mutations present in thyroid tumors (e.g., *BRAF, RAS, TP53*) are not associated with radiation exposure (94–96).

Systemic administration of radioactive iodine for therapeutic purposes can induce changes of similar type but usually of much lesser degree (97). Euthyroid glands usually display a fibrotic atrophic pattern, whereas those from hyperthyroid patients retain hyperplastic and inflammatory (Hashimoto thyroiditis-like) alterations (98). Whether radioactive iodine therapy results in an increased incidence of malignancy in the thyroid gland or other sites remains a controversial issue (99).

AMYLOID GOITER

Amyloid goiter is the term given to the form of thyroid amyloidosis accompanied by clinical enlargement of the gland (fig. 17-37). It may be unilateral or bilateral and nodular or diffuse, and is commonly associated with a foreign

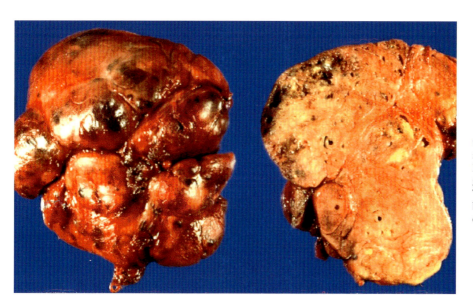

Figure 17-37

AMYLOIDOSIS

The illustration shows the outer aspect and cut surface of localized amyloidosis of the thyroid gland ("amyloid tumor"). The gland is enlarged and bosselated, and has a salmon color on cross section.

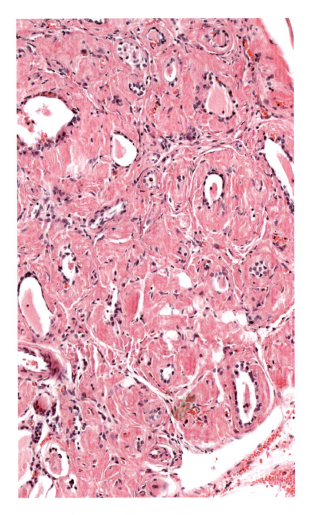

Figure 17-38

AMYLOIDOSIS

The abundant amyloid material surrounds follicles and vessels.

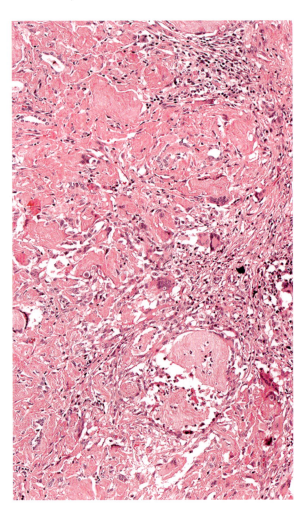

Figure 17-39

AMYLOIDOSIS

The amyloid material has elicited a foreign body-type multinucleated giant cell reaction.

body-type giant cell reaction. The amyloid deposition may be limited to the thyroid gland or, more commonly, accompanied by deposition in other organs (100).

Microscopically, the amyloid deposits are located in the vessel walls and other interfollicular (particularly perifollicular) sites, sometimes massively and diffusely (figs. 17-38, 17-39) (101). Curiously, they are often accompanied by the presence of mature adipose tissue in the stroma. The ultrastructural appearance (nonbranching 9-nm fibrils) and histochemical reactivity (congophilia with apple-green birefringence under polarized light) are typical of amyloid material in general (fig. 17-40). The amyloid deposited in amyloid goiter is usually of the AA type, but cases of the AL type are also on record (102,103).

The differential diagnosis includes amyloid deposition in medullary carcinoma, amyloidosis associated with multiple myeloma (in which the amyloid is of AL type) (104), and conditions resulting in heavy hyalinization (such as hyalinizing trabecular adenoma).

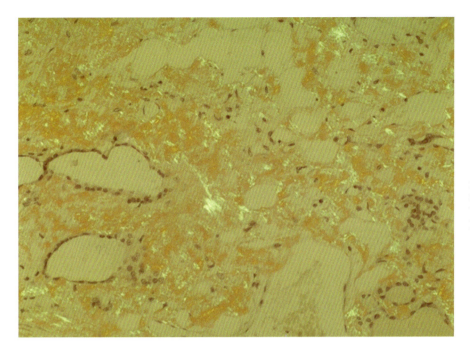

Figure 17-40

AMYLOIDOSIS

Apple-green birefringence is apparent in this Congo red-stained slide of amyloidosis of the thyroid gland seen under polarized light.

REFERENCES

1. Medeiros-Neto G. Iodine deficiency disorders. Thyroid 1990;1:73-82.
2. Pearce EN, Andersson M, Zimmermann MB. Global iodine nutrution: where do we stand in 2013? Thyroid 2013;23:523-8.
3. Zimmermann MB, Jooste PL, Pandav CS. Iodine-deficiency disorders. Lancet 2008;372:1251-62.
4. Mortensen JD, Woolner LB, Bennett WA. Gross and microscopic findings in clinically normal thyroid glands. J Clin Endocrinol Metab 1955;15:1270-80.
5. Tunbridge WM, Evered DC, Hall R, et al. The spectrum of thyroid disease in a community: the Whickham survey. Clin Endocrinol (Oxf) 1977;7:481-93.
6. Derwahl M, Studer H. Nodular goiter and goiter nodules: where iodine deficiency falls short of explaining the facts. Exp Clin Endocrinol Diabetes 2001;109:250-60.
7. Bondeson L, Bondeson AG. Michelangelo's divine goitre. J R Soc Med 2003;96:609-11.
8. Krohn K, Führer D, Bayer Y, et al. Molecular pathogenesis of euthyroid and toxic multinodular goiter. Endocr Rev 2005;26:504-24.
9. Jovanovic L, Delahunt B, McIver B, Eberhardt NL, Grebe SK. Thyroid gland clonality revisited: the embryonal patch size of the normal human thyroid gland is very large, suggesting X-chromosome inactivation tumor clonality studies of thyroid tumors have to be interpreted with caution. J Clin Endocrinol Metab 2003;88:3284-91.
10. Salmon I, Gasperin P, Remmelink M, et al. Ploidy level and proliferative activity measurements in a series of 407 thyroid tumors or other pathologic conditions. Hum Pathol 1993;24:912-20.
11. Belge G, Roque L, Soares J, et al. Cytogenetic investigations of 340 thyroid hyperplasias and adenomas revealing correlations between cytogenetic findings and histology. Cancer Genet Cytogenet 1998;101:42-8.
12. Krohn K, Wohlgemuth S, Gerber H, Paschke R. Hot microscopic areas of iodine-deficient euthyroid goitres contain constitutively activating TSH receptor mutations. J Pathol 2000;192:37-42.
13. Vasko V, Ferrand M, Di Cristofaro J, Carayon P, Henry JF, de Micco C. Specific pattern of RAS oncogene mutations in follicular thyroid tumors. J Clin Endocrinol Metab 2003;88:2745-52.
14. Patchefsky AS, Hoch WS. Psammoma bodies in diffuse toxic goiter. Am J Clin Pathol 1972;57:551-6.
15. Perez-Montiel MD, Suster S. The spectrum of histologic changes in thyroid hyperplasia: a clinicopathologic study of 300 cases. Hum Pathol 2008;39:1080-7.

16. Damiani S, Fratamico F, Lapertosa G, Dina R, Eusebi V. Alcian blue and epithelial membrane antigen are useful markers in differentiating benign from malignant papillae in thyroid lesions. Virchows Arch A Pathol Anat Histopathol 1991;419:131-5.

17. Leoni F, Fabbri R, Pascarella A, et al. Extramedullary haematopoiesis in thyroid multinodular goitre preceding clinical evidence of agnogenic myeloid metaplasia. Histopathology 1996;28:559-61.

18. Lazzi S, Als C, Mazzucchelli L, Kraft R, Kappeler A, Laissue J. Extensive extramedullary hematopoiesis in a thyroid nodule. Mod Pathol 1996;9:1062-5.

19. Weetman AP. Graves' disease. N Engl J Med 2000;343:1236-48.

20. Brent GA. Clinical practice. Graves' disease. N Engl J Med 2008;358:2594-605.

21. Erickson LA, Yousef OM, Jin L, Lohse CM, Pankratz VS, Lloyd RV. p27kip1 expression distinguishes papillary hyperplasia in Graves' disease from papillary thyroid carcinoma. Mod Pathol 2000;13:1014-9.

22. Mizukami Y, Michigishi T, Nonomura A, et al. Histologic changes in Graves' thyroid gland after 131I therapy for hyperthyroidism. Acta Pathol Jpn 1992;42:419-26.

23. Hanson GA, Komorowski RA, Cerletty JM, Wilson SD. Thyroid gland morphology in young adults: normal subjects versus those with prior low-dose neck irradiation in childhood. Surgery 1983;94:984-8.

24. Targovnik HM, Citterio CE, Rivolta CM. Thyroglobulin gene mutations in congenital hypothyroidism. Horm Res Paediatr 2011;75:311-21.

25. Rubio IG, Medeiros-Neto G. Mutations of the thyroglobulin gene and its relevance to thyroid disorders. Curr Opin Endocr Diabetes Obes 2009;16:373-8.

26. Camargo RY, Gross JL, Silveiro SP, Knobel M, Medeiros-Neto G. Pathological findings in dyshormonogenetic goiter with defective iodide transport. Endocr Pathol 1998;9:225-33.

27. Rego KG, Billerbeck AE, Targovnik HM, et al. Clinical, pathological, and molecular studies of two families with iodide organification defect. Endocr Pathol 1997;8:37-47.

28. Kopp P, Bizhanova A. Clinical and molecular characteristics of Pendred syndrome. Ann Endocr (Paris) 2011;72:88-94.

29. Ghossein RA, Rosai J, Heffess C. Dyshormonogenetic goiter: a clinicopathologic study of 56 cases. Endocr Pathol 1997;8:283-92.

30. Fadda G, Baloch ZW, LiVolsi VA. Dyshormonogenetic goiter pathology. Int J Surg Pathol 1999;7:125-31.

31. Kennedy JS. The pathology of dyshormonogenetic goitre. J Pathol 1969;99:251-64.

32. Milles G. Structural features of goiters in sporadic cretins. Am J Pathol 1955;31:997-1003.

33. Smith JF. The pathology of the thyroid in the syndrome of sporadic goitre and congenital deafness. Q J Med 1960;29:297-303.

34. Matos PS, Bisi H, Medeiros-Neto G. Dyshormonogenetic goiter: a morphological and immunohistochemical study. Endocr Pathol 1994;5:49-58.

35. Abs R, Verhelst J, Schoofs E, De Somer E. Hyperfunctioning metastatic follicular thyroid carcinoma in Pendred's syndrome. Cancer 1991;67:2191-3.

36. Vickery AL Jr. The diagnosis of malignancy in dyshormonogenetic goiter. Clin Endocrinol Metab 1981;10:317-35.

37. Cooper DS, Axelrod L, DeGroot LJ, Vickery AL Jr, Maloof F. Congenital goiter and the development of metastatic follicular carcinoma with evidence for a leak of nonhormonal iodide: clinical, pathological, kinetic, and biochemical studies and a review of the literature. J Clin Endocrinol Metab 1981;52:294-306.

38. Pearce EN, Farwell AP, Braverman LE. Thyroiditis. N Engl J Med 2003;348:2646-55.

39. Dayan CM, Daniels GH. Chronic autoimmune thyroiditis. N Engl J Med 1996;335:99-107.

40. Desailloud R, Hober D. Viruses and thyroiditis: an update. Virol J 2009;6:5.

41. Barbesino G, Chiovato L. The genetics of Hashimoto's disease. Endocr Metab Clin North Am 2000;29:357-74.

42. Hsi ED, Singleton TP, Svoboda SM, Schnitzer B, Ross CW. Characterization of the lymphoid infiltrate in Hashimoto thyroiditis by immunohistochemistry and polymerase chain reaction for immunoglobulin heavy chain gene rearrangement. Am J Clin Pathol 1998;110:327-33.

43. Vollenweider I, Hedinger C. Solid cell nests (SCN) in Hashimoto's thyroiditis. Virchows Arch A Pathol Anat Histopathol 1988;412:357-63.

44. Asioli S, Erickson LA, Lloyd RV. Solid cell nests in Hashimoto's thyroiditis sharing features with papillary thyroid microcarcinoma. Endocr Pathol 2009;20:197-203.

45. Chan JK, Albores-Saavedra J, Battifora H, Carcangiu ML, Rosai J. Sclerosing mucoepidermoid carcinoma with eosinophilia. A distinctive low-grade thyroid malignancy arising from the metaplastic follicles of Hashimoto's thyroiditis. Am J Surg Pathol 1991;15:438-48.

46. Caillou B. Ductal metaplasia in chronic lymphocytic thyroiditis as a manifestation of phylogenic regression to an exocrine structure. Am J Surg Pathol 2006;30:774-81.

47. Louis DN, Vickery AL Jr, Rosai J, Wang CA. Multiple branchial cleft-like cysts in Hashimoto's thyroiditis. Am J Surg Pathol 1989;13:45-9.

48. Ryska A, Vokurka J, Michal M, Ludvíková M. Intrathyroidal lymphoepithelial cyst. A report of two cases not associated with Hashimoto's thyroiditis. Pathol Res Pract 1997;193:777-81.

49. Vanni R, Marras-Virdis S, Gerosa C, Lai ML, Tallini G. Cytogenetics of thyroid nodules in Hashimoto thyroiditis. Cancer Genet Cytogenet 2000;120:87-8.

50. Hunt JL, Baloch ZW, Barnes L, et al. Loss of heterozygosity mutations of tumor suppressor genes in cytologically atypical areas in chronic lymphocytic thyroiditis. Endocr Pathol 2002;13:321-30.

51. Rhoden KJ, Unger K, Salvatore G, et al. RET/papillary thyroid cancer rearrangement in nonneoplastic thyrocytes: follicular cells of Hashimoto's thyroiditis share low-level recombination events with a subset of papillary carcinoma. J Clin Endocrinol Metab 2006;91:2414-23.

52. Schmid KW, Ofner C, Ramsauer T, et al. CA 19-9 expression in subacute (de Quervain's) thyroiditis: an immunohistochemical study. Mod Pathol 1992;5:268-72.

53. Harach HR, Williams ED. Fibrous thyroiditis—an immunopathological study. Histopathology 1983;7:739-51.

54. Schwaegerle SM, Bauer TW, Esselstyn CB Jr. Riedel's thyroiditis. Am J Clin Pathol 1988;90:715-22.

55. Chan JK, Carcangiu ML, Rosai J. Papillary carcinoma of thyroid with exuberant nodular fasciitis-like stroma. Report of three cases. Am J Clin Pathol 1991;95:309-14.

56. Papi G, LiVolsi VA. Current concepts on Riedel thyroiditis. Am J Clin Pathol 2004;121:S50-63.

57. Neild GH, Rodriguez-Justo M, Wall C, Connolly JO. Hyper-IgG4 disease: report and characterisation of a new disease. BMC Med 2006;4:23.

58. Dahlgren M, Khosroshahi A, Nielsen GP, Deshpande V, Stone JH. Riedel's thyroiditis and multifocal fibrosclerosis are part of the IgG4-related systemic disease spectrum. Arthritis Care Res (Hoboken) 2010;62:1312-8.

59. Julie C, Vieillefond A, Desligneres S, Schaison G, Grunfeld JP, Franc B. Hashimoto's thyroiditis associated with Riedel's thyroiditis and retroperitoneal fibrosis. Pathol Res Pract 1997;193:573-7; discussion, 578.

60. Baloch ZW, Feldman MD, LiVolsi VA. Combined Riedel's disease and fibrosing Hashimoto's thyroiditis: a report of three cases with two showing coexisting papillary carcinoma. Endocr Pathol 2000;11:157-63.

61. Li Y, Zhou G, Ozakai T, et al. Distinct histopathological features of Hashimoto's thyroiditis with respect to IgG4-related disease. Mod Pathol 2012;25:1086-97.

62. Poli F, Trezzi R, Fellegara G, Rosai J. Multifocal sclerosing thyroiditis. Int J Surg Pathol 2009;17:144.

63. Frank R, Baloch ZW, Gentile C, Watt CD, LiVolsi VA. Multifocal fibrosing thyroiditis and its association with papillary thyroid carcinoma using BRAF pyrosequencing. Endocr Pathol 2013 [Epub ahead of print].

64. Katoh R, Ishizaki T, Tomichi N, Yagawa K, Kurihara H. Malakoplakia of the thyroid gland. Am J Clin Pathol 1989;92:813-20.

65. Larsimont D, Hamels J, Fortunati D. Thyroid-gland malakoplakia with autoimmune thyroiditis. Histopathology 1993;23:491-4.

66. Carney JA, Moore SB, Northcutt RC, Woolner LB, Stillwell GK. Palpation thyroiditis (multifocal granulomatours folliculitis). Am J Clin Pathol 1975;64:639-47.

67. Mizukami Y, Michigishi T, Nonomura A, et al. Postpartum thyroiditis. A clinical, histologic, and immunopathologic study of 15 cases. Am J Clin Pathol 1993;100:200-5.

68. LiVolsi VA. Postpartum thyroiditis. The pathology slowly unravels. Am J Clin Pathol 1993;100:193-5.

69. Manson CM, Cross P, De Sousa B. Post-operative necrotizing granulomas of the thyroid. Histopathology 1992;21:392-3.

70. Mizukami Y, Nonomura A, Michigishi T, Ohmura K, Matsubara S, Noguchi M. Sarcoidosis of the thyroid gland manifested initially as thyroid tumor. Pathol Res Pract 1994;190:1201-5.

71. Schmitz KJ, Baumgaertel MW, Schmidt C, Sheu SY, Betzler M, Schmid KW. Wegener's granulomatosis in the thyroid mimicking a tumour. Virchows Arch 2008;452:571-4.

72. Lima MK, Freitas LL, Montandon C, Filho DC, Silva-Vergara ML. The thyroid in acquired immunodeficiency syndrome. Endocr Pathol 1998;9:217-23.

73. Teja K, Sabio H, Langdon DR, Johanson AJ. Involvement of the thyroid gland in histiocytosis X. Hum Pathol 1981;12:1137-9.

74. Saiz E, Bakotic BW. Isolated Langerhans cell histiocytosis of the thyroid: a report of two cases with nuclear imaging-pathologic correlation. Ann Diagn Pathol 2000;4:23-8.

75. Elliott DD, Sellin R, Egger JF, Medeiros LJ. Langerhans cell histiocytosis presenting as a thyroid gland mass. Ann Diagn Pathol 2005;9:267-74.

76. Coode PE, Shaikh MU. Histiocytosis X of the thyroid masquerading as thyroid carcinoma. Hum Pathol 1988;19:239-41.

77. Yap WM, Chuah KL, Tan PH. Langerhans cell histiocytosis involving the thyroid and parathyroid glands. Mod Pathol 2001;14:111-5.

78. Lassalle S, Hofman V, Santini J, Sadoul JL, Hofman P. Isolated Langerhans cell histiocytosis of the thyroid and Graves' disease: an unreported association. Pathology 2008;40:525-7.

79. Vergez S, Rouquette I, Ancey M, Serrano E, Caron P. Langerhans cell histiocytosis of the thyroid is a rare entity, but an association with a papillary thyroid carcinoma is often described. Endocr Pathol 2010;21:274-6.

80. Goldstein N, Layfield LJ. Thyromegaly secondary to simultaneous papillary carcinoma and histiocytosis X. Report of a case and review of the literature. Acta Cytol 1991;35:422-6.

81. Schofield JB, Alsanjari NA, Davis J, Maclennan KA. Eosinophilic granuloma of lymph nodes associated with metastatic papillary carcinoma of the thyroid. Histopathology 1992;20:181-3.

82. Safali M, McCutcheon JM, Wright DH. Langerhans cell histiocytosis of lymph nodes: draining a papillary carcinoma of the thyroid. Histopathology 1997;30:599-603.

83. Schofield JB, Alsanjari NA, Davis J, MacLennan KA. Eosinophilic granuloma of lymph nodes associated with metastatic papillary carcinoma of the thyroid. Histopathology 1992;20:181-3.

84. Thompson LD, Wenig BM, Adair CF, Smith BC, Heffess CS. Langerhans cell histiocytosis of the thyroid: a series of seven cases and a review of the literature. Mod Pathol 1996;9:145-9.

85. Carpenter RJ III, Banks PM, McDonald RJ, Sanderson DR. Sinus histiocytosis with massive lymphadenopathy (Rosai-Dorfman disease): report of a case with respiratory tract involvement. Laryngoscope 1978;88:1963-9.

86. Larkin DF, Dervan PA, Munnelly J, Finucane J. Sinus histiocytosis with massive lymphadenopathy simulating subacute thyroiditis. Hum Pathol 1986;17:321-4.

87. Powell JG, Goellner JR, Nowak LE, McIver B. Rosai-Dorfman disease of the thyroid masquerading as anaplastic carcinoma. Thyroid 2003;13:217-21.

88. Lee FY, Jan YJ, Chou G, Wang J, Wang CC. Thyroid involvement in Rosai-Dorfman disease. Thyroid 2007;17:471-6.

89. Cocker RS, Kang J, Kahn LB. Rosai-Dorfman disease. Report of a case presenting as a midline thyroid mass. Arch Pathol Lab Med 2003;127:e197-200.

90. Favus MJ, Schneider AB, Stachura ME, et al. Thyroid cancer occurring as a late consequence of head-and-neck irradiation. Evaluation of 1056 patients. N Engl J Med 1976;294:1019-25.

91. Ron E, Brenner A. Non-malignant thyroid diseases after a wide range of radiation exposures. Radiat Res 2010;174:877-88.

92. Carr RF, LiVolsi VA. Morphologic changes in the thyroid after irradiation for Hodgkin's and non-Hodgkin's lymphoma. Cancer 1989;64:825-9.

93. Nikiforov YE, Heffess CS, Korzenko AV, Fagin JA, Gnepp DR. Characteristics of follicular tumors and nonneoplastic thyroid lesions in children and adolescents exposed to radiation as a result of the Chernobyl disaster. Cancer 1995;76:900-9.

94. Bounacer A, Wicker R, Caillou B, et al. High prevalence of activating ret proto-oncogene rearrangements, in thyroid tumors from patients who had received external radiation. Oncogene 1997;15:1263-73.

95. Elisei R, Romei C, Vorontsova T, et al. RET/PTC rearrangements in thyroid nodules: studies in irradiated and not irradiated, malignant and benign thyroid lesions in children and adults. J Clin Endocrinol Metab 2001;86:3211-6.

96. Rabes HM, Demidchik EP, Sidorow JD, et al. Pattern of radiation-induced RET and NTRK1 rearrangements in 191 post-Chernobyl papillary thyroid carcinomas: biological, phenotypic, and clinical implications. Clin Cancer Res 2000;6:1093-103

97. Kennedy JS, Thomson JA. The changes in the thyroid gland after irradiation with 131I or partial thyroidectomy for thyrotoxicosis. J Pathol 1974;112:65-81.

98. Friedman NB, Catz B. The reactions of euthyroid and hyperthyroid glands to radioactive iodine. Arch Pathol Lab Med 1996;120:660-1.

99. Lee SL. Complications of radioactive iodine treatment of thyroid carcinoma. J Natl Compr Canc Netw 2010;8:1277-86.

100. Hamed G, Heffess CS, Shmookler BM, Wenig BM. Amyloid goiter. A clinicopathologic study of 14 cases and review of the literature. Am J Clin Pathol 1995;104:306-12.

101. Goldsmith JD, Lai ML, Daniele GM, Tomaszewski JE, LiVolsi VA. Amyloid goiter: report of two cases and review of the literature. Endocr Pract 2000;6:318-23.

102. Kanoh T, Shimada H, Uchino H, Matsumura K. Amyloid goiter with hypothyroidism. Arch Pathol Lab Med 1989;113:542-4.

103. Moriuchi A, Yokoyama S, Kashima K, Andoh T, Nakayama I, Noguchi S. Localized primary amyloid tumor of the thyroid developing in the course of Hashimoto's thyroiditis. Acta Pathol Jpn 1992;42:210-6.

104. Hirota S, Miyamoto M, Kasugai T, Kitamura Y, Morimura Y. Crystalline light-chain deposition and amyloidosis in the thyroid gland and kidneys of a patient with myeloma. Arch Pathol Lab Med 1990;114:429-31.

18 BENIGN THYROID TISSUE IN ABNORMAL LOCATIONS

There are several situations in which benign thyroid tissue is found outside the anatomic confines of, and anatomically separate from, the thyroid gland. It is important to be aware of them in order to avoid an overdiagnosis of metastatic thyroid carcinoma.

ECTOPIA

A migration failure along the pathway of the thyroglossal duct (see chapter 1) can result in the presence of *ectopic thyroid tissue* anywhere between the foramen cecum at the base of the tongue and the normal site of the gland (fig. 18-1) (1–4). The most common sites for ectopic tissue are: 1) the base of the tongue (lingual thyroid); 2) beneath the tongue (sublingual thyroid); and 3) in or around the hyoid bone (as a component of a thyroglossal duct cyst). On occasion, the opposite phenomenon occurs, in which the thyroglossal duct migrates excessively, resulting in mediastinal thyroid tissue. It is likely, however, that most substernal thyroid glands with features of nodular hyperplasia were originally in their normal cervical position and were pulled down by the hyperplastic nodular transformation that occurred within them.

Lingual thyroid tissue is rare as a clinical problem but common as an incidental microscopic finding (fig. 18-2). In one series, almost 10 percent of tongues examined at autopsy had remnants of thyroid tissue in them (5). When voluminous, lingual thyroid may result in dysphagia, bleeding, and severe respiratory distress (3,6). In most instances, the diagnosis is made during adolescence, and a predominance in women has been noted (5,7,8). In over 75 percent of the cases, the migration failure is total, and no thyroid tissue is present in the normal location; however, some follicles may be found in the hyoid region (8–10). In such cases, removal of the lingual thyroid may result in permanent hypothyroidism.

Microscopically, the ectopic thyroid follicles usually appear normal, but the irregular interface with the surrounding skeletal muscle fibers and the hypercellularity that they may exhibit can result in a pseudomalignant appearance (fig. 18-3) (11). True malignant tumors arising in lingual thyroid tissue are rare. Close to 100 cases have been reported, but not all are convincing (8,12,13). Interestingly, most of them were diagnosed as follicular rather than papillary carcinomas (14). This includes a unique case of poorly differentiated Hürthle cell carcinoma (15).

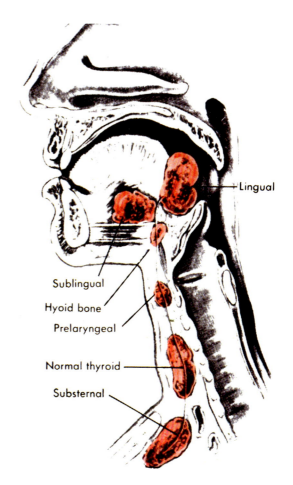

Figure 18-1

LOCATIONS OF ECTOPIC THYROID TISSUE

All of the locations shown in this diagram are in, or close to, the midline, along the course of the thyroglossal duct.

Figure 18-2

ECTOPIC LINGUAL THYROID TISSUE

The ectopic gland presents as a bulge at the base of the tongue.

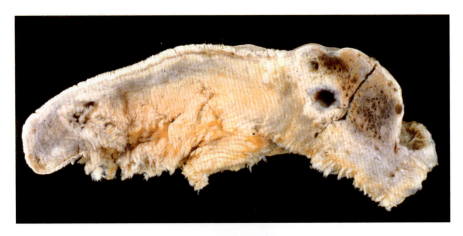

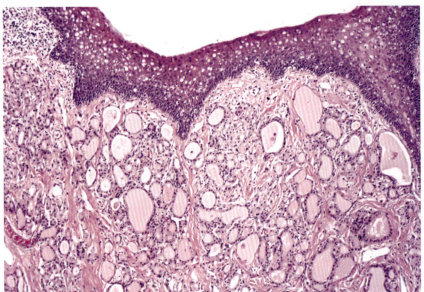

Figure 18-3

ECTOPIC LINGUAL THYROID TISSUE

Normal-looking thyroid follicles are located beneath the squamous epithelium of the tongue.

Thyroglossal duct cyst is nearly always connected with the hyoid bone (1). Upward movement of the mass on swallowing is characteristic of this condition. Most cysts measure from 1 to 2 cm in diameter (fig. 18-4). The original lining epithelium of the duct is cuboidal ("transitional") or columnar, and often ciliated. It tends to become squamous or to disappear altogether as a result of secondary inflammatory changes (16). Thyroid tissue is found in the wall of the cyst in over half of the cases, usually in the form of irregular aggregates of follicles. Immunoreactivity for thyroid transcription factor (TTF)-1 (but not thyroglobulin) is often detectable in the lining epithelium (17).

The treatment of thyroglossal duct cyst is surgical. It includes the removal of the middle third of the hyoid bone and the suprahyoid tract up to the foramen cecum (18). This extended operation prevents most recurrences, although a few still develop (19).

The thyroid tissue in thyroglossal duct cyst may have a normal appearance, exhibit inflammatory or hyperplastic nodular changes, or be the site of a malignancy. The latter event is an unusual but well-documented complication of this condition. Nearly all of the reported malignancies have been papillary thyroid carcinomas (fig. 18-5), but there are also scattered reports of other tumor types, including follicular carcinoma and undifferentiated or squamous carcinoma (20–26). The outstanding absence is medullary carcinoma, and this can be explained by the fact that C-cells have a different embryologic source. The papillary carcinoma arising in a thyroglossal duct cyst is morphologically identical to its

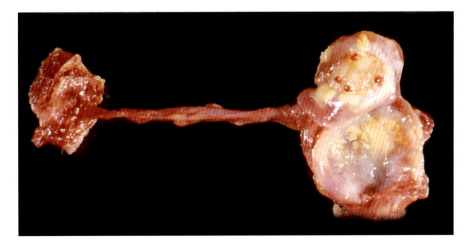

Figure 18-4

ECTOPIC THYROID WITH PAPILLARY CARCINOMA

A large tumor nodule is present at one end of the thyroglossal duct.

Figure 18-5

ECTOPIC THYROID WITH PAPILLARY CARCINOMA

This papillary carcinoma arose from the thyroid epithelium of a thyroglossal duct.

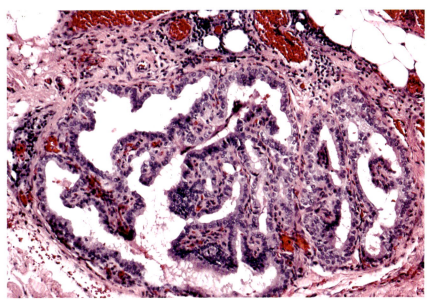

homologue in the orthotopic gland, and its behavior is similar as well. Removal of the cyst containing the tumor is usually curative. The possibility of an independent papillary carcinoma in the thyroid gland itself is remote, and there is, therefore, no need for a prophylactic thyroidectomy if the gland is normal on palpation and scintigraphic examination.

All instances of ectopic thyroid tissue related to the thyroglossal duct appear as midline lesions, in keeping with the path of descent of this embryologic structure. Thyroid tissue located laterally in the neck may still be of benign nature (see Parasitic Nodule below) but cannot be ascribed to the developmental abnormality discussed here.

Other sites of ectopic thyroid tissue have been documented (27). They include larynx (28),

trachea (29), submandibular region (30), aortic arch (31), heart and pericardium (fig. 18-6) (32), mediastinal esophagus (33), stomach (34), diaphragm, region of gallbladder/common bile duct/porta hepatis (35–37), adrenal gland (38, 39), retroperitoneum, inguinal region, vagina (40), and sella turcica (41). There are also isolated reports of ectopic thyroid tissue in the lung (42,43), but it may be difficult to rule out the alternative possibility of a well-differentiated metastasis from an occult thyroid carcinoma.

MECHANICAL IMPLANTATION

Normal or abnormal thyroid tissue disrupted mechanically from the main gland can lodge in the soft tissues of the neck, survive, and thereby result in the formation of a discrete nodule,

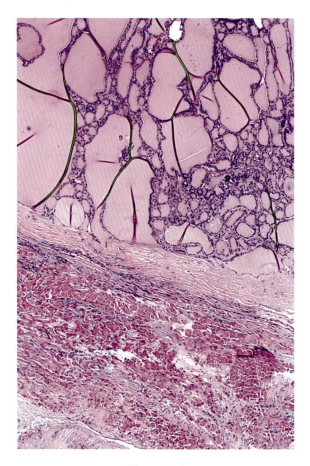

Figure 18-6

PARASITIC THYROID NODULE

This thyroid nodule, which shows features of nodular hyperplasia, was attached to the heart, and intimately admixed with myocardial fibers.

usually of microscopic size. The most common scenario for this event is a previous operation. The *implanted thyroid tissue* is likely to be surrounded by a fibrous reaction, and suture material may be detected nearby (44–46).

Implantation of thyroid tissue may also be the result of accidental trauma. We know of a patient with a thyroid adenoma who had a crush injury to the neck. Months later, an operation disclosed numerous little nodules of adenomatous thyroid tissue scattered throughout the region (E. D. Williams, personal communication, 2004). The event seems analogous to that referred to in the spleen as splenosis, and may therefore be designated *thyroidosis* or *strumosis*.

PARASITIC NODULE

A *parasitic (sequestered) nodule* is the focal expression of nodular hyperplasia (adenomatoid goiter) in which one of the most peripherally located nodules is anatomically separate from the main gland, or so it appears to the surgeon (figs. 18-7, 18-8). It is a much more common process than suggested by the meager number of reports (47–49). Many pathologists and surgeons do not know of its existence and, as a result, often diagnose this innocuous condition as malignant. Many of the cases labeled as aberrant lateral thyroid tissue in the past are examples of parasitic nodules; others represent metastatic well-differentiated carcinomas in cervical lymph nodes (see chapter 7). The parasitic nodule is probably the result of nodular

Figure 18-7

PARASITIC THYROID NODULE

The parasitic nodule is connected to the main gland only by vessels.

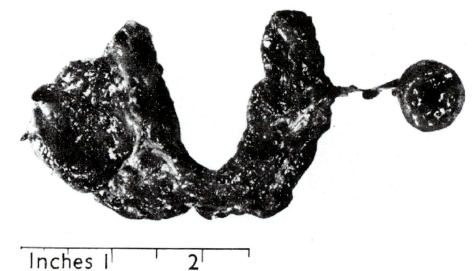

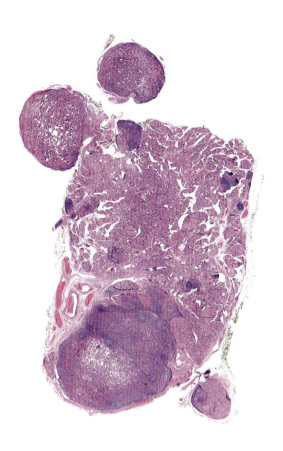

Figure 18-8

PARASITIC THYROID NODULE

Panoramic view of thyroid gland with associated parasitic nodules.

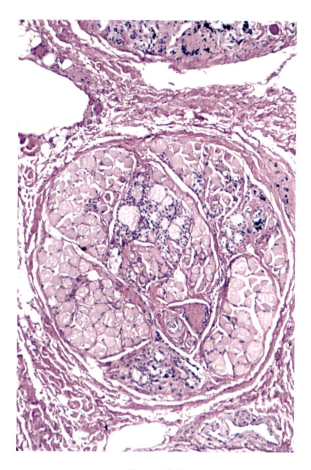

Figure 18-9

NON-NEOPLASTIC THYROID TISSUE INSIDE SKELETAL MUSCLE

This normal finding should not be misinterpreted as extrathyroid extension and muscle invasion by a thyroid carcinoma.

enlargement of thyroid tissue originally located outside the capsule of the gland, a common microscopic finding (fig. 18-9) (50).

At the time of surgery, a thin pedicle is found in some cases, joining the nodule to the thyroid gland (fig. 18-6). In other cases, the original connection with the main organ is lost or was never present, and a new vascular supply may have been acquired. Whatever the mechanism, the result is a detached thyroid nodule. The clue to the diagnosis is the microscopic appearance of a benign hyperplastic process throughout the nodule and similar morphologic features in the orthotopic gland, if it has been removed or sampled (fig. 18-10). No lymph node remnants should be found around the nodule, which

should also be devoid of any of the cytoarchitectural features that characterize conventional papillary carcinoma or its follicular variant.

A particularly treacherous variant of this phenomenon occurs when the parasitic nodule is seen in the context of nodular Hashimoto thyroiditis (Hashimoto thyroiditis plus nodular hyperplasia). In this case, the nodule is likely to feature a prominent lymphoid component that may simulate a residual lymph node, as well as the nuclear features that often accompany Hashimoto thyroiditis, such as partial nuclear clearing or the opposite phenomenon of bizarre hyperchromatic nuclei. Here, too, comparison with the orthotopic gland and realization that the changes present in it are the same as

Figure 18-10

PARASITIC THYROID NODULE

Both the parasitic nodule and the main gland (not shown) were involved by Hashimoto thyroiditis and nodular hyperplasia. This combination results in a particularly treacherous pitfall.

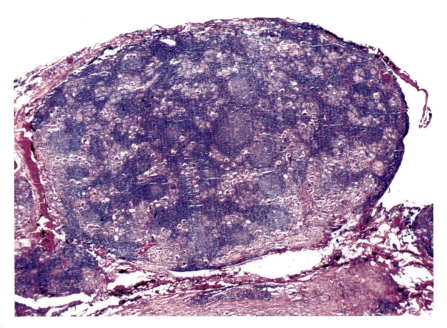

those in the nodule should lead to a correct interpretation of the lesion. The same criteria apply to the unusual cases of parasitic nodules in patients with Graves disease due to diffuse thyroid hyperplasia (51).

Parasitic thyroid nodules are not restricted to the neck. They also occur in the anterosuperior mediastinum, usually as a result of nodular hyperplasia (mediastinal goiter) and through a mechanism analogous to the one described above. Because of their protected and hidden location, mediastinal parasitic nodules may reach a much larger size than those found in the neck.

THYROID INCLUSIONS IN LYMPH NODES

The presence of histologically normal-looking thyroid follicles within the confines of a cervical lymph node is a controversial issue (52). Some authors believe that these formations represent metastatic foci from an occult thyroid primary, regardless of how well differentiated they appear (44,53). There is no question that metastatic thyroid cancer may present initially in a cervical node in the absence of an obvious thyroid nodule and that the microscopic appearance of this metastasis may closely resemble non-neoplastic thyroid tissue. For this reason, the criteria for benign thyroid inclusions need to be stringent. In any case in which the

thyroid tissue has replaced one third or more of the node, several nodes are affected, or the involvement includes the nodal parenchyma (as opposed to being limited to the capsular/subcapsular region) the diagnosis of metastasis is to be favored. This is also true whenever the intranodal thyroid tissue shows any of the cytoarchitectural features of papillary carcinoma (e.g., abortive papillae or ground-glass nuclei). The presence of psammoma bodies is almost proof that the process is metastatic, no matter how benign its microscopic appearance. In summary, for intranodal thyroid tissue to be regarded as benign, it should be restricted to a few small follicles located in or immediately beneath the nodal capsule, and these follicles should have an unremarkable architectural and cytologic (especially nuclear) appearance (54). In doubtful cases, molecular analysis, especially for *BRAF*, may prove useful.

Good evidence in favor of the existence of this phenomenon was provided by Meyer and Steinberg (55). The authors identified five cases at autopsy in which one of the cervical nodes contained thyroid tissue and serially sectioned the entire thyroid gland in those cases in search of an occult primary. Only one tumor was found (a papillary microcarcinoma), and this was located in the thyroid lobe on the side opposite the nodal inclusion.

The fact that this phenomenon does occur should not be surprising. Well-documented examples of ectopic benign tissue in lymph nodes are plentiful. They include salivary gland, müllerian epithelium ("endosalpingiosis"), breast, nevus cells, and mesothelial cells.

THYROID AS A COMPONENT OF TERATOMA (INCLUDING STRUMA OVARII)

Thyroid tissue is a common component of ovarian teratomas, but is seen only exceptionally in teratomas of testis or extragonadal sites. The thyroid tissue may appear normal or exhibit diffuse or nodular hyperplastic changes. Cases of hyperthyroidism resulting from the hyperfunction of teratoma-based thyroid tissue are on record (56,57).

In some instances, the thyroid tissue is the predominant or sole component of the ovarian lesion, a process interpreted as a monodermal form of teratoma and designated as *struma ovarii* (57). An intriguing variation is *strumal carcinoid*, an ovarian neoplasm in which thyroid tissue coexists with a carcinoid tumor, usually in the absence of other teratomatous elements (55). Early suggestions that this tumor represents a medullary carcinoma arising from C-cells located in the thyroid tissue have not been confirmed. The neoplasm is usually devoid of amyloid, usually negative for calcitonin at the immunohistochemical level, and has a morphologic appearance more in keeping with a trabecular carcinoid of pulmonary or gastrointestinal type.

Malignant neoplasms of bonafide thyroid type (i.e., composed of thyroid follicular cells) developing in struma ovarii are rare (56–61).

Most of the cases reported in the old literature have been diagnosed as follicular carcinomas, but using current criteria many of them would qualify as the follicular variant of papillary carcinoma (62,63). Papillary carcinoma of the classic type also occurs (64).

The differential diagnosis is with proliferative struma ovarii, which is regarded as a form of struma ovarii with unusually florid hyperplastic changes (65). In general, the criteria used in the orthotopic thyroid for the identification of papillary carcinoma (including its follicular variant) and poorly differentiated carcinoma (as recommended in the Turin proposal, see chapter 8) apply (66). A more difficult situation arises with well-differentiated follicular neoplasms, since capsular invasion is impossible to evaluate. An unresolved issue concerns cases of struma ovarii associated with peritoneal implants, which can be extensive, and whether they are to be regarded as metastases of extremely well-differentiated carcinomas or as examples of thyroidosis/strumosis (63,67,68). The reader is referred to the Fascicle, Tumors of the Ovary, Maldeveloped Gonads, Fallopian Tube, and Broad Ligament (69), for a more detailed discussion of these issues. Another curious finding with potential histogenetic implications is the recent description of thyroid-type solid nests in association with struma ovarii (70).

The molecular alterations that characterize orthotopic thyroid tumors (e.g. *BRAF V600E*, *RET/PTC, RAS* mutations) have been described in the corresponding carcinomas arising in struma ovarii (71–73), indicating that the same molecular mechanisms of tumorigenesis operate.

REFERENCES

1. Allard RH. The thyroglossal cyst. Head Neck Surg 1982;5:134-46.
2. Guimaraes SB, Uceda JE, Lynn HB. Thyroglossal duct remnants in infants and children. Mayo Clin Proc 1972;47:117-20.
3. Larochelle D, Arcand P, Belzile M, Gagnon NB. Ectopic thyroid tissue—a review of the literature. J Otolaryngol 1979;8:523-30.
4. Guerra G, Cinelli M, Mesolella M, et al. Morphological, diagnostic and surgical features of ectopic thyroid gland: a review of literature. Int J Surg 2014;pii: S1743-9191.
5. Baughman RA. Lingual thyroid and lingual thyroglossal tract remnants. A clinical and histopathologic study with a review of the literature. Oral Surg 1972;34:781-99.
6. Reaume CE, Sofie VL. Lingual thyroid. Review of the literature and report of a case. Oral Surg Oral Med Oral Pathol 1978;45:841-5.
7. Kansal P, Sakati N, Rifai A, Woodhouse N. Lingual thyroid. Diagnosis and treatment. Arch Intern Med 1987;147:2046-8.
8. Neinas FW, Gorman CA, Devine KD, Woolner LB. Lingual thyroid. Clinical characteristics of 15 cases. Ann Intern Med 1973;79:205-10.
9. Strickland AL, Macfie JA, Van Wyk JJ, French FS. Ectopic thyroid glands simulating thyroglossal duct cysts. Hypothyroidism following surgical excision. JAMA 1969;208:307-10.
10. Talib H. Lingual thyroid. Br J Clin Pract 1966;20:322-3.
11. Wapshaw H. Lingual thyroid. Br J Surg 1942;30:160-5.
12. Fish J, Moore RM. Ectopic thyroid tissue and ectopic thyroid carcinoma: a review of the literature and report of a case. Ann Surg 1963;157:212-22.
13. Smithers DW. Carcinoma associated with thyroglossal duct anomalies. In: Smithers DW, ed. Tumours of the thyroid gland. Edinburgh: Livingstone, 1970:155-65.
14. Hari CK, Kumar M, Abo-Khatwa MM, Adams-Williams J, Zeitoun H. Follicular variant of papillary carcinoma arising from lingual thyroid. Ear Nose Throat J 2009;88:E7.
15. Seoane JM, Cameselle-Teijeiro J, Romero MA. Poorly differentiated oxyphilic (Hürthle cell) carcinoma arising in lingual thyroid: a case report and review of the literature. Endocr Pathol 2002;13:353-60.
16. Soucy P, Penning J. The clinical relevance of certain observations on the histology of the thyroglossal tract. J Pediatr Surg 1984;19:506-9.
17. Kreft A, Hansen T, Kirkpatrick CJ. Thyroid transcription factor 1 expression in cystic lesions of the neck: an immunohistochemical investigation of thyroglossal duct cysts, branchial cleft cysts and metastatic papillary thyroid cancer. Virchows Arch 2005;447:9-11.
18. Solomon JR, Rangecroft L. Thyroglossal-duct lesions in childhood. J Pediatr Surg 1984;19:555-61.
19. Ein SH, Shandling B, Stephens CA, Mancer K. The problem of recurrent thyroglossal duct remnants. J Pediatr Surg 1984;19:437-9.
20. Jaques DA, Chambers RG, Oertel JE. Thyroglossal tract carcinoma. A review of the literature and addition of eighteen cases. Am J Surg 1970;120:439-46.
21. Joseph TJ, Komorowski RA. Thyroglossal duct carcinoma. Hum Pathol 1975;6:717-29.
22. LiVolsi VA, Perzin KH, Savetsky L. Carcinoma arising in median ectopic thyroid (including thyroglossal duct tissue). Cancer 1974;34:1303-15.
23. Mobini J, Krouse TB, Klinghoffer JF. Squamous cell carcinoma arising in a thyroglossal duct cyst. Am Surg 1974;40:290-4.
24. Nussbaum M, Buchwald RP, Ribner A, Mori K, Litwins J. Anaplastic carcinoma arising from median ectopic thyroid (thyroglossal duct remnant). Cancer 1981;48:2724-8.
25. Ruppmann E, Georgsson G. Squamous carcinoma of the thyroglossal duct. Ger Med Mon 1966;11:442-7.
26. Villet WT, Kemp CB. Thyroglossal duct carcinoma. A case report and a review of the literature. S Afr Med J 1981;60:795-6.
27. Kaplan M, Kauli R, Lubin E, Grunebaum M, Laron Z. Ectopic thyroid tissue. A clinical study of 30 children and review. J Pediatr 1978;92:205-9.
28. Bone RC, Biller HF, Irwin TM. Intralaryngotracheal thyroid. Ann Otol Rhinol Laryngol 1972;81:424-8.
29. Donegan JO, Wood MD. Intratracheal thyroid—familial occurrence. Laryngoscope 1985;95:6-8.
30. Babazade F, Mortazavi H, Jalalian H, Shahvali E. Thyroid tissue as a submandibular mass: a case report. J Oral Sci 2009;51:655-7.
31. Williams RJ, Lindop G, Butler J. Ectopic thyroid tissue on the ascending aorta: an operative finding. Ann Thorac Surg 2002;73:1642-3.
32. Pollice L, Caruso G. Struma cordis. Ectopic thyroid goiter in the right ventricle. Arch Pathol Lab Med 1986;110:452-3.
33. Postlethwait RW, Detmer DE. Ectopic thyroid nodule in the esophagus. Ann Thorac Surg 1975;19:98-100.

34. Hammers YA, Kelly DR, Muensterer OJ, Hardin WD Jr, Saeed SA, Mroczek-Musulman EC. Giant polypoid gastric heterotopia with ectopic thyroid tissue: unusual cause of jejuno-jejunal intussusception. J Pediatr Gastroenterol Nutr 2007;45:484-7.

35. Cassol CA, Noria D, Asa SL. Ectopic thyroid tissue within the gall bladder: case report and brief review of the literature. Endocr Pathol 2010;21:263-5.

36. Sekine S, Nagata M, Hamada H, Watanabe T. Heterotopic thyroid tissue at the porta hepatis in a fetus with trisomy 18. Virchows Arch 2000;436:498-501.

37. Harach HR. Ectopic thyroid tissue adjacent to the gallbladder. Histopathology 1998;32:90-91.

38. Shiraishi T, Imai H, Fukutome K, Watanabe M, Yatani R. Ectopic thyroid in the adrenal gland. Hum Pathol 1999;30:105-8.

39. Romero-Rojas A, Bella-Cueto MR, Meza-Cabrera IA, et al. Ectopic thyroid tissue in the adrenal gland: a report of two cases with pathogenetic implications. Thyroid 2013;23:1644-50.

40. Kurman RJ, Prabha AC. Thyroid and parathyroid glands in the vaginal wall: report of a case. Am J Clin Pathol 1973;59:503-7.

41. Ruchti C, Balli-Antunes H, Gerber HA. Follicular tumor in the sellar region without primary cancer of the thyroid. Heterotopic carcinoma? Am J Clin Pathol 1987;87:776-80.

42. Simon M, Baczako K. Thyroid inclusion in the lung. Metastasis of an occult papillary carcinoma or ectopia? Pathol Res Pract 1989;184:263-7.

43. Di Mari N, Barbagli L, Mourmouras V, Miracco C. Ectopic thyroid of the lung. An additional case. Pathologica 2010;102:102-3.

44. Block MA, Wylie JH, Patton RB, Miller JM. Does benign thyroid tissue occur in the lateral part of the neck? Am J Surg 1966;112:476-81.

45. Klopp CT, Kirson SM. Therapeutic problems with ectopic non-cancerous follicular thyroid tissue in the neck: 18 case reports according to etiological factors. Ann Surg 1966;163:653-64.

46. Moses DC, Thompson NW, Nishiyama RH, Sisson JC. Ectopic thyroid tissue in the neck. Benign or malignant. Cancer 1976;38:361-5.

47. Hathaway BM. Innocuous accessory thyroid nodules. Arch Surg 1965;90:222-7.

48. Sisson JC, Schmidt RW, Beierwaltes WH. Sequestered nodular goiter. N Engl J Med 1964;270:927-32.

49. Rodriguez J, Rosai J. Parasitic nodules of the thyroid, a metastasis simulator. A study of 76 cases, Lab Invest 2006;86(Suppl.):96A (Abstract)

50. Hanson GA, Komorowski RA, Cerletty JM, Wilson SD. Thyroid gland morphology in young adults: normal subjects versus those with prior low-dose neck irradiation in childhood. Surgery 1983;96:984-8.

51. Shimizu M, Hirokawa M, Manabe T. Parasitic nodule of the thyroid in a patient with Graves' disease. Virchows Arch 1999;434:241-4.

52. Anila KR, Sebastian P, Somanathan T, George NA, Jayasree K. Significance of incidentally detected thyroid tissue in lymph nodes of neck dissections in patients with head and neck carcinoma. Int J Surg Pathol 2012;20:564-9.

53. Ward R. Relation of tumors of lateral aberrant thyroid tissue to malignant disease of the thyroid gland. Arch Surg 1940;40:606-15.

54. Frantz VK, Forsythe R, Hanford JM, Rogers WM. Lateral aberrant thyroids. Ann Surg 1942;115:161-83.

55. Meyer JS, Steinberg LS. Microscopically benign thyroid follicles in cervical lymph nodes. Serial section study of lymph node inclusions and entire thyroid gland in 5 cases. Cancer 1969;24:302-11.

56. Kempers RD, Dockerty MB, Hoffman DL, Bartholomew LG. Struma ovarii—ascitic, hyperthyroid, and asymptomatic syndromes. Ann Intern Med 1970;72:883-93.

57. Woodruff JD, Rauh JT, Markley RL. Ovarian struma. Obstet Gynecol 1966;27:194-202.

58. Robboy SJ, Scully RE. Strumal carcinoid of the ovary: an analysis of 50 cases of a distinctive tumor composed of thyroid tissue and carcinoid. Cancer 1980;46:2019-34.

59. Pardo-Mindán FJ, Vázquez JJ. Malignant struma ovarii. Light and electron microscopic study. Cancer 1983;51:337-43.

60. Rosenblum NG, LiVolsi VA, Edmonds PR, Mikuta JJ. Malignant struma ovarii. Gynecol Oncol 1989;32:224-7.

61. Willemse PH, Oosterhuis JW, Aalders JG, et al. Malignant struma ovarii treated by ovariectomy, thyroidectomy, and 131I administration. Cancer 1987;60:178-82.

62. Brunskill PJ, Rollason TP, Nicholson HO. Malignant follicular variant of papillary struma ovarii. Histopathology 1990;17:574-6.

63. Garg K, Soslow RA, Rivera M, Tuttle MR, Ghossein RA. Histologically bland "extremely well differentiated" thyroid carcinomas arising in struma ovarii can recur and metastasize. Int J Gynecol Pathol 2009;28:222-30.

64. Zhang X, Axiotis C. Thyroid-type carcinoma of struma ovarii. Arch Pathol Lab Med 2010;134:786-91.

65. Devaney K, Snyder R, Norris HJ, Tavassoli FA. Proliferative and histologically malignant struma ovarii: a clinicopathologic study of 54 cases. Int J Gynecol Pathol 1993;12:333-43.

66. Roth LM, Talerman A, Wadsley J, Karseladze AI. Risk factors in thyroid-type carcinoma arising in ovarian struma: a report of 15 cases with comparison to ordinary struma ovarii. Histopathology 2010;57:148-52.

67. Shaco-Levy R, Bean SM, Bentley RC, Robboy SJ. Natural history of biologically malignant struma ovarii: analysis of 27 cases with extraovarian spread. Int J Gynecol Pathol 2010;29:212-27.

68. Robboy SJ, Shaco-Levy R, Peng RY, et al. Malignant struma ovarii: an analysis of 88 cases, including 27 with extraovarian spread. Int J Gynecol Pathol 2009;28:405-22.

69. Scully RE, Young RH, Clement PB. Tumors of the ovary, maldeveloped gonads, fallopian tube, and broad ligament. AFIP Atlas of Tumor Pathology, 3rd Series, Fascicle 23. Washington, DC: American Registry of Pathology; 1998.

70. Cameselle-Teijeiro J, Caramés N, Romero-Rojas A, et al. Thyroid-type solid cell nests in struma ovarii. Int J Surg Pathol 2011;19:627-31.

71. Flavin R, Smyth P, Crotty P, et al. BRAF T1799A mutation occurring in a case of malignant struma ovarii. Int J Surg Pathol 2007;15:116-20.

72. Coyne C, Nikiforov YE. RAS mutation-positive follicular variant of papillary thyroid carcinoma arising in a struma ovarii. Endocr Pathol 2010:21:144-7.

73. Boutross-Tadross O, Saleh R, Asa SL. Follicular variant papillary thyroid carcinoma arising in struma ovarii. Endocr Pathol 2007;18:182-6.

19 MOLECULAR GENETIC ALTERATIONS OF SPECIFIC THYROID TUMORS OF FOLLICULAR CELLS

FOLLICULAR ADENOMA AND VARIANTS

There is no molecular test that currently can be used to distinguish follicular adenoma from follicular carcinoma. Genetic alterations such as chromosomal abnormalities, activating *RAS* mutations, and the *PAX8/PPARγ* rearrangement, often found in carcinoma, are also encountered in adenoma, albeit usually with a lower prevalence (Table 19-1). The main molecular alterations found in follicular adenoma are discussed below with follicular carcinomas.

The available evidence indicates that follicular adenomas and carcinomas share the same tumorigenic pathway, which is different from

Table 19-1

MUTATED GENES AND CHROMOSOMAL ALTERATIONS IN THYROID TUMORS OF FOLLICULAR CELLS

Follicular Adenoma	Follicular Carcinoma	Papillary Carcinoma (Conventional Type)	Encapsulated Follicular Variant of Papillary Carcinoma	Poorly Differentiated Thyroid Carcinoma	Undifferentiated (Anaplastic) Thyroid Carcinoma
RAS (20-40)[a]	*RAS* (30-50)	*BRAF* (30-70)	*RAS* (25-45)	*RAS* (20-50)	*TP53* (50-80)
PAX8/PPARγ (5-20)	*PAX8/PPARγ* (20-50)	*RET/PTC* (10-40)	*BRAF* (5-10)	*TERT* (20-50)	*TERT* (30-50)
TSHR and *GNAS*[b]	*TERT* (10-35)	*TERT* (5-25)	*TERT* (5-10)	*TP53* (15-40)	*RAS* (20-50)
Chromosomal DNA unstable[d], karyotypes with simple abnormalities in 35-65% of cases	*PIK3CA* (0-10)	*RAS* (0-10)	*RET/PTC* (0-10)	*BRAF* (5-15)	*BRAF* (10-50)
	PTEN (0-10)	*NTRKI* rearrangement (0-10)	*PAX8/PPARγ* (0-30)	*PIK3CA* (5-10)	*CTNNB1*[c] (5-65)
	Chromosomal DNA unstable[d], abnormal karyotypes in ~65% of cases	Chromosomal DNA stable[d], karyotypes with simple abnormalities in 10-40% of cases	Chromosomal DNA unstable[d], alterations similar to follicular neoplasms	*CTNNB1*[c] (0-25)	*PIK3CA* (5-25)
				ALK rearrangement (0-10)	*PTEN* (5-15)
				Chromosomal DNA unstable[d], complex karyotypic alterations	*ALK* rearrangement (0-10)
					Chromosomal DNA unstable and highly aneuploid[d], complex karyotypic alterations

[a]In parenthesis the mutation prevalence estimated from the literature, percentage range.
[b]Hyperfunctioning follicular adenomas and hyperplastic nodules have thyroid-stimulating hormone (TSH)-receptor gene (*TSHR*) mutations in ~50-80% of cases and Gsα gene (*GNAS*) mutations in ~5% of cases.
[c]The gene encoding β-catenin.
[d]According to conventional cytogenetics, cytometric measurement of DNA content, comparative genomic hybridization, and loss of heterozygosity.

that of papillary thyroid carcinoma (see chapter 2) (1,2). As a corollary to this, it may be argued that follicular adenomas with a specific molecular alteration, e.g., *PAX8/PPARγ* rearrangement, are in fact noninvasive or preinvasive follicular carcinomas, or that the tumor has not been adequately sampled. This possibility is supported by the more common occurrence of the rearrangement in follicular carcinoma and also by the high cellularity and "atypical" features of some follicular adenomas with the *PAX8/PPARγ* rearrangement (3). A similar argument can be made for *RAS* mutations, since *RAS*-mutated follicular adenomas may progress to *RAS*-mutated follicular carcinomas and undergo further dedifferentiation (2,4).

While *RAS* mutations and even *PAX8/PPARγ* rearrangements occur in follicular adenomas, *PTEN* gene mutations are not usually identified in sporadic adenomas (5). This is somewhat surprising considering that loss of function germline *PTEN* mutations are responsible for the Cowden syndrome, which is characterized by multiple follicular adenomas and adenomatous nodules (see follicular adenoma in Hereditary Syndromes below). Indeed, the PI3K/PTEN/AKT pathway does not appear to play an important role in the development of follicular adenoma not related to Cowden syndrome. Activating *PIK3CA* mutations are rare (up to about 5 percent of cases) and *PIK3CA* gene amplification is not common (up to 10 to 20 percent of cases) (5). The *BRAF* K601E mutation has been reported in rare follicular adenomas (6). Follicular adenoma and benign thyroid nodules express lower levels of full-length *TERT* transcripts, have lower telomerase activity, and have longer telomeres when compared with carcinomas (7–9). Measuring *TERT* expression may be useful to differentiate benign from malignant thyroid nodules, even in fine-needle aspiration samples, but telomerase activity and *TERT* expression in lymphoid cells have to be taken into account (7,8). *TERT* promoter mutations are rare, and when present the adenoma usually has atypical features (10). Rearrangement of the *ALK* gene has not been reported (11).

Follicular adenomas are neoplasms and, as such, are expected to be clonal when analyzed by methods that exploit the random inactivation of genes on the X chromosome to determine the clonality status (clonal versus polyclonal) in samples from female patients. Although most follicular adenomas are clonal when examined with these methods (12–15), several studies have found that a significant proportion of hyperplastic nodules are also clonal (12,16). This may reflect the true clonal origin of nodules that look clearly hyperplastic on histologic grounds. It may also point to some limitations of X chromosome inactivation analysis. In fact, since the size of the embryonal X chromosome inactivation patch in the thyroid gland is large (0.5 to 1.0 cm^2), microdissection of the area of interest before DNA extraction may yield false positive results (17). Conversely, DNA obtained from a larger area may produce results difficult to interpret due to contamination with nonlesional tissue. In either case, X chromosome inactivation analysis should be interpreted with caution and cannot be used as an absolute criterion to distinguish follicular adenomas from hyperplastic thyroid nodules (17).

Conventional karyotyping identifies aberrations in 35 to 65 percent of follicular adenomas, with both numerical changes and structural abnormalities that overlap with those of follicular carcinomas (18–20). Numerical changes are characterized by trisomy 7, with a sequence that begins with an extra copy of chromosome 7, followed by the acquisition of additional copies of other chromosomes. This sequence has been shown to parallel the morphologic transition from hyperplastic to adenomatous nodules (18).

Structural abnormalities typically involve 19q13.4 with a breakpoint at the *ZNF331* gene locus (21) or 2p21 with a breakpoint at the *THADA* (thyroid adenoma associated) gene locus (22). These alterations are mutually exclusive and together are detectable in about 10 percent of cases by karyotyping but in a somewhat higher proportion by fluorescence in situ hybridization (FISH) (23). The genes involved fuse to partners that vary with the translocation (22). Importantly, 19q13.4 and 2p21 rearrangements do not appear to be a feature of follicular carcinoma (24).

Cytometric measurements of DNA content (25–27) and comparative genomic hybridization studies identify aneuploidy in both follicular adenomas and carcinomas (28). Approximately 25 percent of nononcocytic follicular adenomas are aneuploid by flow cytometry (25–27). Although the degree of aneuploidy increases from adenomas to carcinomas and from indolent carcinomas to aggressive tumors, the overlap of DNA content in these groups is too large to be diagnostically or prognostically useful (26). The segmental amplification of chromosomes 7 and 12, and chromosome 22 deletions found in follicular adenoma may help to distinguish the latter from the follicular variant of papillary carcinoma (29).

"Toxic" Adenoma

"Toxic" adenoma, also known as *hyperfunctioning adenoma* or *Plummer adenoma*, is a follicular adenoma that is scintigraphically "hot" and sometimes associated with overt hyperthyroidism (see chapter 5). These tumors typically have activating mutations in the genes encoding for the thyroid stimulating hormone (TSH) receptor (*TSHR*) or its associated *Gsα* subunit protein (*GNAS*), which lead to activation of the cyclic AMP pathway. Mutations in one of the two genes are detected in up to 90 percent of cases (30). *TSHR* mutations are more common and are reported with a prevalence of 50 to 80 percent, compared to about 5 percent for the *Gsα* gene (*GNAS*) (30,31). Despite the variability related to the detection method, the prevalence of *TSHR* and *Gsα* gene mutations is essentially the same in different parts of the world and appears independent of dietary iodine intake (32,33).

Hyalinizing Trabecular Adenoma

Hyalinizing trabecular adenoma does not share *BRAF* mutations with papillary carcinoma or *RAS* mutations with follicular neoplasms (34,35). The *RET/PTC* rearrangement, a marker of papillary carcinoma, has been detected in some studies (34,36,37), but not in others (35). The studies that identified *RET/PTC* used highly sensitive methods to detect the rearrangement and the biologic relevance of this finding is uncertain (2). The fact that miRNAs known to be upregulated in papillary carcinoma (such as miR-146b, -181b, -21, -221, -222) are not overexpressed in hyalinizing trabecular tumors does not support a link between the two (35).

Follicular Adenoma in Hereditary Syndromes

The presence of *multiple follicular adenomas*, particularly in young patients, may be a clue to the diagnosis of Cowden syndrome, an autosomal dominant disorder with germline inactivating mutations of the *PTEN* gene (38). Patients with this syndrome develop multicentric follicular adenomas and hyperplastic nodules (39) with a wide range of cytoarchitectural patterns, including microadenomatous foci, oncocytic and clear cell changes, and sometimes, lesions with the features of hyalinizing trabecular adenoma and adenolipoma. Patients are usually in the third decade of life by the time these thyroid lesions become clinically evident (39). The fact that they also develop follicular carcinoma (see Follicular Carcinoma below) suggests that the carcinoma evolves from a preexisting follicular adenoma, thus supporting the concept that benign and malignant follicular neoplasms share a common pathway.

Hyperplastic nodules and follicular adenomas that are hyperfunctioning are a major feature of the McCune-Albright syndrome, caused by sporadic, postzygotic activating mutations of the *Gsα* gene (*GNAS*) (40). Follicular adenomas and hyperplastic nodules also occur in the Carney complex, a disease due to inactivating germline mutations of the *PRKAR1A* gene (41,42). The occurrence of follicular carcinomas in the background of hyperplastic nodules has been reported in both diseases (41,43,44).

FOLLICULAR CARCINOMA

As stated above, follicular carcinomas share with follicular adenomas a common tumorigenic pathway. This pathway is different from that of a papillary carcinoma, and is characterized by the frequent occurrence of *RAS* mutations and other alterations, including the *PAX8/PPARγ* rearrangement and aneuploidy (see chapter 2). The main genetic alterations of follicular carcinomas are summarized in Table 19-1.

RAS Mutation

RAS mutations are identified in 30 to 50 percent of follicular carcinomas, and represent the most common oncogenic alteration of this tumor type (1,2). *H-RAS, K-RAS,* and *N-RAS* are closely related genes that encode a family of G proteins with a key role in relaying signals originating at the cell membrane to the MAPK and the PI3K/PTEN/AKT pathways (see chapter 2). In follicular carcinoma, as well as in other thyroid tumors, *K-RAS*, *N-RAS*, and *H-RAS* may all be affected, but mutations at codon 61 of *N-RAS* followed by *H-RAS* codon 61 mutations are those most frequently reported (4,45). *RAS* mutations are uncommon in conventional papillary carcinoma. They represent instead a marker for follicular-patterned thyroid lesions since they are usually identified with comparable frequencies in follicular carcinoma, follicular adenoma, and the follicular variant of papillary carcinoma (45,46).

The fact that *RAS* mutations have been associated with unfavorable clinical features and poor outcome, and that they are frequently found in poorly differentiated and undifferentiated (anaplastic) carcinomas, suggests that they have a role in promoting tumor progression (47–49). A meta-analysis of the cases reported in the literature, where the presence of *RAS* mutations was confirmed by direct sequencing, has shown that mutations at codon 61 of *N-RAS* and at codon 61 of *H-RAS* are more frequent in follicular carcinoma than in adenoma or other benign thyroid nodules (p<0.03 for codon 61 of *N-RAS* and p<0.02 for codon 61 of *H-RAS*) (4). Nevertheless, the variability in the prevalence and the specific types of *RAS* mutations reported in the literature is significant. It likely reflects a variety of factors, including specific methodologies for mutation detection and case selection, and the impact of the environment (2,4,50). A higher prevalence of *RAS* mutations has been reported in areas of iodine deficiency (50).

PPARγ Rearrangement

The *PAX8/PPARγ* (*PAX8/PPARG*) rearrangement, the result of the t(2;3)(q13;p25) that fuses the *PPARγ* gene located at 3p25 with *PAX8* at 2q13, is present in about one third of follicular carcinomas (1,2,51). It is unclear whether *PAX8/PPARγ* interacts with the same pathways activated by *RAS*, but the two molecular alterations rarely coexist in the same tumor (45,52). Originally thought to be specific, *PAX8/PPARγ* has also been found in a small proportion of follicular adenomas (5 to 20 percent in most studies) (3) and in a similar proportion of encapsulated follicular variant papillary carcinomas (53). A low prevalence of the rearrangement is generally reported in follicular oncocytic tumors (45,54,55).

The considerable variability in the prevalence of *PAX8/PPARγ* is at least partially due to the methods used for its detection (56). These include conventional karyotyping, reverse transcriptase polymerase chain reaction (RT-PCR), FISH, and immunohistochemistry with antibodies for PPARγ. FISH tends to be more sensitive than RT-PCR, although it is more difficult to standardize. One study based on FISH identified the rearrangement in 45 percent of follicular carcinomas, in 33 percent of follicular adenomas, and in 37 percent of follicular variant papillary carcinomas (52). When immunohistochemistry is used, only strong nuclear immunoreactivity for PPARγ should be scored and confirmation by molecular analysis is recommended (3). Importantly, the rearrangement has not been identified in benign thyroid tissue or hyperplastic nodules (3,55).

PAX8/PPARγ is rare in aggressive tumors such as poorly differentiated or undifferentiated thyroid carcinoma (57,58). In follicular carcinoma, it is associated with female gender, younger patient age, high cellularity, and locally invasive features (45). The risk for distant metastases may be lower for *PAX8/PPARγ* positive follicular carcinomas than for tumors lacking the rearrangement (54). Thus, *PAX8/PPARγ* appears to be a marker for a distinct subset of tumors characterized by follicular growth and invasive potential but lacking overtly aggressive features.

CREB3L2/PPARγ is the second rearranged form of *PPARγ* that has been identified in follicular carcinoma (59). The recombination is the result of the t(3;7)(p25;q34) that fuses the *PPARγ* gene with *CREB3L2* at 7q34. *CREB3L2/PPARγ* is not common and is estimated to be present in less than 3 percent of follicular carcinomas (59). The rearrangement has not been found in benign tumors or non-neoplastic thyroid lesions, including follicular adenoma, oncocytic adenoma, and Hashimoto thyroiditis (59). *PPARγ* rearrangements are not specifically associated with exposure to ionizing radiation, but both *PAX8/PPARγ* (60) and *CREB3L2/PPARγ* (61) have been reported in follicular variants of papillary carcinoma that developed after the Chernobyl nuclear accident.

PI3K/PTEN/AKT Pathway Dysregulation

AKT is a family of serine/threonine protein kinases, activated by PI3K and negatively regulated by PTEN. This signaling pathway regulates many important cellular functions, including proliferation, survival, and metabolism. Activated AKT phosphorylates and interacts with numerous targets, and the subcellular localization of AKT appears to be an important factor in determining its biologic effects (see chapter 2) (62–65). The PI3K/PTEN/AKT pathway becomes aberrantly activated in follicular carcinomas that develop in patients with Cowden syndrome, an inherited disease due to germline loss of function *PTEN* gene mutations (see Follicular Carcinoma in Hereditary Syndromes below).

In sporadic follicular carcinomas, inactivating *PTEN* mutations are usually reported in less than 10 percent of cases (5,65–67). Decreased PTEN mRNA and protein levels appear to be frequent, however (68–70), suggesting that loss of heterozygosity or epigenetic mechanisms, like *PTEN* promoter methylation, are a more common cause for reduced PTEN function (65,69,70).

Activating *PIK3CA* gene mutations have been reported in up to 10 percent of follicular carcinomas (5,65–67). Copy number gain of the *PIK3CA* gene is identified in 20 to 30 percent of cases, which correlates with the immunohistochemical expression of the protein (5), and has little overlap with *PIK3CA* gene mutations (5,66,67). *PTEN* and *PIK3CA* gene mutations, *PIK3CA* copy number gain, and *RAS* mutations rarely coexist in follicular carcinomas, pointing to an independent role for each alteration (5,66). The fact that in aggressive thyroid tumors and undifferentiated (anaplastic) carcinomas these alterations can overlap with each other and also with the *BRAF* mutations suggests a role for the PI3K/PTEN/AKT pathway in promoting tumor progression (5,58,66,71,72).

TERT

TERT is the protein core component with reverse transcriptase activity of the telomerase enzyme complex that maintains telomere length, thus allowing cell replication. It is encoded by the *TERT* gene and is expressed in thyroid tumors, including follicular and papillary carcinomas (see chapter 2). Similar to papillary carcinoma, follicular carcinomas have short telomeres, but express a high proportion of full-length *TERT* transcripts and have high telomerase enzymatic activity (7–9).

Rapidly following their original identification in melanoma in 2013, several groups reported two mutually exclusive oncogenic mutations of the promoter region of *TERT*, *C228T*, and *C250T*, activating its transcription in malignant tumors derived from follicular cells (73–76). *TERT* promoter mutations are present in approximately 20 percent of follicular carcinomas, but rare in follicular adenomas or other benign nodules (10,74–78). They are also uncommon in conventional and minimally invasive oncocytic tumors (73,77). Of the two mutations, *C228T* is the most common in follicular carcinoma, it is approximately 5 to 10 times more frequent than *C250T* (10,74,75,78).

TERT promoter mutations are usually identified in the subset of differentiated thyroid carcinomas, papillary and follicular, with unfavorable clinicopathologic features, and may represent an important prognostic factor (74,77,78). They have been associated with decreased survival in patients with follicular carcinoma (74,77). Poorly and undifferentitated (anaplastic) carcinomas have a higher proportion of *TERT* promoter mutations than conventional follicular carcinoma, suggesting that they support the development of aggressive forms of thyroid cancer (73–77). Cases with *PAX8/PPARγ* do not have *TERT* promoter mutations (77).

Chromosomal DNA and Other Somatic Genetic Alterations

At variance with papillary carcinoma, follicular neoplasms, both benign and malignant, commonly have cytogenetic imbalances that result in aneuploid DNA content and that are detected by loss of heterozygosity (LOH) studies. Progression from clinically benign or indolent to more aggressive tumors is paralleled by a higher prevalence of chromosomal DNA alterations and by an increase in their complexity.

Cytogenetic aberrations are found in about 65 percent of follicular carcinomas by conventional karyotyping, with both numerical changes and structural abnormalities, including the t(2;3)(q13,p25) associated with the *PAX8/PPARγ* rearrangement (see above) (19,20,79). The numerical changes are similar to those of follicular adenomas and include hyperdiploid karyotypes with extra copies of chromosome 7. In follicular carcinoma, however, unbalanced rearrangements and complex karyotypes are common, and chromosomal losses appear to be more frequent (18–20,79,80).

Cytometric measurements of DNA content (20) and comparative genomic hybridization (CGH) also identify aneuploidy in both follicular carcinomas and adenomas (28). Follicular carcinomas tend to have a higher degree of aneuploidy, but differences between benign and malignant tumors are of no diagnostic value in individual cases because of the overlap between the two groups. Based on the pattern of chromosomal DNA alterations and the degree of aneuploidy, Castro et al. (81) have postulated the existence of two groups of follicular neoplasms, independent of their classification as adenomas or carcinomas (81). One group features prominent aneuploidy, chromosomal gains, and microfollicular/trabecular/solid architecture. The other group features diploid or near-diploid DNA content with common chromosomal losses and normofollicular architecture (81). One study found a high rate of LOH in follicular carcinoma, about 20 percent per chromosome arm. This rate was much higher than that found in follicular adenoma (about 5 percent) or papillary carcinoma (about 2.5 percent) (82). Poor outcome in follicular carcinoma has been correlated with LOH at the *VHL* gene locus (83) and with high LOH rates at tumor suppressor gene loci (84).

In follicular carcinoma, receptor tyrosine kinase genes, particularly *EGFR* and *VEGFR1*, frequently have copy number gains, but no mutations have been detected in hot spot regions (66). Rearrangements or mutations of the *ALK* gene have not been reported (11,85).

TSHR and *Gsα* gene (*GNAS*) mutations are generally considered uncommon in follicular carcinoma (86), but their prevalence may be underestimated. Nikiforova et al. identified *TSHR* mutations in 4 of 18 follicular carcinomas using targeted next-generation sequencing (87). *TSHR* mutations have been identified in hyperfunctioning carcinomas, including cases showing poorly differentiated histologic features (88). The possible coexistence in hyperfunctioning carcinomas of *TSHR* mutations with other common mutations, such as those of *RAS,* suggests that in some tumors the latter drive the malignant transformation, while the *TSHR* mutation confers the hyperfunctioning features (89).

Markedly decreased expression of Rap1GAP (a Rap1 GTPase activating protein with putative tumor suppressor functions) has been reported in widely invasive follicular carcinoma, but in only a small proportion of minimally invasive tumors (90). The *BRAF* K601E mutation has been reported in a case of follicular carcinoma (91).

Many studies have analyzed the mRNA expression profile of follicular neoplasms, usually follicular carcinoma, and have shown that it is different from that of papillary carcinoma (92,93). Signatures that reliably distinguish between follicular adenoma and follicular carcinoma have been proposed, but they need validation in larger studies (94,95). Among the proposed markers is HGMA2, which is overexpressed in benign rather than malignant nodules (96–98). Similarly, dysregulated miRNA expression is well documented in follicular neoplasms (99). Expression of miR-197 and miR-346 at levels significantly higher in follicular carcinoma than in follicular adenoma has been reported in one study (100). Since miRNAs can be analyzed in formalin-fixed samples and in fine-needle aspiration specimens, their use appears particularly promising as an effective tool for the preoperative assessment of thyroid nodules (101).

Follicular Carcinoma in Hereditary Syndromes

Follicular carcinoma develops in a familial setting in the context of Cowden syndrome (38). This syndrome, together with other *PTEN* hamartoma tumor syndromes (Bannayan-Riley-Ruvalcaba syndrome, *PTEN*-related Proteus syndrome and Proteus-like syndrome), is part of a set of genetic disorders characterized by benign tumors and hamartomatous proliferations in various organs. It is inherited as an autosomal dominant trait and related to inactivating germline mutations of the *PTEN* tumor suppressor gene at 10q23.31 (102).

Germline *PTEN* mutations are present in up to 85 percent of patients that meet the diagnostic criteria for Cowden syndrome (102). This syndrome is the only *PTEN* hamartoma tumor syndrome with a well-documented link to malignant tumors: breast, thyroid gland, and endometrial carcinomas, in order of frequency. Follicular carcinoma is among the major criteria required for the clinical diagnosis. Patients with Cowden syndrome have a 10 percent lifetime risk of developing follicular carcinoma. Follicular carcinoma is not, however, an important cause of death (102). Reports of papillary carcinoma in patients with Cowden syndrome are most likely coincidental, and there is no association with medullary carcinoma (39). Follicular carcinoma develops in young patients who have multiple follicular adenomas and hyperplastic nodules, thus supporting the concept that follicular carcinoma develops from a preexisting follicular adenoma (39).

Follicular carcinoma has also been reported in patients with McCune-Albright syndrome, Carney complex, and Werner syndrome (adult progeria) (41,43,103).

In contrast with papillary carcinoma, familial aggregation of follicular carcinoma without syndromic extrathyroid pathology is uncommon: follicular carcinomas represent less than 10 percent of familial nonmedullary thyroid carcinomas (FNMTC) (104). In some instances, however, familial occurrence has been documented, including cases with metastatic disease (105).

PAPILLARY CARCINOMA AND VARIANTS

The main genetic alterations of papillary thyroid carcinoma (PTC) are summarized in Table 19-1. The most important feature is activation of the mitogen-activated protein kinase (MAPK) pathway (see chapter 2) (1,2). This activation is the consequence of three events: gene rearrangements (*RET/PTC* or the less common *NTRK1* and *NTRK3* rearrangements), activating mutations of *RAS*, and activating mutations of *BRAF*. These events act sequentially on the MAPK pathway in the order reported above and are therefore mutually exclusive. One or another of them is detected in the majority (70 percent) of the cases (1,2,6,106).

The oncogenic role of *RET/PTC*, *BRAF*, and *RAS* mutations on thyroid follicular cells has been demonstrated by numerous studies, in vitro and using transgenic animal models. As expected, cDNA expression analysis shows that these genetic alterations produce tumors that have similar, yet distinct, transcriptional profiles (107).

PTC is by far the most common type of thyroid carcinoma that develops after exposure to ionizing radiation, as shown in the survivors of the Hiroshima and Nagasaki atomic bombs and in patients exposed to radiation after the Chernobyl nuclear accident. In these tumors oncogenic rearrangements predominate over point mutations like *BRAF* V600E. PTCs with rearrangement tend to occur following higher radiation doses, and to develop after a shorter latency period. Uncommon types of *RET/PTC* and other oncogenic rearrangements like *ETV6/NTRK3* are specifically associated with exposure to ionizing radiation (60,61,108,109).

BRAF Mutations

Activating mutations of *BRAF* are found in about 45 percent of cases of PTC, thus representing the most common genetic alteration of this tumor type (110). Over 95 percent of *BRAF* mutations in PTC are thymine to adenine transversions at the nucleotide 1799 (T1799A) of exon 15. This nucleotide change replaces a valine (V) with a glutamate (E) at residue (codon) 600, leading to the *BRAF* V600E (*BRAF* Val600Glu) mutation (1,2). Although V600E accounts for the majority of mutations in other *BRAF*-mutated tumors (e.g., melanoma), in PTC it accounts for almost all of them (1,2).

Alternative forms of oncogenic *BRAF* are rare and include the K601E mutation (*BRAF* Lys601Glu), small insertion or deletions close to codon 600 (111), and a paracentric inversion of chromosome 7 that juxtaposes *BRAF* (at 7q34) with the gene *AKAP9* located at 7q21-22 (*AKAP9/BRAF*) (112). This chromosomal rearrangement is associated with radiation exposure and is identified in approximately 10 percent of PTCs that developed with short latency, during the first few years following the Chernobyl nuclear accident (112). Another radiation-associated intrachromosomal rearrangement fuses *BRAF* to *AGK* at 7q34, where both genes are located (61). The rearrangement was identified in 1 of 26 thyroid carcinomas that developed in children after the Chernobyl accident. The tumor with *AGK/BRAF* was a conventional (classic) papillary carcinoma, and the rearrangement was not found in control tumors from patients not exposed to radiation (61).

BRAF mutations are easy to identify using a variety of methods. They are reliably detected in nucleic acids extracted from different sources, including paraffin-embedded material, fine-needle aspiration samples, cells scraped from cytology smears after removal of the coverslip, and the peripheral blood of patients with PTC (113,114). A monoclonal antibody specific for the BRAF V600E mutated protein has also been developed (115).

The *BRAF* V600E mutation is essentially diagnostic of PTC, or of those poorly differentiated and undifferentiated carcinomas derived from PTC. A large meta-analysis of the data reported in the literature showed that *BRAF* V600E was absent in medullary and follicular carcinomas, as well as in over 500 benign thyroid nodules (110). The identification of *BRAF* V600E in PTC arising within struma ovarii confirms the specificity of the mutation (116,117). *BRAF* mutations have not been found in Hashimoto thyroiditis, even in cases containing non-neoplastic atypical follicular cells (118).

Among PTCs, the link of *BRAF* V600E is strongest with the tall cell variant and weakest with the follicular variant (53,119–122). The meta-analysis quoted above (110) reported *BRAF* V600E in 77 percent of tall cell PTCs and in 60 percent of conventional PTCs, but only in 12 percent of follicular variant papillary carcinomas (FVPTCs). In some series (122,123), as well as in our experience, *BRAF* V600E is present in virtually all cases of tall cell variant PTC. *BRAF* V600E-mutated tumors that do not fulfill all the criteria for the tall cell variant are often characterized by cells that are more polygonal but share with the tall cell variant several features, including the fully developed nuclear PTC alterations and the eosinophilic "oncocytoid" cytoplasm (124). *BRAF* activation is uncommon in the follicular variant, but *BRAF* mutations other than the V600E are usually found only in this tumor type (111,120). *BRAF* K601E has been reported in up to 7 percent of cases (120), as well as in rare follicular adenomas (6) and follicular carcinomas (91).

The proportion of conventional (classic) PTCs positive for *BRAF* V600E may have increased over time (125,126). In a large study of Chinese patients with PTC, the mutation was associated with high iodine levels in natural drinking water (127). Unlike *RET/PTC* and *AKAP9/BRAF* rearrangements, *BRAF* point mutations are not a feature of PTC related to radiation exposure (60,61,112,128).

The prognostic relevance of the *BRAF* V600E mutation in PTC is a matter of debate. A significant body of evidence indicates that *BRAF* V600E is a very important marker for aggressive behavior. Numerous reports, including meta-analyses of data collected from the literature (129), have correlated the V600E mutation with older age at diagnosis, male gender, extrathyroid invasion, lymph node or distant metastases, and unfavorable outcome (110,119,129–133). Experimental models have indicated that *BRAF* V600E promotes tumor progression (134,135). Decreased expression of the sodium iodide symporter (NIS), which is responsible for iodide uptake in the follicular cell, as well as of other iodide-metabolizing enzymes, has been shown in *BRAF* V600E-mutated PTCs (129,136,137). These data and the high prevalence of *BRAF* V600E in poorly differentiated radioactive iodine-refractory thyroid carcinomas (58) support the concept that the V600E-mutated tumors are more likely to become aggressive, loose their functional differentiation, and become unresponsive to treatment. In fact, in some studies *BRAF* V600E has been associated with recurrent or persistent disease (even in patients with low stage tumors) (138–140), as well as with reduced survival (132), independent of other clinicopathologic parameters. Based on this evidence, the *BRAF* V600E mutation has been proposed as a decisive prognostic factor for risk stratification (141). The *BRAF* mutational status can reliably be tested preoperatively on fine-needle aspiration samples, and according to some endocrinologists it may be very useful to plan the extent of initial surgery, as well as to make postoperative choices on the most appropriate radioiodine treatment, thyroid-stimulating hormone suppression, and surveillance modalities to manage patients with thyroid carcinoma (141).

Other evidence does not support a major prognostic relevance for the *BRAF* V600E mutation. In the first place, the mutation is very common among small tumors, including microcarcinomas (120,142), indicating that other factors are also important in determining the prognosis of patients with PTC. Furthermore, not all the reports have demonstrated a relationship between *BRAF* V600E and aggressive clinical features or poor prognosis (120,143–147). Some studies have raised the possibility that *BRAF* V600E may not be present in all neoplastic cells within a given tumor, but only in neoplastic cell subclones (148). This finding is controversial (149,150) and its prognostic relevance unclear (151,152). In a large retrospective study that included PTC cases from 13 medical centers in the United States, Europe, Australia, and Japan, *BRAF* V600E was statistically associated with increased cancer-related mortality, but the association was not independent of conventional clinicopathologic parameters (153).

The available data indicate that *BRAF* V600E-mutated PTCs may have a greater potential for an unfavorable outcome, but additional studies are needed to fully define the prognostic relevance of the mutation. At present there is no general consensus on whether and how utilize *BRAF* mutational status to improve patient management.

A clinical response to BRAF kinase inhibitors that target the V600E mutation, like Vemurafenib has been demonstrated in patients with aggressive *BRAF* V600E-mutated thyroid carcinomas (154), and *BRAF* mutational analysis may become necessary to select patients for treatment with molecularly targeted antineoplastic agents.

RAS Mutations

In the thyroid gland, oncogenic *H-RAS*, *K-RAS*, and *N-RAS* mutations are markers of follicular-patterned thyroid lesions, being typically associated with follicular adenomas and carcinomas. *H-RAS*, *K-RAS*, and *N-RAS* have been identified in PTC, but the overall prevalence is about 10 percent, i.e., much lower than in follicular tumors (4). The important exception is the encapsulated FVPTC, where *RAS* mutations are detected in about 35 percent of cases, a percentage similar to that for follicular adenoma and carcinoma. The most common mutation is at codon 61 of *N-RAS*, followed by codon 61 *H-RAS* (53,122). If the FVPTC is not encapsulated but infiltrative, the prevalence of the *RAS* mutation is significantly lower, analogous to that of classic PTC (53).

RET/PTC Rearrangements

RET/PTCs are rearranged forms of the gene encoding the RET receptor tyrosine kinase (see chapter 2). *RET/PTC1* (*CCDC6/RET*) and *RET/PTC3* (*NCOA4/RET*) represent the large majority (over 90 percent) of the rearrangements, with *RET/PTC1* being detected in approximately two thirds and *RET/PTC3* in approximately one third of *RET/PTC*-positive cases (155). *RET/PTC2* (*PRKAR1A/RET*) represents less than 5 percent of all *RET/PTC* variants (155).

The *RET* rearrangement is usually identified by RT-PCR. FISH and immunohistochemistry are also be used, but the latter depends on the availability of reliable antibodies and therefore should be confirmed by other methods (155).

The reported prevalence of *RET/PTC* in PTC is highly variable due to geographic variations but also to the different sensitivities of the methods used for its detection. It is, therefore, often difficult to compare the data reported in the literature (155). Very sensitive methods detect *RET/PTC* in the peripheral blood of patients with PTC (156), but they should be avoided for routine molecular diagnosis (157,158). In fact, low level *RET/PTC* recombination can be identified by highly sensitive techniques in PTC (157,159), with or without other mutational events (e.g., *BRAF*) due to genetic heterogeneity (158). Low level recombination is also seen in hyperplastic thyroid nodules, particularly if they show focal nuclear irregularities similar to those seen in PTC (160,161) and Hashimoto thyroiditis (157). With appropriate methods, *RET/PTC* is now detected in approximately 20 percent of PTCs (range, 10 to 40 percent) (1,2,162).

The rearrangement usually occurs in young patients and children (122,163), and in tumors that show classic papillary histology with psammoma bodies (122,164,165). *RET/PTC*-positive PTCs often present with lymph node metastases. Because of the young patient age, however, they are usually low-stage tumors (122,163–166). *RET* rearrangements are common in microcarcinomas (167,168), and several studies (164–166) have failed to correlate *RET/PTC* with increased morbidity and mortality. The rearrangement, in particular *RET/PTC1* that largely predominates among cases not associated with radiation exposure, is generally found in indolent tumors showing little propensity to progress to poorly differentiated and undifferentiated carcinomas (164,165).

RET/PTC is strongly associated with therapeutic or environmental radiation exposure (169,170). Most of the PTCs that occurred after the Chernobyl nuclear disaster of 1986 had *RET/PTC* rearrangements, with figures reported as high as 80 percent (171). *RET/PTC3* was common (169,171,172), particularly in tumors that developed after exposure to high radioactivity levels, that were of short latency, more aggressive (larger size, extrathyroidal extension), and classified as solid variants of PTC (172,173). These data suggest that *RET/PTC3* may have a higher oncogenic potential than *RET/PTC1*, but a correlation between *RET/PTC3* and aggressive features is not well documented in tumors from patients not exposed to radiation, possibly due to the low prevalence of *RET/PTC3* (155). *RET* rearrangement variants different from *RET/PTC1*, *RET/PTC2*, and *RET/PTC3* have been described in a few papillary carcinomas that developed after radiation exposure, but they are rare in nonradiation-associated tumors (155,170).

The prevalence of the *RET/PTC* rearrangement among nonradiation-associated tumors appears to be decreasing (126).

NTRK1 and NTRK3 Rearrangements

NTRK1 is another gene rearranged and activated in PTC as a result of intrachromosomal or interchromosomal recombination. Like RET, NTRK1 is a tyrosine kinase receptor protein, and the mechanisms responsible for oncogenic *NTRK1* activation are the same as those described for *RET/PTC*. *NTRK1* rearrangements are also known as the *TRK* oncogenes: *TRK (TPM3/NTRK1)* (174), *TRK-T1/T2 (TPR/NTRK1)* (175), and *TRK-T3 (TFG/NTRK1)* (see chapter 2) (176). They are much less common than *RET/PTC*. In some series the *NTRK1* rearrangement has been identified in 10 to 15 percent of PTCs (163,177), while other studies have failed to identify it (178,179). The prevalence of the rearrangement is probably about 5 percent. In one study (177), tumors with the *NTRK1* rearrangement were more aggressive than those with *RET/PTC*, but their overall clinicopathologic features did not seem to be much different (163). *NTRK1* rearrangements, usually *TPM3/NTRK1*, have been reported in a minority of radiation-associated PTCs (61,172).

Fusion of NTRK3, a neurotrophic tyrosine kinase receptor closely related to NTRK1, to the *ETV6* gene has been reported in PTC (see chapter 2). *ETV6/NTRK3*, detected cytogenetically as the t(12;15)(p13;q25), is typically associated with congenital fibrosarcoma, congenital mesoblastic nephroma, and secretory carcinomas of the breast and salivary glands. In the thyroid, *ETV6/NTRK3* (with *ETV6* exon 4-*NTRK3* exon 14 fusion points) is linked to radiation exposure (61,109).The rearrangement has been identified in approximately 15 percent of PTCs

that developed after the Chernobyl nuclear accident, but in only 2 percent of tumors not related to radiation (109). *ETV6/NTRK3* appears to be associated with a follicular architecture, particularly among radiation-associated tumors, and cases carrying the rearrangement are often classified as follicular variant PTC or classic PTC with a component of follicular growth. Areas of solid growth pattern are present in the radiation-associated tumors, but are not found in those unrelated to radiation exposure (61,109). *ETV6/NTRK3*, after *RET/PTC*, may be the most common form of oncogenic rearrangement in radiation-associated PTCs (61,109).

ALK

ALK rearrangements have been identified in a small minority of PTCs (approximately 1 to 5 percent of cases) (11,85). In virtually all tumors the rearrangement results in the fusion of the exon 3 of the *STRN* gene (located at 2p22.2) to the exon 10 of *ALK* (located at 2p23), causing upregulation of the ALK tyrosine kinase domain (see chapter 2) (11,85). *STRN/ALK* can be detected using the same FISH probes and antibodies used to identify *ALK* rearrangement in lung carcinomas. Cases with *STRN/ALK* show a predominantly follicular growth pattern, but some have been reported as classic PTC (11,85). They may present with aggressive features (extrathyroidal extension, lymph node metastases) and develop in PTCs undergoing dedifferentiation (180), consistent with the higher prevalence of *STRN/ALK* in tumors that are poorly differentiated or undifferentiated (85). *STRN/ALK* positive cases may respond to ALK inhibitor drugs (crizotinib) (180).

EML4/ALK rearrangements of the type encountered in lung carcinomas are rare in PTC not associated to radiation, or in cases that developed after the Chernobyl nuclear accident (61,85). They have, however, been reported in PTCs that developed among patients exposed to Hiroshima and Nagasaki atomic bomb radiation. In these cases, the *ALK* rearrangement was associated with solid/trabecular tumor growth, exposure to high radiation levels, and younger age (181).

TERT

TERT, encoded by the *TERT* gene, is the protein core component with reverse transcriptase activity of the telomerase enzyme complex that maintains telomere length, allowing cell replication (see chapter 2). Activation of telomerase has been demonstrated in PTCs that, like follicular carcinomas, have short telomeres, but express a high proportion of full-length *TERT* transcripts and have high telomerase enzymatic activity (7–9). *C228T* and *C250T*, two mutually exclusive oncogenic mutations in the promoter region of *TERT,* which activate transcription of the gene, were originally demonstrated in melanoma in 2013. In the same year they were also reported in several other tumor types, including malignant tumors derived from follicular cells (although not in medullary carcinoma) (see chapter 2) (73–76).

TERT promoter mutations are present in approximately 15 percent of PTCs. They have not been identified in normal thyroid parenchyma, lymphocytic thyroiditis, or hyperplastic thyroid nodules, and are rarely detected in follicular adenomas (10,73–78). The prevalence of mutations is higher in conventional PTC compared with follicular variant PTC (75,77). *C228T* is the most frequent mutation, and in most series its prevalence in PTCs at least 5 times that of the *C250T* mutation (74,75,78).

TERT promoter mutations are more prevalent among differentiated thyroid carcinomas, papillary and follicular, with unfavorable clinicopathologic features, and may represent a very important prognostic marker (74,77,78). In differentiated thyroid carcinomas (follicular or papillary), the mutations are associated with older age, large tumor size, extrathyroidal extension, high stage at presentation, distant metastases, and persistent disease (74,77,78). In some series, they were an independent predictor of disease-specific mortality for patients with differentiated thyroid carcinomas, and, specifically, for those with PTC (74,77).

As *TERT* promoter mutations are identified with higher prevalence in poorly and undifferentiated (anaplastic) carcinomas, they appear to support the progression to aggressive forms of thyroid cancer (73–77). *BRAF* V600E and *TERT* promoter mutations may coexist in the same tumor, and the association supports the possibility that MAPK-induced expression of transcription factors of the ETS family may further enhance the expression of *TERT* (see chapter 2) (75,77,78). The coexistence of *BRAF* V600E and *TERT* mutations does not appear to correlate with more aggressive clinicopathologic features or worse outcome (77). Cases with *RET/PTC* do not usually have *TERT* promoter mutations (77). *TERT* mutations have not been associated with PTCs that developed after exposure to ionizing radiation (74,77).

Chromosomal DNA and Other Somatic Genetic Alterations

PTCs, unlike follicular neoplasms, typically have a diploid karyotype, euploid chromosomal DNA content, and low LOH rates (19,20,80,82,182). Conventional cytogenetic analysis identifies chromosomal alterations in 20 to 40 percent of cases (19,20). These alterations are usually simple, with few numeric or balanced structural abnormalities (20,183). Structural abnormalities have been detected in about 20 percent of cases in a large series of PTCs (184). They often (but not always) involve the long arm of chromosome 10, where the inv(10)(q11.2q21.2) reflects the occurrence of the *RET/PTC1* rearrangement (20,80,182,184). Structural changes of the long arm of chromosome 1 at the site of the gene *NTRK1* (1q21-22) are rarely detected, and molecular diagnosis is necessary to identify most intrachromosomal rearrangements (185). Other chromosomal breakpoint loci have been reported at 1p32-36, 1p11-13 3p25-26, and 7q34-36 (184).

Complex karyotypic alterations by conventional cytogenetics (80,184) and aneuploidy, detected by flow cytometric DNA content analysis (186–188) or comparative genomic hybridization (189–191), have been linked to aggressive disease (189) and poor prognosis (186–188). They are associated with unfavorable characteristics, such as high grade or poorly differentiated features (80,184,190), or the tall cell variant of PTC (191). Specifically, comparative genomic hybridization shows that some chromosomal sites have gains (1q, 9q33-qter, 17q, X) or losses (9q21.3-q32, 22q) more frequently than others (189,192). Gains at 1q and loss of 9q21.3-32 have been correlated with aggressive behavior (189) and are also reported among the chromosomal DNA alterations specifically associated with the tall cell variant of PTC (191).

Unlike follicular carcinoma, dysregulation of the PI3K/PTEN/AKT pathway is uncommon in PTC (65). Markedly decreased expression of Rap1GAP has been correlated with invasive growth (90).

Microarray analysis has shown that PTC has a distinct mRNA profile, different from follicular carcinoma and other thyroid tumors (92,193,194). The expression signature has been correlated to specific subtypes, including the follicular and tall cell variants, and to distinct oncogenic events, like *RET/PTC*, *BRAF*, and *RAS* mutations (107). Among the genes overexpressed in PTC are the oncogene *MET*, as well as some of the immunohistochemical markers currently used for diagnostic purposes, including galectin 3, keratin 19, and CITED1 (193). Overexpression of *MUC1* has been demonstrated in aggressive PTC, validated by immunohistochemistry, and shown to predict poor prognosis independently of histologic typing and clinicopathologic parameters (191). The analysis of mRNA expression signatures can be a useful diagnostic tool for the preoperative diagnosis of thyroid nodules (93,195).

Dysregulated expression of miRNA has been documented in PTC. Upregulation of miR-146b, miR-221, and miR-222 has been consistently reported (196). MiRNAs can be analyzed on formalin-fixed samples and in fine-needle aspiration specimens (99,197), and their use as diagnostic markers (99,197–200) is being evaluated with promising results (101). The prognostic role of miRNA is also being actively investigated. Upregulation of miR-146b and miR-222 and downregulation of miR-34b and miR-130b have been linked to aggressive behavior (199,200). MiR-146b has been associated with *BRAF* V600E and with aggressive behavior in *BRAF* V600E-mutated tumors (199,200).

Papillary Microcarcinoma

It is difficult to analyze the genetic alterations in microcarcinomas due to their small size. However, several studies have shown that they carry the same changes found in larger tumors, including *BRAF* V600E, *RET/PTC*, and *RAS* mutations (142,165,201). Most studies have shown that the prevalence of *BRAF* V600E in microcarcinomas is lower compared with larger tumors. One study identified *BRAF* V600E in 17 percent of tumors smaller than 5 mm found incidentally, versus 38 percent of microcarcinomas diagnosed preoperatively and 45 percent of PTCs that were clinically evident (142). In a study where the prevalence of the mutation was

adjusted for the growth pattern and only tumors exhibiting papillary architecture were compared, however, *BRAF* V600E was found in 43 percent of microcarcinomas versus 46 percent of the larger tumors (120). The prevalence of the *RET/PTC* rearrangement in microcarcinomas has been reported to be higher compared with larger, clinically evident tumors (168).

It is uncertain whether the correlation between *BRAF* V600E and the aggressive features shown by many studies for larger tumors (see above) applies to microcarcinomas as well. Some studies suggest that this might be the case. A group from Korea, a country where the prevalence of the mutation appears to be particularly high, has found that *BRAF* V600E is independently correlated with size greater than 5 mm and extrathyroidal extension (202). A large study from Italy has shown a similar correlation between the *BRAF* mutation and tumor size, extrathyroidal extension, and lymph node metastasis in PTCs smaller than 2 cm (133). In one series of microcarcinomas from the United States (203) the V600E mutation was correlated with lymph node metastases and extrathyroidal extension. Nevertheless, it is difficult to reconcile the association between *BRAF* V600E and unfavorable prognostic features with the indolent behavior of the vast majority of microcarcinomas. It is logical to surmise that other factors must be at play in addition to the V600E mutation. Niemeier et al. (201) have proposed a scoring system (molecular pathologic [MP] score) that takes into account not only *BRAF* status but also three histologic parameters (subcapsular tumor location, intraglandular spread, tumor fibrosis) to predict the likelihood of lymph node metastases or tumor recurrence in microcarcinomas.

Follicular Variant

The molecular profile of the follicular variant in its prototypical "infiltrative" form is more similar to that of conventional PTC (mutated *BRAF* and *RET/PTC*) than to that of follicular neoplasms or the encapsulated follicular type of the tumor (mutated *RAS* and *PAX8/PPARγ*) (see below). Rivera et al. (53) found *BRAF* V600E in 26 percent and *RET/PTC* in 10 percent of 19 FVPTCs with infiltrative growth. Both mutations were absent in 28 encapsulated tumors, which showed instead a higher prevalence of *RAS* mutations

(36 percent in the encapsulated tumors versus 10 percent in the infiltrative ones) and one case with the *PAX8/PPARγ* rearrangement.

Follicular growth patterns predominate in PTCs with *STRN/ALK* (85), and follicular growth is also associated with tumors carrying the *ETV6/NTRK3* rearrangement (61,109). Radiation-associated tumors with *PPARγ* rearrangements (both *PAX8/PPARγ* and *CREB3L2/PPARγ*) are classified as follicular variant PTC (60,61).

Encapsulated Follicular Variant and the "Uncertain Malignant Potential" Concept

It is very difficult to determine exactly how many of the numerous cases of FVPTC in which genetic alterations have been analyzed were encapsulated. Reflecting their higher prevalence over overtly invasive forms (204), most of the data on genetic alterations reported in the literature likely refer to encapsulated tumors with little or no invasion. These tumors have molecular alterations that are clearly different from those of conventional PTC. *RET/PTC* and the *BRAF* V600E mutation are infrequent (122,165), *BRAF* K601E has been reported in up to 7 percent of cases (120), and other rare *BRAF* mutants are usually found only in encapsulated FVPTCs (111).

In contrast with conventional PTC, *RAS* mutations are common, most frequently at *N-RAS* codon 61 followed by H-RAS codon 61 (46). Adeniran et al. (122) found *RAS* mutations in 46 percent of 30 cases. The *PAX8/PPARγ* rearrangement also occurs, being present in 37 percent of the cases in one series (52). One cytogenetic study has associated isolated trisomy 17 with encapsulated FVPTCs (205) and, at variance with conventional PTC, comparative genomic hybridization detected unbalanced chromosomal DNA profiles in a significant proportion of cases (28).

The mRNA expression profile is also clearly different in encapsulated FVPTC from that of classic PTC (107). FVPTC, but not encapsulated thyroid nodules with partial features of PTC, show overexpression of miR-146b (198).

It is important to note that the profile of molecular alterations found in the encapsulated FVPTC is statistically speaking, "intermediate" between that of follicular neoplasms (*RAS* mutation, *PAX8/PPARγ*, aneuploidy), and that of conventional PTC (*BRAF* mutation, *RET/PTC*, euploidy) (28,52,53,122). In fact, the molecular profile of some encapsulated FVPTCs appears more similar to that of follicular neoplasms (adenomas and carcinomas) than to that of conventional PTC. This observation, together with the difficulty in making a reproducible histologic diagnosis of carcinoma (see chapter 7), suggest that at least some encapsulated FVPTCs are follicular carcinomas (when invasive) or adenomas (when noninvasive) (206).

Solid/Trabecular Variant

The solid variant of PTC represented a high proportion (about 35 percent) of the tumors that occurred in children during the first years after the Chernobyl nuclear disaster of 1986 (171,207). In one study, *RET* was found to be rearranged in 70 percent of the radiation-associated solid variant of PTC (172) and *RET/PTC3* was the predominant recombination, reported in about 80 percent of the *RET*-rearranged cases (171,172). *RET/PTC1* predominated in the more conventional PTCs that developed with longer latency after radiation exposure (169,172,173). The association between *RET/PTC3* and the solid variant has not been reported among adult patients without a history of radiation (208). Areas of solid growth are present in radiation-associated PTCs with *ETV6/NTRK3*, but absent in cases unrelated to radiation (109). *BRAF* mutations, including a rare *BRAF* VK600-1E variant, also have been reported in solid/trabecular PTC (131,209).

Diffuse Sclerosing Variant

A pronounced reduction of membrane E-cadherin expression, accompanied by a relocation of the protein to the cytoplasm, has been noted in the diffuse sclerosing variant of PTC. These changes have been linked to mutations of the *CDH1* gene encoding the E-cadherin protein, or to methylation of its promoter (210). Both *RET/PTC1* and *RET/PTC3* have been identified (211). *BRAF* mutations appear to be rare (211).

Oncocytic and Warthin-Like Variants

Both *BRAF* V600E (120) and *RET/PTC* (212) have been identified in Warthin-like PTCs, supporting the close correlation of this variant with conventional PTC. The molecular alterations of oncocytic tumors are discussed in chapter 10.

Tall and Columnar Cell Variants

The main molecular alteration of tall cell PTCs is the *BRAF* V600E mutation. Among all thyroid tumor subtypes, this mutation shows its highest prevalence in the tall cell variant, where it can be found in more than 90 percent of cases (122,123).

The *BRAF* mutation is considered important not only for tumor initiation, but also for its role in promoting invasion and progression. Deregulation of cell adhesion, remodeling of extracellular matrix, and changes consistent with epithelial-mesenchymal transition have been linked to the V600E mutation and demonstrated during progression of *BRAF* V600E-mutated PTC to poorly differentiated thyroid carcinoma (135). Overexpression of MMP-2 (matrix metalloproteinase 2), a neutral metalloproteinase that initiates the degradation of type IV collagen in basement membranes (213), and of MUC1, a membrane glycoprotein that can promote cellular dissociation by interfering with cell-cell and cell-matrix adhesion, have been specifically linked to tall cell PTC (191). MUC1 has also been shown by Wreesmann et al. (191) to be an independent predictor of poor survival for patients with PTC and is encoded by a gene at 1q21, a chromosomal site that the authors found frequently amplified in tall cell carcinoma. In the same study, gains at 1q and loss of 9q21.3-32 were among the chromosomal DNA alterations specifically associated with the tall cell variant (191). Both chromosomal sites were correlated with aggressive behavior in PTC in a previous report from a different group (189).

Little is known about the molecular alterations of the columnar cell variant of PTC. Expression of the intestinal transcription factor CDX2 has been identified in 6 of 11 cases (55 percent), but not in any other benign or malignant thyroid lesions, including the tall cell variant of PTC (214). *BRAF* V600E has been detected in 3 of 8 columnar cell PTCs analyzed by Chen et. al (215), a proportion much lower than that reported in the tall cell variant. Both findings argue against a close relationship between the two tumor types.

Cribriform-Morular Variant

The cribriform-morular variant of PTC can occur as an extraintestinal manifestation of the familial adenomatous polyposis (FAP) syndrome or in a sporadic form. It is a very rare tumor, representing 0.1 to 0.2 percent of all PTCs (216,217), but its recognition is important because it can be the first manifestation of the hereditary polyposis syndrome (216).

The main molecular feature of the tumor is aberrant activation of the Wnt signaling pathway. This leads to cytoplasmic overexpression and nuclear accumulation of β-catenin, detectable immunohistochemically (218). Aberrant Wnt signaling is a consequence of loss of function germline mutations of the *APC* (adenomatous polyposis coli) gene in patients with the FAP syndrome (219). In sporadic cases it is associated either with somatic mutations in exon 3 of the β-catenin gene (*CTNNB1*) that stabilizes β-catenin, preventing its cytoplasmic degradation and promoting its accumulation in the nucleus, or with somatic *APC* mutations (218,220). *RET/PTC* (219,221), but not *BRAF* (222) mutations have been reported.

Papillary Carcinoma in Hereditary Syndromes

PTC may be seen in a familial setting, both in cases where the predominant pathology is in the thyroid gland, as well as in hereditary conditions where PTC is a component of a syndrome dominated by extrathyroidal pathology (103,223–225). The latter situation includes mainly cases of FAP and Gardner syndromes, where patients develop the cribriform-morular variant of PTC (see above). PTC is uncommon in Cowden and other PTEN hamartoma tumor syndromes, where the most frequent thyroid malignancy is follicular carcinoma (39), but it has been reported in patients with Carney complex type I, McCune-Albright syndrome, and Werner syndrome (adult progeria) (44,103,224–227).

Up to approximately 5 percent of PTCs show familial aggregation that meets the criteria for a hereditary condition in which the dominant pathology is in the thyroid gland. This condition, generically referred to as familial nonmedullary thyroid carcinoma (FNMTC), shows an autosomal dominant pattern of inheritance with reduced penetrance (103,224,225). In a study based on the Swedish Family-Cancer Database (228), the risks for first-degree relatives compared with the general population were 3.21

and 6.21 if a parent or a sibling were diagnosed with thyroid carcinoma, respectively. The same study showed that the risk was even higher (11.9) among sisters.

Among these familial PTCs are cases with (229) or without (230) oncocytic features that have been linked to a locus at 19p13.2, cases associated with papillary renal cell carcinoma linked to a susceptibility locus at 1q21 (231), cases associated with nodular hyperplasia linked to a susceptibility locus at 2q21 (232), and cases linked to a susceptibility locus at 8q24 (233). These familial PTCs often develop in the background of parenchymal hyperplasia with hyperplastic and adenomatous nodules (232,234). Most of the tumors are classic PTC, although FVPTCs represented at least half of the malignant tumors in the familial cases linked to the 2q21 locus (232). No causative germline mutations have been identified. Genes that are commonly the site of somatic alterations in sporadic thyroid tumors (e.g. *BRAF*, *RET*) do not appear to be involved (103,224,225).

The impact of the above quoted loci on PTC susceptibility in the general population, however, is small, and most of the familial risk remains unexplained. This risk is likely to result from the coinheritance of multiple alleles with low to moderate penetrance. Genome-wide association studies (GWAS) have identified several single nucleotide polymorphisms (SNPs) that affect the predisposition to develop PTC, including rs944289 located at 14q.13.3 in proximity of the *NKX2-1* gene encoding the thyroid transcription factor-1 (TTF1) protein, rs965513 at 9q22.33 near the *FOXE1* gene encoding the thyroid transcription factor-2 (TTF2) protein, rs2439302 in an intron of the *NGR1* gene located at 8p12, and rs966423 in an intron of the *DIRC3* gene at 2q35 (235,236).

The histologic features and the pattern of somatic mutations in familial tumors are similar to those of sporadic cases, but they tend to develop at an earlier age (237). Several reports have indicated that familial cases are often multifocal and have a higher rate of recurrence (238,239). In other studies no significant differences in the clinicopathologic features were observed between familial and sporadic cases (237). A worse outcome has been observed in some series (238,240), but not in others (239).

POORLY DIFFERENTIATED CARCINOMA

The pattern of genetic alterations present in thyroid carcinomas supports the concept of a group of tumors with features that are intermediate between conventional papillary and follicular carcinomas, and undifferentiated (anaplastic) carcinoma (1,2). Despite some of the inconsistencies in the way the term "poorly differentiated" has been used (see chapter 8), it is clear that genetic alterations tend to sequentially accumulate in the progression from clinically indolent to highly aggressive tumors. This progression is also apparent from the data published on the immunohistochemical expression of markers for the cell cycle (e.g. p53, p27, p21, cyclin D1) and apoptosis (BCL-2, BAX) (241–245). Tumors that are poorly differentiated have features intermediate between those of well-differentiated carcinoma (papillary and follicular) and undifferentiated carcinoma. In poorly differentiated carcinomas, cell cycle inhibitors (p27, p21) have reduced expression and p53 is commonly overexpressed, as is cyclin D1. The expression of BCL-2 is retained (unlike the case of undifferentiated carcinoma) and BAX immunoreactivity is present (241–245).

The main genetic alterations reported in poorly differentiated carcinomas are summarized in Table 19-1. Complex chromosomal changes are a feature of insular carcinoma (79,246), and it is likely that many of the follicular carcinomas with complex karyotypes reported in the past were poorly differentiated (182). Aneuploidy is very common, with a number of chromosomal DNA alterations detectable by CGH, intermediate between that found in undifferentiated and well-differentiated tumors (190). Inactivating *TP53* mutations occur in about 25 percent of cases (247,248), a lower proportion than that of undifferentiated carcinomas, but high enough to link loss of p53 function with thyroid carcinoma progression. Nuclear accumulation of p53, which correlates, at least in part, with the presence of gene mutations, is more evident in areas of infiltrative growth or at the periphery of the tumor (241).

The *C228T* and *C250T* mutations in the promoter region of the *TERT* gene, which encodes the protein core component of the telomerase complex, are found in approximately 35 percent of poorly differentiated carcinomas (73,75–77), often coexisting with the *BRAF* V600E mutation (73,75,77). *C228T* and *C250T* are mutually exclusive, and *C228T* is the mutation observed most frequently. Both promoter mutations activate transcription of the *TERT* gene and thus support cellular proliferation (see chapter 2). They are detected with a higher prevalence in poorly (or undifferentiated) tumors compared with conventional papillary and follicular carcinomas, where they are usually identified in association with unfavorable clinicopathologic features and poor outcome. They may promote tumor progression and are emerging as an important marker for aggressive behavior in thyroid carcinoma (73–78).

Fusion of *ALK* to the *STRN* gene, resulting in the *STRN/ALK* rearrangement (see chapter 2), has been identified in approximately 9 percent of poorly differentiated carcinomas (85). Tumors with *STRN/ALK* appear to develop from PTCs undergoing dedifferentiation. The rearrangement can be detected with the same FISH probes and antibodies used to detect *ALK* rearrangements in lung carcinomas, and patients with *STRN/ALK* may respond to molecular treatment with ALK inhibitors (11,85,180).

Mutations of the *CTNNB1* β-catenin gene, which stabilizes the protein leading to its accumulation in the nucleus, have been detected in up to approximately 25 percent of cases (and in a higher proportion of undifferentiated carcinomas), but not in well-differentiated papillary or follicular carcinomas, indicating that they also play a role in the progression of thyroid tumors (249). The accumulation of β-catenin in the nucleus is demonstrated in tumor sections by immunofluorescence or conventional immunohistochemistry, but the latter is less reliable (249).

Mutations commonly found in conventional papillary and follicular carcinomas also occur in poorly differentiated tumors, a fact that is consistent with the origin of many of the latter from well-differentiated precursors. The prevalence of these mutations varies. *RAS* mutations, which are common (47,48,250), are associated with poor prognosis (47,48) and with the less-differentiated components in mixed tumors (48). *BRAF* mutations occur in cases that originate from PTC (119). *RET/PTC* (165,166) is uncommon and *PAX8/PPARγ* is rare (54,58), suggesting that neither promotes tumor dedifferentiation

(54,166). Volante et al. (49) have shown that in tumors that strictly fulfill the diagnostic criteria of the "Turin proposal" for poorly differentiated carcinoma (see chapter 8), *RAS* mutations (virtually all of which in codon 61 of *NRAS*) are the most common alteration and correlate with poor prognosis. In the study, *BRAF* mutations were infrequent, and no *RET/PTC* or *PAX8/PPARγ* rearranged cases were identified (49).

Ricarte-Filho et al. found activating *AKT1* mutations in 17 percent of aggressive radioactive iodine-refractory tumors, and *PIK3CA* mutations in 6 percent of poorly differentiated tumors defined on the basis of mitotic activity and necrosis (58). In both cases, the mutations often coexisted with *BRAF* V600E (58), indicating that concomitant activation of both PI3K/PTEN/AKT and MAPK pathways is a feature of aggressive thyroid carcinoma (5,58,66,71,72).

The patterns of gene expression as well as miRNA alterations show that tumors with poorly differentiated histologic features have profiles that are different from those of well-differentiated and undifferentiated carcinomas (251–253).

UNDIFFERENTIATED (ANAPLASTIC) CARCINOMA

The main genetic alterations of undifferentiated carcinomas are summarized in Table 19-1. Undifferentiated carcinoma represents the final stage of thyroid tumor progression. As such, it typically has a complex karyotype by conventional cytogenetics (182) and a high LOH rate (254). A high degree of aneuploidy is found by both flow cytometric DNA content analysis (255,256) and comparative genomic hybridization (190,257). Using comparative genomic hybridization, Wressman et al. (190) found 10 as the median number of chromosomal DNA alterations per case with detectable abnormalities, compared with 5.5 for poorly differentiated and 1.0 for well-differentiated PTCs.

A high prevalence of copy number gains of receptor tyrosine kinase genes like *EGFR*, *VEGFR2*, *PDGFRα* and -β, and *KIT* has been reported in undifferentiated carcinoma, but no activating mutations are usually identified (66). While no specific chromosomal loci have been linked to the development of undifferentiated carcinoma, a higher rate of chromosomal DNA alterations has been shown in undifferentiated tumors derived from a preexisting follicular carcinoma (257).

Expression mRNA profiling shows that undifferentiated carcinoma has a distinctive molecular signature, with overexpression of specific genes that promote chromosomal instability in addition to cell proliferation (258).

Marked dysregulation of the mechanisms that normally control proliferation and survival is demonstrated by immunohistochemical analysis of cell cycle proteins (p53, p27, p21, cyclin D1) and of those that regulate apoptosis (BCL2, BAX) (241–245). The pattern of immunohistochemical reactivity has possible diagnostic applications. In undifferentiated carcinomas, p27 and p21 expression is markedly reduced (243,245,259), p53 and cyclin D1 are often strongly expressed (244), while BCL2 (unlike BAX) is usually absent (241,242).

Loss of function mutations of *TP53* are present in 50 to 80 percent of undifferentiated carcinomas, a fact that sets them apart from most well-differentiated follicular and papillary tumors, where these mutations are rarely found (247,248,260,261). Although inactivating *TP53* mutations also occur in poorly differentiated carcinomas, widespread nuclear accumulation of the p53 protein is a typical feature of undifferentiated carcinomas. Importantly, in tumors where undifferentiated carcinoma coexists with a better-differentiated component, *TP53* mutations and nuclear accumulation of the protein are not usually detected in the better-differentiated component but are restricted to the anaplastic foci (241,247,262). This indicates that the mutations occur after the initial development of the tumor, and points to their important role in the progression to undifferentiated carcinoma.

The *TERT* promoter gene mutations *C228T* and *C250T* are found in approximately 40 percent of undifferentiated carcinomas, a percentage similar to that reported in poorly differentiated tumors, and higher than that of well-differentiated carcinomas (73–77). The two mutations are mutually exclusive, and *C228T* is the most common. Both promoter mutations activate transcription of the *TERT* gene, resulting in increased telomerase activity and unrestricted cellular proliferation (see chapter 2). In addition to poorly differentiated and undifferentiated carcinomas, these *TERT* muta-

tions are identified in a subset of conventional papillary and follicular carcinomas that often have unfavorable clinicopathologic features and poor outcome. *TERT* promoter mutations frequently coexist with *BRAF* V600E, support tumor progression, and are emerging as an important marker for aggressive behavior in thyroid carcinoma (73–78).

Mutations of the *CTNNB1* gene encoding for β-catenin have been detected in up to approximately two thirds of undifferentiated carcinomas, and in a smaller proportion of high-grade, poorly differentiated tumors (249,263). These mutations stabilize β-catenin and allow the protein to accumulate in the nucleus, where it functions as a transcription factor with oncogenic properties. Nuclear reactivity for β-catenin is demonstrated by immunofluorescence, but not always by conventional immunohistochemistry (249,264). Inactivating mutations of *APC* and *Axin*, genes controlling two proteins essential for β-catenin degradation, have been reported in some undifferentiated carcinomas (264).

The *STRN/ALK* rearrangement that juxtaposes *ALK* to the *STRN* gene has been identified in a subset of undifferentiated carcinomas that appear to develop from PTC. Pérot et al. (11) found the rearrangement in an undifferentiated carcinoma with a PTC component and lung metastases (180). *STRN/ALK* was detected both in the PTC and in the undifferentiated carcinoma, and the patient responded to treatment with the ALK kinase inhibitor crizotinib (11,180). Kelly et al. (85) reported the rearrangement in 1 of 24 undifferentiated carcinomas with a follicular variant PTC component. The rearrangement can be detected with the same FISH probes and antibodies used to detect *ALK* rearrangements in lung carcinomas. Activating point mutations in *ALK* exon 23 encoding the tyrosine kinase domain of the protein were identified in two tumors, in one series that included a total of 18 undifferentiated cases (265). One case harbored the *C3592T* mutation, the second the *G3602A* mutation, both different from the *ALK* mutations found in neuroblastoma. No point mutations were identified in well-differentiated papillary or follicular carcinomas (265). Two mutations in exon 4 of the *IDH1* gene encoding the isocitrate dehydrogenase 1 have been reported by the same investigators in a few undifferentiated carcinomas (266). One mutation was *IDH1* G367A, the other *IDH1* V71I, both different from the exon 4 *IDH1* mutation hot spots in glial neoplasms (266).

Mutations commonly found in differentiated thyroid tumors are also present in undifferentiated ones, a clue to the evolution of many such cases from preexisting low-grade lesions. In particular, *RAS* mutations are common (47,48,58), as is the *BRAF* V600E mutation, which is usually detected in cases where a PTC component is identified (58,119). *RET/PTC* and *PAX8/PAPRγ* are not frequent, indicating that these rearrangements (unlike *RAS* and *BRAF* mutations) do not promote tumor progression and dedifferentiation (58,165,166,267).

The PI3K/PTEN/AKT pathway is frequently altered and the following data suggest that activation of this pathway plays a role in the progression of thyroid tumors to undifferentiated carcinoma. A high prevalence of copy number gains of *PIK3CA* and *AKT* has been reported in undifferentiated carcinomas (5,66), compared with well-differentiated (follicular) ones. In one study, *PIK3CA* copy gain was present in 39 percent of cases and was infrequently found in the part of the tumor where a differentiated component could

be demonstrated (72). Both loss of function *PTEN* mutations as well as activating mutations of the *PIK3CA* gene (exons 9 and 20) have been identified in up to 15 percent and up to 25 percent of cases, respectively (5,66,71). *PIK3CA* gene mutations can be focal within the tumor, but they are associated with the anaplastic areas in tumors with a better-differentiated component (71). While *PTEN* and *PIK3CA* genetic alterations infrequently coexist in well-differentiated carcinomas, they often overlap with each other and with either *BRAF* or *RAS* mutations in undifferentiated tumors. Thus, the simultaneous activation of both PI3K/PTEN/AKT and MAPK pathways appears to be an attribute of aggressive forms of thyroid carcinoma (5,58,66,71,72).

Analysis of the miRNA profile has shown a significant decrease in miR-30d, miR-30a-5p, miR-125b, and miR-26a expression, with a possible pathogenic role for miR-125b and miR-26a (268).

OTHER TUMORS

The molecular genetic alterations of medullary carcinoma, oncocytic tumors, sarcomas, and malignant lymphomas of the thyroid gland are discussed in their respective chapters.

REFERENCES

1. Kondo T, Ezzat S, Asa SL. Pathogenetic mechanisms in thyroid follicular-cell neoplasia. Nat Rev Cancer 2006;6:292-306.

2. Nikiforov YE, Nikiforova MN. Molecular genetics and diagnosis of thyroid cancer. Nat Rev Endocrinol 2011;7:569-80.

3. Nikiforova MN, Biddinger PW, Caudill CM, Kroll TG, Nikiforov YE. PAX8-PPARgamma rearrangement in thyroid tumors: RT-PCR and immunohistochemical analyses. Am J Surg Pathol 2002;26:1016-23.

4. Vasko V, Ferrand M, Di Cristofaro J, Carayon P, Henry JF, de Micco C. Specific pattern of RAS oncogene mutations in follicular thyroid tumors. J Clin Endocrinol Metab 2003;88:2745-52.

5. Hou P, Liu D, Shan Y, et al. Genetic alterations and their relationship in the phosphatidylinositol 3-kinase/Akt pathway in thyroid cancer. Clin Cancer Res 2007;13:1161-70.

6. Soares P, Trovisco V, Rocha AS, et al. BRAF mutations and RET/PTC rearrangements are alternative events in the etiopathogenesis of PTC. Oncogene 2003;22:4578-80.

7. Saji M, Xydas S, Westra WH, et al. Human telomerase reverse transcriptase (hTERT) gene expression in thyroid neoplasms. Clin Cancer Res 1999;5:1483-9.

8. Wang Y, Kowalski J, Tsai HL, et al. Differentiating alternative splice variant patterns of human telomerase reverse transcriptase in thyroid neoplasms. Thyroid 2008;18:1055-63.

9. Wang Y, Meeker AK, Kowalski J, et al. Telomere length is related to alternative splice patterns of telomerase in thyroid tumors. Am J Pathol 2011;179:1415-24.

10. Wang N, Liu T, Sofiadis A, et al. TERT promoter mutation as an early genetic event activating telomerase in follicular thyroid adenoma (FTA) and atypical FTA. Cancer 2014;120:2965-79.

11. Pérot G, Soubeyran I, Ribeiro A, et al. Identification of a recurrent STRN/ALK fusion in thyroid carcinomas. PLoS One 2014;9:e87170.

12. Namba H, Matsuo K, Fagin JA. Clonal composition of benign and malignant human thyroid tumors. J Clin Invest 1990;86:120-5.

13. Hicks DG, LiVolsi VA, Neidich JA, Puck JM, Kant JA. Clonal analysis of solitary follicular nodules in the thyroid. Am J Pathol 1990;137:553-62.

14. Krohn K, Fuhrer D, Holzapfel HP, Paschke R. Clonal origin of toxic thyroid nodules with constitutively activating thyrotropin receptor mutations. J Clin Endocrinol Metab 1998;83:130-4.

15. Chung DH, Kang GH, Kim WH, Ro JY. Clonal analysis of a solitary follicular nodule of the thyroid with the polymerase chain reaction method. Mod Pathol 1999;12:265-71.

16. Apel RL, Ezzat S, Bapat BV, Pan N, LiVolsi VA, Asa SL. Clonality of thyroid nodules in sporadic goiter. Diagn Mol Pathol 1995;4:113-21.

17. Jovanovic L, Delahunt B, McIver B, Eberhardt NL, Grebe SK. Thyroid gland clonality revisited: the embryonal patch size of the normal human thyroid gland is very large, suggesting X-chromosome inactivation tumor clonality studies of thyroid tumors have to be interpreted with caution. J Clin Endocrinol Metab 2003;88:3284-91.

18. Belge G, Roque L, Soares J, et al. Cytogenetic investigations of 340 thyroid hyperplasias and adenomas revealing correlations between cytogenetic findings and histology. Cancer Genet Cytogenet 1998;101:42-8.

19. Herrmann M. Standard and molecular cytogenetics of endocrine tumors. Am J Clin Pathol 2003;119(Suppl):S17-38.

20. Ribeiro FR, Meireles AM, Rocha AS, Teixeira MR. Conventional and molecular cytogenetics of human nonmedullary thyroid carcinoma: characterization of eight cell line models and review of the literature on clinical samples. BMC Cancer 2008;8:371.

21. Belge G, Rippe V, Meiboom M, Drieschner N, Garcia E, Bullerdiek J. Delineation of a 150-kb breakpoint cluster in benign thyroid tumors with 19q13.4 aberrations. Cytogenet Cell Genet 2001;93:48-51.

22. Rippe V, Drieschner N, Meiboom M, et al. Identification of a gene rearranged by 2p21 aberrations in thyroid adenomas. Oncogene 2003;22:6111-4.

23. Drieschner N, Rippe V, Laabs A, et al. Interphase fluorescence in situ hybridization analysis detects a much higher rate of thyroid tumors with clonal cytogenetic deviations of the main cytogenetic subgroups than conventional cytogenetics. Cancer Genet 2011;204:366-74.

24. Meiboom M, Murua Escobar H, Pentimalli F, Fusco A, Belge G, Bullerdiek J. A 3.4-kbp transcript of ZNF331 is solely expressed in follicular thyroid adenomas. Cytogenet Genome Res 2003;101:113-7.

25. Greenebaum E, Koss LG, Elequin F, Silver CE. The diagnostic value of flow cytometric DNA measurements in follicular tumors of the thyroid gland. Cancer 1985;56:2011-8.

26. Hruban RH, Huvos AG, Traganos F, Reuter V, Lieberman PH, Melamed MR. Follicular neoplasms of the thyroid in men older than 50 years of age. A DNA flow cytometric study. Am J Clin Pathol 1990;94:527-32.

27. Joensuu H, Klemi P, Eerola E. DNA aneuploidy in follicular adenomas of the thyroid gland. Am J Pathol 1986;124:373-6.

28. Wreesmann VB, Ghossein RA, Hezel M, et al. Follicular variant of papillary thyroid carcinoma: genome-wide appraisal of a controversial entity. Genes Chromosomes Cancer 2004;40:355-64.

29. Liu Y, Cope L, Sun W, et al. DNA copy number variations characterize benign and malignant thyroid tumors. J Clin Endocrinol Metab 2013; 98:E558-66.

30. Parma J, Duprez L, Van Sande J, et al. Diversity and prevalence of somatic mutations in the thyrotropin receptor and Gs alpha genes as a cause of toxic thyroid adenomas. J Clin Endocrinol Metab 1997;82:2695-701.

31. Trulzsch B, Krohn K, Wonerow P, et al. Detection of thyroid-stimulating hormone receptor and Gs alpha mutations: in 75 toxic thyroid nodules by denaturing gradient gel electrophoresis. J Mol Med (Berl) 2001;78:684-91.

32. Gozu HI, Bircan R, Krohn K, et al. Similar prevalence of somatic TSH receptor and Gsalpha mutations in toxic thyroid nodules in geographical regions with different iodine supply in Turkey. Eur J Endocrinol 2006;155:535-45.

33. Vanvooren V, Uchino S, Duprez L, et al. Oncogenic mutations in the thyrotropin receptor of autonomously functioning thyroid nodules in the Japanese population. Eur J Endocrinol 2002;147:287-91.

34. Salvatore G, Chiappetta G, Nikiforov YE, et al. Molecular profile of hyalinizing trabecular tumours of the thyroid: high prevalence of RET/PTC rearrangements and absence of B-raf and N-ras point mutations. Eur J Cancer 2005;41:816-21.

35. Sheu SY, Vogel E, Worm K, Grabellus F, Schwertheim S, Schmid KW. Hyalinizing trabecular tumour of the thyroid-differential expression of distinct miRNAs compared with papillary thyroid carcinoma. Histopathology 2010;56:632-40.

36. Cheung CC, Boerner SL, MacMillan CM, Ramyar L, Asa SL. Hyalinizing trabecular tumor of the thyroid: a variant of papillary carcinoma proved by molecular genetics. Am J Surg Pathol 2000;24:1622-6.

37. Papotti M, Volante M, Giuliano A, et al. RET/PTC activation in hyalinizing trabecular tumors of the thyroid. Am J Surg Pathol 2000;24:1615-21.

38. Liaw D, Marsh DJ, Li J, et al. Germline mutations of the PTEN gene in Cowden disease, an inherited breast and thyroid cancer syndrome. Nat Genet 1997;16:64-7.

39. Harach HR, Soubeyran I, Brown A, Bonneau D, Longy M. Thyroid pathologic findings in patients with Cowden disease. Ann Diagn Pathol 1999;3:331-40.

40. Mastorakos G, Mitsiades NS, Doufas AG, Koutras DA. Hyperthyroidism in McCune-Albright syndrome with a review of thyroid abnormalities sixty years after the first report. Thyroid 1997;7:433-9.

41. Stratakis CA, Courcoutsakis NA, Abati A, et al. Thyroid gland abnormalities in patients with the syndrome of spotty skin pigmentation, myxomas, endocrine overactivity, and schwannomas (Carney complex). J Clin Endocrinol Metab 1997;82:2037-43.

42. Kirschner LS, Carney JA, Pack SD, et al. Mutations of the gene encoding the protein kinase A type I-alpha regulatory subunit in patients with the Carney complex. Nat Genet 2000;26:89-92.

43. Yang GC, Yao JL, Feiner HD, Roses DF, Kumar A, Mulder JE. Lipid-rich follicular carcinoma of the thyroid in a patient with McCune-Albright syndrome. Mod Pathol 1999;12:969-73.

44. Collins MT, Sarlis NJ, Merino MJ, et al. Thyroid carcinoma in the McCune-Albright syndrome: contributory role of activating Gs alpha mutations. J Clin Endocrinol Metab 2003;88:4413-7.

45. Nikiforova MN, Lynch RA, Biddinger PW, et al. RAS point mutations and PAX8-PPAR gamma rearrangement in thyroid tumors: evidence for distinct molecular pathways in thyroid follicular carcinoma. J Clin Endocrinol Metab 2003;88:2318-26.

46. Zhu Z, Gandhi M, Nikiforova MN, Fischer AH, Nikiforov YE. Molecular profile and clinical-pathologic features of the follicular variant of papillary thyroid carcinoma. An unusually high prevalence of ras mutations. Am J Clin Pathol 2003;120:71-7.

47. Basolo F, Pisaturo F, Pollina LE, et al. N-ras mutation in poorly differentiated thyroid carcinomas: correlation with bone metastases and inverse correlation to thyroglobulin expression. Thyroid 2000;10:19-23.

48. Garcia-Rostan G, Zhao H, Camp RL, et al. Ras mutations are associated with aggressive tumor phenotypes and poor prognosis in thyroid cancer. J Clin Oncol 2003;21:3226-35.

49. Volante M, Rapa I, Gandhi M, et al. RAS mutations are the predominant molecular alteration in poorly differentiated thyroid carcinomas and bear prognostic impact. J Clin Endocrinol Metab 2009;94:4735-41.

50. Shi YF, Zou MJ, Schmidt H, et al. High rates of ras codon 61 mutation in thyroid tumors in an iodide-deficient area. Cancer Res 1991;51:2690-3.

51. Eberhardt NL, Grebe SK, McIver B, Reddi HV. The role of the PAX8/PPARgamma fusion oncogene in the pathogenesis of follicular thyroid cancer. Mol Cell Endocrinol 2010;321:50-6.

52. Castro P, Rebocho AP, Soares RJ, et al. PAX8-PPAR-gamma rearrangement is frequently detected in the follicular variant of papillary thyroid carcinoma. J Clin Endocrinol Metab 2006;91:213-20.

53. Rivera M, Ricarte-Filho J, Knauf J, et al. Molecular genotyping of papillary thyroid carcinoma follicular variant according to its histological subtypes (encapsulated vs infiltrative) reveals distinct BRAF and RAS mutation patterns. Mod Pathol 2010;23:1191-200.

54. Sahin M, Allard BL, Yates M, et al. PPARgamma staining as a surrogate for PAX8/PPARgamma fusion oncogene expression in follicular neoplasms: clinicopathological correlation and histopathological diagnostic value. J Clin Endocrinol Metab 2005;90:463-8.

55. Algeciras-Schimnich A, Milosevic D, McIver B, et al. Evaluation of the PAX8/PPARG translocation in follicular thyroid cancer with a 4-color reverse-transcription PCR assay and automated high-resolution fragment analysis. Clin Chem 2010;56:391-8.

56. Klemke M, Drieschner N, Laabs A, et al. On the prevalence of the PAX8-PPARG fusion resulting from the chromosomal translocation t(2;3)(q13;p25) in adenomas of the thyroid. Cancer Genet 2011;204:334-9.

57. Dwight T, Thoppe SR, Foukakis T, et al. Involvement of the PAX8/peroxisome proliferator-activated receptor gamma rearrangement in follicular thyroid tumors. J Clin Endocrinol Metab 2003;88:4440-5.

58. Ricarte-Filho JC, Ryder M, Chitale DA, et al. Mutational profile of advanced primary and metastatic radioactive iodine-refractory thyroid cancers reveals distinct pathogenetic roles for BRAF, PIK3CA, and AKT1. Cancer Res 2009;69:4885-93.

59. Lui WO, Zeng L, Rehrmann V, et al. CREB3L2-PPARgamma fusion mutation identifies a thyroid signaling pathway regulated by intramembrane proteolysis. Cancer Res 2008;68:7156-64.

60. Leeman-Neill RJ, Brenner AV, Little MP, et al. RET/PTC and PAX8/PPARγ chromosomal rearrangements in post-Chernobyl thyroid cancer and their association with iodine-131 radiation dose and other characteristics. Cancer 2013;119:1792-9.

61. Ricarte-Filho JC, Li S, Garcia-Rendueles ME, et al. Identification of kinase fusion oncogenes in post-Chernobyl radiation-induced thyroid cancers. J Clin Invest 2013;123:4935-44.

62. Sansal I, Sellers WR. The biology and clinical relevance of the PTEN tumor suppressor pathway. J Clin Oncol 2004;22:2954-63.

63. Cully M, You H, Levine AJ, Mak TW. Beyond PTEN mutations: the PI3K pathway as an integrator of multiple inputs during tumorigenesis. Nat Rev Cancer 2006;6:184-92.

64. Engelman JA, Luo J, Cantley LC. The evolution of phosphatidylinositol 3-kinases as regulators of growth and metabolism. Nat Rev Genet 2006;7:606-19.

65. Paes JE Ringel MD. Dysregulation of the phosphatidylinositol 3-kinase pathway in thyroid neoplasia. Endocrinol Metab Clin North Am 2008;37:375-87, viii-ix.

66. Liu Z, Hou P, Ji M, et al. Highly prevalent genetic alterations in receptor tyrosine kinases and phosphatidylinositol 3-kinase/akt and mitogen-activated protein kinase pathways in anaplastic and follicular thyroid cancers. J Clin Endocrinol Metab 2008;93:3106-16.

67. Wang Y, Hou P, Yu H, et al. High prevalence and mutual exclusivity of genetic alterations in the phosphatidylinositol-3-kinase/akt pathway in thyroid tumors. J Clin Endocrinol Metab 2007;92:2387-90.

68. Bruni P, Boccia A, Baldassarre G, et al. PTEN expression is reduced in a subset of sporadic thyroid carcinomas: evidence that PTEN-growth suppressing activity in thyroid cancer cells mediated by p27kip1. Oncogene 2000;19:3146-55.

69. Gimm O, Perren A, Weng LP, et al. Differential nuclear and cytoplasmic expression of PTEN in normal thyroid tissue, and benign and malignant epithelial thyroid tumors. Am J Pathol 2000;156:1693-700.

70. Alvarez-Nunez F, Bussaglia E, Mauricio D, et al. PTEN promoter methylation in sporadic thyroid carcinomas. Thyroid 2006;16:17-23.

71. Garcia-Rostan G, Costa AM, Pereira-Castro I, et al. Mutation of the PIK3CA gene in anaplastic thyroid cancer. Cancer Res 2005;65:10199-207.

72. Santarpia L, El-Naggar AK, Cote GJ, Myers JN, Sherman SI. Phosphatidylinositol 3-kinase/akt and ras/raf-mitogen-activated protein kinase pathway mutations in anaplastic thyroid cancer. J Clin Endocrinol Metab 2008;93:278-84.

73. Landa I, Ganly I, Chan TA, et al. Frequent somatic TERT promoter mutations in thyroid cancer: higher prevalence in advanced forms of the disease. J Clin Endocrinol Metab 2013;98:1562-6.

74. Liu T, Wang N, Cao J, et al. The age- and shorter telomere-dependent TERT promoter mutation in follicular thyroid cell-derived carcinomas. Oncogene 2014;33:4978-84.

75. Liu X, Bishop J, Shan Y, et al. Highly prevalent TERT promoter mutations in aggressive thyroid cancers. Endocr Relat Cancer 2013;20:603-10.

76. Vinagre J, Almeida A, Pópulo H, et al. Frequency of TERT promoter mutations in human cancers. Nat Commun 2013;4:2185.

77. Melo M, da Rocha AG, Vinagre J, et al. TERT promoter mutations are a major indicator of poor outcome in differentiated thyroid carcinomas. J Clin Endocrinol Metab 2014;99:E754-65.

78. Liu X, Qu S, Liu R, et al. TERT promoter mutations and their association with BRAF V600E mutation and aggressive clinicopathological characteristics of thyroid cancer. J Clin Endocrinol Metab 2014;99:E1130-6.

79. Roque L, Clode A, Belge G, et al. Follicular thyroid carcinoma: chromosome analysis of 19 cases. Genes Chromosomes Cancer 1998;21:250-5.

80. Herrmann MA, Hay ID, Bartelt DH Jr, et al. Cytogenetic and molecular genetic studies of follicular and papillary thyroid cancers. J Clin Invest 1991;88:1596-604.

81. Castro P, Eknaes M, Teixeira MR, et al. Adenomas and follicular carcinomas of the thyroid display two major patterns of chromosomal changes. J Pathol 2005;206:305-11.

82. Ward LS, Brenta G, Medvedovic M, Fagin JA. Studies of allelic loss in thyroid tumors reveal major differences in chromosomal instability between papillary and follicular carcinomas. J Clin Endocrinol Metab 1998;83:525-30.

83. Hunt JL, Yim JH, Tometsko M, Finkelstein SD, Swalsky P, Carty SE. Loss of heterozygosity of the VHL gene identifies malignancy and predicts death in follicular thyroid tumors. Surgery 2003;134:1043-7; discussion 1047-8.

84. Hunt JL, Yim JH, Carty SE. Fractional allelic loss of tumor suppressor genes identifies malignancy and predicts clinical outcome in follicular thyroid tumors. Thyroid 2006;16:643-9.

85. Kelly LM, Barila G, Liu P, et al. Identification of the transforming STRN-ALK fusion as a potential therapeutic target in the aggressive forms of thyroid cancer. Proc Natl Acad Sci U S A 2014;111:4233-8.

86. Spambalg D, Sharifi N, Elisei R, Gross JL, Medeiros-Neto G, Fagin JA. Structural studies of the thyrotropin receptor and Gs alpha in human thyroid cancers: low prevalence of mutations predicts infrequent involvement in malignant transformation. J Clin Endocrinol Metab 1996;81:3898-901.

87. Nikiforova MN, Wald AI, Roy S, Durso MB, Nikiforov YE. Targeted next-generation sequencing panel (ThyroSeq) for detection of mutations in thyroid cancer. J Clin Endocrinol Metab 2013;98:E1852-60.

88. Russo D, Tumino S, Arturi F, et al. Detection of an activating mutation of the thyrotropin receptor in a case of an autonomously hyperfunctioning thyroid insular carcinoma. J Clin Endocrinol Metab 1997;82:735-8.

89. Niepomniszcze H, Suarez H, Pitoia F, et al. Follicular carcinoma presenting as autonomous functioning thyroid nodule and containing an activating mutation of the TSH receptor (T620I) and a mutation of the Ki-RAS (G12C) genes. Thyroid 2006;16:497-503.

90. Zuo H, Gandhi M, Edreira MM, et al. Downregulation of Rap1GAP through epigenetic silencing and loss of heterozygosity promotes invasion and progression of thyroid tumors. Cancer Res 2010;70:1389-97.

91. Pennelli G, Vianello F, Barollo S, et al. BRAF(K601E) mutation in a patient with a follicular thyroid carcinoma. Thyroid 2011;21:1393-6.

92. Aldred MA, Huang Y, Liyanarachchi S, et al. Papillary and follicular thyroid carcinomas show distinctly different microarray expression profiles and can be distinguished by a minimum of five genes. J Clin Oncol 2004;22:3531-9.

93. Griffith OL, Melck A, Jones SJ, Wiseman SM. Meta-analysis and meta-review of thyroid cancer gene expression profiling studies identifies important diagnostic biomarkers. J Clin Oncol 2006;24:5043-51.

94. Weber F, Shen L, Aldred MA, et al. Genetic classification of benign and malignant thyroid follicular neoplasia based on a three-gene combination. J Clin Endocrinol Metab 2005;90:2512-21.

95. Stolf BS, Santos MM, Simao DF, et al. Class distinction between follicular adenomas and follicular carcinomas of the thyroid gland on the basis of their signature expression. Cancer 2006;106:1891-900.

96. Chiappetta G, Ferraro A, Vuttariello E, et al. HMGA2 mRNA expression correlates with the malignant phenotype in human thyroid neoplasias. Eur J Cancer 2008;44:1015-21.

97. Belge G, Meyer A, Klemke M, et al. Upregulation of HMGA2 in thyroid carcinomas: a novel molecular marker to distinguish between benign and malignant follicular neoplasias. Genes Chromosomes Cancer 2008;47:56-63.

98. Prasad NB, Somervell H, Tufano RP, et al. Identification of genes differentially expressed in benign versus malignant thyroid tumors. Clin Cancer Res 2008;14:3327-37.

99. Nikiforova MN, Tseng GC, Steward D, Diorio D, Nikiforov YE. MicroRNA expression profiling of thyroid tumors: biological significance and diagnostic utility. J Clin Endocrinol Metab 2008;93:1600-8.

100. Weber F, Teresi RE, Broelsch CE, Frilling A, Eng C. A limited set of human microRNA is deregulated in follicular thyroid carcinoma. J Clin Endocrinol Metab 2006;91:3584-91.

101. Nikiforova MN, Chiosea SI, Nikiforov YE. MicroRNA expression profiles in thyroid tumors. Endocr Pathol 2009;20:85-91.

102. Hobert JA Eng C. PTEN hamartoma tumor syndrome: an overview. Genet Med 2009;11:687-94.

103. Bonora E, Tallini G, Romeo G. Genetic predisposition to familial nonmedullary thyroid cancer: an update of molecular findings and state-of-the-art studies. J Oncol 2010;2010:385206.

104. Loh KC. Familial nonmedullary thyroid carcinoma: a meta-review of case series. Thyroid 1997;7:107-13.

105. Cooper DS, Axelrod L, DeGroot LJ, Vickery AL Jr, Maloof F. Congenital goiter and the development of metastatic follicular carcinoma with evidence for a leak of nonhormonal iodide: clinical, pathological, kinetic, and biochemical studies and a review of the literature. J Clin Endocrinol Metab 1981;52:294-306.

106. Kimura ET, Nikiforova MN, Zhu Z, Knauf JA, Nikiforov YE, Fagin JA. High prevalence of BRAF mutations in thyroid cancer: genetic evidence for constitutive activation of the RET/PTC-RAS-BRAF signaling pathway in papillary thyroid carcinoma. Cancer Res 2003;63:1454-7.

107. Giordano TJ, Kuick R, Thomas DG, et al. Molecular classification of papillary thyroid carcinoma: distinct BRAF, RAS, and RET/PTC mutation-specific gene expression profiles discovered by DNA microarray analysis. Oncogene 2005;24:6646-56.

108. Hamatani K, Eguchi H, Ito R, et al. RET/PTC rearrangements preferentially occurred in papillary thyroid cancer among atomic bomb survivors exposed to high radiation dose. Cancer Res 2008;68:7176-82.

109. Leeman-Neill RJ, Kelly LM, Liu P, et al. ETV6-NTRK3 is a common chromosomal rearrangement in radiation-associated thyroid cancer. Cancer 2014;120:799-807.

110. Xing M. BRAF mutation in thyroid cancer. Endocr Relat Cancer 2005;12:245-62.

111. De Falco V, Giannini R, Tamburrino A, et al. Functional characterization of the novel T599I-VKSRdel BRAF mutation in a follicular variant papillary thyroid carcinoma. J Clin Endocrinol Metab 2008;93:4398-402.

112. Ciampi R, Knauf JA, Kerler R, et al. Oncogenic AKAP9-BRAF fusion is a novel mechanism of MAPK pathway activation in thyroid cancer. J Clin Invest 2005;115:94-101.

113. Cohen Y, Rosenbaum E, Clark DP, et al. Mutational analysis of BRAF in fine needle aspiration biopsies of the thyroid: a potential application for the preoperative assessment of thyroid nodules. Clin Cancer Res 2004;10:2761-5.

114. Cradic KW, Milosevic D, Rosenberg AM, Erickson LA, McIver B, Grebe SK. Mutant BRAF(T1799A) can be detected in the blood of papillary thyroid carcinoma patients and correlates with disease status. J Clin Endocrinol Metab 2009;94:5001-9.

115. Koperek O, Kornauth C, Capper D, et al. Immunohistochemical detection of the BRAF V600E-mutated protein in papillary thyroid carcinoma. Am J Surg Pathol 2012;36:844-50.

116. Flavin R, Smyth P, Crotty P, et al. BRAF T1799A mutation occurring in a case of malignant struma ovarii. Int J Surg Pathol 2007;15:116-20.

117. Schmidt J, Derr V, Heinrich MC, et al. BRAF in papillary thyroid carcinoma of ovary (struma ovarii). Am J Surg Pathol 2007;31:1337-43.

118. Sargent R, LiVolsi V, Murphy J, Mantha G, Hunt JL. BRAF mutation is unusual in chronic lymphocytic thyroiditis-associated papillary thyroid carcinomas and absent in non-neoplastic nuclear atypia of thyroiditis. Endocr Pathol 2006;17:235-41.

119. Nikiforova MN, Kimura ET, Gandhi M, et al. BRAF mutations in thyroid tumors are restricted to papillary carcinomas and anaplastic or poorly differentiated carcinomas arising from papillary carcinomas. J Clin Endocrinol Metab 2003;88:5399-404.

120. Trovisco V, Soares P, Preto A, et al. Type and prevalence of BRAF mutations are closely associated with papillary thyroid carcinoma histotype and patients' age but not with tumour aggressiveness. Virchows Arch 2005;446:589-95.

121. Trovisco V, Vieira de Castro I, Soares P. BRAF mutations are associated with some histological types of papillary thyroid carcinoma. J Pathol 2004;202:247-51.

122. Adeniran AJ, Zhu Z, Gandhi M, et al. Correlation between genetic alterations and microscopic features, clinical manifestations, and prognostic characteristics of thyroid papillary carcinomas. Am J Surg Pathol 2006;30:216-22.

123. Rivera M, Ricarte-Filho J, Tuttle RM, et al. Molecular, morphologic, and outcome analysis of thyroid carcinomas according to degree of extrathyroid extension. Thyroid 2010;20:1085-93.

124. Finkelstein A, Levy GH, Hui P, et al. Papillary thyroid carcinomas with and without BRAF V600E mutations are morphologically distinct. Histopathology 2012;60:1052-9.

125. Mathur A, Moses W, Rahbari R, et al. Higher rate of BRAF mutation in papillary thyroid cancer over time: a single-institution study. Cancer 2011;117:4390-5.

126. Jung CK, Little MP, Lubin JH, et al. The increase in thyroid cancer incidence during the last four decades is accompanied by a high frequency of BRAF mutations and a sharp increase in RAS mutations. J Clin Endocrinol Metab 2014;99:276-85.

127. Guan H, Ji M, Bao R, et al. Association of high iodine intake with the T1799A BRAF mutation in papillary thyroid cancer. J Clin Endocrinol Metab 2009;94:1612-7.

128. Lima J, Trovisco V, Soares P, et al. BRAF mutations are not a major event in post-Chernobyl childhood thyroid carcinomas. J Clin Endocrinol Metab 2004;89:4267-71.

129. Xing M. BRAF mutation in papillary thyroid cancer: pathogenic role, molecular bases, and clinical implications. Endocr Rev 2007;28:742-62.

130. Kim TY, Kim WB, Rhee YS, et al. The BRAF mutation is useful for prediction of clinical recurrence in low-risk patients with conventional papillary thyroid carcinoma. Clin Endocrinol (Oxf) 2006;65:364-8.

131. Lupi C, Giannini R, Ugolini C, et al. Association of BRAF V600E mutation with poor clinicopathological outcomes in 500 consecutive cases of papillary thyroid carcinoma. J Clin Endocrinol Metab 2007;92:4085-90.

132. Elisei R, Ugolini C, Viola D, et al. BRAF(V600E) mutation and outcome of patients with papillary thyroid carcinoma: a 15-year median follow-up study. J Clin Endocrinol Metab 2008;93:3943-9.

133. Basolo F, Torregrossa L, Giannini R, et al. Correlation between the BRAF V600E mutation and tumor invasiveness in papillary thyroid carcinomas smaller than 20 millimeters: analysis of 1060 cases. J Clin Endocrinol Metab 2010;95:4197-205.

134. Nucera C, Porrello A, Antonello ZA, et al. B-Raf(V600E) and thrombospondin-1 promote thyroid cancer progression. Proc Natl Acad Sci U S A 2010;107:10649-54.

135. Knauf JA, Sartor MA, Medvedovic M, et al. Progression of BRAF-induced thyroid cancer is associated with epithelial-mesenchymal transition requiring concomitant MAP kinase and TGFbeta signaling. Oncogene 2011;30:3153-62.

136. Durante C, Puxeddu E, Ferretti E, et al. BRAF mutations in papillary thyroid carcinomas inhibit genes involved in iodine metabolism. J Clin Endocrinol Metab 2007;92:2840-3.

137. Riesco-Eizaguirre G, Gutierrez-Martinez P, Garcia-Cabezas MA, Nistal M, Santisteban P. The oncogene BRAF V600E is associated with a high risk of recurrence and less differentiated papillary thyroid carcinoma due to the impairment of Na+/I- targeting to the membrane. Endocr Relat Cancer 2006;13:257-69.

138. Xing M, Westra WH, Tufano RP, et al. BRAF mutation predicts a poorer clinical prognosis for papillary thyroid cancer. J Clin Endocrinol Metab 2005;90:6373-9.

139. Kebebew E, Weng J, Bauer J, et al. The prevalence and prognostic value of BRAF mutation in thyroid cancer. Ann Surg 2007;246:466-70; discussion 470-1.

140. Elisei R, Viola D, Torregrossa L, et al. The BRAF(V600E) mutation is an independent, poor prognostic factor for the outcome of patients with low-risk intrathyroid papillary thyroid carcinoma: single-institution results from a large cohort study. J Clin Endocrinol Metab 2012;97:4390-8.

141. Xing M. Prognostic utility of BRAF mutation in papillary thyroid cancer. Mol Cell Endocrinol 2010;321:86-93.

142. Ugolini C, Giannini R, Lupi C, et al. Presence of BRAF V600E in very early stages of papillary thyroid carcinoma. Thyroid 2007;17:381-8.

143. Fugazzola L, Puxeddu E, Avenia N, et al. Correlation between B-RAFV600E mutation and clinico-pathologic parameters in papillary thyroid carcinoma: data from a multicentric Italian study and review of the literature. Endocr Relat Cancer 2006;13:455-64.

144. Ito Y, Yoshida H, Maruo R, et al. BRAF mutation in papillary thyroid carcinoma in a Japanese population: its lack of correlation with high-risk clinicopathological features and disease-free survival of patients. Endocr J 2009;56:89-97.

145. Eloy C, Santos J, Soares P, Sobrinho-Simões M. The preeminence of growth pattern and invasiveness and the limited influence of BRAF and RAS mutations in the occurrence of papillary thyroid carcinoma lymph node metastases. Virchows Arch 2011;459:265-76.

146. Pelttari H, Schalin-Jäntti C, Arola J, Löyttyniemi E, Knuutila S, Välimäki MJ. BRAF V600E mutation does not predict recurrence after long-term follow-up in TNM stage I or II papillary thyroid carcinoma patients. APMIS 2012;120:380-6.

147. Sancisi V, Nicoli D, Ragazzi M, Piana S, Ciarrocchi A. BRAFV600E mutation does not mean distant metastasis in thyroid papillary carcinomas. J Clin Endocrinol Metab 2012;97:E1745-9.

148. Guerra A, Sapio MR, Marotta V, et al. The primary occurrence of BRAF(V600E) is a rare clonal event in papillary thyroid carcinoma. J Clin Endocrinol Metab 2012;97:517-24.

149. Ghossein RA, Katabi N, Fagin JA. Immunohistochemical detection of mutated BRAF V600E supports the clonal origin of BRAF-induced thyroid cancers along the spectrum of disease progression. J Clin Endocrinol Metab 2013;98: E1414-21.

150. de Biase D, Cesari V, Visani M, et al. High sensitivity brafmutation Analysis: BRAF V600E is acquired early during tumor development but is heterogeneously distributed in a subset of papillary thyroid carcinomas. J Clin Endocrinol Metab 2014;99:E1530-8.

151. Guerra A, Fugazzola L, Marotta V, et al. A high percentage of BRAFV600E alleles in papillary thyroid carcinoma predicts a poorer outcome. J Clin Endocrinol Metab 2012;97:2333-40.

152. Gandolfi G, Sancisi V, Torricelli F, et al. Allele percentage of the BRAF V600E mutation in papillary thyroid carcinomas and corresponding lymph node metastases: no evidence for a role in tumor progression. J Clin Endocrinol Metab 2013;98:E934-42.

153. Xing M, Alzahrani AS, Carson KA, et al. Association between BRAF V600E mutation and mortality in patients with papillary thyroid cancer. JAMA 2013;309:1493-501.

154. Rosove MH, Peddi PF, Glaspy JA. BRAF V600E inhibition in anaplastic thyroid cancer. N Engl J Med 2013;368:684-5.

155. Tallini G, Asa SL. RET oncogene activation in papillary thyroid carcinoma. Adv Anat Pathol 2001;8:345-54.

156. Tallini G, Ghossein RA, Emanuel J, et al. Detection of thyroglobulin, thyroid peroxidase, and RET/PTC1 mRNA transcripts in the peripheral blood of patients with thyroid disease. J Clin Oncol 1998;16:1158-66.

157. Rhoden KJ, Unger K, Salvatore G, et al. RET/papillary thyroid cancer rearrangement in nonneoplastic thyrocytes: follicular cells of Hashimoto's thyroiditis share low-level recombination events with a subset of papillary carcinoma. J Clin Endocrinol Metab 2006;91:2414-23.

158. Zhu Z, Ciampi R, Nikiforova MN, Gandhi M, Nikiforov YE. Prevalence of RET/PTC rearrangements in thyroid papillary carcinomas: effects of the detection methods and genetic heterogeneity. J Clin Endocrinol Metab 2006;91:3603-10.

159. Rhoden KJ, Johnson C, Brandao G, Howe JG, Smith BR, Tallini G. Real-time quantitative RT-PCR identifies distinct c-RET, RET/PTC1 and RET/PTC3 expression patterns in papillary thyroid carcinoma. Lab Invest 2004;84:1557-70.

160. Ishizaka Y, Kobayashi S, Ushijima T, Hirohashi S, Sugimura T, Nagao M. Detection of retTPC/PTC transcripts in thyroid adenomas and adenomatous goiter by an RT-PCR method. Oncogene 1991;6:1667-72.

161. Fusco A, Chiappetta G, Hui P, et al. Assessment of RET/PTC oncogene activation and clonality in thyroid nodules with incomplete morphological evidence of papillary carcinoma:

162. Santoro M, Carlomagno F, Hay ID, et al. Ret oncogene activation in human thyroid neoplasms is restricted to the papillary cancer subtype. J Clin Invest 1992;89:1517-22.

163. Bongarzone I, Vigneri P, Mariani L, Collini P, Pilotti S, Pierotti MA. RET/NTRK1 rearrangements in thyroid gland tumors of the papillary carcinoma family: correlation with clinicopathological features. Clin Cancer Res 1998;4:223-8.

164. Soares P, Fonseca E, Wynford-Thomas D, Sobrinho-Simoes M. Sporadic ret-rearranged papillary carcinoma of the thyroid: a subset of slow growing, less aggressive thyroid neoplasms? J Pathol 1998;185:71-8.

165. Tallini G, Santoro M, Helie M, et al. RET/PTC oncogene activation defines a subset of papillary thyroid carcinomas lacking evidence of progression to poorly differentiated or undifferentiated tumor phenotypes. Clin Cancer Res 1998;4:287-94.

166. Santoro M, Papotti M, Chiappetta G, et al. RET activation and clinicopathologic features in poorly differentiated thyroid tumors. J Clin Endocrinol Metab 2002;87:370-9.

167. Viglietto G, Chiappetta G, Martinez-Tello FJ, et al. RET/PTC oncogene activation is an early event in thyroid carcinogenesis. Oncogene 1995;11:1207-10.

168. Corvi R, Martinez-Alfaro M, Harach HR, Zini M, Papotti M, Romeo G. Frequent RET rearrangements in thyroid papillary microcarcinoma detected by interphase fluorescence in situ hybridization. Lab Invest 2001;81:1639-45.

169. Nikiforov YE. Radiation-induced thyroid cancer: what we have learned from Chernobyl. Endocr Pathol 2006;17:307-17.

170. Castellone MD, Santoro M. Dysregulated RET signaling in thyroid cancer. Endocrinol Metab Clin North Am 2008;37:363-74, viii.

171. Nikiforov YE, Rowland JM, Bove KE, Monforte-Munoz H, Fagin JA. Distinct pattern of ret oncogene rearrangements in morphological variants of radiation-induced and sporadic thyroid papillary carcinomas in children. Cancer Res 1997;57:1690-4.

172. Rabes HM, Demidchik EP, Sidorow JD, et al. Pattern of radiation-induced RET and NTRK1 rearrangements in 191 post-Chernobyl papillary thyroid carcinomas: biological, phenotypic, and clinical implications. Clin Cancer Res 2000;6:1093-103.

173. LiVolsi VA, Abrosimov AA, Bogdanova T, et al. The Chernobyl thyroid cancer experience: pathology. Clin Oncol (R Coll Radiol) 2011;23:261-7.

174. Radice P, Sozzi G, Miozzo M, et al. The human tropomyosin gene involved in the generation of the TRK oncogene maps to chromosome 1q31. Oncogene 1991;6:2145-8.

175. Greco A, Miranda C, Pagliardini S, Fusetti L, Bongarzone I, Pierotti MA. Chromosome 1 rearrangements involving the genes TPR and NTRK1 produce structurally different thyroid-specific TRK oncogenes. Genes Chromosomes Cancer 1997;19:112-23.

176. Greco A, Mariani C, Miranda C, et al. The DNA rearrangement that generates the TRK-T3 oncogene involves a novel gene on chromosome 3 whose product has a potential coiled-coil domain. Mol Cell Biol 1995;15:6118-27.

177. Musholt TJ, Musholt PB, Khaladj N, Schulz D, Scheumann GF, Klempnauer J. Prognostic significance of RET and NTRK1 rearrangements in sporadic papillary thyroid carcinoma. Surgery 2000;128:984-93.

178. Delvincourt C, Patey M, Flament JB, et al. Ret and trk proto-oncogene activation in thyroid papillary carcinomas in French patients from the Champagne-Ardenne region. Clin Biochem 1996;29:267-71.

179. Kuo CS, Lin CY, Hsu CW, Lee CH, Lin HD. Low frequency of rearrangement of TRK protooncogene in Chinese thyroid tumors. Endocrine 2000;13:341-4.

180. Godbert Y, Henriques de Figueiredo B, Bonichon F, et al. Remarkable response to crizotinib in woman with anaplastic lymphoma kinase-rearranged anaplastic thyroid carcinoma. J Clin Oncol 2014. [Epub ahead of print]

181. Hamatani K, Mukai M, Takahashi K, Hayashi Y, Nakachi K, Kusunoki Y. Rearranged anaplastic lymphoma kinase (ALK) gene in adult-onset papillary thyroid cancer amongst atomic bomb survivors. Thyroid 2012;22:1153-9.

182. Jenkins RB, Hay ID, Herath JF, et al. Frequent occurrence of cytogenetic abnormalities in sporadic nonmedullary thyroid carcinoma. Cancer 1990;66:1213-20.

183. Antonini P, Venuat AM, Linares G, Caillou B, Berger R, Parmentier C. A translocation (7;10)(q35;q21) in a differentiated papillary carcinoma of the thyroid. Cancer Genet Cytogenet 1989;41:139-44.

184. Roque L, Nunes VM, Ribeiro C, Martins C, Soares J. Karyotypic characterization of papillary thyroid carcinomas. Cancer 2001;92:2529-38.

185. Sozzi G, Bongarzone I, Miozzo M, et al. Cytogenetic and molecular genetic characterization of papillary thyroid carcinomas. Genes Chromosomes Cancer 1992;5:212-8.

186. Cohn K, Backdahl M, Forsslund G, et al. Prognostic value of nuclear DNA content in papillary thyroid carcinoma. World J Surg 1984;8:474-80.

187. Joensuu H, Klemi P, Eerola E, Tuominen J. Influence of cellular DNA content on survival in differentiated thyroid cancer. Cancer 1986;58:2462-7.

188. Smith SA, Hay ID, Goellner JR, Ryan JJ, McConahey WM. Mortality from papillary thyroid carcinoma. A case-control study of 56 lethal cases. Cancer 1988;62:1381-8.

189. Kjellman P, Lagercrantz S, Hoog A, Wallin G, Larsson C, Zedenius J. Gain of 1q and loss of 9q21.3-q32 are associated with a less favorable prognosis in papillary thyroid carcinoma. Genes Chromosomes Cancer 2001;32:43-9.

190. Wreesmann VB, Ghossein RA, Patel SG, et al. Genome-wide appraisal of thyroid cancer progression. Am J Pathol 2002;161:1549-56.

191. Wreesmann VB, Sieczka EM, Socci ND, et al. Genome-wide profiling of papillary thyroid cancer identifies MUC1 as an independent prognostic marker. Cancer Res 2004;64:3780-9.

192. Singh B, Lim D, Cigudosa JC, et al. Screening for genetic aberrations in papillary thyroid cancer by using comparative genomic hybridization. Surgery 2000;128:888-93;discussion 893-4.

193. Huang Y, Prasad M, Lemon WJ, et al. Gene expression in papillary thyroid carcinoma reveals highly consistent profiles. Proc Natl Acad Sci U S A 2001;98:15044-9.

194. Chevillard S, Ugolin N, Vielh P, et al. Gene expression profiling of differentiated thyroid neoplasms: diagnostic and clinical implications. Clin Cancer Res 2004;10:6586-97.

195. Alexander EK, Kennedy GC, Baloch ZW, et al. Preoperative diagnosis of benign thyroid nodules with indeterminate cytology. N Engl J Med 2012;367:705-15.

196. He H, Jazdzewski K, Li W, et al. The role of microRNA genes in papillary thyroid carcinoma. Proc Natl Acad Sci U S A 2005;102:19075-80.

197. Pallante P, Visone R, Croce CM, Fusco A. Deregulation of microRNA expression in follicular-cell-derived human thyroid carcinomas. Endocr Relat Cancer 2010;17:F91-104.

198. Chen YT, Kitabayashi N, Zhou XK, Fahey TJ 3rd, Scognamiglio T. MicroRNA analysis as a potential diagnostic tool for papillary thyroid carcinoma. Mod Pathol 2008;21:1139-46.

199. Chou CK, Chen RF, Chou FF, et al. miR-146b is highly expressed in adult papillary thyroid carcinomas with high risk features including extrathyroidal invasion and the BRAF(V600E) mutation. Thyroid 2010;20:489-94.

200. Yip L, Kelly L, Shuai Y, et al. MicroRNA signature distinguishes the degree of aggressiveness of papillary thyroid carcinoma. Ann Surg Oncol 2011;18:2035-41.

201. Niemeier LA, Kuffner Akatsu H, Song C, et al. A combined molecular-pathologic score improves risk stratification of thyroid papillary microcarcinoma. Cancer 2012;118:2069-77.

202. Kwak JY, Kim EK, Chung WY, Moon HJ, Kim MJ, Choi JR. Association of BRAFV600E mutation with poor clinical prognostic factors and US features in Korean patients with papillary thyroid microcarcinoma. Radiology 2009;253:854-60.

203. Virk RK, Van Dyke AL, Finkelstein A, et al. BRAFV600E mutation in papillary thyroid microcarcinoma: a genotype-phenotype correlation. Mod Pathol 2013;26:62-70.

204. Liu J, Singh B, Tallini G, et al. Follicular variant of papillary thyroid carcinoma: a clinicopathologic study of a problematic entity. Cancer 2006;107:1255-64.

205. Frau DV, Lai ML, Caria P, et al. Trisomy 17 as a marker for a subset of noninvasive thyroid nodules with focal features of papillary carcinoma: cytogenetic and molecular analysis of 62 cases and correlation with histological findings. J Clin Endocrinol Metab 2008;93:177-81.

206. Daniels GH. What if many follicular variant papillary thyroid carcinomas are not malignant? A review of follicular variant papillary thyroid carcinoma and a proposal for a new classification. Endocr Pract 2011;17:768-87.

207. Nikiforov Y, Gnepp DR. Pediatric thyroid cancer after the Chernobyl disaster. Pathomorphologic study of 84 cases (1991-1992) from the Republic of Belarus. Cancer 1994;74:748-66.

208. Nikiforov YE, Erickson LA, Nikiforova MN, Caudill CM, Lloyd RV. Solid variant of papillary thyroid carcinoma: incidence, clinical-pathologic characteristics, molecular analysis, and biologic behavior. Am J Surg Pathol 2001;25:1478-84.

209. Trovisco V, Soares P, Soares R, Magalhaes J, Sa-Couto P, Sobrinho-Simões M. A new BRAF gene mutation detected in a case of a solid variant of papillary thyroid carcinoma. Hum Pathol 2005;36:694-7.

210. Rocha AS, Soares P, Seruca R, et al. Abnormalities of the E-cadherin/catenin adhesion complex in classical papillary thyroid carcinoma and in its diffuse sclerosing variant. J Pathol 2001;194:358-66.

211. Sheu SY, Schwertheim S, Worm K, Grabellus F, Schmid KW. Diffuse sclerosing variant of papillary thyroid carcinoma: lack of BRAF mutation but occurrence of RET/PTC rearrangements. Mod Pathol 2007;20:779-87.

212. D'Antonio A, De Chiara A, Santoro M, Chiappetta G, Losito NS. Warthin-like tumour of the thyroid gland: RET/PTC expression indicates it is a variant of papillary carcinoma. Histopathology 2000;36:493-8.

213. Campo E, Merino MJ, Liotta L, Neumann R, Stetler-Stevenson W. Distribution of the 72-kd type IV collagenase in nonneoplastic and neoplastic thyroid tissue. Hum Pathol 1992;23:1395-401.

214. Enriquez ML, Baloch ZW, Montone KT, Zhang PJ, LiVolsi VA. CDX2 expression in columnar cell variant of papillary thyroid carcinoma. Am J Clin Pathol 2012;137:722-6.

215. Chen JH, Faquin WC, Lloyd RV, Nose V. Clinicopathological and molecular characterization of nine cases of columnar cell variant of papillary thyroid carcinoma. Mod Pathol 2011;24:739-49.

216. Tomoda C, Miyauchi A, Uruno T, et al. Cribriform-morular variant of papillary thyroid carcinoma: clue to early detection of familial adenomatous polyposis-associated colon cancer. World J Surg 2004;28:886-9.

217. Ito Y, Miyauchi A, Ishikawa H, et al. Our experience of treatment of cribriform morular variant of papillary thyroid carcinoma; difference in clinicopathological features of FAP-associated and sporadic patients. Endocr J 2011;58:685-9.

218. Xu B, Yoshimoto K, Miyauchi A, et al. Cribriform-morular variant of papillary thyroid carcinoma: a pathological and molecular genetic study with evidence of frequent somatic mutations in exon 3 of the beta-catenin gene. J Pathol 2003;199:58-67.

219. Soravia C, Sugg SL, Berk T, et al. Familial adenomatous polyposis-associated thyroid cancer: a clinical, pathological, and molecular genetics study. Am J Pathol 1999;154:127-35.

220. Cameselle-Teijeiro J, Ruiz-Ponte C, Loidi L, Suarez-Penaranda J, Baltar J, Sobrinho-Simões M. Somatic but not germline mutation of the APC gene in a case of cribriform-morular variant of papillary thyroid carcinoma. Am J Clin Pathol 2001;115:486-93.

221. Cameselle-Teijeiro J, Menasce LP, Yap BK, et al. Cribriform-morular variant of papillary thyroid carcinoma: molecular characterization of a case with neuroendocrine differentiation and aggressive behavior. Am J Clin Pathol 2009;131:134-42.

222. Schuetze D, Hoschar AP, Seethala RR, Assaad A, Zhang X, Hunt JL. The T1799A BRAF mutation is absent in cribriform-morular variant of papillary carcinoma. Arch Pathol Lab Med 2009;133:803-5.

223. Lote K, Andersen K, Nordal E, Brennhovd IO. Familial occurrence of papillary thyroid carcinoma. Cancer 1980;46:1291-7.
224. Kebebew E. Hereditary non-medullary thyroid cancer. World J Surg 2008;32:678-82.
225. Nose V. Familial non-medullary thyroid carcinoma: an update. Endocr Pathol 2008;19:226-40.
226. Plail RO, Bussey HJ, Glazer G, Thomson JP. Adenomatous polyposis: an association with carcinoma of the thyroid. Br J Surg 1987;74:377-80.
227. Ishikawa Y, Sugano H, Matsumoto T, Furuichi Y, Miller RW, Goto M. Unusual features of thyroid carcinomas in Japanese patients with Werner syndrome and possible genotype-phenotype relations to cell type and race. Cancer 1999;85:1345-52.
228. Hemminki K, Eng C, Chen B. Familial risks for nonmedullary thyroid cancer. J Clin Endocrinol Metab 2005;90:5747-53.
229. Canzian F, Amati P, Harach HR, et al. A gene predisposing to familial thyroid tumors with cell oxyphilia maps to chromosome 19p13.2. Am J Hum Genet 1998;63:1743-8.
230. Bevan S, Pal T, Greenberg CR, et al. A comprehensive analysis of MNG1, TCO1, fPTC, PTEN, TSHR, and TRKA in familial nonmedullary thyroid cancer: confirmation of linkage to TCO1. J Clin Endocrinol Metab 2001;86:3701-4.
231. Malchoff CD, Sarfarazi M, Tendler B, et al. Papillary thyroid carcinoma associated with papillary renal neoplasia: genetic linkage analysis of a distinct heritable tumor syndrome. J Clin Endocrinol Metab 2000;85:1758-64.
232. McKay JD, Lesueur F, Jonard L, et al. Localization of a susceptibility gene for familial non-medullary thyroid carcinoma to chromosome 2q21. Am J Hum Genet 2001;69:440-6.
233. He H, Nagy R, Liyanarachchi S, et al. A susceptibility locus for papillary thyroid carcinoma on chromosome 8q24. Cancer Res 2009;69:625-31.
234. Harach HR, Lesueur F, Amati P, et al. Histology of familial thyroid tumours linked to a gene mapping to chromosome 19p13.2. J Pathol 1999;189:387-93.
235. de la Chapelle A. Unraveling the genetic predisposition to differentiated thyroid carcinoma. J Clin Endocrinol Metab 2013;98:3974-6.
236. Köhler A, Chen B, Gemignani F, et al. Genome-wide association study on differentiated thyroid cancer. J Clin Endocrinol Metab 2013;98:1674-81.
237. Moses W, Weng J, Kebebew E. Prevalence, clinicopathologic features, and somatic genetic mutation profile in familial versus sporadic nonmedullary thyroid cancer. Thyroid 2011;21:367-71.
238. Capezzone M, Marchisotta S, Cantara S, et al. Familial non-medullary thyroid carcinoma displays the features of clinical anticipation suggestive of a distinct biological entity. Endocr Relat Cancer 2008;15:1075-81.
239. Ito Y, Kakudo K, Hirokawa M, et al. Biological behavior and prognosis of familial papillary thyroid carcinoma. Surgery 2009;145:100-5.
240. McDonald TJ, Driedger AA, Garcia BM, et al. Familial papillary thyroid carcinoma: a retrospective analysis. J Oncol 2011;2011:948786.
241. Pilotti S, Collini P, Del Bo R, Cattoretti G, Pierotti MA, Rilke F. A novel panel of antibodies that segregates immunocytochemically poorly differentiated carcinoma from undifferentiated carcinoma of the thyroid gland. Am J Surg Pathol 1994;18:1054-64.
242. Manetto V, Lorenzini R, Cordon-Cardo C, et al. Bcl-2 and Bax expression in thyroid tumours. An immunohistochemical and western blot analysis. Virchows Arch 1997;430:125-30.
243. Tallini G, Garcia-Rostan G, Herrero A, et al. Downregulation of p27KIP1 and Ki67/Mib1 labeling index support the classification of thyroid carcinoma into prognostically relevant categories. Am J Surg Pathol 1999;23:678-85.
244. Wang S, Lloyd RV, Hutzler MJ, Safran MS, Patwardhan NA, Khan A. The role of cell cycle regulatory protein, cyclin D1, in the progression of thyroid cancer. Mod Pathol 2000;13:882-7.
245. Saltman B, Singh B, Hedvat CV, Wreesmann VB, Ghossein R. Patterns of expression of cell cycle/apoptosis genes along the spectrum of thyroid carcinoma progression. Surgery 2006;140:899-905; discussion 905-6.
246. Roque L, Castedo S, Clode A, Soares J. Deletion of 3p25—>pter in a primary follicular thyroid carcinoma and its metastasis. Genes Chromosomes Cancer 1993;8:199-203.
247. Donghi R, Longoni A, Pilotti S, Michieli P, Della Porta G, Pierotti MA. Gene p53 mutations are restricted to poorly differentiated and undifferentiated carcinomas of the thyroid gland. J Clin Invest 1993;91:1753-60.
248. Dobashi Y, Sugimura H, Sakamoto A, et al. Stepwise participation of p53 gene mutation during dedifferentiation of human thyroid carcinomas. Diagn Mol Pathol 1994;3:9-14.
249. Garcia-Rostan G, Camp RL, Herrero A, Carcangiu ML, Rimm DL, Tallini G. Beta-catenin dysregulation in thyroid neoplasms: downregulation, aberrant nuclear expression, and CTNNB1 exon 3 mutations are markers for aggressive tumor phenotypes and poor prognosis. Am J Pathol 2001;158:987-96.

250. Costa AM, Herrero A, Fresno MF, et al. BRAF mutation associated with other genetic events identifies a subset of aggressive papillary thyroid carcinoma. Clin Endocrinol (Oxf) 2008;68:618-34.

251. Pita JM, Banito A, Cavaco BM, Leite V. Gene expression profiling associated with the progression to poorly differentiated thyroid carcinomas. Br J Cancer 2009;101:1782-91.

252. Schwertheim S, Sheu SY, Worm K, Grabellus F, Schmid KW. Analysis of deregulated miRNAs is helpful to distinguish poorly differentiated thyroid carcinoma from papillary thyroid carcinoma. Horm Metab Res 2009;41:475-81.

253. Dettmer MS, Perren A, Moch H, Komminoth P, Nikiforov YE, Nikiforova MN. MicroRNA profile of poorly differentiated thyroid carcinomas: new diagnostic and prognostic insights. J Mol Endocrinol 2014;52:181-9.

254. Hunt JL, Tometsko M, LiVolsi VA, Swalsky P, Finkelstein SD, Barnes EL. Molecular evidence of anaplastic transformation in coexisting well-differentiated and anaplastic carcinomas of the thyroid. Am J Surg Pathol 2003;27:1559-64.

255. Klemi PJ, Joensuu H, Eerola E. DNA aneuploidy in anaplastic carcinoma of the thyroid gland. Am J Clin Pathol 1988;89:154-9.

256. Galera-Davidson H, Bibbo M, Dytch HE, Gonzalez-Campora R, Fernandez A, Wied GL. Nuclear DNA in anaplastic thyroid carcinoma with a differentiated component. Histopathology 1987;11:715-22.

257. Miura D, Wada N, Chin K, et al. Anaplastic thyroid cancer: cytogenetic patterns by comparative genomic hybridization. Thyroid 2003;13:283-90.

258. Salvatore G, Nappi TC, Salerno P, et al. A cell proliferation and chromosomal instability signature in anaplastic thyroid carcinoma. Cancer Res 2007;67:10148-58.

259. Erickson LA, Jin L, Wollan PC, Thompson GB, van Heerden J, Lloyd RV. Expression of p27kip1 and Ki-67 in benign and malignant thyroid tumors. Mod Pathol 1998;11:169-74.

260. Ito T, Seyama T, Mizuno T, et al. Unique association of p53 mutations with undifferentiated but not with differentiated carcinomas of the thyroid gland. Cancer Res 1992;52:1369-71.

261. Fagin JA, Matsuo K, Karmakar A, Chen DL, Tang SH, Koeffler HP. High prevalence of mutations of the p53 gene in poorly differentiated human thyroid carcinomas. J Clin Invest 1993;91:179-84.

262. Quiros RM, Ding HG, Gattuso P, Prinz RA, Xu X. Evidence that one subset of anaplastic thyroid carcinomas are derived from papillary carcinomas due to BRAF and p53 mutations. Cancer 2005;103:2261-8.

263. Garcia-Rostan G, Tallini G, Herrero A, D'Aquila TG, Carcangiu ML, Rimm DL. Frequent mutation and nuclear localization of beta-catenin in anaplastic thyroid carcinoma. Cancer Res 1999;59:1811-5.

264. Kurihara T, Ikeda S, Ishizaki Y, et al. Immunohistochemical and sequencing analyses of the Wnt signaling components in Japanese anaplastic thyroid cancers. Thyroid 2004;14:1020-9.

265. Murugan AK, Xing M. Anaplastic thyroid cancers harbor novel oncogenic mutations of the ALK gene. Cancer Res 2011;71:4403-11.

266. Murugan AK, Bojdani E, Xing M. Identification and functional characterization of isocitrate dehydrogenase 1 (IDH1) mutations in thyroid cancer. Biochem Biophys Res Commun 2010;393:555-9.

267. Marques AR, Espadinha C, Catarino AL, et al. Expression of PAX8-PPAR gamma 1 rearrangements in both follicular thyroid carcinomas and adenomas. J Clin Endocrinol Metab 2002;87:3947-52.

268. Visone R, Pallante P, Vecchione A, et al. Specific microRNAs are downregulated in human thyroid anaplastic carcinomas. Oncogene 2007;26:7590-5.

20 CYTOPATHOLOGY OF THYROID TUMORS

Fine-needle aspiration biopsy (FNAB) has become an integral component of the evaluation of patients with thyroid lesions. It is regarded as the initial biopsy method in the workup of a palpable or ultrasound-detected thyroid nodule, following the clinical history, physical examination, and serum measurement of thyroid-stimulating hormone (TSH) (1,2). As the first diagnostic test to be performed for the preoperative evaluation of the solitary thyroid nodule, FNAB has proven to be efficient and cost effective (3,4). While of lesser value, FNAB may also be helpful in evaluating the multinodular or diffusely enlarged thyroid gland, particularly when there is a dominant nodule.

FNAB of the thyroid gland is the most effective method for determining whether a given thyroid nodule is actually a true neoplasm, and in most cases, whether that neoplasm is malignant. This procedure acts as a screening examination to determine surgical versus nonsurgical therapy. Thyroid nodules develop at an estimated rate of 0.06 to 0.08 percent per year in the United States, but only a small percentage of these are malignant (25/million people/year) (5). Prior to the use of FNAB, surgery was the only effective diagnostic procedure available to patients with a thyroid nodule. FNAB is also useful for documenting a malignant thyroid tumor in those patients where surgery is contraindicated, such as in undifferentiated (anaplastic) carcinoma and malignant lymphoma.

Tables 20-1 and 20-2 list the indications for FNAB of the thyroid gland, focusing on the thyroid nodule (6). Other clinical indications include a rapidly enlarging dominant nodule and a family history of medullary carcinoma. In the presence of a diffusely enlarged gland, subacute or chronic lymphocytic thyroiditis may need to be confirmed. Malignant lymphoma and undifferentiated (anaplastic) carcinoma presenting as rapidly enlarging glands where there is no specific mass are diagnoses easily confirmed by FNAB.

The technical aspects of FNAB of the thyroid gland are important for obtaining a good sample for interpretation, but are beyond the scope of this Fascicle. There are a number of excellent monographs and papers describing the most important technical and clinical considerations (7,8,13). Because of the increasing use of ultrasound by radiologists, endocrinologists, and other clinicians, who also procure aspiration biopsies, the importance of skill in obtaining the sample and making high quality smears cannot

Table 20-1

INDICATIONS FOR FNAB[a] OF A THYROID NODULE USING PALPATION GUIDANCE

Nodule >1.0 cm in diameter confirmed by ultrasound examination

Nodule is discrete and readily identified on physical examination

Nodule is primarily solid (<25% cystic) on ultrasound

Patient has no other head or neck disease or prior head or neck surgery that may affect the thyroid anatomy

A prior nondiagnostic biopsy of the nodule has not occurred

Obtaining ultrasound guidance for the FNAB is logistically difficult or not readily available

[a]FNAB = fine-needle aspiration biopsy.

Table 20-2

INDICATIONS FOR FNAB OF THE THYROID GLAND USING ULTRASOUND GUIDANCE

Nodules that are not palpable

Nodules that have a greater than 25% cystic component

A prior aspiration contained insufficient cells/colloid for interpretation

As an alternative to palpation localization:
to be certain that the nodule of interest is aspirated
to insure that a discrete nodule is present before aspiration
to avoid passing the needle into critical structures in the neck

Table 20-3

PROPOSED THYROID FNAB CLASSIFICATION SCHEME, NCI CONSENSUS CONFERENCE[a]

Proposed Categories	Alternate Category(ies)/Terms	Risk of Malignancy
Benign		< 1%
Follicular lesion of undetermined significance	Atypia of undetermined significance Atypical follicular lesion Cellular follicular lesion	5-10%

Neoplasm
  Follicular neoplasm
  Hürthle cell neoplasm
	Suspicious for neoplasm
	Suspicious for follicular neoplasm
	Suspicious for Hürthle cell neoplasm
		20-30%

Suspicious for malignancy		50-75%
Malignant		100%
Nondiagnostic	Unsatisfactory	

[a]FNAB = fine-needle aspiration biopsy; NCI = National Cancer Institute.

be overemphasized. Many of these practitioners are marginal in the performance of these two very important techniques. This leads the pathologist, often uninformed of the clinical and ultrasound findings, to an unsatisfactory interpretation of "insufficient sample," "indeterminate findings," or "atypical." As a response, some pathologists have learned the technique of ultrasound and added this technology to their aspiration biopsy practice, the most notable example in North America being the Outpatient Pathology Associates in Sacramento, California (9). The National Cancer Institute (NCI) Consensus Conference on Thyroid FNAB failed to fully come to terms with this reality (10).

The terminology used for reporting FNAB findings is important, particularly when clinicians are performing the procedure and sending the sample for evaluation by a pathologist unfamiliar with the patient and the history of the lesion, or unaware of the ultrasound findings. It is imperative that complete clinical information be provided to the pathologist, including location, duration, size, and any change in the size of the thyroid lesion; associated symptoms; results of ultrasound examination and scans if they have been performed; and results of any thyroid hormone studies.

Guidelines from the NCI Consensus Conference on Thyroid FNAB, also known as the Bethesda System for Reporting Thyroid Cytopathology, have been published, and the recommended terminology is presented in Table 20-3 (10). Alternative terms are provided since a complete consensus on terminology could not be reached

at this conference. There are a variety of terms that generally convey uncertainty, particularly "atypical" and "suspicious."

Cytologic atypia in benign thyroid nodules is not unusual. In most cases it is limited to a few cells and reflects the ebb and flow of hyperplasia and involution with microhemorrhages, fibrosis, and sometimes calcification that create the benign nodule(s) in the first place. This atypia is that of tissue repair, including squamous metaplasia, which is also common in the thyroid gland.

The most important component of the NCI-proposed terminology is the risk assessment for malignancy estimated for each category. This can be determined over time in one's own laboratory or it can be derived from the literature. Doing the latter may be problematic when correlating the terminology that an individual reporting laboratory may be using, the clinical and technical aspects of the procedure, and the cytologic criteria being used. In the final publication of the Bethesda System, however, reporting of risk of malignancy was optional, as were management recommendations (10). Abele et al. (11), with their large and consistent series, provide some sound statistics in this respect (Table 20-4). Microscopic criteria for adequacy are summarized in Table 20-5.

Unsatisfactory specimens also result from a lack of patient or specimen identification, irreparably broken slide(s), and poor quality smears (the result of fixation and staining artifacts, poor smear preparation technique, or excessive obscuring blood). This last feature is common

Table 20-4

FACTORS REDUCING EXCESS OF INDETERMINATE DIAGNOSES

Hypercellularity due to perfect monolayered sheets does not imply microfollicular neoplasm

Artifactual pseudocomplexity does not imply microfollicular neoplasm

Proper biopsy and smearing techniques minimize artifactual pseudocomplexity

Atrophic follicles of small diameter do not imply microfollicular neoplasm

Nonpapillary microfollicles in chronic thyroiditis do not imply microfollicular neoplasm

Table 20-5

GUIDELINES FOR MICROSCOPIC EVALUATION OF SPECIMEN ADEQUACY

Number of Cells	Amount of Colloid	Interpretation
Numerous	Variable	Adequate for interpretation, diagnosis depends on cellular features
Few	Scanty or absent	Unsatisfactory[a]
Few follicular cells	Abundant	Benign colloid nodule[b]
Few follicular cells, numerous histiocytes	Variable	Probably benign cystic goiter[b,c]

[a]If malignant cells, irrespective of the number, are identified in an aspirate, it should automatically be considered satisfactory. If too few malignant cells are present for a definitive diagnosis, a "suspicious" diagnosis or a repeat aspiration may be suggested.
[b]The report should contain a qualifier stating that the interpretation is limited by the paucity of follicular cells.
[c]Occasionally, a cystic papillary carcinoma may present with a similar pattern. Check clinically for a residual solid area, and reaspirate if palpable. The risk of malignancy is higher in large (> 4.0 cm), hemorrhagic cysts and in cysts that recur rapidly or repeatedly.

among practitioners without proper training, practice, and skills. As reported in papers from the NCI Thyroid FNAB State of the Science Conference, technical excellence in obtaining the aspirate and preparing smears can largely eliminate the unsatisfactory and indeterminate categories of cases without increasing the risk that a thyroid malignancy is missed (12,13).

THE NORMAL THYROID GLAND

FNAB of a clinically normal thyroid gland is rarely performed. However, the constellation of non-neoplastic cytologic features found in thyroid nodules or enlargements that are not neoplastic provides the background to compare differences when a neoplasm is actually present.

The normal thyroid gland consists of small uniform sheets of follicular epithelial cells with faintly discernable cell borders and evenly spaced, uniform, small round nuclei (fig. 20-1). Material is often scant, with small fragments or whole thyroid follicles (fig. 20-2) that may (but usually do not) contain colloid. Both the sheets and follicles have smooth borders that are gently curved or in a straight line, without indentations, referred to as "scalloping." The outer border of a single whole thyroid follicle is very even and the entire follicle appears symmetrical. Air-dried smears stained by the Diff-Quik method (a Romanowsky stain variation) demonstrate follicular cell nuclei that are deep purple, uniform, round, and sharply defined. The nucleoli are typically not visible. Thyroid follicle epithelial cells, after fixation and staining with the Papanicolaou method, appear more tightly clustered, with a slight degree of three dimensionality, which becomes apparent by focusing the specimen up or down. Occasional large follicular cell nuclei are found. They represent examples of endocrine organ cytomegaly. The cytoplasm of the follicular cells, when intact, has a gray-blue tinge with the Diff-Quik stain, and pastel, almost translucent green with the Papanicolaou stain. Lysosomal (paravacuolar) granules may be prominent in occasional cells, staining intensely cobalt blue with the Diff-Quik stain.

Colloid has a variety of appearances in aspiration smears and often dominates the

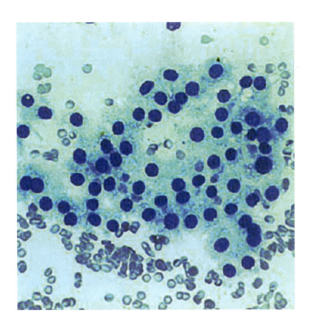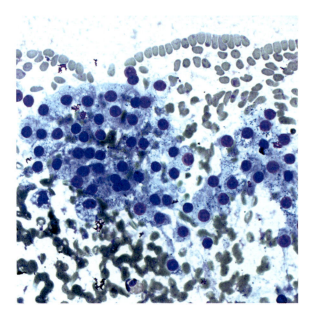

Figure 20-1

NORMAL THYROID GLAND

Left: Normal follicular cells are in sheets, within which nuclei are evenly placed. The outer border of the sheet is smooth and gently curved (Diff-Quik stain).

Right: At higher magnification, uniformly spaced nuclei are found throughout the sheet, which has a smooth outer border. Follicular cell nuclei are round. No dense colloid is seen in this field but the red blood cells are in rouleau formation, suggesting there is thin colloid between them (Diff-Quik stain).

Figure 20-2

NORMAL THYROID GLAND

A sheet of normal follicular cells is in a complete circle that represents a whole thyroid follicle. No colloid is visible within the follicle. There are some faint blue hemosiderin granules in the cytoplasm of the follicular cells, an early degenerative change that is often present (Diff-Quik stain).

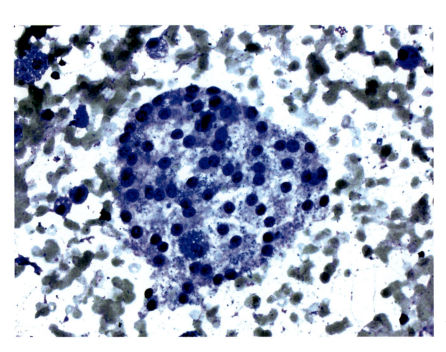

aspirates from nodular hyperplasia or the rare macrofollicular adenoma. It occurs in sheets with "cracks," like a broken pane of glass (fig. 20-3). It may appear very dense (fig. 20-4), both separated from (fig. 20-5) and with collections of thyroid follicular cells. It can appear as a pale-staining thin watery background that gives a rouleau appearance to the often-associated

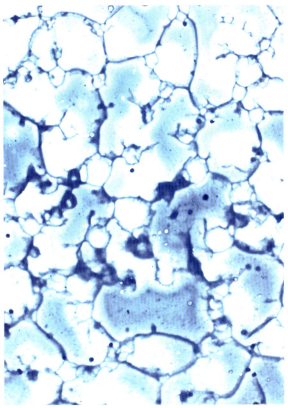

Figure 20-3

PATTERN OF COLLOID

At high magnification, the colloid has a cracked windowpane appearance (Diff-Quik stain).

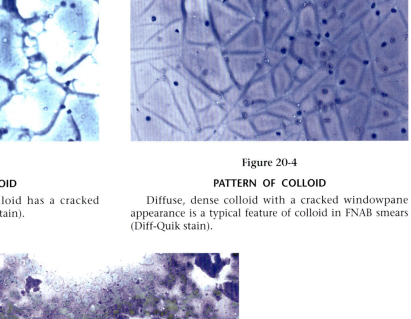

Figure 20-4

PATTERN OF COLLOID

Diffuse, dense colloid with a cracked windowpane appearance is a typical feature of colloid in FNAB smears (Diff-Quik stain).

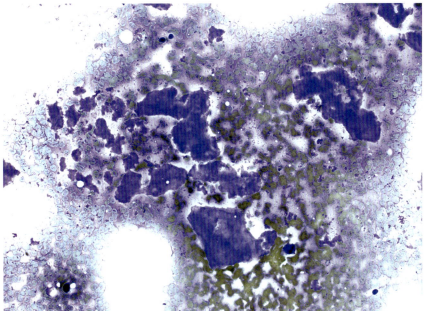

Figure 20-5

PATTERN OF COLLOID

Fragments of dense blue-violet-staining colloid in a very thin, essentially clear pattern makes up the background of the smear. The rouleau formation of the red blood cells is seen around the thin colloid (Diff-Quik stain).

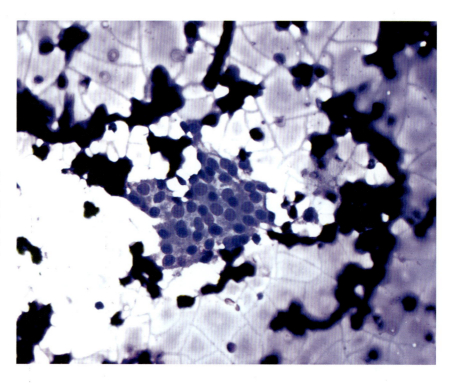

Figure 20-6

NODULAR HYPERPLASIA WITH EARLY ONCOCYTIC CHANGE

There is a small sheet of thyroid follicular cells with abundant surrounding colloid. The follicular cells are beginning to demonstrate more cytoplasm, with a granular metaplastic appearance that represents oncocytic change (Diff-Quik stain).

red blood cells (fig. 20-6). The proportion of colloid to follicular epithelium is one criterion used when judging the presence of a true neoplasm versus a non-neoplastic thyroid process. Abundant follicular epithelium accompanied by scant or little colloid favors a true neoplasm, while the reverse is true for a non-neoplastic goiter. Fragments of "normal" thyroid parenchyma are often encountered in aspirations of non-neoplastic lesions (6).

CYTOLOGY OF THYROID TUMORS AND TUMOR-LIKE CONDITIONS

Nodular Hyperplasia

A dominant nodule as part of a multinodular goiter is the most frequent FNAB thyroid specimen. As the term multinodular goiter implies, patients often develop several thyroid nodules during the course of their disease. When reporting the benign cytology/histology of these nodules and the absence of a true follicular neoplasm, the terms *nodular hyperplasia*, *nodular goiter*, *multinodular goiter*, or *non-neoplastic goiter* are used. The recommended terminology from the NCI Consensus Conference is *benign thyroid nodule*. This interpretation usually allows the clinician to recommend a conservative approach,

i.e., either no treatment or thyroid suppression therapy (6,10).

A diversity of cytologic patterns using this generic terminology indicates little risk of a true thyroid neoplasm. The nodules of nodular hyperplasia may be solid, cystic, or complex, and vary widely in size. Cystic degeneration or hemorrhage into the nodules, increasing symptoms from compression of the trachea, or change in voice is often what brings them to the attention of the patient and the clinician.

This variation, or lack of a consistent pattern, is perhaps the fundamental feature that indicates the presence of a benign non-neoplastic thyroid lesion (figs. 20-6–20-11). Benign follicular cells are arranged in irregular flat sheets, slightly three-dimensional clusters, or as whole follicles. Abundant colloid is usually present, most often as a diffuse background mixed with blood and giving a rouleau pattern to the red blood cells.

Cystic degeneration within these non-neoplastic nodules results in the presence of debris, cholesterol crystals, and histiocytes/macrophages, often containing hemosiderin pigment (fig. 20-7). Fluid from areas of degeneration of thyroid cysts should be examined by either cytocentrifugation or one of the liquid-based monolayer preparation methods to recover any

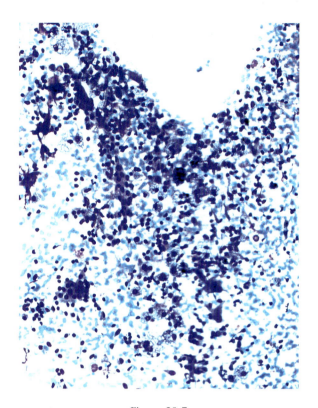

Figure 20-7

NODULAR HYPERPLASIA

The thyroid follicular cells are in a loose irregular pattern with intermingling of small fragments of dense blue colloid. While this field is fairly cellular, there is no consistent pattern of the follicular cells that might suggest a true follicular neoplasm. Many of the rest of the smears in this case showed colloid with a few histiocytes (Diff-Quik stain).

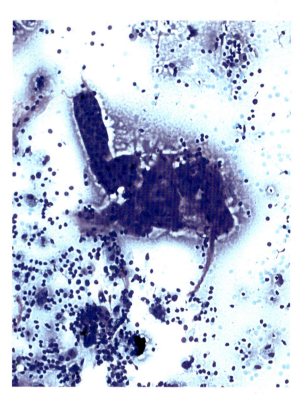

Figure 20-8

NODULAR HYPERPLASIA

Scattered thyroid follicular cells are mixed with large fragments of dense colloid and surrounding thin colloid. The follicular cell nuclei are round and lack evidence of pilling up or any consistent pattern to suggest a true follicular neoplasm (Diff-Quik stain).

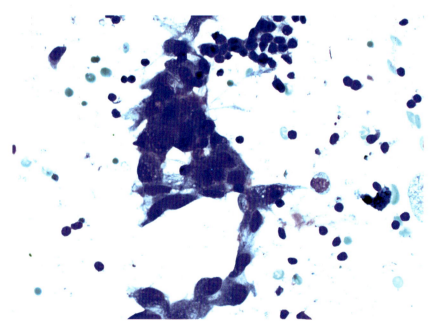

Figure 20-9

NODULAR HYPERPLASIA

A small group of normal follicular cells are at the top of the figure with a sheet of spindle-shaped cells which represent either stromal fibroblasts associated with goiter or degenerative changes in thyroid follicular cells. These spindle-shaped cells, either in small sheets as seen here or as single cells, are found in aspirates of nodular hyperplasia. They do not indicate malignancy but are part of the repair pattern in the evolution of the nodules of nodular hyperplasia (Diff-Quik stain).

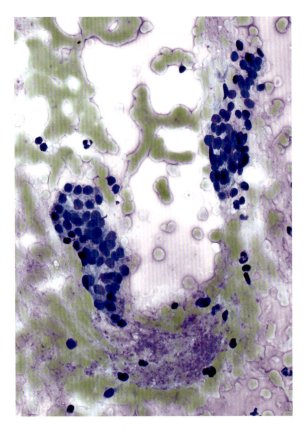

Figure 20-10

NODULAR HYPERPLASIA

Two groups of follicular cells are in a compact pattern, with some overlap of the follicular cell nuclei. Abundant colloid is seen in the background. The follicular cell nuclei are not enlarged. Multiple groups of follicular cells like these seen together in a scalloping pattern suggest a true follicular neoplasm. That pattern is not present in this figure (Diff-Quik stain).

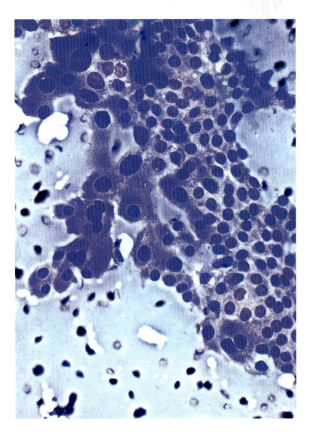

Figure 20-11

**NODULAR HYPERPLASIA
WITH FOCAL ONCOCYTIC CHANGE**

A large flat sheet of thyroid follicular cells with surrounding colloid. The cells at the bottom edge of the sheet are larger, with more granular cytoplasm and larger nuclei. These are oncocytes commonly found in aspirates from nodular hyperplasia (Diff-Quik stain).

follicular cells that might be present. Hemosiderin within macrophages in these aspirates appears as dark blue granules of varying sizes with the Diff-Quik stain, and as golden brown slightly refractive granules with the Papanicolaou stain. Cholesterol crystals are usually dissolved during staining by the Papanicolaou method but they are visible against the gray-blue background of the Diff-Quik stain.

The benign follicular cells in degenerating non-neoplastic thyroid nodules often have frayed cytoplasm and indistinct nuclear features. Tissue repair in the form of squamous metaplasia and spindle cell proliferation may occur within these nodules, resulting in cytologic atypia (fig. 20-9). There are rarely more than

a few atypical cells, a presentation completely different from the cytologic features of poorly differentiated or undifferentiated thyroid carcinoma (6,14).

When only abundant colloid with minimal numbers of follicular cells is present in a thyroid FNAB, the term *colloid nodule* may be used. Some of these nodules may have been present for a long time, and may be difficult to aspirate since the colloid becomes dense and inspissated, with a very sticky consistency and sometimes nearly water-clear. This material has a strong tendency to fall off slides during the staining process. To overcome this problem, the smears are fixed in 95 percent alcohol for Papanicolaou staining or methyl alcohol for Diff-Quik staining. The

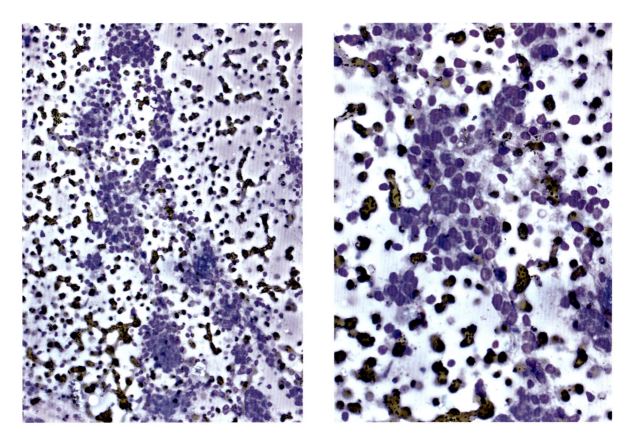

Figure 20-12

CELLULAR FOLLICULAR LESION

Left: Many follicular cells in a background of abundant colloid. The follicular cells show some clustering. The outer border of the follicular cell groups suggests some indentations (scalloping) rather than a straight or gently curved line. There is also a suggestion of crowding of the follicular cells with nuclear overlap. If this pattern is consistent in several smears or fields, the term cellular follicular lesion is used in the report. A true follicular neoplasm cannot be ruled out. Depending on the clinical circumstances, a trial of thyroid suppression therapy may be undertaken (Diff-Quik stain).

Right: At higher magnification, some crowding and overlap of follicular cell nuclei are seen. The follicular cell nuclei are slightly larger than normal, although this is difficult to judge in aspiration biopsy smears. The follicular cell groups have indented and irregular borders and a monotonous pattern of cells (Diff-Quik stain).

smears are then allowed to dry completely before proceeding with the next steps of the staining procedure.

When the thyroid nodule is dominated by a proliferation of follicular epithelial cells, the aspirate appears cellular and composed of sheets, dispersed single cells, or loose follicles (figs. 20-12, 20-13). These single cells often lack cytoplasm and look like lymphocytes, but no lymphoglandular bodies are found. The stripped follicular cell nuclei also have a great uniformity in features in comparison to lymphocytes. Oncocytic-appearing follicular cells have abundant granular cytoplasm, large nuclei, and prominent, centrally placed nucleoli.

They may be present in hyperplastic nodules with intermediate forms, i.e., follicular cells of smaller size with an early granular appearance in the cytoplasm (figs. 20-6, 20-11).

Smears with numerous follicular cells that overlap in the absence of abundant colloid result in the differential diagnosis between a hyperplastic nodule and a true follicular neoplasm. The NCI Consensus Conference recommends reporting these aspirates as "follicular lesion of undetermined significance," "atypia of undetermined significance," "atypical follicular lesion," and "cellular follicular lesion" (10). The author prefers "cellular follicular lesion," followed by a statement favoring either a non-neoplastic

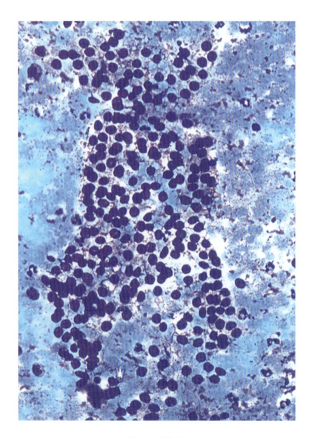

Figure 20-13

CELLULAR FOLLICULAR LESION

A large sheet of evenly spaced follicular cells with abundant background colloid. The borders of the sheets are smooth and straight. The configuration of the follicular cells is monotonous. Despite the abundant colloid, the aspirates were cellular. This pattern can be seen in a true follicular neoplasm of the macrofollicular type. It is difficult to separate from aspirates of nodular hyperplasia. There is a faint red granularity at the edge of the cell cytoplasm of many of the follicular cells, a finding seen in some aspirates of toxic hyperplasia (Diff-Quik stain).

goiter (hyperplastic nodule) or a follicular neoplasm (fig. 20-13).

Depending on the clinical features (including ultrasound findings), cases are managed according to the guidelines put forth by the American Thyroid Association, which usually recommends surgery if a follicular neoplasm is favored (1). The risk of a malignant thyroid neoplasm should not be more than 5 to 10 percent for this category (10). A trial of suppression therapy may also be used with a patient compliant for both therapy and follow-up. The cytologic features of nodular hyperplasia are summarized in Table 20-6.

Table 20-6

CYTOLOGIC FEATURES OF NODULAR HYPERPLASIA

Colloid
  Inspissated or smooth/cracked (light green with
    Papanicolaou stain; purple with Diff-Quik stain)
Follicular cells
  May be arranged as follicles, sheets, or single cells
  Bland nuclear features
  Indistinct nucleoli/chromocenters
  Frayed cytoplasm (degeneration)
Hemosiderin-laden macrophages

Diffuse Hyperplasia

FNAB is rarely used to diagnose *diffuse hyperplasia* (*Graves disease*) since the clinical and biochemical findings are usually sufficient in patients with typical hyperthyroidism. Evidence of increased uptake of radioactive iodine completes the diagnosis. If imaging studies locate a solitary "hot" nodule, FNAB becomes a safe and rapid confirmatory test by identifying a functioning follicular neoplasm. More often, such a nodule is found de novo as a localized form of hyperplasia (toxic nodule). This may be encountered unexpectedly when FNAB is used as the first step in the diagnostic workup of a solitary thyroid mass (fig. 20-14, left).

Hyperplasia is easily recognized if the follicular cells show distinctive cytoplasmic features on Diff-Quik–stained smears (15,16). These include marginal cytoplasmic vacuoles and fraying or blebs in the cytoplasmic edges ("colloid suds") having a magenta tinge ("fire flares") (fig. 20-14, right). These cytoplasmic features are often not seen with Papanicolaou-stained preparations. Cellularity may be high in hyperplasia, with the presence of little or no colloid, suggesting a true follicular neoplasm (6). Table 20-7 summarizes the cytologic findings of diffuse hyperplasia.

Hashimoto Thyroiditis

The cytologic findings on FNAB in typical cases of *Hashimoto thyroiditis* present no difficulty in interpretation. Smears are fairly cellular and composed of a mixed lymphocytic population of plasma cells intermingled with scattered oncocytic and nononcocytic follicular cells, some arranged in small groups (fig. 20-15).

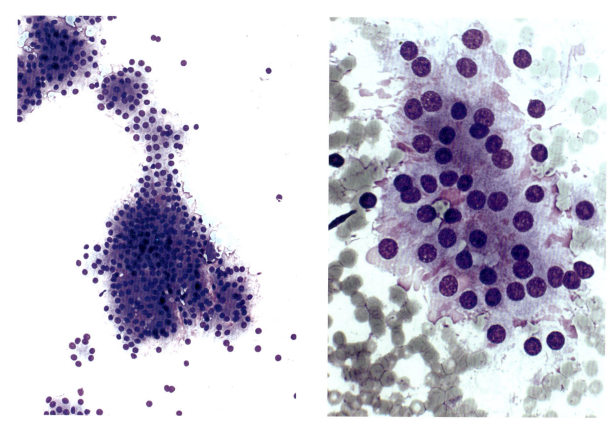

Figure 20-14

TOXIC HYPERPLASIA

Left: This cellular aspirate shows sheets and groups of uniform follicular cells. Some microfollicles and some suggestion of a scalloped outline to the large sheet suggest a true follicular neoplasm. The faint metachromatic edge to the follicular cell cytoplasm along the upper border of the largest sheet appears to flare out from the cell surface. This "fire flare" appearance, also referred as "toxic suds," is a cytologic manifestation of toxic hyperplasia, but is not entirely specific for it (Diff-Quik stain).

Right: Higher magnification of the follicular cells shows the flare-like metachromatic cytoplasm (Diff-Quik stain).

Germinal center fragments with tingible body macrophages also may be identified.

Hashimoto thyroiditis, however, may present as a dominant nodule, without the typical clinical features. The dominant nodule may be composed of oncocytes, squamous-appearing cells, or papillary clusters, the latter sometimes showing nuclear changes that raise the possibility of papillary thyroid carcinoma (fig. 20-16). A predominance of oncocytes suggests either a benign or malignant oncocytic neoplasm. Large squamoid cells suggest one of the neoplasms described in chapter 12 (especially papillary carcinoma), while papillary clusters having the nuclear changes of papillary carcinoma should be readily interpreted as such. In the absence of the typical mixed inflammatory background, it

Table 20-7
CYTOLOGIC FEATURES OF DIFFUSE HYPERPLASIA (HYPERTHYROIDISM)
Abundant blood
Minimal free colloid
Moderate to high cellularity
Follicular cells 　　Occasional oncocytic cell change 　　Loose groupings; pseudopapillary clusters 　　Fire flares/colloid suds/marginal vacuoles

may be difficult to avoid making a false positive interpretation. Ultrasound examination may reveal additional nodules in the thyroid gland, not clinically evident, and sampling of these

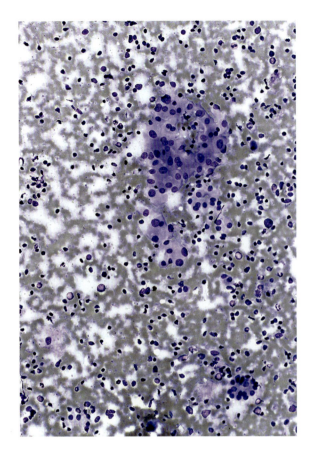

Figure 20-15

HASHIMOTO THYROIDITIS

A sheet of oncocytes, a small atrophic follicle on the right side of the field, and an inflammatory infiltrate of lymphocytes and some plasma cells are seen (Diff-Quik stain).

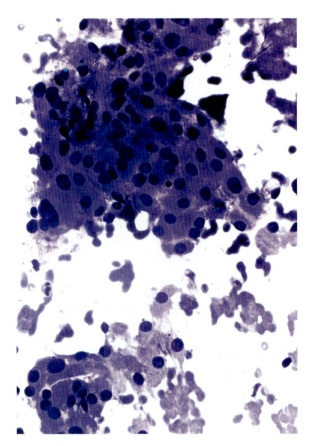

Figure 20-16

HASHIMOTO THYROIDITIS

A large irregular sheet of oncocytes is the dominant finding in this case. Other fields showed a mixture of lymphocytes and plasma cells. Differentiating between Hashimoto thyroiditis and true oncocytic neoplasm may be difficult (Diff-Quik stain).

may reveal the more typical pattern of Hashimoto thyroiditis.

The differential diagnosis also includes true thyroid neoplasms, as they can coexist within a thyroid gland with Hashimoto thyroiditis. Confronted with this dilemma, it is prudent to report such aspirates as being at least suspicious for a thyroid neoplasm, thus avoiding delay in therapy.

Patients with Hashimoto thyroiditis are at increased risk for developing a primary thyroid lymphoma. Most lymphomas are of large B-cell type and present as rapid, usually unilateral, thyroid enlargement in a patient with a long history of Hashimoto thyroiditis. On-site evaluation of adequacy by the cytopathology team ensures the proper triage of the FNAB sample for flow cytometric analysis, which provides a detailed immunophenotypic analysis of the lymphoma-

tous process. Lymphomas are easily diagnosed on FNAB and can be classified accurately using immunohistochemical or molecular methods (clonality and gene rearrangement studies) on the aspiration sample. Low-grade lymphomas, which typically present with subtle thyroid enlargement over time, are more difficult to recognize. The aspirates tend to show a uniform population of small lymphocytes, few or no plasma cells, and only rare or no oncocytic cells.

Follicular Neoplasms

The NCI Consensus Conference recommends the term "follicular lesion of undetermined significance" to reflect the difficulty of FNAB to distinguish among follicular lesions that may represent nodular hyperplasia, follicular adenoma, or follicular carcinoma (10). The risk of malignancy in this group is estimated at 5 to 10 percent (10).

The interpretation of a follicular neoplasm as malignant is based on capsule penetration or vascular space invasion by the tumor, features usually not identifiable on FNAB smears. The greatest difficulty is in distinguishing between adenoma (including the macrofollicular type), low-grade follicular carcinoma, and nodules of nodular hyperplasia (17). The clinical features and ultrasound findings may facilitate these diagnoses and aid in assessing risk that a malignant follicular neoplasm may be present and require surgical excision. Under these circumstances, FNAB represents a screening rather than a diagnostic procedure (18). In a multi-institutional study, the "indeterminate" category has not performed well in correlation with histologic or clinical follow-up (19).

There are two important features that help to distinguish between a true follicular neoplasm and nodular hyperplasia: the ratio between the follicular cells and the colloid, and the presence of a consistent pattern of follicular cells arranged in aggregates ("follicular arrays") with scalloping of the outer borders of the aggregates (figs. 20-17–20-20). The more follicular cells that are present and the less colloid identified in a solitary thyroid nodule, the more likely that it is a true follicular neoplasm. This is not true for those follicular neoplasms (almost invariably adenomas) that are composed predominantly of macrofollicles. These neoplasms have abundant colloid within their follicles that dominates the smear pattern, providing a low ratio of follicular cells to colloid (fig. 20-21). They also undergo degeneration, as do other follicular neoplasms, and this may confuse the aspiration smear pattern with findings of hemosiderin-laden macrophages, variations in follicular cell size, and individual follicular cell atypia (fig. 20-22). One report notes that the presence of hemosiderin-laden macrophages and hemosiderin within follicular cells in an aspiration smear is a strong predictor of a benign thyroid lesion (20).

While the ratio of follicular cells to colloid is an important criterion for true follicular neoplasia in an aspiration smear, the arrangement of the follicular cells is probably more helpful

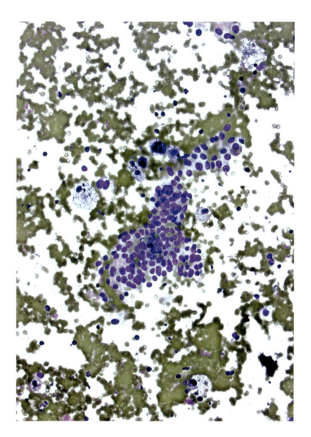

Figure 20-17

FOLLICULAR NEOPLASM

A sheet of thyroid follicular cells shows some overlap of nuclei. The outer border of the cell group is indented (scalloped) rather than straight or gently curved. A small fragment of dense colloid is present. The cellularity of the aspirate must be increased, and this pattern of monotonous follicular cells with overlapping of nuclei and a scalloped border must be repetitious, before the biopsy can be reported as a follicular neoplasm. Without a consistent pattern but only a few fields like the one illustrated here, it is more appropriate to interpret the aspirate as "cellular follicular lesion," favoring either non-neoplastic goiter or follicular neoplasm, dependent in some respects on the clinical presentation (Diff-Quik stain).

in identifying the presence of a true follicular neoplasm. It is important to study the configuration of the follicular cell groups. A scalloped pattern at their outer border, in contrast to a gentle curve or straight line with an abrupt angle to edges of the sheet of follicular cells (figs. 20-18–20-20), suggests true neoplastic follicles piled up on one another in a somewhat haphazard pattern of growth. In contrast, aspirate smears of nodular hyperplasia contain sheets of follicular cells with no evidence of scalloping

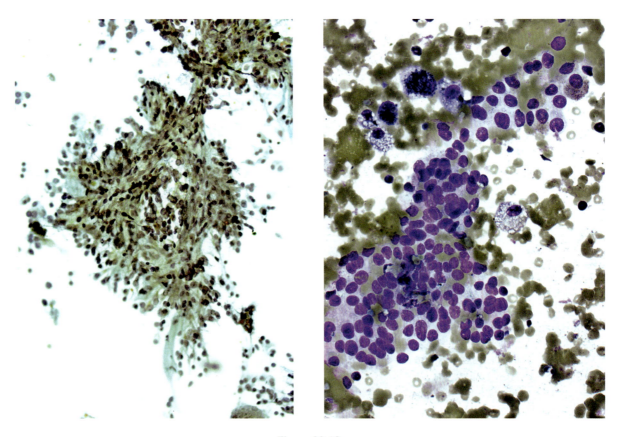

Figure 20-18

FOLLICULAR NEOPLASM

Left: The cellular aspirate has uniform follicular cells but a piling up of cell nuclei and an irregular outer border of the large group of follicular cells (same case as fig. 20-17). No colloid is visible in this figure. The aspirate overall was quite cellular, with a repetition of the pattern illustrated (Papanicolaou stain).

Right: At higher magnification, the piling up and overlap of the follicular cell nuclei are seen. These nuclei are larger than normal and there is some pleomorphism. The latter finding has no meaning with respect to malignancy. The border of the cell aggregate is scalloped, particularly along the upper aspect of the cell grouping (Diff-Quik stain).

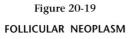

Figure 20-19

FOLLICULAR NEOPLASM

An aggregate of thyroid follicle cells has a microfollicular pattern. The outer border of the entire group also demonstrates a scalloped pattern (Diff-Quik stain).

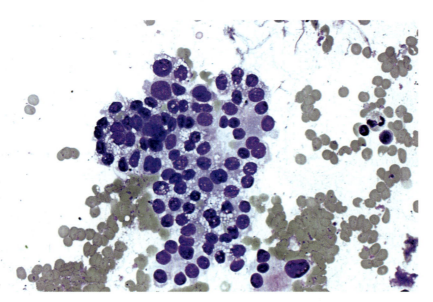

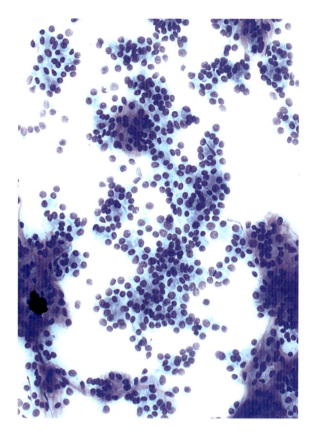

Figure 20-20

FOLLICULAR NEOPLASM

Many microfollicles, a well-developed scalloping pattern, and overlap of follicular cells with nuclei that are uniform and slightly enlarged are seen. A consistent pattern like this in a thyroid aspiration smear is interpreted as a follicular neoplasm (Diff-Quik stain).

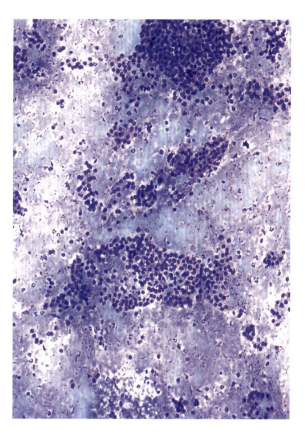

Figure 20-21

NODULAR HYPERPLASIA WITH FOLLOW-UP DIAGNOSIS OF MACROFOLLICULAR ADENOMA

Abundant colloid and sheets of follicular cells without a scalloped pattern. The uniformity of the sheets and the abundant colloid favor nodular hyperplasia. Excision of the nodule revealed a macrofollicular adenoma (Diff-Quik stain).

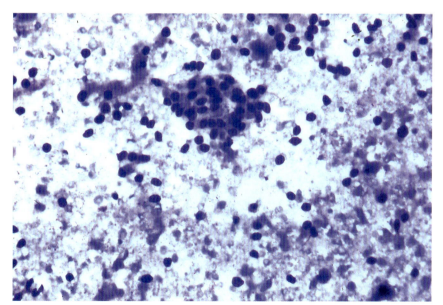

Figure 20-22

FOLLICULAR NEOPLASM WITH DEGENERATION

A small cluster of degenerated follicular cells and many free follicular cell nuclei in a background of colloid and degenerated blood make it difficult to recognize as a true follicular neoplasm (Diff-Quik stain).

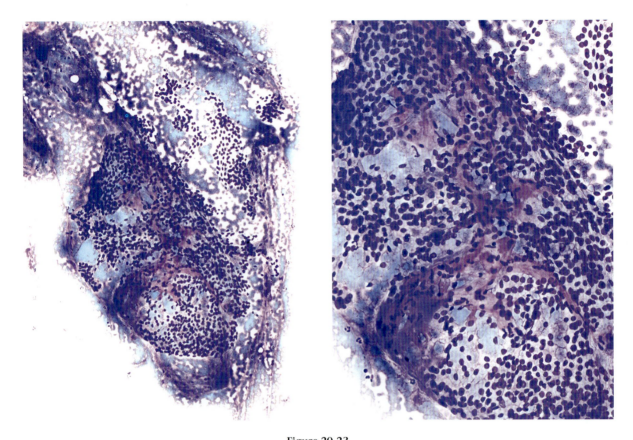

Figure 20-23

FOLLICULAR NEOPLASM

Left: The large follicular cell group is divided into compartments by metachromic stroma. Even at this low magnification, the cellularity, overlap of follicular cell nuclei, and irregular outline of the entire cell group suggest a follicular neoplasm (Diff-Quik stain).

Right: At higher magnification, the large cellular fragment shows a uniform pattern of follicular cells bonded into groupings by metachromatic stroma. The follicular cell nuclei overlap, a feature similar to the histologic appearance of a true follicular neoplasm (Diff-Quik stain).

of their border. The piling up of follicular cells in true neoplasia results in the overlapping of nuclei (figs. 20-23, 20-24), while in smears of nodular hyperplasia, the nuclei in cell sheets or groups are evenly spaced, with no or little overlap (14). The appearance of single microfollicles is of little value in this differential interpretation and the reproducibility of identification of microfollicles in aspiration smears is problematic (21).

In some cases of follicular carcinoma, the nuclear characteristics commonly associated with malignancy (increased nuclear/cytoplasmic ratio, coarse chromatin, and nucleoli) may suggest that carcinoma is present based on the aspiration smear alone (figs. 20-25, 20-26). This cannot be relied upon exclusively, however,

since significant nuclear atypia can be present in some follicular adenomas, while some low-grade follicular carcinomas are cytologically bland (fig. 20-27).

The NCI Consensus Conference terminology uses the category "neoplasm" when the cytology seems to indicate that a definite neoplasm is present. This category is further subdivided into follicular neoplasm and Hürthle cell neoplasm. Alternative terms are "suspicious for neoplasm," "suspicious for follicular neoplasm," and "suspicious for Hürthle cell neoplasm." The risk of malignancy in this group is estimated at 20 to 30 percent (10). The clinician may consider suppression therapy for an interpretation favoring nodular hyperplasia. If no response occurs within several months, the FNAB may

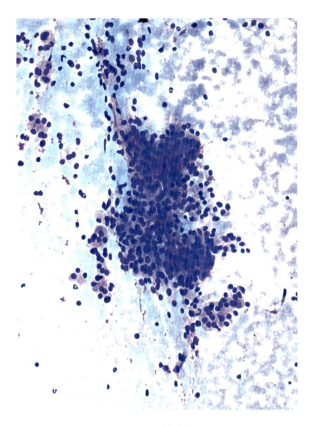

Figure 20-24

FOLLICULAR NEOPLASM WITH FOLLOW-UP DIAGNOSIS OF FOLLICULAR CARCINOMA, MINIMALLY INVASIVE

A cellular aspirate has a well-developed scalloping pattern. The follicular cells are uniform. While a firm interpretation of a follicular neoplasm can be made, there are no cytologic features that predict that this lesion is a minimally invasive follicular carcinoma (Diff-Quik stain).

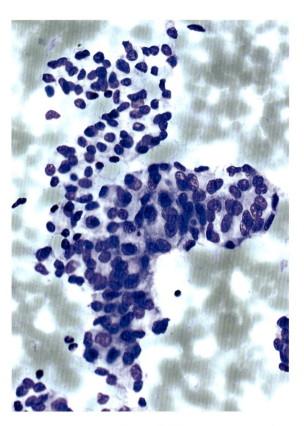

Figure 20-25

FOLLICULAR NEOPLASM WITH FOLLOW-UP DIAGNOSIS OF FOLLICULAR CARCINOMA

The compact group of follicular cells mimic the trabecular arrangement that is found in some adenomas. No cytologic features of the aspirate suggest a low-grade malignancy. Histologically, the tumor demonstrates capsular and vascular invasion (Diff-Quik stain).

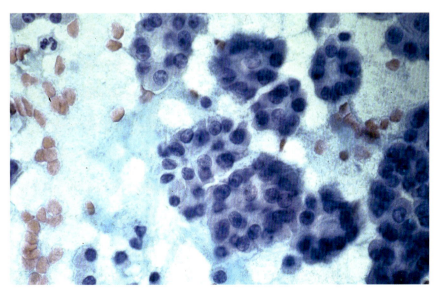

Figure 20-26

FOLLICULAR NEOPLASM WITH FOLLOW-UP DIAGNOSIS OF FOLLICULAR CARCINOMA

Enlarged follicular cells have a striking microfollicular pattern. Some of the follicular cell nuclei appear convoluted and have an empty appearance. These are features of follicular adenoma/carcinoma that overlap with papillary carcinoma. No grooves or intranuclear inclusions are detected (Papanicolaou stain).

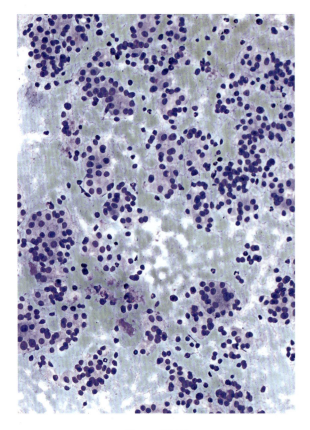

Figure 20-27

**FOLLICULAR NEOPLASM WITH
FOLLOW-UP DIAGNOSIS OF FOLLICULAR
CARCINOMA, MINIMALLY INVASIVE**

Another field from the case illustrated in figure 20-24. The smear is cellular, with many individual microfollicles. There is only minimal variation in nuclear size and shape, not a reliable indicator of malignancy (Diff-Quik stain).

Table 20-8
CYTOLOGIC FEATURES OF FOLLICULAR NEOPLASMS

Scant to absent colloid

Hypercellularity
   Monotonous follicular cells
      Micro or macrofollicles, trabeculae, syncytial
        fragments, scalloping
      Enlarged bland nuclei, overlapping (except in
        higher-grade carcinomas)
      Fine to coarse, dispersed nuclear chromatin
      Distinct nucleoli

be repeated or surgical excision carried out. In the category reported as neoplasm, surgical excision is advised.

The authors' experience, as well as that of Layfield and others, indicate that over 80 percent of thyroid nodules diagnosed as follicular neoplasms by FNAB are correctly identified (22,23). Histologic evaluation confirms that the majority of these nodules are adenomas, while a small percentage are well-differentiated follicular carcinomas. DeMay (24) has commented on the low incidence of true follicular carcinomas, indicating a minimal risk to patients when a diagnosis of "follicular neoplasm, favor adenoma" is made on FNAB. The cytologic features of follicular neoplasms are summarized in Table 20-8.

While most FNAB reports of follicular lesions are concerned with distinguishing true follicular neoplasms from nodular hyperplasia, occasionally it is possible to state more definitively that a follicular carcinoma is present. As there is a spectrum of subtle cytologic changes from adenoma to carcinoma, clinical and ultrasound features become significant for a definitive report of follicular carcinoma (figs. 20-28–20-33). These tumors are usually large and of the widely invasive variety, so that they have at least some partial fixation within the thyroid gland and neck area. If the cytopathologist does not examine the patient and perform the aspirate, he is at a great disadvantage in attempting to make a definite interpretation of follicular carcinoma from the aspiration smears alone.

Among the various subtypes of follicular adenoma, special mention should be made of *hyalinizing trabecular adenoma*. This rare lesion may be difficult to recognize on an aspiration biopsy smear (25). The pattern is that of loose cell aggregates or syncytial fragments with a trabecular pattern (fig. 20-34). The cells are either oval or spindle shaped, while the nuclei have a fine, evenly distributed chromatin pattern, giving them an empty appearance similar to the nuclei of papillary thyroid carcinoma. The presence of nuclear grooves and nuclear pseudoinclusions reinforces the similarity to papillary carcinoma and leads to an almost unavoidable misinterpretation of the aspirate (fig. 20-35). The amorphous hyaline material that helps identify this adenoma variant in histologic sections can be seen cytologically. It can mimic the amyloid found in medullary carcinoma but is negative with amyloid stains. The hyaline material may look like the dense colloid that is found in some

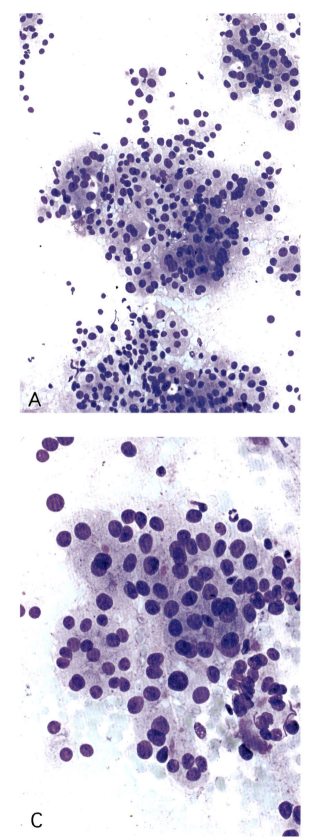

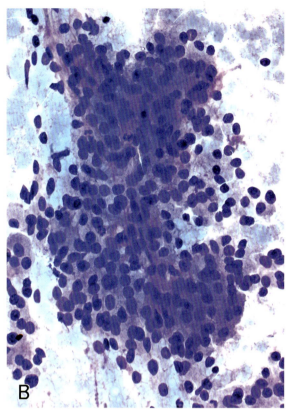

Figure 20-28

FOLLICULAR NEOPLASM WITH FOLLOW-UP DIAGNOSIS OF FOLLICULAR CARCINOMA, MINIMALLY INVASIVE

A: The monotonous-appearing follicular cells demonstrate a microfollicular pattern. Some variation in nuclear size and shape is present. This feature does not predict malignancy (Diff-Quik stain).

B: At higher magnification, the cellular group of follicular cells illustrates a microacinar pattern but without cellular pleomorphism (Diff-Quik stain).

C: Another cell group shows some variation in size and shape of the follicular cell nuclei. There is also some increase in the volume of cytoplasm and a suggestion of granularity that may indicate oncocytic change. There are no specific cytologic features of malignancy (Diff-Quik stain).

Figure 20-29

FOLLICULAR NEOPLASM WITH FOLLOW-UP DIAGNOSIS OF FOLLICULAR CARCINOMA

The trabecular pattern of this follicular neoplasm is demonstrated with a Papanicolaou stain. A microfollicular pattern is evident within some trabecular groups. No cytologic features of malignancy are seen. Histologically, the tumor was clearly invasive.

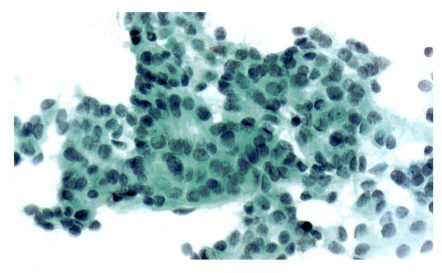

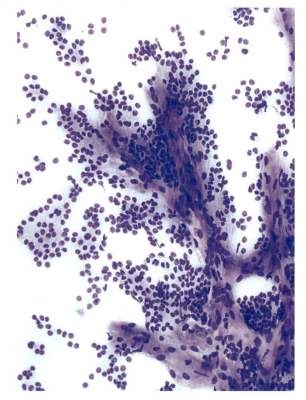
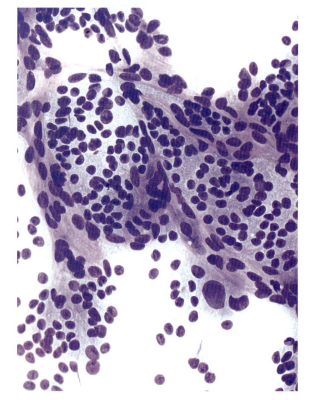

Figure 20-30

FOLLICULAR NEOPLASM WITH FOLLOW-UP DIAGNOSIS OF FOLLICULAR CARCINOMA

Left: A cellular aspirate from the same case as figure 20-23, with better definition of the metachromatically staining stroma. The fibrovascular cores are also found in aspirates from papillary carcinoma. The follicular cell nuclei are round, whereas those from papillary carcinoma are usually elongated. Higher magnification is required to determine the presence of intranuclear inclusions or nuclear grooves, important cytologic features of papillary carcinoma. None were present in the follicular cells in this aspirate. Histologically, this neoplasm was definitely invasive (Diff-Quik stain).

Right: At higher magnification, some pleomorphism of the follicular cell nuclei and a microacinar pattern are seen. Pleomorphism is not independently predictive of the presence of follicular carcinoma, but may be correlated with the clinical features to support such an interpretation. The metachromatic stroma contains capillaries lined by flattened endothelial cells that are visible in this field (Diff-Quik stain).

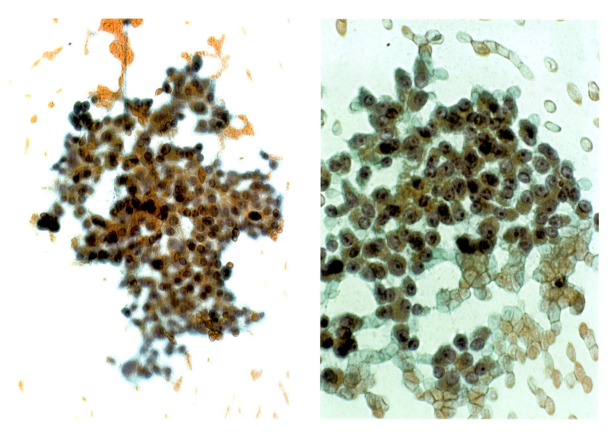

Figure 20-31

FOLLICULAR NEOPLASM WITH FOLLOW-UP DIAGNOSIS OF FOLLICULAR CARCINOMA

Left: Papanicolaou-stained aspiration smear of the same case illustrated in figures 20-30 and 20-33. Overlapping round follicular cell nuclei are seen without the definitive cytologic features of malignancy. Alcohol fixation creates some depth of focus or a tridimensional appearance to the follicular cell groups in a true follicular neoplasm.

Right: At higher magnification, round follicular cell nuclei with some coarse granularity of the chromatin are seen. Small nucleoli are visible in most of the nuclei. Their presence, along with the somewhat coarse granular chromatin pattern, favors the interpretation of follicular carcinoma.

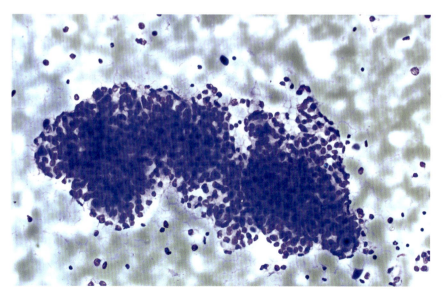

Figure 20-32

FOLLICULAR NEOPLASM WITH FOLLOW-UP DIAGNOSIS OF FOLLICULAR CARCINOMA

A large group of overlapping follicular cells have a scalloped edge to the cell aggregate. No pleomorphism of individual cells is noted at this magnification. Histologically, the tumor demonstrated vascular and capsular invasion (Diff-Quik stain).

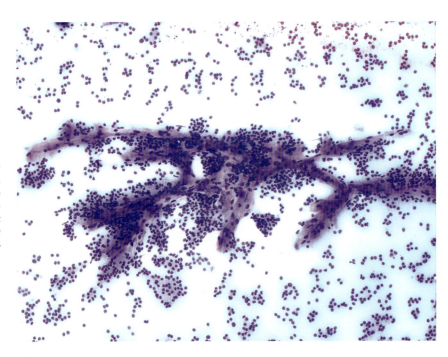

Figure 20-33

FOLLICULAR NEOPLASM WITH FOLLOW-UP DIAGNOSIS OF FOLLICULAR CARCINOMA

The large group of follicular cells is partly defined by a metachromatic stroma. In the background are many micro-follicular aggregates. No specific cytologic features indicate that this follicular neoplasm is malignant (Diff-Quik stain).

aspirates of papillary carcinoma (fig. 20-35). The tumor cells are also negative for calcitonin, another important feature distinguishing this adenoma from medullary carcinoma.

Since the report of five cases interpreted on FNAB as either suspect or outright papillary or medullary carcinoma by Goellner and Carney (33), there have been 18 additional cases where an aspiration biopsy has been reported for cases that ultimately were diagnosed histologically as hyalinizing trabecular adenoma (26–32). In only one had the correct unequivocal interpretation been made on FNAB (25). In two other cases, the diagnosis was suggested from the FNAB (27). There were four false positive interpretations of papillary carcinoma, and four of medullary carcinoma. The remaining cases had nonspecific generic interpretations, such as follicular lesion suggestive of thyroiditis, neoplasm of uncertain type, or no statement as to the aspiration biopsy diagnosis provided in the reports (26–33). These results are not surprising. One report noted the distinctive purplish red stromal deposits seen on May-Grunwald-Giemsa-stained smears that help identify hyalinizing trabecular adenoma. These deposits correspond to accumulations of basement membrane material (30). A more recent report (34) documents the use of MIB-1 immunostaining of aspiration smears in cases of hyalinizing trabecular adenoma (see chapter

3). A peripheral staining pattern of the tumor cell cytoplasm was seen in 17 of 24 cases. Three other cases demonstrated equivocal staining, while the remaining 4 cases were negative. Five specimens each of papillary carcinoma, medullary carcinoma, follicular carcinoma, and oncocytoma showed no staining with MIB-1.

Papillary Carcinoma

Papillary carcinoma (PTC) is perhaps the easiest neoplasm to diagnose cytologically from an FNAB of the thyroid gland. It is the most common thyroid malignancy, and usually presents as a discrete and solitary thyroid nodule. As already stated, it has distinctive nuclear features that are key to its recognition in both cytologic and histologic preparations (10).

The solitary nodule of PTC usually feels firmer than a nodule of nodular hyperplasia, but this is far from a reliable clinical finding. A rather distinctive "scritching" sound may accompany the FNAB of a firm thyroid nodule. Correlation with the histology of PTC suggests the needle is contacting either psammoma bodies or dense fibrous tissue, the latter being found prominently in sclerotic PTC.

Other important cytologic features of PTC are summarized below and include three-dimensional papillary fragments (fig. 21-36), multinucleated giant cells (particularly in follicular

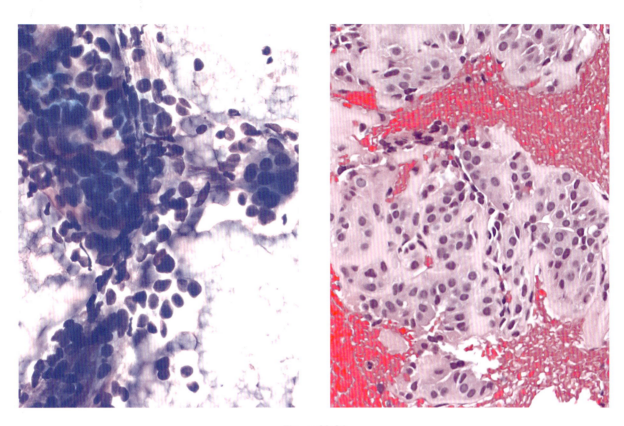

Figure 20-34

HYALINIZING TRABECULAR ADENOMA

Left: Follicular cells with consistently elongated nuclei are bounded by strands of slightly metachromatic stroma. The elongated nuclei suggest the possibility of hyalinizing trabecular adenoma but this feature, along with nuclear grooves and intranuclear inclusions, favors the much more common neoplasm, papillary carcinoma (Diff-Quik stain).

Right: The cell block fragment shows the compact pattern of elongated follicular cells with elongated nuclei. Although there is no definite hyaline material seen, the overall pattern of the cells suggests the possibility of hyalinizing trabecular adenoma (hematoxylin and eosin [H&E] stain). (Left and right: Courtesy of Dr. C. N. Powers, Richmond, VA.)

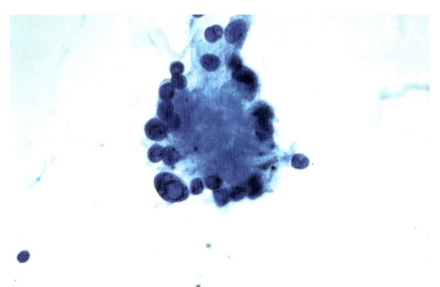

Figure 20-35

HYALINIZING TRABECULAR ADENOMA

A group of follicular cells surrounds homogeneous material that could represent the hyaline or dense colloid sometimes seen in papillary carcinoma. One cell has a large intranuclear inclusion. The cytologic features of hyalinizing trabecular adenoma are essentially identical to those of conventional papillary carcinoma (Papanicolaou stain).

417

variant PTC [FVPTC]) (figs. 20-37, 20-38), and dense "ropy" colloid described as being twisted like bubble gum (35). This dense and irregular colloid is often metachromatically stained with Diff-Quik (figs. 20-39–20-41). The identification of this peculiar colloid is subjective, particularly its metachromatic staining quality. On the whole, it is not a strong indicator of PTC. Rather, its presence indicates the need for a careful search for follicular cells having the diagnostic nuclear features (6).

Kini et al. (14) analyzed 329 surgically confirmed cases of PTC and found four features of aspiration biopsy smears that were important in order to reach the correct cytologic diagnosis: 1) syncytial-type tissue fragments (figs. 20-42–20-44); 2) powdery nuclear chromatin (fig. 21-45); 3) micronucleoli or macronucleoli (figs. 20-46, 20-47); and 4) intranuclear cytoplasmic inclusions (figs. 20-48–20-50) (14). Psammoma bodies, often a part of the histopathologic diagnosis of PTC, are infrequently encountered in FNAB specimens (20 percent of the cases in Kini's series) (figs. 20-51, 20-52). This may be due to the inability of the very thin needle bore to aspirate the entire psammoma body or the inability of the needle tip to fracture the psammoma body into smaller fragments (6). Ellison et al. (36) reviewed the frequency of psammoma bodies in 313 FNABs and found them 50 percent predictive as a single feature for PTC; nuclear features combined with psammoma bodies were 100 percent predictive; and nuclear features alone were 80 percent predictive.

Nuclear grooves occur in aspirates from thyroid diseases, both neoplastic and non-neoplastic. Francis et al. (37) counted the number of cells with nuclear grooves in cases of PTC, follicular neoplasm, oncocytic neoplasm, medullary carcinoma, thyrotoxic goiter, chronic lymphocytic and subacute thyroiditis, and colloid goiter. Nuclear grooves were present in 100 percent of cases of PTC but also in small numbers in 75 to 100 percent of the other thyroid disorders. Eighty-eight percent of PTCs in this study had 20 percent or more of tumor cells with nuclear grooves. This finding has been recently confirmed (38). Nuclear grooves were much easier to identify in either Papanicolaou- or hematoxylin and eosin-stained smears than in air-dried smears stained with Diff-Quik or a Romanowsky type of stain (figs. 20-45, 20-46

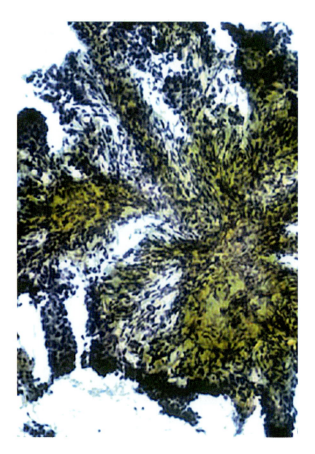

Figure 20-36

PAPILLARY CARCINOMA

Although no cellular detail can be seen in this large papillary fragment, the fibrovascular pattern with elongated cells covering it is suggestive of papillary carcinoma (Papanicolaou stain).

left; 20-53) (37). This suggests that the grooves are accentuated by or may represent a fixation artifact. Nuclear grooves should, in at least some examples, extend over the length of the nucleus, most often along the longitudinal axis (figs. 20-45, right; 20-53). When incomplete grooves are found they should not be ignored, but it is important that other criteria supporting the diagnosis of PTC be identified (6,40–42).

Smears from PTC most often lack any evidence of colloid and are cellular, with sheets and clusters of thyroid follicular cells. These cells may not always appear in three-dimensional papillary formations but rather as flat sheets, especially in air-dried smears stained with the Diff-Quik stain. The presence of concentrically organized aggregates of "cellular swirls" helps in

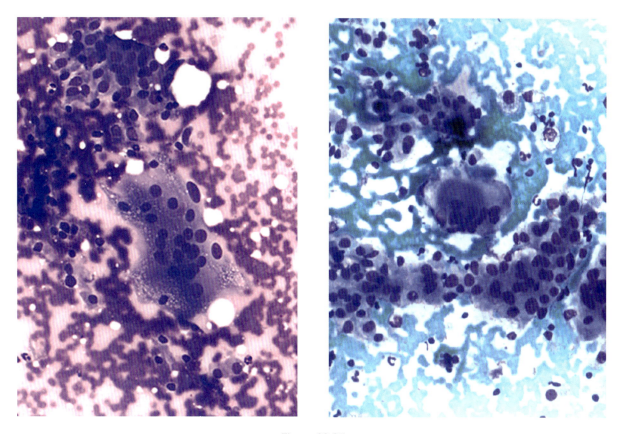

Figure 20-37

PAPILLARY CARCINOMA: FOLLICULAR VARIANT

Left: Loose sheet of follicular cells to the left with a large multinucleated giant cell present in the center of the figure. The presence of the giant cells suggests the follicular variant of papillary carcinoma (Diff-Quik stain).

Right: A multinucleated giant cell is seen at higher magnification. The pattern of the other follicular cells is trabecular, a feature more suggestive of follicular adenoma or follicular carcinoma (Diff-Quik stain).

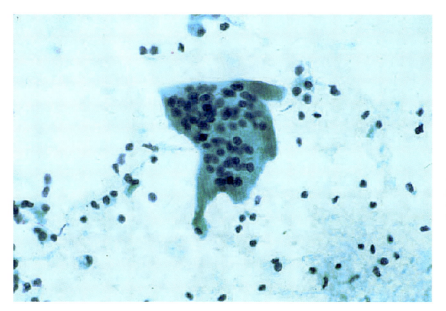

Figure 20-38

PAPILLARY CARCINOMA: FOLLICULAR VARIANT

Higher magnification of a single, large, multinucleated giant cell in an aspirate from a follicular variant of papillary carcinoma (Papanicolaou stain).

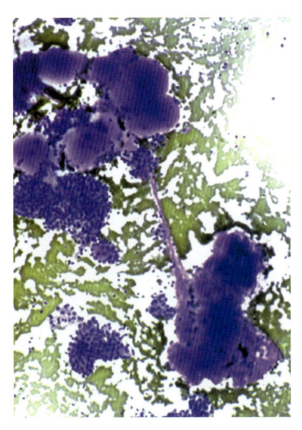

Figure 20-39

PAPILLARY CARCINOMA

The follicular cells have large rounded and irregular masses of dense metachromatic colloid, sometimes referred to as "chewing gum" colloid (Diff-Quik stain).

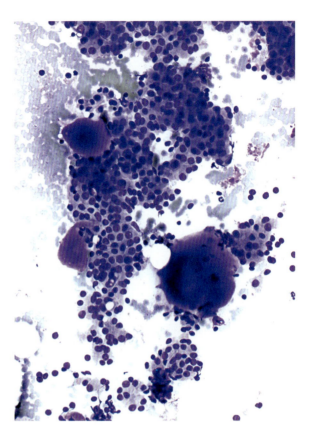

Figure 20-40

PAPILLARY CARCINOMA

A follicular-like arrangement of cells with dense round masses of colloid that may suggest a follicular adenoma ; however, the presence of this dense metachromatic colloid is more in keeping with papillary carcinoma (Diff-Quik stain).

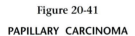

Figure 20-41

PAPILLARY CARCINOMA

The dense cracked pattern of colloid indicative of papillary carcinoma is seen in a Papanicolaou stained smear.

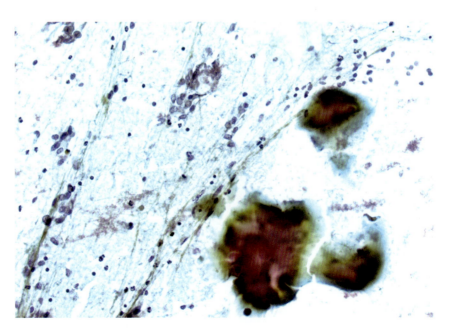

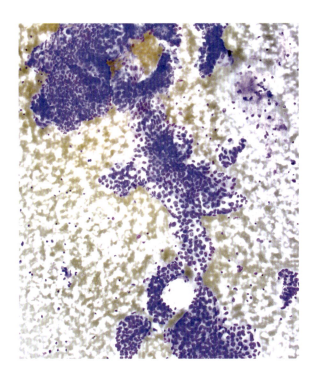

Figure 20-42

PAPILLARY CARCINOMA

The elongated follicular cells are in irregular branching fragments. Even without cellular detail at this magnification, this is highly suggestive of papillary carcinoma (Diff-Quik stain).

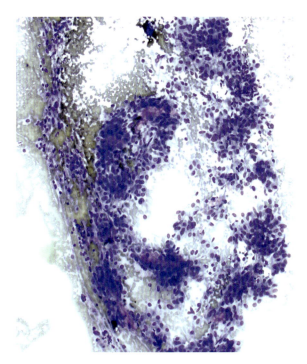

Figure 20-43

PAPILLARY CARCINOMA

The clustering and scalloping simulate a follicular neoplasm. Additional cytologic features of papillary carcinoma would have to be found to make that interpretation (Diff-Quik stain).

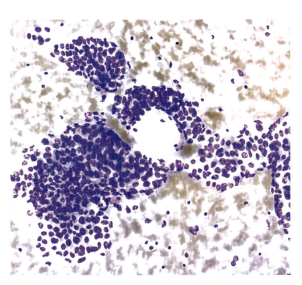

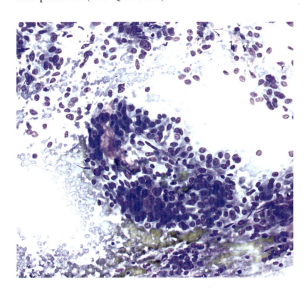

Figure 20-44

PAPILLARY CARCINOMA

Left: Irregular branching pattern of a large fragment of follicular cells. Most of the nuclei are elongated. The pattern plus the elongated follicular cell nuclei are highly indicative of papillary carcinoma (Diff-Quik stain).

Right: The clustering of follicular cells and follicular cell nuclei that are elongated and enlarged are features strongly indicating papillary carcinoma (Diff-Quik stain).

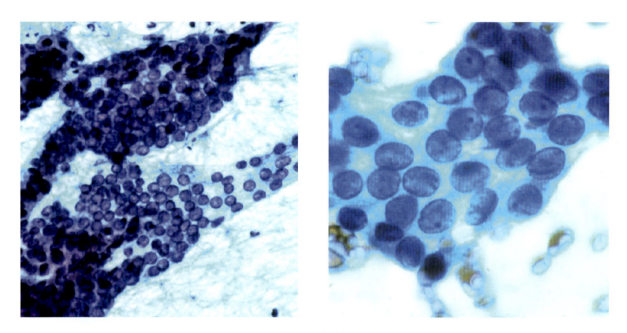

Figure 20-45

PAPILLARY CARCINOMA

Left: A sheet of follicular cells shows generally rounded nuclei and nuclear overlapping. The nuclei have an empty appearance. This is the cytologic counterpart of the optically clear nuclei of papillary carcinoma seen histologically (Papanicolaou stain).

Right: Higher magnification shows the extremely fine nuclear chromatin pattern that results in the empty appearance of the nuclei. There are also several cells with nuclear grooves (Papanicolaou stain).

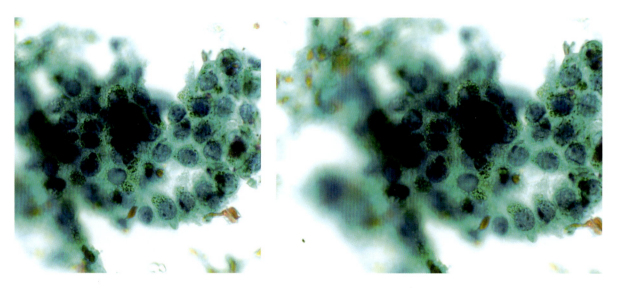

Figure 20-46

PAPILLARY CARCINOMA

Left: A tridimensional cluster of a group of follicular cells is present in a papillary carcinoma. Not all of the cells are in focus in a single plane. A large intranuclear inclusion is just below the center of the field. The nuclei appear empty (Papanicolaou stain).

Right: A different focal plane demonstrates the tridimensional quality of the cell group commonly found in papillary carcinoma when the smears are alcohol fixed and stained with the Papanicolaou method.

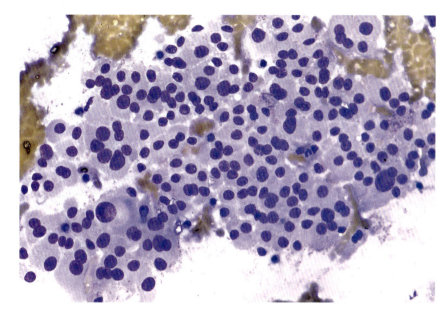

Figure 20-47

PAPILLARY CARCINOMA

The cells demonstrate nuclear pleomorphism, macronucleoli, and oncocytic features (Diff-Quik stain).

Figure 20-48

PAPILLARY CARCINOMA

One evident intranuclear inclusion is found in a sheet of follicular cells just below and to the left of the center of the field. Note that the color of the inclusion reflects the color of the cytoplasm projecting into and through the nucleus (Diff-Quik stain).

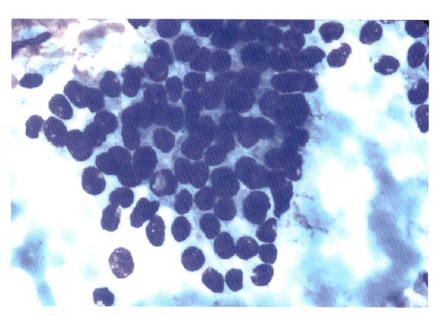

the correct cytologic interpretation of PTC (figs. 20-44, 20-53) (39). Also, the consistent appearance of some cells with glassy intranuclear inclusions is extremely important for the cytologic diagnosis of PTC. Along with nuclear grooves, they are the most reliable and consistent feature cytologically and histologically for its diagnosis.

Intranuclear pseudoinclusions are invaginations of cytoplasm into the nucleus and therefore should stain like the cell cytoplasm, in contrast to the staining quality of the remainder of the nucleus (figs. 20-47, 20-49, 20-50). They should have a very distinct border or edge, which is more prominent in alcohol-fixed Papanicolaou-stained smears (figs. 20-49, left; 20-50). Vague or even relatively sharp holes in nuclei should not be accepted as intranuclear pseudoinclusions as they represent artifacts that are more likely to be found in air-dried Diff-Quik-stained smears (10).

As originally reported, the optically clear nucleus is a strong criterion for a diagnosis of PTC in hematoxylin and eosin-stained histologic sections (43). This feature is not nearly as distinctive

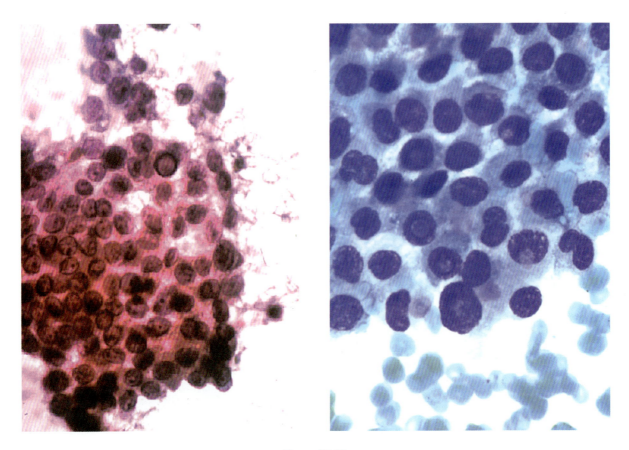

Figure 20-49

PAPILLARY CARCINOMA

Left: A sheet of follicular cells with an obvious intranuclear inclusion. The inclusion has a distinct border and the color of the cell cytoplasm is seen projecting through the nucleus (Papanicolaou stain).

Right: At higher magnification, several nuclei having intranuclear inclusions are seen. This is an important feature for the interpretation of the aspirate as papillary carcinoma (Diff-Quik stain).

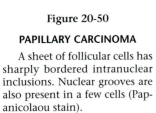

Figure 20-50

PAPILLARY CARCINOMA

A sheet of follicular cells has sharply bordered intranuclear inclusions. Nuclear grooves are also present in a few cells (Papanicolaou stain).

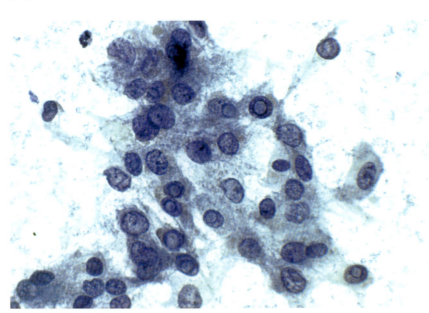

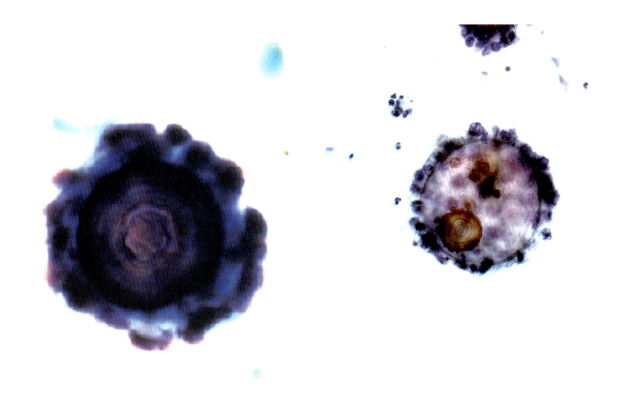

Figure 20-51

PAPILLARY CARCINOMA

A psammoma body is a rare finding in aspirates of thyroid papillary carcinoma, probably because these structures are too large to fit through the very thin needle (Papanicolaou stain).

Figure 20-52

PAPILLARY CARCINOMA

A small psammoma body is surrounded by follicular cells. The characteristics of the attached follicular cells do not lead to an interpretation of papillary carcinoma, but the presence of the psammoma body is highly supportive of that interpretation (Papanicolaou stain).

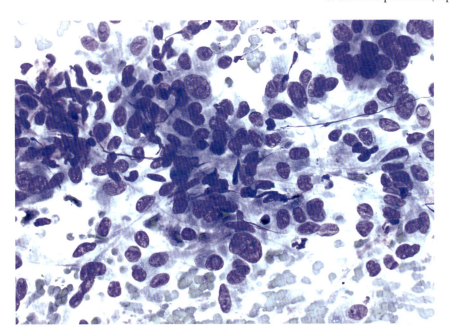

Figure 20-53

PAPILLARY CARCINOMA

The follicular cell nuclei are enlarged and elongated, and overlap with each other. There is a large intranuclear inclusion in a cell at the right edge of the field (Diff-Quik stain).

425

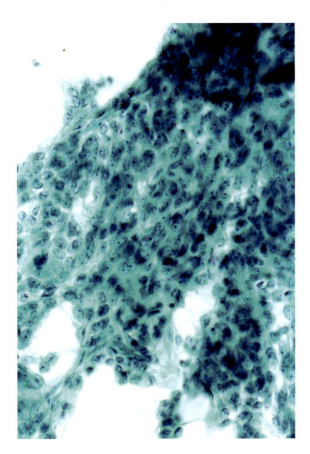

Figure 20-54

PAPILLARY CARCINOMA

The sheet of follicular cells has elongated nuclei. The follicular cell nuclei in the thinner areas of the cell sheet have an empty appearance (Papanicolaou stain).

Table 20-9
CYTOLOGIC FEATURES OF PAPILLARY CARCINOMA

Smear Composition
  Cellular
  Monolayered cell sheets
  Three-dimensional tissue fragments
  Multinucleated giant cells (follicular variant)
  Ropy (chewing gum) colloid
  Psammoma bodies (infrequent)
Cytoplasm
  Metaplastic cytoplasm (oncocytic)
  Distinct cell borders
Nuclei
  Pale nuclei (Papanicolaou stain)
  Definitive nucleoli
  Intranuclear inclusions
  Nuclear grooves
  Variation in nuclear size
  Enlarged nuclei

in cytologic smears. In Papanicolaou-stained smears of PTC, the nuclei appear quite bland, almost empty, but clearly have an extremely fine and even chromatin structure (fig. 20-45, right). This is believed to be the cytologic counterpart of the completely clear nucleus found in tissue sections of PTC. The difference is presumed to be the result of formalin fixation of tissue versus alcohol fixation of cytologic smears.

In the preparation of aspiration biopsy smears, follicular cells are pulled away from the fibrovascular cores of finger-like projections of "stroma." When closely evaluated, this homogenous stromal material may demonstrate small endothelial-lined vessels or simply a row of elongated oval nuclei that represent endothelial cells (figs. 20-53, 20-54) (6). The cytologic features of PTC are summarized in Table 20-9.

Cystic degeneration in PTC can significantly alter the above-described cytologic pattern and make the diagnosis impossible. However, there are some important gross findings of the aspirate and clinical features of the behavior of the cyst that point toward the correct diagnosis. Aspiration of a cyst where the fluid has the appearance of fresh blood should be considered suspicious for cystic PTC even though no tumor cells are identified. An aspirated cyst of the thyroid gland that rapidly refills, often almost immediately after the aspiration is completed, also indicates the presence of cystic PTC. It is important after aspiration of a thyroid cyst to reexamine the area for any residual mass and to reaspirate that area if feasible. The use of ultrasound allows the repeat aspiration to be targeted more specifically.

Cystic PTC has few follicular cells, mostly hemosiderin-laden macrophages, with degenerative features on aspiration biopsy smears. More cells are recovered and evaluated by using a cytospin preparation. Small numbers of follicular cells may be nondescript. Actual papillary fragments or follicular cells with intranuclear pseudoinclusions and grooves are rare. These nuclear features, along with clusters of cells that appear as three-dimensional groups, are seen in some aspirates of nodular hyperplasia with cystic degeneration (fig. 20-55). In those cases, there is rarely any residual mass. If the cyst refills, it does

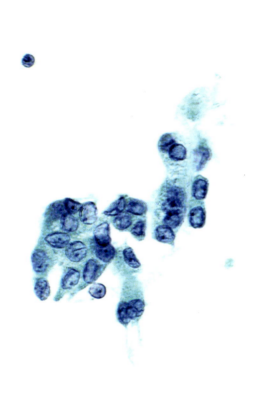

Figure 20-55

CYSTIC PAPILLARY CARCINOMA

A single cluster of follicular cells from an aspirate of a thyroid cyst shows nuclear grooves and clear nuclei. While the interpretation was probable cystic papillary carcinoma, the excised lesion proved to be a thyroid cyst after extensive sectioning of the cyst wall (Papanicolaou stain).

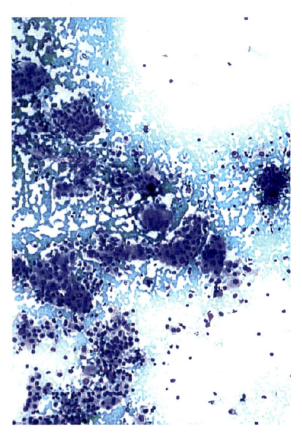

Figure 20-56

PAPILLARY CARCINOMA: FOLLICULAR VARIANT

A multinucleated giant cell is seen in the middle of a cellular aspirate with the follicular pattern of overlapping cells. There were several others on the aspiration smears, a finding that suggests the follicular variant of papillary carcinoma (Diff-Quik stain).

so very slowly. A trial of thyroid suppression is clinically useful in such cases to reduce the incidence of recurrence of the cyst.

Variants of Papillary Thyroid Carcinoma

As indicated elsewhere in this chapter, there are a number of histologic variants of PTC (43). These variations impact on the standard cytologic criteria listed above. The major diagnostic problem is separating these variants from other thyroid lesions that have some of the cytologic criteria of PTC.

FVPTC is the most frequent subtype of PTC encountered in FNAB of the thyroid gland. With a good sample, the cellularity and overlapping follicle pattern (scalloping) within groups of follicular cells immediately indicates the presence of a thyroid neoplasm. Several studies empha-

size the difficulty of recognizing this variant of PTC on aspirate smears (44–48). Many authors have remarked on the increased cellularity, with monolayered sheets and syncytial clusters without an acinar formation rather than a microfollicular pattern (figs. 20-37, 20-56) (45). One report found the standard cytologic features of PTC, intranuclear pseudoinclusions, nuclear grooves, and nuclei having powdery chromatin, to be common in FNAB smears of the FVPTC (45). In contrast, Baloch et al. (44) found these features in only 5 of 17 cases in their series of FVPTCs. In a more recent series, the sensitivity of FNAB for the diagnosis of FVPTC was only 9 percent (47).

Two other components of the aspiration smears of FVPTC are suggestive enough to initiate the search for nuclear grooves and

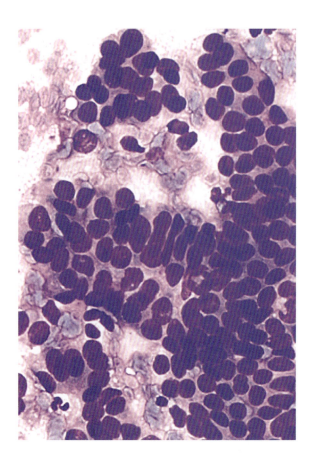
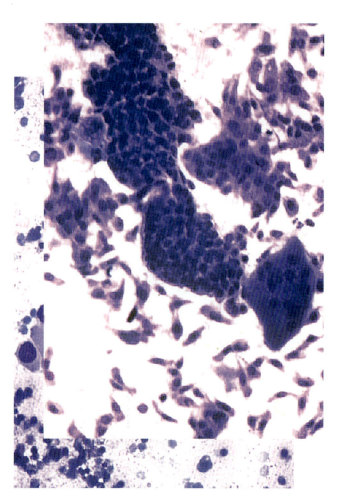

Figure 20-57

PAPILLARY CARCINOMA: ONCOCYTIC VARIANT

Left: A large sheet of follicular cells has lightly metachromatic, fine granular cytoplasm and somewhat elongated dark nuclei. Oncocytic features are evident but there are no nuclear features or pattern suggesting papillary carcinoma. Aspirates of this variant of papillary carcinoma are easily interpreted as oncocytoma or carcinoma with oncocytic features (Diff-Quik stain).

Right: At higher magnification, another sheet of oncocytic-appearing follicular cells is seen. No nuclear features of papillary carcinoma are present in this smear (Diff-Quik stain).

intranuclear pseudoinclusions. They are the presence of multinucleated giant cells and small fragments of dense metachromatic colloid (figs. 20-37, right; 20-38; 20-56). Zacks et al. (49) point out that FVPTC is difficult to distinguish from a colloid nodule in some aspirates. From their analysis, three elements were important for the diagnosis: large nuclei, high nuclear to cytoplasmic ratio, and the more frequent presence of intranuclear pseudoinclusions. Comparing FVPTC with the conventional type of PTC, the usual smear pattern of PTC has less cellular cohesion, less architectural polarity, and a greater number of papillary groups of cells. It is important to find good examples of nuclear grooves and intranuclear pseudoinclusions before the diagnosis of FVPTC is made unequivocally. It may be necessary in

some cases to report the aspiration biopsy as "follicular neoplasm with features suggestive of the FVPTC." This allows the surgeon to proceed with the excision of the nodule (6).

A tumor difficult to recognize on aspiration biopsy smears is the *oncocytic variant of PTC*, perhaps an important distinction, as some authors believe that this variant has a more aggressive course (50–52). The aspirates are typically cellular, with flat sheets and single cells having granular eosinophilic cytoplasm when seen with the Papanicolaou stain, and granular and faintly metachromatic cytoplasm with the Diff-Quik stain (fig. 20-57). Nuclear pleomorphism is found, as is typical of oncocytic neoplasms of the thyroid gland. Any presence of three-dimensional papillary groups is minimal or not apparent.

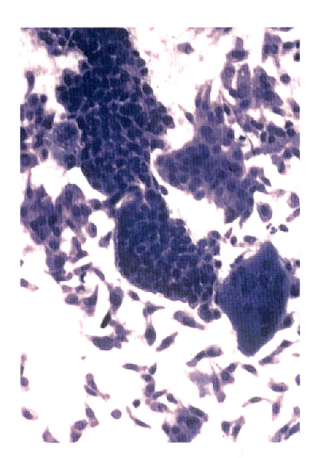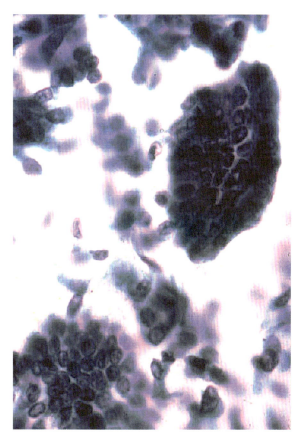

Figure 20-58

PAPILLARY CARCINOMA: TALL CELL VARIANT

Left: There are large clusters of enlarged and very elongated follicular cells. The nuclei are small relative to the length of the entire cell, a feature suggesting the tall cell variant of papillary carcinoma. Such tumors usually have prominent nucleoli, a feature not present in this smear (Diff-Quik stain).

Right: The clusters of elongated follicular cells have a marked tridimensional arrangement (Papanicolaou stain).

Unfortunately, nuclear grooves and intranuclear pseudoinclusions are also sparse in some cases (53). This is in contrast to the histology of the oncocytic variant of PTC, which usually has obvious papillary areas with large oncocytic-appearing cells. The nuclear features of PTC seem to be much more evident in histologic sections of this variant than they are in FNAB smears (54).

There are two reports of the cytologic features of a *Warthin-like variant of PTC*. The presence of oncocytic cells with the sparse nuclear features of typical PTC and accompanying lymphocytes is a pattern that closely simulates a Warthin tumor (55–57).

There are other variants of PTC that appear to have more aggressive behavior. They include *tall cell* (fig. 20-58), *columnar cell, solid/trabecu-lar*, and *diffuse sclerosing PTC* (fig. 20-59). Some authors believe that these variations cannot be distinguished cytologically (58). Others maintain that the tall cell variant of PTC can be identified based on the larger cell size, more frequent intranuclear pseudoinclusions, and greater degree of nuclear pleomorphism (59–63).

Kini (14) describes the solid variant of PTC as having both isolated cells and syncytial tissue fragments without any follicular or papillary pattern (fig. 20-60). No monolayered sheets are found. The nuclear morphology is characteristic of PTC. Histologically, in addition to the solid areas, there may be papillary and follicular areas and evidence of squamous metaplasia.

One case examined by Kini (14), and two other case reports (64) describe the cytology

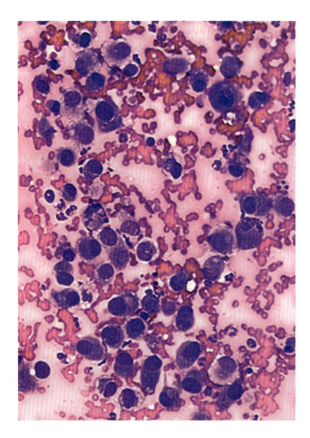 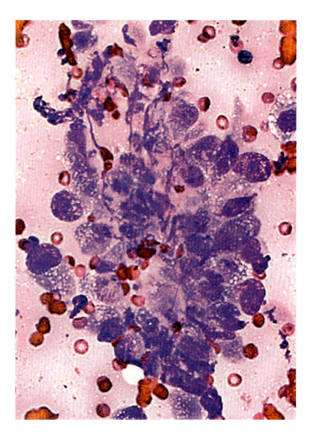

Figure 20-59

PAPILLARY CARCINOMA WITH NODULAR FASCIITIS-LIKE STROMA

Left: Single enlarged atypical follicular cells in a loose pattern. The aspirate is highly cellular, with a background of acute inflammatory cells. The degree of acute inflammation is unusual for a typical aspiration smear of papillary carcinoma (Diff-Quik stain).

Right: In another field, a sheet of some spindle-shaped and enlarged thyroid follicular cells, with blood and some inflammatory cells in the background, is seen (Diff-Quik stain). (Left and right: courtesy of Dr. G. deBlois, Richmond, VA.)

of the diffuse sclerosing variant of PTC. FNAB preferentially samples the tumor cells and lymphocytes, giving rise to a diagnosis of PTC within lymphocytic thyroiditis. Other features include sheets of squamous-appearing tumor cells, many psammoma bodies, and an absence of stringy colloid. A recent report described the ultrasound and computerized tomography (CT) findings in eight cases of diffuse sclerosing PTC, with successful interpretation by aspiration biopsy (65). The ultrasound findings were a heterogeneous echo texture, solid composition, and ill-defined margins in the majority of cases. CT scan showed a "snow storm" of microcalcifications in six of the eight cases. The cytologic features included tumor cells mixed with lymphocytes, squamous metaplastic cells,

psammoma bodies, and the typical nuclear features of PTC (65). Two additional cases of this variant have been reported by Kumaraskinhe et al. (66). Both were recognized by some sheets of follicular cells with the typical nuclear features of PTC.

A case of *PTC with exuberant nodular fasciitis-like stroma* has been illustrated cytologically. Kini (14) comments that the FNAB smears showed the cytologic features of either conventional PTC or its follicular variant.

Albores-Saavedra et al. (67) reported a *macrofollicular variant of PTC*. It was confusing both cytologically and histologically because of the abundant colloid and macrofollicles that simulated nodular hyperplasia or a macrofollicular adenoma. Six of their patients had FNAB,

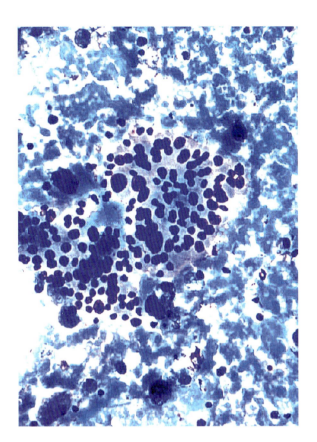 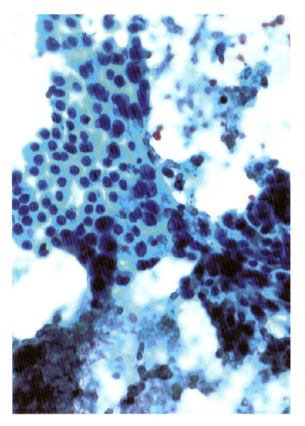

Figure 20-60

PAPILLARY CARCINOMA: SOLID VARIANT WITH PLEOMORPHIC CELLS

Left: A large irregular cluster of follicular cells shows great variation in nuclear size and shape. The nuclear features of papillary carcinoma are not seen in this field but were present in other fields. This degree of nuclear pleomorphism is unusual for typical papillary carcinoma but does not seem to have prognostic implications and does not indicate the presence of anaplastic thyroid carcinoma (Diff-Quik stain).

Right: With the Papanicolaou stain, there is much less nuclear pleomorphism. Air-dried smears that are stained by the Romanowsky method tend to accentuate differences in the size and configuration of the cells and nuclei.

with four diagnosed as colloid or hyperplastic nodule, and two reported as a follicular neoplasm. The key nuclear features of this type of PTC were those of its follicular variant, but were difficult to find (67,68).

Five cases of an *adenoid cystic variant* (or at least a pattern resembling that of adenoid cystic carcinoma) within a FVPTC have been reported (69,70). This pattern was recognized in four cases, based largely on the presence of hyaline globules that did not stain for thyroglobulin (70).

Insular Carcinoma

Insular carcinoma and its cytologic characteristics have only been encountered sporadically in FNAB specimens (71–75). The diagnosis from an aspiration biopsy remains difficult.

The important cytologic features are high cellularity, with cells occurring singly, or in clusters, nests, and trabeculae (figs. 20-61–20-63). The pattern of the neoplastic cells is uniform and monotonous. Cytologic pleomorphism is deceptively minimal but can be found in some cases (fig. 21-62). Grooved nuclei and intranuclear pseudoinclusions are identified, but are infrequent. Small red granules in the cytoplasm of tumor cells, similar to those of medullary carcinoma, are rarely seen. Immunocytochemistry identifies thyroglobulin-positive cytoplasmic vacuoles. This tumor has many cytologic features that overlap with medullary thyroid carcinoma, particularly those cases with a carcinoid-like appearance, including isolated cells with melanin pigment (figs. 20-64, 20-65).

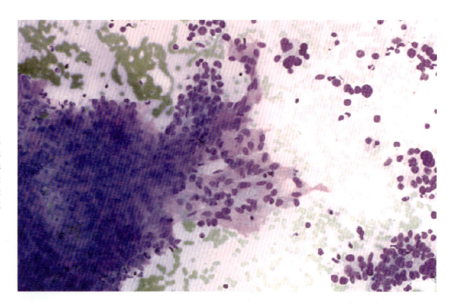

Figure 20-61

INSULAR CARCINOMA

Loose clusters, single cells, and nonspecific stromal fragments are seen. The homogeneous staining pattern and light red blush of the cytoplasm suggest medullary carcinoma (Diff-Quik stain).

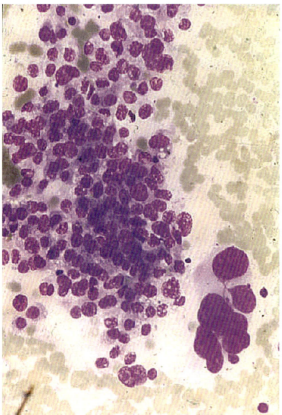

Figure 20-62

INSULAR CARCINOMA

The tumor cells are clustered in a nested or follicular pattern. Some nuclei are very large, similar to those seen in some cases of medullary carcinoma. Some intermediate-sized nuclei on the right of the main group of cells have large nucleoli (Diff-Quik stain).

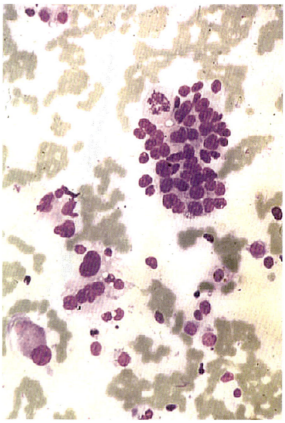

Figure 20-63

INSULAR CARCINOMA

A small island-like cluster of tumor cells and scattered cells with larger nuclei (Diff-Quik stain).

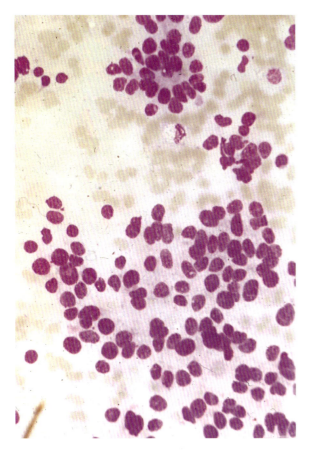

Figure 20-64

INSULAR CARCINOMA

The pattern of many uniform small cells with absent or scant cytoplasm suggests a carcinoid-like neuroendocrine tumor (Diff-Quik stain).

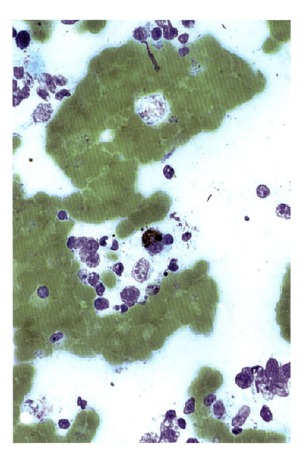

Figure 20-65

INSULAR CARCINOMA

Scattered, somewhat pleomorphic tumor cells with a single heavily melanin-pigmented cell in the center of the field (Diff-Quik stain).

Undifferentiated (Anaplastic) Carcinoma

FNAB provides a rapid diagnosis in cases of *undifferentiated (anaplastic) carcinoma*, allowing clinicians to institute treatment prior to a definitive histologic diagnosis or even without it, since the differential diagnosis is usually with malignant lymphoma (6).

Smears of this carcinoma are highly cellular, dominated by large, often bizarre cells, and with background necrosis and inflammation (figs. 20-66, 20-67) (76,77). Within the cytoplasm of the tumor cells are phagocytized neutrophils (figs. 20-67, right; 20-68, left) (6). These may be most obvious in tumor giant cells. Tumor cells with enlarged, pleomorphic nuclei having coarse chromatin and prominent nucleoli clearly identify this neoplasm as a high-grade carcinoma (figs. 20-

68–20-71). Table 20-10 summarizes the cytologic findings of undifferentiated thyroid carcinoma.

Tumors with Oncocytic Features

A common type of neoplasm of follicular cells is the *oncocytic (oxyphilic, Hürthle cell) variant*. Oncocytic cell change or metaplasia is a common finding in many thyroid lesions: hyperplastic nodules in nodular hyperplasia, chronic lymphocytic thyroiditis, Graves disease, and PTC. Differentiating the various entities that can contain oncocytes from a true oncocytic neoplasm is difficult when oncocytic cell metaplasia dominates the sample.

The most important cytologic features for a true oncocytic neoplasm are many large follicular cells with abundant granular cytoplasm and

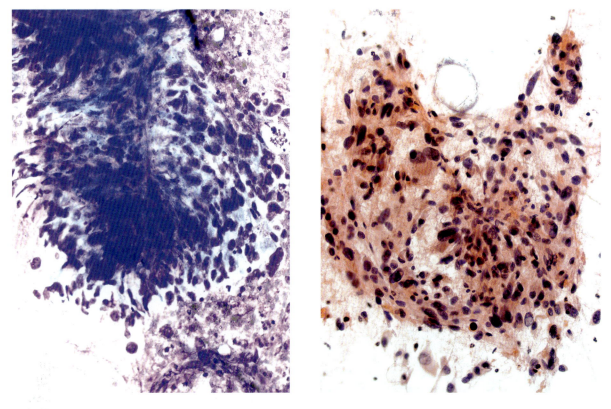

Figure 20-66

UNDIFFERENTIATED (ANAPLASTIC) CARCINOMA

Left: A highly cellular fragment of spindle-shaped tumor cells. The nuclei at the edges of the fragment are enlarged and irregular (Diff-Quik stain).

Right: A similar fragment of pleomorphic spindle-shaped tumor cells (Papanicolaou stain).

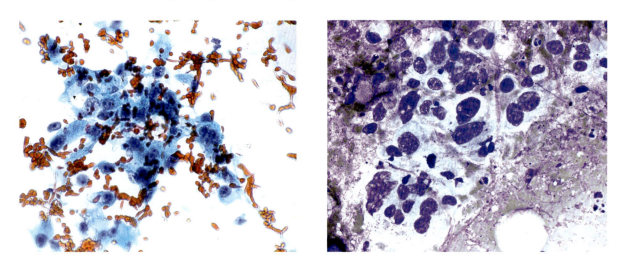

Figure 20-67

UNDIFFERENTIATED (ANAPLASTIC) CARCINOMA

Left: A cluster of poorly differentiated, more epithelial-appearing tumor cells from same case as figure 20-66 (Papanicolaou stain).

Right: At higher magnification, the enlarged anaplastic tumor cells show coarse chromatin and variation in size and shape of the nuclei. Obvious malignant features of these very cellular smears were found throughout the aspirate (Diff-Quik stain).

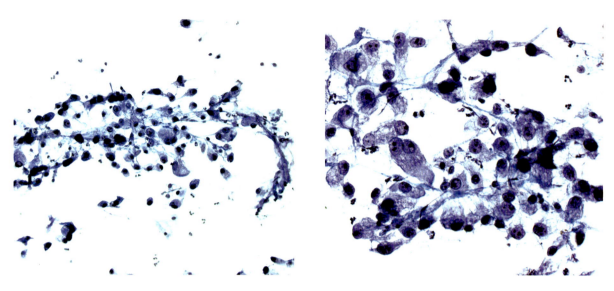

Figure 20-68

UNDIFFERENTIATED (ANAPLASTIC) CARCINOMA

Left: A loose cell group of poorly differentiated tumor cells is seen (Papanicolaou stain).

Right: At higher magnification, the large tumor cell size can be compared to the neutrophils in the background. Some nuclei have prominent nucleoli (Papanicolaou stain).

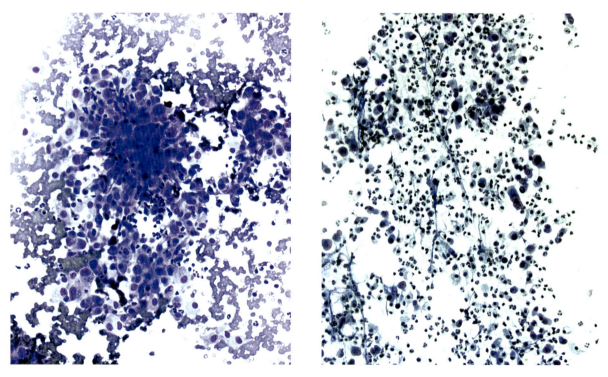

Figure 20-69

UNDIFFERENTIATED (ANAPLASTIC) CARCINOMA

Left: The enlarged tumor cells have a predominant epithelial pattern. The tumor cells are large in relation to the red blood cells in the background (Diff-Quik stain).

Right: Loose, enlarged, poorly differentiated tumor cells with a background of acute inflammatory cells, a feature often seen in aspirates from undifferentiated carcinoma (Papanicolaou stain).

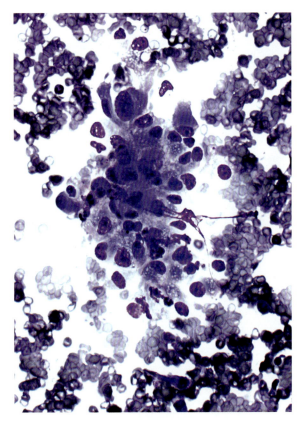

Figure 20-70

UNDIFFERENTIATED (ANAPLASTIC) CARCINOMA

High magnification of group of pleomorphic tumor cells (Diff-Quik stain).

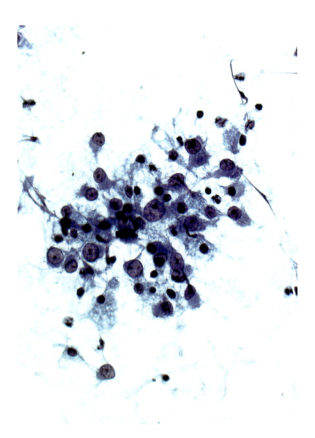

Figure 20-71

UNDIFFERENTIATED (ANAPLASTIC) CARCINOMA

Some cells have prominent nucleoli and others are undergoing apoptosis (Papanicolaou stain).

nuclei that are round, oval, or irregular (figs. 20-72–20-77). The tumor cells have readily visible nucleoli. Oncocytic cells presenting as isolated cells or small cohesive clusters usually represent metaplasia. This finding is particularly common in Hashimoto thyroiditis and nodular hyperplasia. Aspiration smears from true oncocytic neoplasms are highly cellular, with a monomorphic population of discohesive cells or syncytia. These smears lack lymphocytes, plasma cells, and macrophages (10,78). Colloid is scant or inspissated.

The recognition of typical oncocytic cells is not color dependent. The cytoplasm of these cells may stain green, orange, or blue with the Papanicolaou method (figs. 20-74, 20-75) and appear blue, gray or purple with the Diff-Quik stain (figs. 20-73, 20-74, 20-76).

An uncommon papillary variant of oncocytic follicular neoplasm has been reported by Kaur et al. (50). Five tumors were encountered on aspi-

Table 20-10
CYTOLOGIC FEATURES OF UNDIFFERENTIATED (ANAPLASTIC) CARCINOMA
Absent colloid
High cellularity
Acute inflammation
Necrosis

Bizarre, pleomorphic/giant cells
    Isolated cells, syncytial fragments
    Sarcomatoid appearance
    Neutrophils within the cytoplasm
    Coarse chromatin
    Macronucleoli (often multiple)
    Mitoses, many atypical

ration biopsy and subsequently interpreted from histologic sections to represent carcinomas. This variant was composed entirely of oncocytic cells

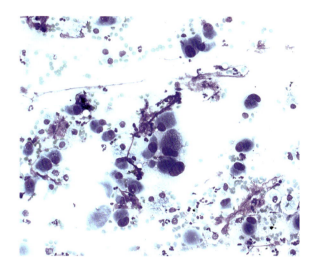

Figure 20-72

FOLLICULAR NEOPLASM WITH ONCOCYTIC FEATURES

Some of the follicular cells in small clusters have enlarged irregular nuclei and dense granular cytoplasm (lower edge of the group of follicular cells in the center of the figure). The pattern seen in this field is not specific for a follicular neoplasm (Diff-Quik stain).

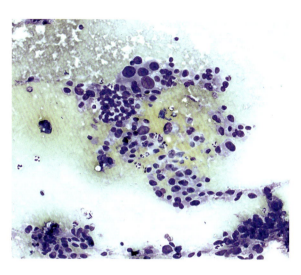

Figure 20-73

FOLLICULAR NEOPLASM WITH ONCOCYTIC FEATURES

A cluster of oncocytic follicular cells has enlarged irregular nuclear outlines and abundant granular cytoplasm. The outer border of the cell group is scalloped, a feature favoring a true follicular neoplasm. One cell has a clear intranuclear inclusion. This finding may indicate the oncocytic variant of papillary carcinoma. It may be necessary in some of these cases to interpret the aspirate as a follicular neoplasm with oncocytic features versus the oncocytic variant of papillary carcinoma (Diff-Quik stain).

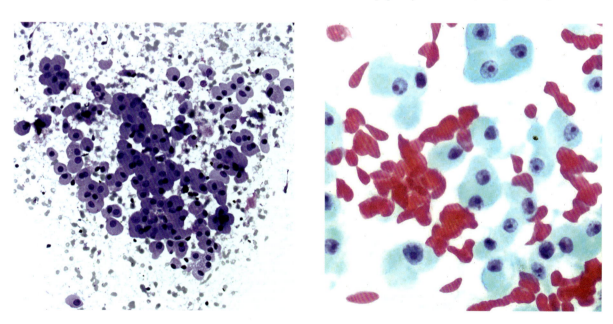

Figure 20-74

FOLLICULAR NEOPLASM WITH ONCOCYTIC FEATURES

Left: Typical field of follicular cells with a prominent oncocytic appearance. This pattern of clustered follicular cells with oncocytic features was consistent throughout the smears (Diff-Quik stain).

Right: With a Papanicolaou stained smear, the granularity of the follicular cell cytoplasm is evident. Prominent nucleoli are visible.

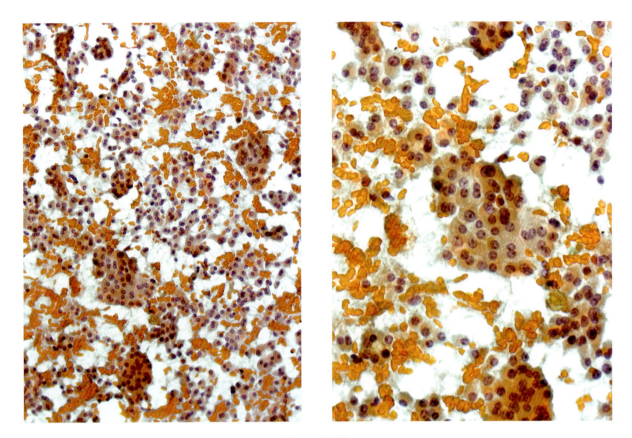

Figure 20-75

FOLLICULAR NEOPLASM WITH ONCOCYTIC FEATURES

Left: A highly cellular aspirate of oncocytic-appearing follicular cells. While no specific cytologic features of malignancy are seen at this magnification, the high cellularity plus the clinical features in this case indicated a malignant thyroid neoplasm.

Right: At higher magnification, the oncocytic features of the follicular cells are obvious. In addition, some cells have prominent nucleoli, although the chromatin is bland. The clinical features indicated that this neoplasm was malignant (left and right: Papanicolaou stain).

Figure 20-76

FOLLICULAR NEOPLASM WITH ONCOCYTIC FEATURES

A highly cellular smear with variation in nuclear size and some prominent nucleoli shows the typical pattern of an oncocytic thyroid neoplasm with cells having abundant, finely granular blue-gray cytoplasm (Diff-Quik stain).

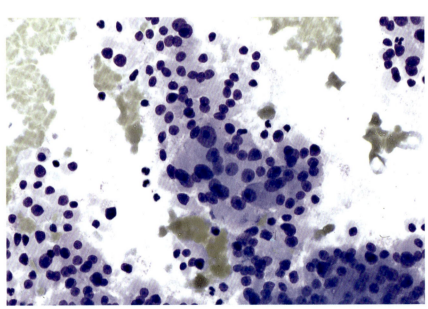

Table 20-11

**CYTOLOGIC FEATURES OF
ONCOCYTIC CELL TUMORS**

Hypercellularity

Monomorphic population of oncocytic cells
    Large polygonal cells
    Granular cytoplasm
    Enlarged nuclei, binucleation
    Prominent nuclei

Scant to absent colloid

Absent inflammation

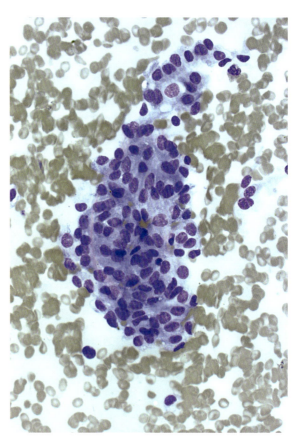

Figure 20-77

PAPILLARY CARCINOMA: CLEAR CELL VARIANT

A sheet of follicular cells is in the form of a small papillary-like fragment. The nuclei are irregular and elongated. The cytoplasm is very delicate and pale, which probably corresponds to the clear cell appearance seen in the histologic sections. These features are not specific enough to recognize with the Romanowsky stain (Diff-Quik stain).

in papillary arrays. True papillae with fibrovascular cores were identified but no nuclear features of classic PTC were present. Distinguishing these cases from bonafide PTC is difficult since the characteristic nuclear features are sparse or absent in the oncocytic variant of PTC. A true PTC with oncocytic features has been reported associated with Hashimoto thyroiditis (79).

Like nononcocytic follicular neoplasms, the malignant potential of oncocytic follicular lesions is best assessed histologically. Unlike the deceptively bland PTCs that make the distinction from adenomas challenging, the opposing problem of cytologic atypia, commonly encountered in oncocytic cells, makes a precise interpretation of a malignant versus a benign oncocytic neoplasm difficult. The clinical features of age over 40 years, male sex, and tumor size 2 cm or greater favor a malignant oncocytic tumor (80,81).

Cytologic pleomorphism and atypia are frequently encountered in oncocytic follicular neoplasms that are subsequently classified histologically as adenomas. In contrast, two studies found that small oncocytic tumor cells having poorly defined cytoplasm and prominent nucleoli with an arrangement in syncytial fragments and with abundant naked tumor cell nuclei favored a diagnosis of oncocytic carcinoma (fig. 20-75) (82,83). The small size of the tumor cell has recently been confirmed by morphometry (84). Interobserver variability for the interpretation of oncocytic features in thyroid aspiration biopsies remains problematic (85). Table 20-11 summarize the cytologic features of oncocytic follicular neoplasms.

Tumors with Clear Cell Features

Kini (14) reported an example of *clear cell change* in a PTC of the thyroid gland at the cytologic level, describing the cytoplasm of the cells as very pale in the aspiration smear stained by the Papanicolaou method (figs. 20-77, 20-78). She noted a possible misinterpretation as medullary carcinoma on aspiration smears because of the dominant single cell pattern; however, the nuclei in her case had the typical features of PTC.

Nine additional cases of this change appreciated in FNAB smears of the thyroid gland have been reported: five follicular adenomas, one moderately differentiated follicular

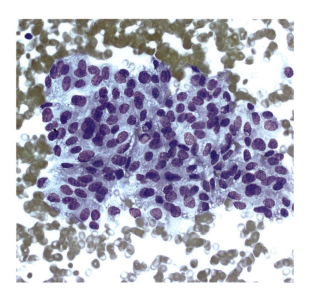

Figure 20-78

PAPILLARY CARCINOMA: CLEAR CELL VARIANT

A papillary-like grouping of cells has pale light blue cytoplasm. Some nuclei demonstrate intranuclear inclusions, which supports the interpretation of papillary carcinoma (Diff-Quik stain).

carcinoma, and one poorly differentiated follicular carcinoma. Two adenomas with a signet cell pattern have been recognized on aspiration smears (86,87). All other cases were non-neoplastic thyroid conditions in which clear cell change was evident in some follicular cells (87).

The author (WJF) has seen a similar case that also had the typical nuclear features of PTC (fig. 20-79). The cytoplasm in both the Papanicolaou- and Romanowsky-stained smears was pale or not visible.

Tumors with Squamous Features

Squamous metaplasia is common in PTC and gives rise to the metaplastic appearance of thyroid follicular cells that has been described as a feature of PTC in FNAB smears. The morphology of thyroid tumors with squamous features overlaps with the oncocytic appearance of the follicular cells, particularly when viewed on Diff-Quik-stained aspiration smears that are taken from the PTC (see fig. 20-57, right). The nuclear features of PTC can be sparse in aspirates with this pattern of tumor cells.

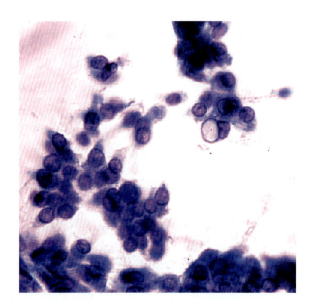 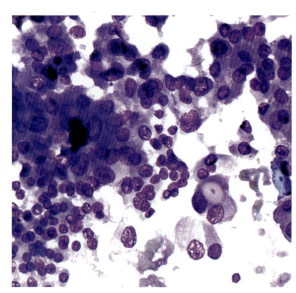

Figure 20-79

PAPILLARY CARCINOMA WITH SIGNET RING CELL FEATURES

Left: Overlapping clusters of follicular cells have enlarged nuclei. In a few cells, the cytoplasmic vacuoles look like "magenta bodies" (target appearance). These features suggest a signet ring cell pattern of papillary carcinoma, a rare finding (Diff-Quik stain).

Right: A sharply defined cytoplasmic vacuole (magenta body) is present, suggesting the signet ring cell pattern of papillary carcinoma. A rare small intranuclear inclusion is seen (Diff-Quik stain).

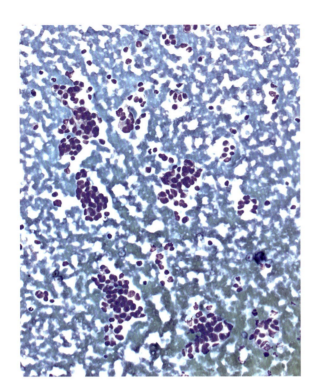 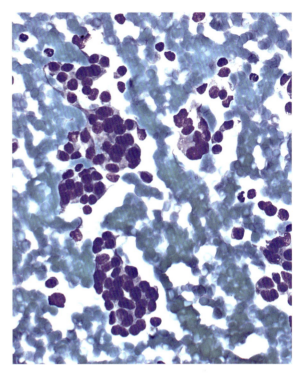

Figure 20-80

MEDULLARY CARCINOMA

Left: Clusters of small follicular cells in a background of red blood cells. The pattern is nonspecific for medullary carcinoma but does suggest a follicular neoplasm (Diff-Quik stain).

Right: At higher magnification, the tight clusters of follicular cells in a bloody background are evident. The very tight clustering gives the appearance of a neuroendocrine neoplasm (Diff-Quik stain).

Mucoepidermoid carcinoma of the thyroid has been described in a few FNABs as has pure squamous cell carcinoma (88–90). In one report of two cases of mucoepidermoid carcinoma, the dominant smear pattern was that of obvious squamous cells, with only scattered mucin-producing cells, usually with a large vacuole and a signet ring cell appearance. These two reported cases were clinically aggressive, in contrast to the mucoepidermoid carcinomas of the thyroid reported in the surgical pathology literature (88).

Medullary Carcinoma

FNAB of *medullary carcinoma* is variably cellular, depending on the amount of stromal fibrosis and the extent of amyloid deposition (6). Several patterns are seen. Most specimens are composed of dispersed large polygonal cells with ample cytoplasm having one or more nuclei and relatively inconspicuous nucleoli (figs. 20-80; 20-81, left) (91). Cell borders tend to be poorly defined.

Nuclear chromatin is coarse and granular (92). The tumor cells of medullary carcinoma may resemble plasma cells (figs. 20-81, right–20-83) (93), oncocytes, and the cells of malignant melanoma, carcinoid tumors, and undifferentiated carcinoma (94,95). A melanotic variant of medullary carcinoma with melanin pigment and positive staining of some of the tumor cells with HMB-45 has been identified by FNAB (96).

The cells in aspirates typically appear pleomorphic, and while some cells are small and round, others are cuboidal, polyhedral, or spindle shaped (figs. 20-84–20-86, left). Occasional tumors are dominated by one cell type. Nuclear pseudoinclusions may be present (6).

The cytoplasm is generally pale and fibrillary in Papanicolaou-stained preparations, with occasional areas of process formation. In Diff-Quik-stained slides, cytoplasmic granularity may be evident, and in some instances, the granules appear metachromatic (fig. 20-86). The

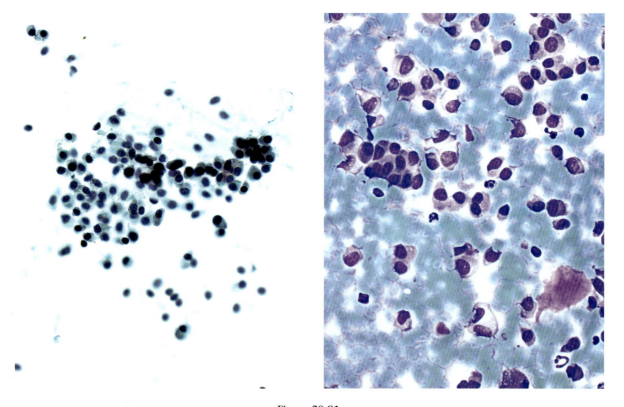

Figure 20-81

MEDULLARY CARCINOMA

Left: The small round cells have a granular nuclear chromatin pattern that is very distinctive. Small nucleoli are seen. The Papanicolaou stain accentuates the neuroendocrine appearance of medullary carcinoma in this aspirate. (Same case as fig. 20-80).

Right: At higher magnification, there is some clustering of follicular cells and the aspirate does not represent an inflammatory process. The eccentric position of the nuclei in the tumor cells is consistent, another variation of the cells of medullary carcinoma. A small fragment of metachromatic material is seen, most probably representing amyloid stroma (Diff-Quik stain).

Figure 20-82

MEDULLARY CARCINOMA

The clustering of tumor cells is apparent, as is the plasma-cytoid appearance of some of the individual tumor cells (Papanicolaou stain).

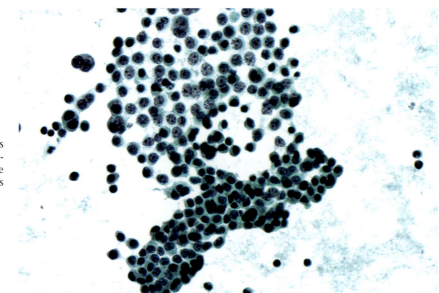

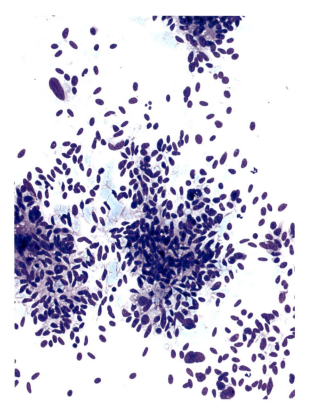

Figure 20-83

MEDULLARY CARCINOMA

The spindle cell pattern is a more typical aspiration pattern of medullary carcinoma. There is a small amount of metachromatic, probably amyloid-like, stroma at the very top of the figure juxtaposed to the tumor cells. Some large irregular nuclei of medullary carcinoma are seen (Diff-Quik stain).

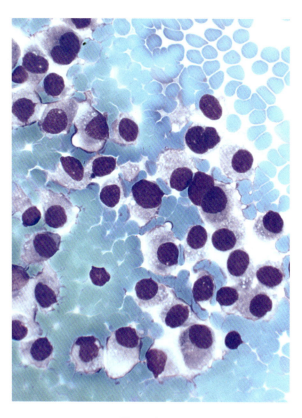

Figure 20-84

MEDULLARY CARCINOMA

The plasmacytoid appearance of the tumor cells and a faint red blush of the cytoplasm rather than distinct red granules that represent calcitonin are seen (Diff-Quik stain).

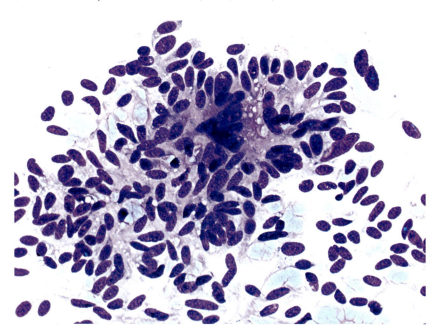

Figure 20-85

MEDULLARY CARCINOMA

Higher magnification of case pictured in figure 20-84 shows the marked spindle cell pattern. The faint scattered red granularity to the cytoplasm is helpful in identifying medullary carcinoma (Diff-Quik stain).

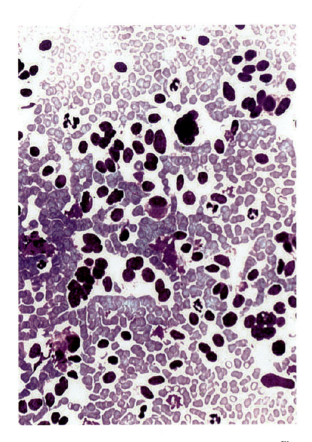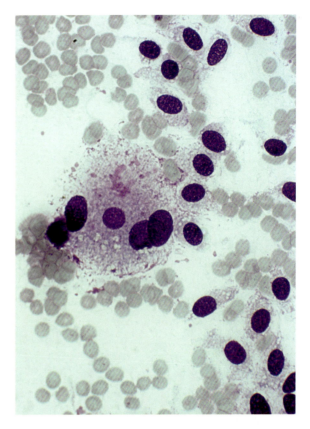

Figure 20-86

MEDULLARY CARCINOMA

Left: Seen in the center of the figure is the distinctive cell full of red granules in the cytoplasm (Diff-Quik stain).

Right: Higher magnification illustrates the faint red granules in the cytoplasm that can be found in aspirates from medullary carcinoma. The nuclei have a monotonous oval appearance (Diff-Quik stain).

granules represent the neurosecretory product of calcitonin. This is confirmed with immunohistochemistry on smears and or cell blocks of the aspirate (6).

Amyloid may be indistinguishable from colloid in Papanicolaou-stained smears, but appears as a light green, almost cyanophilic material that may blend into the background of the smear. The Congo red stain confirms its presence. With the Diff-Quik stain, amyloid appears as dense, acellular, metachromatic material that is somewhat fibrillary on close examination (figs. 20-81, right; 20-87) (6). The amyloid is seen as ill-defined pink to violet masses easily noticed, if present, at low magnification. The diagnosis of medullary carcinoma should be confirmed with immunostains for calcitonin or chromogranin.

While most cases of medullary carcinoma have classic cytomorphologic features, some of the variants may be difficult to diagnose in the absence of calcitonin immunohistochemistry (97). When there is a predominant pattern of small and uniform cells, the impression is that of neuroendocrine tumor and not a typical follicular or papillary thyroid neoplasm. Rare cytologic findings seen in FNAB smears of medullary carcinoma include grape-like cell clusters, cytoplasmic nippling and elongated cytoplasmic processes, carrot-shaped nuclei (fig. 20-85), nuclear buddings (fig. 20-81, right), mast cell-like cells (an appearance simulating Burkitt lymphoma), and a pseudoangiosarcomatous pattern (98,99).

An aspirate smear of medullary carcinoma can at times resemble papillary or follicular

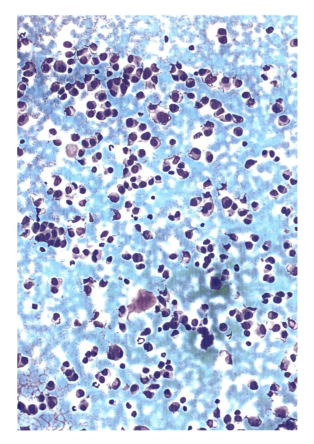

Figure 20-87

MEDULLARY CARCINOMA

At this magnification, the loose pattern of the follicular cells resembles and can be confused with an inflammatory process. There is a single small fragment of metachromatic stroma that may represent amyloid (Diff-Quik stain).

Table 20-12
CYTOLOGIC FEATURES OF MEDULLARY CARCINOMA
Scant to absent colloid
Moderate to high cellularity

Monomorphic population of tumor cells (C-cells)
    Discohesive or loosely cohesive (plasmacytoid) cells
    Polygonal cells, ample finely granular cytoplasm
    Neurosecretory granules (Diff-Quik stain)
    Binucleation and multinucleation
    Eccentric nuclei
    Coarse chromatin
    Intranuclear inclusions (occasional)
    Nucleoli, small, generally inconspicuous

Amyloid

Malignant Lymphoma

The aspiration smears of *high-grade large B-cell lymphomas* of the thyroid gland are cellular and composed of a population of large lymphoid cells with lymphoglandular bodies easily identified in the background (figs. 20-88–20-92).

Aspirations from *low-grade mucosal-associated lymphoid tissue (MALT) lymphomas* may demonstrate a dominant pattern of small lymphocytes but may also have larger follicular center cells, macrophages, plasma cells, and even some oncocytes, in keeping with the aspiration smear pattern of chronic lymphocytic thyroiditis (103). In these situations, ancillary studies such as flow cytometry and immunocytochemistry are used to detect monoclonality.

Flow cytometry has been applied by Zeppo et al. (104) to study the composition of the thyroid lymphocytic infiltrate. They found two patterns, which they designated "lymphocytic" and "lymph node-like." There was a predominance of CD3- and CD5-positive lymphocytes in 30 of 34 cases studied, while there was a predominance of CD19-positive cells in 4 cases. Evaluation of the lambda/kappa ratio demonstrated a light chain ratio of greater than 3.7 in 5 cases. Even with the presence of significant T cells, 22 cases in their study had a B-cell population (CD19 positive) of greater than 20 percent. Statistically, Zeppo et al. found a definite association between the lymphocytic cytologic pattern and the T-cell phenotype, and between the lymph node-like pattern and the B-cell phenotype. At the time of the report

carcinoma. It is also difficult to recognize the spindle cell variant of medullary carcinoma as a thyroid primary. FNAB samples are used to identify calcitonin gene transcripts, to screen new nodules of the thyroid in patients with a family history of medullary carcinoma (92,100), and in at least one case, to diagnose C-cell hyperplasia in the absence of a family history of multiple endocrine neoplasias (101). The cytologic features of medullary carcinoma are summarized in Table 20-12.

For reporting cytopathology of medullary carcinoma, see the NCI scheme for reporting thyroid cytopathology (the Bethesda System for Reporting Thyroid Cytopathology) (102).

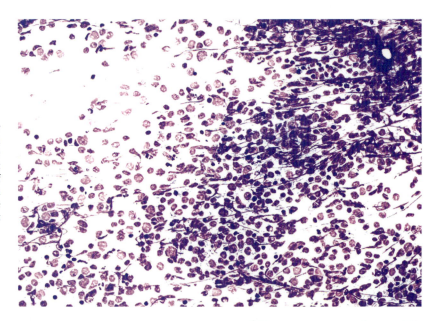

Figure 20-88

NON-HODGKIN LYMPHOMA

A diffuse pattern of irregular lymphoid-appearing cells in an aspirate from a 49-year-old female presenting with an enlarged left thyroid lobe and a past history of chronic lymphocytic thyroiditis. High cellularity and consistency of the pattern indicate this is a malignant lymphoma (Diff-Quik stain).

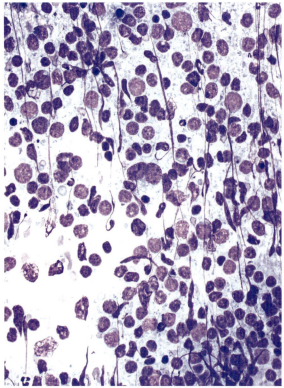

Figure 20-89

NON-HODGKIN LYMPHOMA

The diffuse pattern of enlarged lymphoid cells with somewhat irregular nuclear contours and visible nucleoli is seen. Small gray bodies in the background represent lymphoglandular bodies, which identify the cells as lymphoid. Most of the thyroid lymphomas are of large B-cell type, as was this case (Diff-Quik stain).

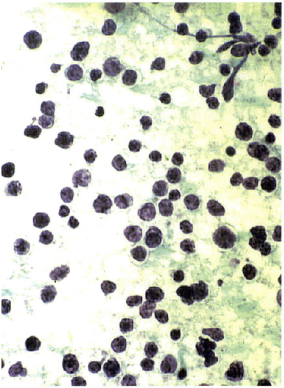

Figure 20-90

NON-HODGKIN LYMPHOMA

Many large, individual, poorly differentiated cells are seen. The diffuse individual presentation of the cells and fragments of cytoplasm (lymphoglandular bodies) in the background indicate a large cell lymphoma. Several of the cells have multiple large nucleoli (Papanicolaou stain).

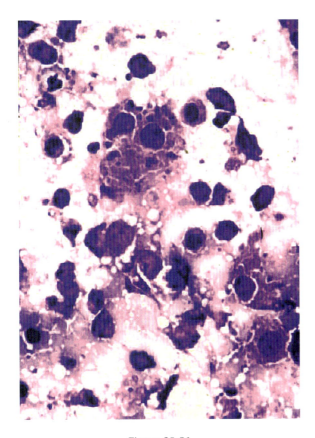

Figure 20-91

NON-HODGKIN LYMPHOMA

The cellular aspirate from the same case as figure 20-90 shows a diffuse individual cell pattern with large cells, a high nuclear to cytoplasmic ratio, and fragments of cytoplasm (lymphoglandular bodies), supporting the diagnosis of large cell lymphoma (Diff-Quik stain).

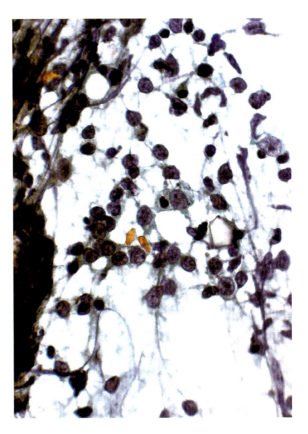

Figure 20-92

NON-HODGKIN LYMPHOMA

At high power, the prominent nucleoli, often multiple, and scant fragmented cytoplasm of a large cell lymphoma are seen (Papanicolaou stain).

none of the patients had developed lymphoma although the follow-up period was short (35 months) (104).

Chan et al. (105) also studied 21 patients with Hashimoto thyroiditis by flow cytometry to determine the kappa/lambda ratio of germinal center B cells. They found a ratio of greater than 3.07 in 18 cases. Cases tested further by polymerase chain reaction (PCR) showed no clonal proliferation. No patients developed lymphoma in 3 years of follow-up. The follow-up periods in both these series are short as generally patients who develop lymphoma in a background of Hashimoto thyroiditis have had the disease for many years.

Some malignant lymphomas of the thyroid gland are of the *follicular type* (106,107). These cases are usually difficult to diagnose from FNAB smears. A case of *Burkitt lymphoma*, presenting as a rapidly growing thyroid mass, has been recognized by FNAB as suspicious for lymphoma, leading to emergency chemotherapy (108).

Secondary/Metastatic Tumors

Renal cell carcinoma and *adenocarcinomas of lung and breast* are the most frequent metastatic tumors to the thyroid gland while *squamous cell carcinoma* represents the most frequent tumor with direct extension involving the thyroid gland (see chapter 16). In most cases, the primary carcinoma has been located and diagnosed previously (figs. 20-93–20-95) (6). Comparing the primary tumor's cytology/histology with the aspirate smears obtained from the thyroid mass is important in identifying the thyroid lesion as a metastasis. An immunohistochemical profile is useful in some cases.

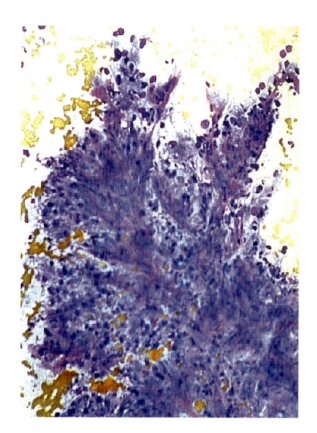
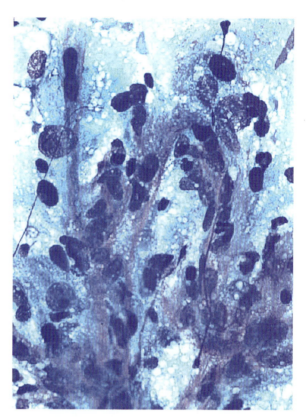

Figure 20-93

METASTATIC RENAL CELL CARCINOMA

Left: The cell groups are divided by metachromatic fibrous bands. There are some penetrating vascular structures not visible at this magnification. The pattern would be most unusual for a primary thyroid neoplasm. Clinically, the patient presented with several recently noted thyroid nodules, which seemed to be enlarging. A radical nephrectomy for a conventional renal cell carcinoma had been performed 11 years previously (Diff-Quik stain).

Right: Higher magnification illustrates some pleomorphism of the tumor cells and a finely vacuolated cytoplasm that probably represents the clear cell areas found when the metastatic nodules were resected as part of a total thyroidectomy. The thyroid involvement was the only area of detected metastasis from the original conventional renal cell carcinoma (Diff-Quik stain).

Figure 20-94

METASTATIC RENAL CELL CARCINOMA

A sheet of pleomorphic tumor cells from metastatic renal cell carcinoma is visualized with the Papanicolaou stain. Pleomorphic, large and very hyperchromatic nuclei are depicted. Other cytologic details are lacking.

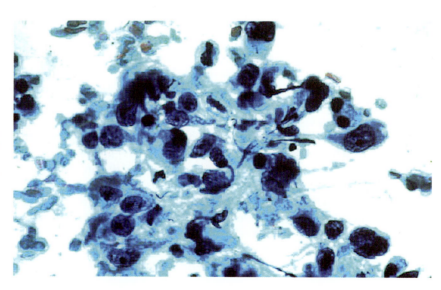

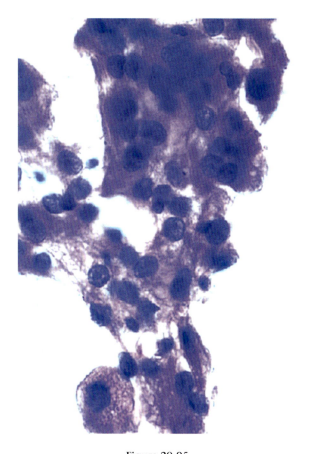

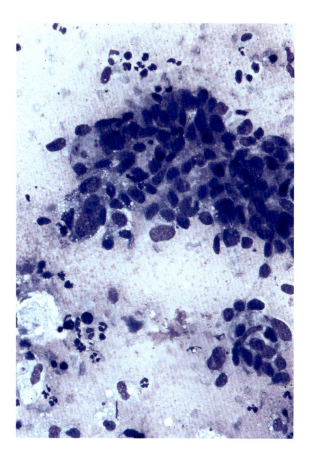

Figure 20-95

METASTATIC RENAL CELL CARCINOMA

A sheet of tumor cells with granular cytoplasm is seen in conventional renal cell carcinoma. The original tumor and the metastases to the thyroid both had areas of clear cell and granular cell renal cell carcinoma (Diff-Quik stain).

Figure 20-96

SQUAMOUS CELL CARCINOMA

The tumor extended from the larynx to present as a thyroid mass. The patient had no symptoms of hoarseness (Diff-Quik stain).

Aspirates of metastatic renal cell carcinoma often appear as discohesive cells with only a slightly increased nuclear to cytoplasmic ratio and minimal nuclear atypia. It is the recognition of slightly atypical cells with abundant clear, vacuolated, or granular cytoplasm that identifies renal cell carcinoma metastatic to the thyroid gland. Rare primary neoplasms of the thyroid, both benign and malignant, have an aspiration pattern dominated by clear cells (see chapter 9). Vigorous smearing may result in cytoplasmic disruption and the release of cytoplasmic vacuoles into the background, making the identification of the clear cell appearance difficult. A cohesive fragment of tumor cells with a peripheral vascular structure may help identify metastatic renal cell carcinoma, since this is an exceedingly rare finding in primary thyroid neoplasms (6). Two cases of metastatic epithelioid angiosarcoma to the thyroid gland have been correctly interpreted by FNAB (109).

Of the metastatic tumors that demonstrate squamous features, the lung and larynx are the usual primary sites (110). The author (WJF) has aspirated a single case of squamous cell carcinoma extending from the larynx to produce a solitary thyroid mass as the clinical presentation (fig. 20-96). Remarkably, the patient had no laryngeal symptoms. The undifferentiated nature of the tumor on aspiration led to an incorrect interpretation of primary undifferentiated (anaplastic) thyroid carcinoma.

DIAGNOSTIC MOLECULAR PATHOLOGY OF FNAB

The nature of fine needle aspiration samples makes them ideal for molecular analysis for several reasons. In thyroid tumors there is a remarkable correlation between between phenotype (i.e., tumor type) and genotype (i.e., genetic alterations), a correlation that is more robust than for many other epithelial tumors (see chapter 2). Specifically, carcinomas with a papillary architecture (classic PTC or its tall cell variant) are characterized by a high prevalence of the *BRAF* V600E mutation and by the *RET/PTC* rearrangement. Encapsulated tumors with follicular architecture (follicular adenoma, follicular carcinoma, and FVPTC) are characterized by *RAS* mutations (usually at codon 61) or by the *PAX8/PPARγ* rearrangement.

Despite the considerable variability in their reported prevalence, the above genetic alterations tend to be mutually exclusive, and one of them is present in about 70 percent of carcinomas of follicular cell origin. They are also easy to detect with assays based on DNA (for *BRAF* and *RAS*) or on RNA (for *RET/PTC* and *PAX8/PPARγ*) analysis.

FNAB samples are an ideal source for molecular studies because the cells can be immediately placed in special solutions to preserve nucleic acids at the time of the procedure, and even the lavage fluid obtained from rinsing the needles after smear preparation can give adequate results. Moreover, the alcohol-based fixation and stains (e.g., Papanicolaou) used for diagnosis preserve nucleic acids well, so that molecular analysis can be easily performed after removal of the coverslip (111).

Many studies have shown that molecular diagnosis can complement FNAB by providing additional information in cases with equivocal cytologic findings (111–137). Early studies indicated that the detection of molecular alterations in FNAB material is both useful and technically feasible. Recent work has shown the utility of molecular techniques as applied to the defined diagnostic categories of the National Cancer Institute's six-tiered Bethesda System for Reporting Thyroid Cytopathology (102), and has been prospective rather than retrospective (114,117,118,120–123,125,128). These studies support the idea that molecular analysis used in conjunction with cytologic diagnosis increases the ability to identify malignant thyroid nodules.

Several excellent reviews have addressed the use of molecular markers to complement the cytologic diagnosis (138–145). The issue is particularly relevant for cases that belong to the indeterminate categories of the Bethesda system, namely the atypia of undetermined significance/follicular lesion of undetermined significance (AUS/FLUS) and follicular neoplasm/suspicious for follicular neoplasm lesions (FN/SFN) groups; such use of molecular markers can be used to improve the preoperative prognostic assessment of patients with thyroid carcinoma.

Using histologic evaluation of the resected specimen as the gold standard, a molecular test can be used to "rule in" malignancy in the preoperative diagnosis of a thyroid nodule if it has high specificity and positive predictive value; it can be used to "rule out" malignancy when the sensitivity and the negative predictive values are high. One general approach relies on the identification in the FNAB material of the above genetic markers (mutations or rearrangements) that presumably drive the development of the thyroid carcinoma. A second approach utilizes molecular markers that are found differentially expressed in benign versus malignant thyroid nodules, regardless of whether they have a pathogenic role in tumor development.

Much work has focused on the analysis of the *BRAF* gene (120,123,125,141), in part because testing for *BRAF* mutations is very cost-effective. Virtually all mutations in thyroid cancer are the result of a T to A transversion in exon 15, at nucleotide 1799 (codon 600), that results in substitution of a Valine with a Glutamate residue (Val600Glu, V600E) (141). The mutation is easily detected, at low cost, even in laboratories with limited equipment, using a variety of methods (113). Even more importantly, *BRAF* V600E is highly specific PTC. A meta-analysis of data on thyroid FNAB samples tested for *BRAF* has shown that out of more than 1,000 nodules positive for the mutation, there were only 8 "false positive" cases where no PTC was found after the thyroidectomy, corresponding to a specificity of 99.3 percent (141). In *BRAF* V600E mutated cases with undetermined cytologic diagnosis due to atypical findings, some authors have recommended a thyroidectomy without the need to repeat the FNAB, while in those that are diagnosed as suspicious for PTC, others have recommended a total thyroidectomy without the need for a frozen section diagnosis (123,125). In case of *BRAF* V600E-positive samples in specimens diagnosed as inadequate, benign or follicular neoplasm, all slides should be reviewed carefully with the ultrasound data. If the initial cytologic diagnosis is confirmed, a repeat FNAB should be prioritized for inadequate or benign specimens while a thyroidectomy instead of a lobectomy may be considered for cases diagnosed as follicular neoplasms.

Testing of FNAB for *BRAF* has also been advocated to improve the management of patients with a malignant (or suspicious) cytologic diagnosis. Changes in the surgical approach to include central compartment lymph node dissection, as well as postoperative decisions concerning radioiodine treatment, TSH suppression, and post-surgical follow up, have been suggested (139,140,142,144). Nevertheless, definitive data regarding the prognostic role of the *BRAF* V600E mutation, and a consensus on how to utilize *BRAF* mutational analysis for patient management still need to be established (142).

Nikiforov et al. (117,128,133) have shown that RAS mutations, *RET/PTC1* and *RET/PTC1*, and *PAX8/PPARγ* can be tested in a panel together with *BRAF*. They have demonstrated that FNABs provide enough material for all the tests to be performed, and that accuracy can be significantly improved by adding markers like *RAS* mutations and the *PAX8/PPARγ* rearrangement, that are particularly relevant for follicular-patterned lesions i.e. follicular adenoma, follicular carcinoma and the FVPTC. Similar results have been shown by other investigators (118,121). In the largest study by Nikiforov et al. (128) the risk of malignancy (positive predictive value) was 88 percent for the AUS/FLUS, 87 percent for the FN/SFN, and 95 percent for the "suspicious for malignant cells" categories of the Bethesda system. Due to their high positive predictive value, molecular tests that rely on a panel of pathogenic cancer-related alterations are most effective to "rule in" cancer and may be best utilized to guide the extent of surgery (lobectomy versus total thyroidectomy) for nodules that have a high risk of malignancy (128,144). The commercial

company Asuragen has developed test platforms that can identify these cancer-related changes in FNAB samples (135,136).

The search of markers that are differentially expressed in malignant nodules versus benign ones, independent of a pathogenic role, has identified several that can be diagnostically useful, including MET, TFF3, SERPINA1, TIMP1, FN1, and TPO (138). One marker that has been validated in a large prospective study is galectin-3, analyzed by immunocytochemistry in FNAB cell-block preparations (114) Another that appears consistently overexpressed in malignant thyroid nodules is HMGA2 (124,146,147). The analysis of micro RNA (miRNA) expression is a new and promising method that can be applied to the preopreative diagnosis of thyroid nodules. The overexpression of some miRNA, like miR-146b, miR-221, miR-222, has been consistently associated with papillary carcinoma, and specific miRNA profiles can be utilized to distinguish benign from malignant nodules in FNAB samples (115,116,127,132).

Affirma®, a gene expression classifier test based on the analysis of 142 proprietary mRNAs has been recently developed, and proposed as a complement to conventional cytologic evaluation of FNABs to "rule out" malignancy (119,129,131,134). The test was designed to achieve high sensitivity with a negative predictive value that allows clinicians to confidently defer diagnostic surgery in patients with indeterminate FNABs diagnoses, for whom the overall risk of malignancy is relatively low (inferior to 30 percent). The authors claim that for a thyroid nodule with an indeterminate cytologic diagnosis corresponding to the AUS/FLUS and FN/SFN categories of the Bethesda system, and a negative ("benign") gene expression classifier result, the risk of malignancy is about 5 percent, comparable to that of a thyroid nodule with a benign cytologic diagnosis (6 to 8 percent) (129,145). The gene expression classifier test does not have enough specificity to "rule in" malignancy (129,145), and may give false positive results in cytologically benign FNABs with a high proportion of blood (134), but its potential clinical utility has been shown by several studies (126,130,137,143).

Molecular analysis of FNAB samples with the panel of cancer-related alterations developed by Nikiforov et al. (133) and the Affirma® gene expression classifier test (126) may be cost-effective tools for the management of patients with thyroid nodules. The American Thyroid Association (ATA) Guidelines Task Force is currently reviewing the data on the use of genetic markers for the diagnosis and management of patients with thyroid nodules. Until that review is completed the ATA recommends a cautious clinical approach to the use of these tests (148).

ACCURACY OF CYTOLOGY: WHAT CAN BE EXPECTED

A number of studies have reported the sensitivity, specificity, and diagnostic accuracy of FNABs of the thyroid gland. A large recent series of 6,226 cases examined over a period of 16 years found a sensitivity of 93 percent for the presence of a neoplasm, and a specificity of 96 percent for the absence of a neoplasm (149). There were 7 false positive cases and 11 false negative interpretations of the aspirates. The results were calculated on the basis that the aspirate was considered sufficient for diagnosis. The criteria for a sufficient aspirate were the presence of at least 6 to 8 tissue fragments of well-preserved follicular epithelium on two slides. Aspirates consisting of cyst fluid were considered unsatisfactory, a decision that cytopathologists who perform the aspiration themselves and are able to evaluate the patient postaspirate for any residual mass, would challenge as unduly restrictive.

The aspirates in this series (149) were all performed by clinicians, more than 20 in this report, with variable degrees of experience. Therefore, the rigid criteria for an acceptable aspirate seem justified. The predictive value for a positive report of a neoplasm was 92 percent but fell to 42 percent when the interpretation was just "suspicious" for the presence of a neoplasm. The range of sensitivities reported in the literature is from 65 to 98 percent, and specificities from 73 to 100 percent. The differences appeared to be how the various reports handle the "suspicious for a neoplasm" category.

A similar large series in which the aspiration biopsies were all performed with ultrasound guidance focused on the reliability of a benign interpretation for nodules larger than 3 cm (150). From 6,921 aspirates performed at the Mayo Clinic over a 4-year period, 742 were interpret-

ed as benign in nodules 3 cm or larger. Only 20 percent, 145 patients, underwent thyroidectomy. There was only 1 false negative case (0.7 percent). No additional malignancies were found in 550 index cases that had 3 years of follow-up.

A number of studies have attempted to refine criteria or use other parameters to improve the sensitivity of FNAB of the thyroid gland to distinguish between follicular adenoma and follicular carcinoma. The overall results show limited success but they do emphasize the importance of either the cytopathologist or experienced radiologist performing the aspiration and evaluating the clinical situation or that information being provided in detail to the cytopathologist by the clinician performing this procedure (151,152). The basic goal of FNAB of the thyroid is to separate true follicular neoplasms from non-neoplastic thyroid nodules (153). Sensitivity and specificity can be significantly improved by repeat aspiration of the nodule when the original interpretation is equivocal (154).

Several papers have examined the use of frozen section in the evaluation of thyroid nodules at the time of surgery in comparison with the original aspiration biopsy report. Three reports concluded that intraoperative frozen section added little to the management of a thyroid nodule when the preoperative FNAB report was positive for cancer (155–157). Two studies concluded that there may be a role for intraoperative frozen section in cases where the FNAB report is only suspicious for malignancy (158,159). A more recent study that reviewed the literature comparing FNAB and frozen section for the evaluation of thyroid nodules found that FNAB was much more sensitive but less specific and had a lower positive predictive value than frozen section (160). Both had essentially the same accuracy in evaluating thyroid nodules that are not follicular lesions.

One recent contrary opinion has been raised about the accuracy of thyroid FNAB in detecting thyroid carcinoma. Reporting from an audit of the National Pathology Data Base in the Netherlands, Giard and Hermans (161) found that with an application rate of 66 percent and a sensitivity rate for the most recent aspirate performed on the patient of 70 percent, only 47 percent of the malignancies were detected by FNAB of the thyroid gland. In an accompanying editorial to this study, Cramer (162) pointed out two important reasons for the poor results of that series. One hundred different laboratories interpreted the FNABs, and 33 percent of the patients with thyroid cancer did not have an FNAB. This latter finding strongly suggests that clinicians lacked experience or confidence in the procedure.

The consensus terminology from the NCI Thyroid State of the Art Conference is presented in Table 20-3. As an option, the risk assessment for the presence of a thyroid malignancy can be included in the report (10). Data can be used from the literature or from results in one's own laboratory. The two reporting categories that have, subsequent to this classification scheme, generated the most controversy are "follicular lesion of undetermined significance" and "neoplasm," the latter subdivided into follicular neoplasm and Hürthle cell neoplasm (10). In a series of 241 patients who underwent FNAB and thyroidectomy and had a report of nondiagnostic biopsy, the use of ultrasound did not reduce the likelihood of a nondiagnostic biopsy (163). Nodules greater than 3 cm had more nondiagnostic interpretations. Malignant disease was present in 14 percent of patients with nondiagnostic FNABs, even after repeat aspirations. Patient age, sex, thyroid function, gland size, number of nodules, and final pathology were not related to a nondiagnostic biopsy.

Banks et al. (164) developed a predictor model to determine the risk of malignancy for an indeterminate or suspicious thyroid aspiration biopsy report. After evaluating 639 patients with an indeterminate or suspicious FNAB, they found that patients at the extremes of age, with large nodule size, and whose FNAB interpretation was suspicious for PTC were at an increased risk for the presence of malignancy. In another series of reports of suspicious for follicular or Hürthle cell neoplasm, the risk of malignancy was higher in male patients and in nodules measuring 2 cm or greater (165).

How well has The Bethesda System for Reporting Thyroid Cytopathology (TBSRTC) been accepted? Results were recently reported of a survey questionnaire on this topic sent to 2,063 laboratories participating in the College of American Pathologists cytopathology interlaboratory comparison program. Seven hundred and seventy-seven laboratories returned the survey of which 451 were using the TBSRTC and 127 were planning to use it in the near future; 70 laboratories were unaware of this reporting system. Most responding laboratories reported that TBSRTC had made little or no change in their practice of thyroid cytopathology (166).

Since the first publications of TBSRTC in 2008 and its formal publication in 2010 (10), a large body of literature has accumulated analyzing the performance of the six diagnostic categories. Most studies have focused on the indeterminate category, AUS/FLUS. In one review, the incidence of this category varied from 2.1 to 20.5 percent of cases in comparison to the anticipated use of the category as noted in the publications on TBSRTC of 7.0 percent or less. For patients having surgical resection with the AUS/FLUS interpretation, a malignancy was found in 15 to 46 percent of cases (167). Seven series were reviewed for this study and demonstrated a surgical resection rate from 30.0 to 52.5 percent. In these same seven series, for patients with a benign diagnosis followed by surgical excision, a malignant lesion was found in 1 to 31 percent.

Bongiovanni et al. (168) from a literature review that totaled 25,445 thyroid aspirations, of which 6,362 (25 percent) had surgical excision, found a sensitivity of 97 percent, a specificity of 50.7 percent, and a diagnostic accuracy of 68.8 percent based on the histologic findings of the resected cases. They excluded the nondiagnostic category from their calculations. Their analysis determined a positive predictive value of 55.9 percent and a negative predictive value of 96.3 percent for FNAB. They found AUS/FLUS rates from 3 to 25 percent for 2,491 cases. Nine-hundred fifty-seven patients had surgical excision with an average rate of malignancy of 15.9 percent. This rate of malignancy for this category is at the upper level of that anticipated by the TBSRTC Consensus Conference (10).

Bose and Walts (169) evaluated the literature for the interpretation of follicular neoplasms of undetermined significance, follicular neoplasm, and suspicious for follicular neoplasm. The range of use of these indeterminant categories varied from 5 to 42 percent within laboratories and from 2.5 to 28.1 percent among individual cytopathologists. Realizing that there is less than universal agreement on the interpretation of follicular patterned lesions among expert surgical pathologists, they noted an interobserver agreement from 17 to 100 percent among six experts reviewing 15 follicular patterned lesions histologically.

In a recent study of 44 thyroid FNABs with an AUS/FLUS interpretation by eight cytopathologists, Collins and Collins (170) used whole slide imaging to attempt to refine results. They found that a nuclear to cytoplasmic ratio of 5 or greater but with fewer than 20 cell groups in the sample had an odds ratio of malignancy of 4.64 while a ratio of 5 or greater and more than 20 cell groups had a odds ratio for malignancy of 7.0. Given the large percentage of cases reported in many series as AUS/FLUS, using whole slide imaging to refine this category does not seem practical.

Wong and Baloch (171), from an extensive literature search for evidence-based studies, reviewed 13 that fulfilled their criteria as acceptable. They included only those with a tiered thyroid FNAB classification scheme of at least four tiers and follow-up histology. Excluded were studies with limited or no surgical pathology follow-up, those focusing on a single thyroid FNAB diagnosis, and those using ancillary techniques. Seven pre-TBSRTC and six post¬TBSRTC studies were analyzed further. Three of the seven pre-TBSRTC studies calculated sensitivity with the following results: 94.0 and 91.5 percent sensitivity, excluding neoplasm/adenoma diagnoses, and 88.2 percent excluding the indeterminant diagnosis. Specificity was correspondingly 98.5, 99.1, and 98.2 percent with the same exclusions. Calculations of sensitivity for the two series with the interpretation of neoplasm/adenoma included dropped to 89.4 and 80.3 percent while specificity was reduced to 70.4 and 79.8 percent. Two of the six post-TBSRTC studies calculated sensitivity, which was 84.4 percent, or 100 percent (neoplasm/adenoma included or excluded). Specificity was 98.7 (neoplasm/adenoma interpretations excluded) and 98.2 percent (included), while specificity for the remaining post-TBSRTC cases was only 36.4 percent. The data are obviously variable and the authors noted a major limitation of the study was selection bias for patients referred for surgery.

Onder et al. (172) focused their study from their own practice on the experience with the outcome for the indeterminant category in TBSRTC. From a total of 6,310 thyroid FNABs, 655 were reported as indeterminant. They subclassified their AUS/FLUS cases into four patterns: papillary thyroid carcinoma, microfollicle pattern, atypical cell pattern, and Hürthle cell pattern. Malignancy rates for AUS/FLUS were 18.9 percent; for follicular neoplasm/suspicious for follicular neoplasm, 45.7 percent; and for suspicious for malignancy, 71 percent. For the AUS/FLUS subcategories, malignancy rates were as follows: papillary thyroid carcinoma pattern, 28 percent; microfollicle pattern, 6.9 percent; atypical cell pattern, 22.2 percent; and Hürthle cell pattern, 0 percent.

VanderLann et al. (173) reviewed both the literature and two large FNAB practices, both of which spanned pre- and post-TBSRTC reporting. In one practice, all of the aspirates were performed by an endocrinologist under ultrasound guidance and the specimens were processed using a liquid-based technique, while for the other practice, approximately one third of the aspirates were performed in an office setting without ultrasound while two thirds were performed by radiologists using ultrasound with immediate cytologic evaluation. The combined series totaled more than 15,000 cases. The focus of this study was the nondiagnostic and AUS categories. The authors found a consistent negative correlation between nondiagnostic and AUS rates analyzed by year, aspirator, and cytologist. The strongest correlation was noted for cytologists. Furthermore, nondiagnostic rates decreased by 1 percent for every 3.5 percent increase in AUS. The conclusion of the authors is that there exists a discrete population of cases that cytologists will classify as nondiagnostic or AUS.

Recently Renshaw and Gould (174) evaluated 9,080 thyroid FNABs to determine the impact of size of the nodule, less than 1 cm, on the indeterminant, AUS/FLUS, and suspicious for follicular/Hürthle cell neoplasm categories. Of 1,393 cases surgically excised, 17 percent were interpreted originally as AUS and 18 percent were interpreted as suspicious for follicular/Hürthle cell neoplasm. Fifty-two incidental papillary carcinomas were identified in the resected specimens. Nodules smaller than 1 cm comprised 16 percent of the reported AUS cases and 8 percent of the suspicious cases. The authors concluded that nodules smaller than

Table 20-13

PITFALLS IN DIAGNOSIS: OVERLAPPING CYTOLOGIC CRITERIA

Cystic Change	Oncocytic Cells
Degeneration in nodular hyperplasia	Oncocytic cell tumor
Papillary carcinoma	Hashimoto thyroiditis
Follicular carcinoma	Nodular hyperplasia
Thyroglossal duct cysts	Papillary carcinoma
Metastatic carcinomas	Hyperplasia
Papillary Formations	**Intranuclear Inclusions**
Papillary carcinoma	Papillary carcinoma
Papillary hyperplasia in nodular hyperplasia	Medullary carcinoma
Pregnancy-induced hyperplasia	Oncocytic cell tumor
Oncocytic cell tumor, papillary variant	Follicular neoplasm
Follicular carcinoma	Metastatic malignant melanoma

1 cm with indeterminant results on FNAB and without features of papillary carcinoma, have the same risk of malignancy as a benign aspirate.

The results of all of these series emphasize the difficulty and variability of the indeterminant thyroid FNAB and increase the importance of using ancillary testing, most obviously molecular. This would substantially improve the positive predictive value for a neoplasm in this group of cases.

Questions have been raised about the validity of thyroid FNAB in children. The argument against this procedure has been the high incidence of true neoplasms in the pediatric age group, as high as 50 percent of all solitary nodules. The obvious counter argument is that 50 percent of these nodules are not neoplastic. Therefore, reasonable results of a thyroid aspiration biopsy can reduce significantly the need for surgery. Two recent studies support this conclusion. One reported a sensitivity rate of 87 percent for identifying a lesion and a diagnostic specificity rate of 92 percent for FNAB (175). The second study reported a sensitivity of 100 percent for malignancy relative to the final histologic diagnosis, thus reducing unnecessary surgery in the pediatric age group (176).

PITFALLS OF THYROID FNAB

The interpretation of FNAB for most thyroid lesions is straightforward. It is important to have adequate material, high quality smears, and an understanding of the cytologic criteria and differential interpretation for at least the most common thyroid lesions. Concise clinical information and radiology studies, if they have been performed, are also important pieces of information.

Stringent adequacy criteria are needed if the cytopathologist only interprets the aspirate and does not see the patient and perform the aspiration. Cytopathologists performing the aspirate may be more liberal with adequacy criteria, particularly in the face of thyroid cysts, colloid nodules, and multinodular goiters. Cysts either show no follicular epithelium or very little of it. While many laboratories report these specimens as unsatisfactory or limited, the complete evacuation of the cyst, with no residual palpable mass, correlates well with a benign follow-up, confirming that these specimens are telling the physician that the lesion is a cyst and therefore the specimen is adequate in that sense (6). Ultrasound imaging following the aspiration can also indicate that the mass is no longer visible.

The overlapping criteria presented in Table 20-13 best summarize the potential pitfalls in thyroid aspiration cytology. It is important to avoid placing too much emphasis on a single criterion for diagnosis. Almost any cytologic finding associated with a specific interpretation can be detected to a lesser degree in other thyroid lesions. There is no single feature that distinguishes a benign from a malignant neoplasm, and therefore no criteria for differentiating follicular adenoma from follicular carcinoma (177,178).

During pregnancy, the thyroid gland may enlarge from an elevation of the basal metabolic rate. Aspirates of a hyperplastic thyroid gland provide smears with exuberant papillary formations that mimic the architectural pattern of PTC. The nuclear features of enlargement, inclusions, and grooves are not found in abundance with hyperplasia of the thyroid gland in general or as a result of pregnancy (179). The incidence of thyroid carcinoma in pregnancy does not appear to be higher than in the nonpregnant woman of similar age. A diagnosis of PTC in pregnant women should only be cautiously rendered.

HISTOLOGIC ALTERATIONS FOLLOWING FNAB

An area of some concern is the potential for aspiration biopsy to cause tissue damage that hinders or precludes subsequent histologic interpretation. Despite the fact that many core needle biopsies have been performed on many tumors over many years, this problem seems to have surfaced among surgical pathologists only with the growing use of FNAB of the thyroid gland. Obviously, since the core needle biopsies are larger, they can do much more damage, so why the concern now? Most of the reported cases focus on histologic alterations in thyroid gland, lymph nodes, and salivary gland, organs easily sampled using FNAB techniques.

Two major types of histologic alterations follow superficial FNAB. One is a reactive proliferation along the needle tract that may produce atypical cells. The other is a total or near-total infarction of the lesion being sampled. Oncocytic neoplasms seem particularly vulnerable to infarction (180).

LiVolsi (181) characterized the spectrum of histologic reactions that occur following FNAB of a thyroid lesion. Postaspiration thyroid histology is similar to that of a healing wound, with reactive fibroblastic proliferation, acute inflammation, hemorrhage, fibrin deposition, and the formation of new capillary blood vessels in the acute phase, from a few days to 3 weeks. This is followed by the chronic phase, with maturation of the fibrous tissue, organization of areas of hemorrhage, and squamous metaplasia of entrapped or adjacent epithelium, occurring approximately 3 to 12 weeks postaspiration. The difficulty for the surgical pathologist is interpreting follicular lesions having follicular cells or metaplastic appearing from reactive atypical epithelial cells within an altered capsule. It is important for the pathologist to have the history with the time interval of the prior FNABs and to recognize the histologic features of the needle tract. The latter is not difficult if one is thinking about it (181).

The author (WJF) has personally reviewed two cases where a microscopic collection of cells from a follicular adenoma was detected within and just outside the capsule following an aspiration biopsy and subsequent surgical excision of the thyroid tumor (182). The association of these cells with the puncture of the capsule and the underlying needle tract was obvious. A rarely encountered morphologic change, papillary endothelial hyperplasia, in a thyroid gland examined histologically after aspiration, may mimic angiosarcoma (183,184). This alteration is considered an unusual proliferation within an organizing hematoma and can usually be distinguished from a true vascular neoplasm, a rare primary tumor of the thyroid gland.

COMPLICATIONS OF FNAB

FNAB of the thyroid gland may be followed, rarely, by minor complications. These include local bleeding, vasovagal episodes, and tracheal puncture. Their numbers are insignificant when compared to the large number of FNABs performed. Bleeding is controlled by the application of pressure to the puncture site. Rarely, delayed bleeding within the thyroid gland causes some enlargement and patient anxiety. This resolves within a short period of time. The potential for tracheal puncture is greatest when aspirating midline lesions. It is immediately apparent by loss of negative pressure within the syringe barrel if suction is used, or the lack of any material appearing in the hub of the needle when using the needle-only method to obtain a sample. Cytologically, tracheal aspiration is confirmed by the presence of bronchial cells on the smears. Patients feel nothing, or minimal discomfort of a tickling sensation that may induce a cough response. The use of ultrasound-guided aspiration minimizes placement of the needle in the incorrect location.

There have been only three reports of acute enlargement of the thyroid gland (185–187) and delayed swelling of the prethyroidal soft tissues (188) following FNAB. The author has personally seen one case of acute thyroid swelling immediately following an aspiration biopsy. All patients were women but there is no other common denominator. The cause of this problem remains obscure. Pre-FNAB anesthesia was given in only one case (185). One aspiration was interrupted when the patient swallowed (186). Enlargement of the thyroid gland was rapid, yet transient. There was no ecchymoses or airway obstruction. Cold packs were applied to the swollen area and reduced the gland enlargement within hours. In a third reported case, swelling was noticed at least 24 hours postaspiration (188). Ultrasound examination indicated edema of the prethyroidal soft tissues. Corticosteroids were administered, with gradual reduction of the swelling within 48 hours.

Kobayashi et al. (189) reported a phenomenon referred to as postaspiration thyrotoxicosis. A retrospective 4-year review noted 5 patients out of 500 who developed transient thyrotoxicosis following FNAB of thyroid cysts using 21-23 gauge needles. All of these patients had large cysts. None developed significant symptoms of hyperthyroidism following the aspiration.

This study was preceded by a brief report by Shulkin (190) who noted the development of a "hot" nodule following FNAB of a thyroid cyst. A hot nodule developing within the same region as the cyst suggested that some follicular disruption or leakage accounted for the changes.

Needle tract seeding during a FNAB of the thyroid gland has yet to be unequivocally documented (22 gauge or higher gauge needle) (191). In 1990, Hales and Hsu (192) reported implantation of cells from a PTC in the cutaneous portion of the needle tract. The patient had undergone three aspiration biopsies of the thyroid using 20-, 21-, and finally 25-gauge needles over a 7-year period. The location, amount of fibrosis, and size of the implant suggested that this slow-growing deposit was seeded during one of the first two aspirations. Despite an initial diagnosis of PTC, the patient refused surgical excision, clearly contributing to the clinical findings of the implant 7 years later.

REFERENCES

1. Cooper DS, Doherty GM, Haugen BR, et al. Management guidelines for patients with thyroid nodules and differentiated thyroid cancer. Thyroid 2006;16:109-42.
2. Layfield LJ, Cibas ES, Gharib H, Mandel SJ. Thyroid aspiration cytology: current status. CA Cancer J Clin 2009;59:99-110
3. Castro MR, Gharib H. Thyroid fine-needle aspiration biopsy: progress, practice, and pitfalls. Endocr Pract 2003;9:128-36.
4. Eedes CR, Wang HH. Cost-effectiveness of immediate specimen adequacy assessment of thyroid fine-needle aspirations. Am J Clin Pathol 2004;121:64-9.
5. Powers CN, Frable WJ. Fine Needle aspiration biopsy of the head and neck. Boston: Butterworth-Heinemann; 1996.
6. Cibas ES, Alexander EK, Benson CB, et al. Indications for thyroid FNA and pre-FNA requirements: a synopsis of the National Cancer Institute Thyroid Fine-needle Aspiration State of the Science Conference. Diagn Cytopathol 2008;36:390-9.
7. Stanley MW, Lowhagen T. Fine needle aspiration of palpable masses. Boston: Butterworth-Heinemann; 1993.
8. Ljung BM. Part II. Techniques of aspiration and smear preparation. In: Koss LG, Woyke S, Olszewski W, eds. Aspiration biopsy: cytologic interpretation and histologic bases. New York: Igaku-Shoin; 1992:12-38.
9. Abele JS. The case for pathologist ultrasound-guided fine-needle aspiration biopsy. Cancer 2008;114:463-8.
10. Ali SZ, Cibas ES, eds. The Bethesda system for reporting thyroid cytopathology: definitions, criteria, and explanatory notes. New York: Springer; 2010.
11. Abele JS, Levine RA. Diagnostic criteria and risk-adapted approach to indeterminate thyroid cytodiagnosis. Cancer Cytopathol 2010;118:415-22.

12. Ljung BM, Langer J, Mazzaferri EL, et al. Training, credentialing and re-credentialing for the performance of a thyroid FNA: a synopsis of the National Cancer Institute Thyroid Fine-Needle Aspiration State of the Science Conference. Diagn Cytopathol 2008;36:400-6.

13. Pitman MB, Abele J, Ali SZ, et al. Techniques for thyroid FNA: a synopsis of the National Cancer Institute Thyroid Fine-needle Aspiration State of the Science Conference. Diagn Cytopathol 2008;36:407-24.

14. Kini SR. Guides to clinical aspiration biopsy. In: Thyroid. New York: Igaku-Shoin; 1987.

15. Nilsson G. Marginal vacuoles in fine needle aspiration biopsy smears of toxic goiters. Acta Pathol Microbiol Scand A 1972;80:289-93.

16. Jayaram G, Singh B, Marwaha RK. Graves' disease. Appearance in cytologic smears from fine needle aspirates of the thyroid gland. Acta Cytol 1989;33:36-40.

17. Frable WJ. Controversies in the pathology and cytology of well-differentiated thyroid carcinoma. Head Neck 1990;2:170-5.

18. Ravinsky E, Safneck JR. Fine needle aspirations of follicular lesions of the thyroid gland. The intermediate-type smear. Acta Cytol 1990;34:813-20.

19. Layfield LJ, Morton MJ, Cramer HM, Hirschowitz S. Implications of the proposed thyroid fine-needle aspiration category of "follicular lesion of undetermined significance": a five year multi-institutional analysis. Diagn Cytopathol 2009;37:710-4.

20. Jaffar R, Mohanty SK, Khan A, Fischer AH. Hemosiderin laden macrophages and hemosiderin within follicular cells distinguish benign follicular lesions from follicular neoplasms. Cytojournal 2009 diu:10.4103/1742.

21. Renshaw AA, Wang E, Wilbur D, et al. Interobserver agreement on microfollicles in thyroid fine-needle aspirates. Arch Pathol Lab Med 2006;130:148-52.

22. Layfield L. Fine-needle aspiration evaluation of the solitary thyroid nodule-the imprecision of diagnostic criteria. Diagn Cytopathol 1993;9:355-7 (editorial).

23. Yassa L, Cibas ES, Benson CB, et al. Long-term assessment of a multidisciplinary approach to thyroid nodule diagnostic evaluation. Cancer 2007;111:508-16.

24. DeMay RM. Follicular lesions of the thyroid. Whither follicular carcinoma? Am J Clin Pathol 2000;114:681-3.

25. Boccato P, Mannara GM, La Rosa F, Rinaldo A, Ferlito A. Hyalinizing trabecular adenoma of the thyroid diagnosed by fine-needle aspiration biopsy. Ann Otol Rhinol Laryngol 2000;109:235-8.

26. Jayaram G. Fine needle aspiration cytology of hyalinizing trabecular adenoma of the thyroid. Acta Cytol 1999;43:978-80.

27. Akin MR, Nguyen GK. Fine-needle aspiration biopsy cytology of hyalinizing trabecular adenomas of the thyroid. Diagn Cytopathol 1999; 20:90-4.

28. Karak AK, Sahoo M, Bhatnagar D. Hyalinizing trabecular adenoma—a case report with FNAC histologic, MIB-1 proliferative index and immunohistochemical findings. Indian J Pathol Microbiol 1998;41:479-84.

29. Kaleem Z, Davila RM. Hyalinizing trabecular adenoma of the thyroid. A report of two cases with cytologic, histologic and immunohistochemical findings. Acta Cytol 1997;41:883-8.

30. Bondeson L, Bondeson AG. Clue helping to distinguish hyalinizing trabecular adenoma from carcinoma of the thyroid in fine-needle aspirates. Diagn Cytopathol 1994;10:25-9.

31. Cerasoli S, Tabarri B, Farabegoli P, et al. Hyalinizing trabecular adenoma of the thyroid. Report of two cases, with cytologic, immunohistochemical and ultrastructural studies. Tumori 1992;8:274-9.

32. Strong CJ, Garcia BM. Fine needle aspiration cytologic characteristics of hyalinizing trabecular adenoma of the thyroid. Acta Cytol 1990;34:359-62.

33. Goellner JR, Carney JA. Cytologic features of fine-needle aspirates of hyalinizing trabecular adenoma of the thyroid. Am J Clin Pathol 1989; 91:115-9.

34. Casey MB, Sebo TJ, Carney JA. Hyalinizing trabecular adenoma of the thyroid gland identification through MIB-1 staining of fine-needle aspiration biopsy smears. Am J Clin Pathol 2004;122:506-10.

35. Akhtar M, Ali MA, Huq M, Bakry M. Fine-needle aspiration biopsy of papillary thyroid carcinoma: cyytologic, histologic and ultrastructural correlations. Diagn Cytopathol 1991;7:373-9.

36. Ellison E, Lapuerta P, Martin SE. Psammoma bodies in fine-needle aspirates of the thyroid: predictive value for papillary carcinoma. Cancer 1998;84:169-75.

37. Francis IM, Das DK, Sheikh ZA, Sharma PN, Gupta SK. Role of nuclear grooves in the diagnosis of papillary thyroid carcinoma. A quantitative assessment on fine needle aspiration smears. Acta Cytol 1995;39:409-15.

38. Alkuwari E, Khetani K, Dendukuri N, Wang L, Auger M. Quantitative assessment of nuclear grooves in fine needle aspirations of the thyroid: a retrospective cytohistologic study of 94 cases. Anal Quant Cytol Histol 2009;31:161-9.

39. Szporn AH, Yuan S, Wu M, Burstein DE. Cellular swirls in fine needle aspirates of papillary thyroid carcinoma: a new diagnostic criterion. Mod Pathol 2006;19:1470-3.

40. Gould E, Watzak L, Chamizo W, Albores-Saavedra J. Nuclear grooves in cytologic preparations. A study of the utility of this feature in the diagnosis of papillary carcinoma. Acta Cytol 1988;33:16-20.

41. Shurbaji MS, Gupta PK, Frost JK. Nuclear grooves: a useful criterion in the cytopathologic diagnosis of papillary thyroid carcinoma. Diagn Cytopathol 1988;4:91-4.

42. Lubitz CC, Faquin WC, Yang J, et al. Clinical and cytological features predictive of malignancy in thyroid follicular neoplasms. Thyroid 2010;20:25-31.

43. Rosai J, Carcangiu ML, DeLellis RA. Tumors of the thyroid gland. AFIP Atlas of Tumor Pathology, 3rd Series, Fascicle 5. Washington, DC: American Registry of Pathology; 1992.

44. Baloch ZW, Gupta PK, Yu GH, Sack MJ, LiVolsi VA. Follicular variant of papillary carcinoma. Cytologic and histologic correlation. Am J Clin Pathol 1999;111:216-22.

45. Martinez-Parra D, Campos Fernandez J, Hierro-Guilmain CC, Sola-Perea J, Perez-Guillermo M. Follicular variant of papillary carcinoma of the thyroid: to what extent is fine needle aspiration reliable? Diagn Cytopathol 1996;15:12-6.

46. Wu HH, Jones JN, Grzybicki DM, Elsheikh TM. Sensitive cytologic criteria for the identification of follicular variant of papillary thyroid carcinoma in fine-needle aspiration biopsy. Diagn Cytopathol 2003;29:262-6.

47. Kesmodel SB, Terhune KP, Canter RJ, et al. The diagnostic dilemma of follicular variant of papillary thyroid carcinoma. Surgery 2003;134:1005-12.

48. El Hag IA, Kollur SM. Benign follicular thyroid lesions versus follicular variant of papillary carcinoma: differentiation by architectural pattern. Cytopathology 2004;15:200-5.

49. Zacks JF, de las Morenas A, Beazley RM, O'Brien MJ. Fine-needle aspiration cytology diagnosis of colloid nodule versus follicular variant of papillary carcinoma of the thyroid. Diagn Cytopathol 1998;18:87-90.

50. Kaur A, Jayaram G. Thyroid tumors: cytomorphology of Hurthle cell tumors, including an uncommon papillary variant. Diagn Cytopathol 1993;9:135-7.

51. Beckner ME, Heffess CS, Oertel JE. Oxyphilic papillary thyroid carcinoma. Am J Clin Pathol 1995;103:280-7.

52. Herrera MF, Hay ID, Wu PS, et al. Hürthle cell (oxyphilic) papillary thyroid carcinoma: a variant with more aggressive biologic behavior. World J Surg 1992;16:669-74.

53. Doria MI Jr, Attal H, Wang HH, Jensen JA, DeMay RM. Fine needle aspiration cytology of the oxyphil variant of papillary carcinoma of the thyroid. A report of three cases. Acta Cytol 1996; 40:1007-11.

54. Das DK, Khanna CM, Tripathi RP, et al. Solitary nodular goiter. Review of cytomorphologic features in 441 cases. Acta Cytol 1999;43:563-74.

55. Apel RL, Asa SL, LiVolsi VA, Papillary Hürthle cell carcinoma with lymphocytic stroma. "Warthin-like tumor" of the thyroid. Am J Surg Pathol 1995;19:810-4.

56. Yousef O, Dichard A, Bocklage T. Aspiration cytology features of the Warthin tumor-like variant of papillary thyroid carcinoma. A report of two cases. Acta Cytol 1997;41(Suppl):1361-8.

57. Vasei M, Kumar PV, Malekhoseini SA, Kadivar M. Papillary Hürthle cell carcinoma (Warthin-like tumor) of the thyroid. Report of a case with fine needle aspiration findings. Acta Cytol 1998;42:1437-40.

58. Leung CS, Hartwick RW, Bedard YC. Correlation of cytologic and histologic features in variants of papillary carcinoma of the thyroid. Acta Cytol 1993;37:645-50.

59. Damiani S, Dina R, Eusebi V. Cytologic grading of aggressive and nonaggressive variants of papillary thyroid carcinoma. Am J Clin Pathol 1994; 101:651-5.

60. Gamboa-Dominguez A, Candanedo-Gonzalez F, Uribe-Uribe NO, Angeles-Angeles A. Tall cell variant of papillary thyroid carcinoma. A cyto-histologic correlation. Acta Cytol 1997; 41:672-6.

61. Harach HR, Zusman SB. Cytopathology of the tall cell variant of thyroid papillary carcinoma. Acta Cytol 1992;36:895-9.

62. Hui PK, Chan JK, Cheung PS, Gwi E. Columnar cell carcinoma of the thyroid. Fine needle aspiration findings in a case. Acta Cytol 1990;34:355-8.

63. Das DK, Mallik MK, Sharma P, et al. Papillary thyroid carcinoma and its variants in fine needle aspiration smears. A cytomorphologic study with special reference to the tall cell variant. Acta Cytol 2004;48:325-36.

64. Caruso G, Tabarri B, Lucchi I, Tison V. Fine needle aspiration cytology in a case of diffuse sclerosing carcinoma of the thyroid. Acta Cytol 1990;34:352-4.

65. Lee JY, Shin JH, Han, BK, et al. Diffuse sclerosing variant of papillary carcinoma of the thyroid: imaging and cytologic findings. Thyroid 2007;17:567-73.

66. Kumarasinghe MP. Cytomorphologic features of diffuse sclerosing variant of papillary carcinoma of the thyroid. A report of two cases in children. Acta Cytol 1998;42:983-6.

67. Albores-Saavedra J, Gould E, Vardaman C, Vuitch F. The macrofollicular variant of papillary thyroid carcinoma: a study of 17 cases. Hum Pathol 1991;22:1195-205.

68. Chung D, Ghossein RA, Lin O. Macrofollicular variant of papillary carcinoma: a potential thyroid FNA pitfall. Diagn Cytopathol 2007;35:560-4.

69. Haji BE, Ahmed MS, Prasad A, Omar MS, Das DK. Papillary thyroid carcinoma with an adenoid cystic pattern: report of a case with fine-needle aspiration cytology and immunocytochemistry. Diagn Cytopathol 2004;30:418-21.

70. Mandal S, Jain S. Adenoid cystic pattern in follicular variant of papillary thyroid carcinoma: a report of four cases. Cytopathology 2010;21:93-6.

71. Pietribiasi F, Sapino A, Papotti M, Bussolati G. Cytologic features of poorly differentiated 'insular' carcinoma of the thyroid, as revealed by fine-needle aspiration biopsy. Am J Clin Pathol 1990;94:687-92.

72. Sironi M, Collini P, Cantaboni A. Fine needle aspiration cytology of insular thyroid carcinoma. A report of four cases. Acta Cytol 1992;36:435-9.

73. Nguyen GK, Akin MR. Cytopathology of insular carcinoma of the thyroid. Diagn Cytopathol 2001;25:325-30.

74. Layfield LJ, Gopez EV. Insular carcinoma of the thyroid: report of a case with intact insulae and microfollicular structures. Diagn Cytopathol 2000;23:409-13.

75. Guiter GE, Auger M, Ali SZ, Allen EA, Zakowski MF. Cytopathology of insular carcinoma of the thyroid. Cancer 1999;87:196-202.

76. Us-Krasovec M, Golouh R, Auersperg M, Besic N, Ruparcic-Oblak L. Anaplastic thyroid carcinoma in fine needle aspirates. Acta Cytol 1996;40:953-8.

77. Kumar PV, Torabinejad S, Omrani GH. Osteoclastoma-like anaplastic carcinoma of the thyroid gland diagnosed by fine needle aspiration cytology. Report of two cases. Acta Cytol 1997;41(Suppl):1345-8.

78. Gonzalez JL, Wang HH, Ducatman BS. Fine-needle aspiration of Hurthle cell lesions. A cytomorphologic approach to diagnosis. Am J Clin Pathol 1993;100:231-5.

79. Lee J, Hasteh F. Oncocytic variant of papillary thyroid carcinoma associated with Hashimoto's thyroiditis: a case report and review of the literature. Diagn Cytopathol 2009;37:600-6.

80. Giorgadze T, Rossi ED, Fadda G, Gupta PK, LiVolsi VA, Beloch Z. Does the fine-needle aspiration diagnosis of "Hürthle-cell neoplasm/follicular neoplasm with oncocytic features" denote increased risk of malignancy? Diagn Cytopathol 2004;31:307-12.

81. Pu RT, Yang J, Wasserman PG, Bhulya T, Griffithe KA, Michael CS. Does Hurthle cell lesion/neoplasm predict malignancy more than follicular lesion/neoplasm on thyroid fine-needle aspiration? Diagn Cytopathol 2006;34:330-4.

82. Nguyen GK, Husain M, Akin MR. Cytodiagnosis of benign and malignant Hürthle cell lesions of the thyroid by fine-needle aspiration biopsy. Diagn Cytopathol 1999;20:261-5.

83. Wu HH, Clouse J, Ren R. Fine-needle aspiration cytology of Hürthle cell carcinoma of the thyroid. Diagn Cytopathol 2008;36:149-54.

84. Zeppa P, Benincasa G, Troncone G, et al. Quantitative assessment of oxyphilic cell lesions of the thyroid gland on fine needle aspiration samples. Anal Quant Cytol Histol 2001;23:178-84.

85. Stelow EB, Woon C, Atkins KA, et al. Interobserver variability with the interpretation of thyroid FNA specimens showing predominantly Hürthle cells. Am J Clin Pathol 2006;126:580-3.

86. el-Sahrigy D, Zhana XM, Elhosseiny A, Melamed MR. Signet-ring follicular adenoma of the thyroid diagnosed by fine needle aspiration. Report of a case with cytologic description. Acta Cytol 2004;48:87-90.

87. Harach HR, Virgili E, Soler G, Zusman SB, Saravia Day E. Cytopathology of follicular tumours of the thyroid with clear cell change. Cytopathology 1991;2:125-35.

88. Vazquez Ramirez F, Otal Salaverri C, Argueta Manzano O, Galera Ruiz H, Gonzalez-Campora R. Fine needle aspiration cytology of high grade mucoepidermoid carcinoma of the thyroid. A case report. Acta Cytol 2000;44:259-64.

89. Mai KT, Yazdi HM, MacDonald L. Fine needle aspiration biopsy of primary squamous cell carcinoma of the thyroid gland. Acta Cytol 1999;43:1194-6.

90. Kumar PV, Malekhusseini SA, Talei AR. Primary squamous cell carcinoma of the thyroid diagnosed by fine needle aspiration cytology. A report of two cases. Acta Cytol 1999;43:659-62.

91. Yang GC, Fried K, Levine PH. Detection of medullary thyroid microcarcinoma using ultrasound-guided fine needle aspiration cytology. Cytopathology 2013;24:92-8.

92. Papaparaskeva K, Nagel H, Droese M. Cytologic diagnosis of medullary carcinoma of the thyroid gland. Diagn Cytopathol 2000;22:351-8.

93. Bourtsos EP, Bedrossian CW, De Frias DV, Nayar R. Thyroid plasmacytoma mimicking medullary carcinoma: a potential pitfall in aspiration cytology. Diagn Cytopathol. 2000;23:354-8.

94. Us-Krasovec M, Auersperg M, Bergant D, Golouh R, Kloboves-Prevodnik V. Medullary carcinoma of the thyroid gland: diagnostic cytopathological characteristics. Pathologica 1998;90:5-13.

95. Green I, Ali SZ, Allen EA, Zakowski MF. A spectrum of cytomorphologic variations in medullary thyroid carcinoma. Fine-needle aspiration findings in 19 cases. Cancer 1997;81:40-44.

96. de Lima MA, Dias Medeiros J, Rodrigues Da Cunha L, et al. Cytological aspects of melanotic variant of medullary thyroid carcinoma. Diagn Cytopathol 2001;24:206-8.

97. Kaushal S, Iyer VK, Mathur SR, Ray R. Fine needle aspiration cytology of medullary carcinoma of the thyroid with a focus on rare variants: a review of 78 cases. Cytopathology 2011;22:95-105.

98. Kumar PV, Hodjati H, Monabati A, Talei A. Medullary thyroid carcinoma. Rare cytologic findings. Acta Cytol 2000;44:181-4.

99. Laforga JB, Aranda FI. Pseudoangiosarcomatous features in medullary thyroid carcinoma spindle-cell variant. Report of a case studied by FNA and munohistochemistry. Diagn Cytopathol 2007;35:424-8.

100. Forrest CH, Frost FA, de Boer WB, Spagnolo DV, Whitaker D, Sterrett BF. Medullary carcinoma of the thyroid: accuracy of diagnosis of fine-needle aspiration cytology. Cancer 1998;84:295-302.

101. Aulicino MR, Szporn AH, Dembitzer R, et al. Cytologic findings in the differential diagnosis of C-cell hyperplasia and medullary carcinoma by fine needle aspiration. A case report. Acta Cytol 1998;42:963-7.

102. Cibas ES, Ali SZ. The Bethesda System for Reporting Thyroid Cytopathology. Thyroid 2009;19:1159-65.

103. Kaba S, Hirokawa M, Kuma S, et al. Cytologic findings of primary thyroid MALT lymphoma with extreme plasma cell differentiation: FNA cytology of two cases. Diagn Cytopathol 2009;37:815-9.

104. Zeppo P, Cozzolino I, Peluse AL, et al. Cytologic, flow cytometry, and molecular assessment of lymphoid infiltrate in fine-needle cytology samples of Hashimoto thyroiditis. Cancer 2009:117:174-84.

105. Chan HI, Akpolat I, Mody D, et al. Restricted kappa/lambda light chain ratio by flow cyometry in germinal center B cells in Hasimoto thyroidits. Am J Clin Pathol 2006:125:42-8.

106. Van den Bruel A, Drijkoningen M, Oyen R, Vanfleteren E, Bouillon R. Diagnostic fine-needle aspiration cytology and immunocytochemistry analysis of a primary thyroid lymphoma presenting as an anatomic emergency. Thyroid 2002;12:169-71.

107. Takashima S, Takayama F, Saito A, Wang Q, Hidaka K, Sone S. Primary thyroid lymphoma: diagnosis of immunoglobulin heavy chain gene rearrangement with polymerase chain reaction in ultrasound-guided fine-needle aspiration. Thyroid 2000;10:507-10.

108. Kalinyak JE, Kong CS, McDougall IR. Burkitt's lymphoma presenting as a rapidly growing thyroid mass. Thyroid 2006;16:1053-7.

109. Fulciniti F, Di Mattia D, Bove P, et al. Fine needle aspiration of metastatic epithelioid angiosarcoma: a report of two cases. Acta Cytol 2008;52:612-8.

110. Michelow PM, Leiman G. Metastases to the thyroid gland: diagnosis by aspiration cytology. Diagn Cytopathol 1995;13:209-13.

111. Cohen Y, Rosenbaum E, Clark DP, et al. Mutational analysis of BRAF in fine needle aspiration biopsies of the thyroid: a potential application for the preoperative assessment of thyroid nodules. Clin Cancer Res 2004;10:2761-5.

112. Salvatore G, Giannini R, Faviana P, et al. Analysis of BRAF point mutation and RET/PTC rearrangement refines the fine-needle aspiration diagnosis of papillary thyroid carcinoma. J Clin Endocrinol Metab 2004;89:5175-80.

113. Jin L, Sebo TJ, Nakamura N, et al. BRAF mutation analysis in fine needle aspiration (FNA) cytology of the thyroid. Diagn Mol Pathol 2006;15:136-43.

114. Bartolazzi A, Orlandi F, Saggiorato E, et al. Galectin-3-expression analysis in the surgical selection of follicular thyroid nodules with indeterminate fine-needle aspiration cytology: a prospective multicentre study. Lancet Oncol 2008;9:543-9.

115. Chen YT, Kitabayashi N, Zhou XK, Fahey TJ 3rd, Scognamiglio T. MicroRNA analysis as a potential diagnostic tool for papillary thyroid carcinoma. Mod Pathol 2008;21:1139-46.

116. Nikiforova MN, Tseng GC, Steward D, Diorio D, Nikiforov YE. MicroRNA expression profiling of thyroid tumors: biological significance and diagnostic utility. J Clin Endocrinol Metab 2008;93:1600-8.

117. Nikiforov YE, Steward DL, Robinson-Smith TM, et al. Molecular testing for mutations in improving the fine-needle aspiration diagnosis of thyroid nodules. J Clin Endocrinol Metab 2009;94:2092-8.

118. Cantara S, Capezzone M, Marchisotta S, et al. Impact of proto-oncogene mutation detection in cytological specimens from thyroid nodules improves the diagnostic accuracy of cytology. J Clin Endocrinol Metab 2010;95:1365-9.

119. Chudova D, Wilde JI, Wang ET, et al. Molecular classification of thyroid nodules using high-dimensionality genomic data. J Clin Endocrinol Metab 2010;95:5296-304.

120. Kim SW, Lee JI, Kim JW, et al. BRAFV600E mutation analysis in fine-needle aspiration cytology specimens for evaluation of thyroid nodule: a large series in a BRAFV600E-prevalent population. J Clin Endocrinol Metab 2010;95:3693-700.

121. Moses W, Weng J, Sansano I, et al. Molecular testing for somatic mutations improves the accuracy of thyroid fine-needle aspiration biopsy. World J Surg 2010;34:2589-94.

122. Ohori NP, Nikiforova MN, Schoedel KE, et al. Contribution of molecular testing to thyroid fine-needle aspiration cytology of "follicular lesion of undetermined significance/atypia of undetermined significance." Cancer Cytopathol 2010;118:17-23.

123. Adeniran AJ, Theoharis C, Hui P, et al. Reflex BRAF testing in thyroid fine-needle aspiration biopsy with equivocal and positive interpretation: a prospective study. Thyroid 2011;21:717-23.

124. Jin L, Lloyd RV, Nassar A, et al. HMGA2 expression analysis in cytological and paraffin-embedded tissue specimens of thyroid tumors by relative quantitative RT-PCR. Diagn Mol Pathol 2011;20:71-80.

125. Kim SK, Hwang TS, Yoo YB, et al. Surgical results of thyroid nodules according to a management guideline based on the BRAF(V600E) mutation status. J Clin Endocrinol Metab 2011;96:658-64.

461

126. Li H, Robinson KA, Anton B, Saldanha IJ, Ladenson PW. Cost-effectiveness of a novel molecular test for cytologically indeterminate thyroid nodules. J Clin Endocrinol Metab 2011;96:E1719-26.

127. Mazeh H, Mizrahi I, Halle D, et al. Development of a microRNA-based molecular assay for the detection of papillary thyroid carcinoma in aspiration biopsy samples. Thyroid 2011;21:111-8.

128. Nikiforov YE, Ohori NP, Hodak SP, et al. Impact of mutational testing on the diagnosis and management of patients with cytologically indeterminate thyroid nodules: a prospective analysis of 1056 FNA samples. J Clin Endocrinol Metab 2011;96:3390-7.

129. Alexander EK, Kennedy GC, Baloch ZW, et al. Preoperative diagnosis of benign thyroid nodules with indeterminate cytology. N Engl J Med 2012;367:705-15.

130. Duick DS, Klopper JP, Diggans JC, et al. TheImpact of benign gene expression classifier test results on the endocrinoloigst-patient decision to operate on patients with thyroid nodules with indeterminate fine-needle aspiration cytopathology. Thyroid 2012;22:996-1001.

131. Jameson JL. Minimizing unnecessary surgery for thyroid nodules. N Engl J Med 2012;367:765-7.

132. Keutgen XM, Filicori F, Crowley MJ, et al. A panel of four miRNAs accurately differentiates malignant from benign indeterminate thyroid lesions on fine needle aspiration. Clin Cancer Res 2012;18:2032-8.

133. Yip L, Farris C, Kabaker AS, et al. Cost impact of molecular testing for indeterminate thyroid nodule fine-needle aspiration biopsies. J Clin Endocrinol Metab 2012;97:1905-12.

134. Walsh PS, Wilde JI, Tom EY, et al. Analytical performance verification of a molecular diagnostic for cytology-indeterminate thyroid nodules. J Clin Endocrinol Metab 2012;97:E2297-306.

135. Hadd AG, Houghton J, Choudhary A, et al. Targeted, high depth, next-generation sequencing of cancer genes in formalin-fixed, praffin-embedded and fine-needle aspiration tumor specimens. J Mol Diagn 2013;15:234-47.

136. Smith DL, Lamy A, Beaudenon-Huibregtse S, et al. A multiplex technology platform for the rapid analysis of clinically actionable genetic alterations and validation for BRAF p.V600E detection in 1549 cytologic and histologic specimens. Arch Pathol Lab Med 2014;138:371-8.

137. Alexander EK, Schorr M, Klopper J, et al. Multicenter clinical experience with the afirma gene expression classifier. J Clin Endocrinol Metab 2014;99:119-25.

138. Griffith OL, Melck A, Jones SJ, Wiseman SM. Meta-analysis and meta-review of thyroid cancer gene expression profiling studies identifies important diagnostic biomarkers. J Clin Oncol 2006;24:5043-51.

139. Xing M. Prognostic utility of BRAF mutation in papillary thyroid cancer. Mol Cell Endocrinol 2010;321:86-93.

140. Ferraz C, Eszlinger M, Paschke R. Current state and future perspective of molecular diagnosis of fine-needle aspiration biopsy of thyroid nodules. J Clin Endocrinol Metab 2011;96:2016-26.

141. Nikiforov YE, Nikiforova MN. Molecular genetics and diagnosis of thyroid cancer. Nat Rev Endocrinol 2011;7:569-80.

142. Theoharis C, Roman S, Sosa JA. The molecular diagnosis and management of thyroid Neoplasms. Curr Opin Oncol 2012;24:35-41.

143. Ali SZ, Fish SA, Lanman R, Randolph GW, Sosa JA. Use of the afirma® gene expression classifier for preoperative identification of benign thyroid nodules with indeterminate fine needle aspiration cytopathology. PLoS Curr 2013;5.

144. Xing M, Haugen BR, Schlumberger M. Progress in molecular-based management of differentiated thyroid cancer. Lancet 2013;381:1058-69.

145. Ward LS, Kloos TR. Molecular markers in the diagnosis of thyroid nodules. Arq Bras Endocrinol Metabol 2013;57:89-97.

146. Chiappetta G, Ferraro A, Vuttariello E, et al. HMGA2 mRNA expression correlates with the malignant phenotype in human thyroid neoplasias. Eur J Cancer 2008;44:1015-21.

147 Prasad NB, Kowalski J, Tsai HL, et al. Three-gene molecular diagnostic model for thyroid cancer. Thyroid 2012;22:275-84.

148. Hodak SP, Rosenthal DS, American Thyroid Association Clinical Affairs Committee. Information for clinicians: commercially available molecular diagnosis testing in the evaluation of thyroid nodule fine-needle aspiration specimens. Thyroid 2013;23:131-4.

149. Amrikachi M, Ramzy I, Rubenfeld S, Wheeler, TM. Accuracy of fine-needle aspiration of thyroid. Arch Pathol Lab Med 2001;125:484-8.

150. Porterfield JR Jr, Grant CS, Dean DS, et al. Reliability of benign fine needle aspiration cytology of large thyroid nodules. Surgery 2008;144:963-8.

151. Baloch ZW, Fleisher S, LiVolsi VA, Gupta PK. Diagnosis of "follicular neoplasm": a gray zone in thyroid fine-needle aspiration cytology. Diagn Cytopathol 2002;26:41-4.

152. Ghofrani M, Beckman D, Rimm DL. The value of onsite adequacy assessment of thyroid fine-needle aspirations is a function of operator experience. Cancer 2006;108:110-3.

153. Oertel YC, Oertel JE. Diagnosis of malignant epithelial thyroid lesions: fine needle aspiration and histopathologic correlation. Ann Diagn Pathol 1998;2:377-400.

154. Flanagan MB, Ghori NP, Carty SE, Hunt JL. Repeat thyroid nodule fine-needle aspiration in patients with initial benign cytologic results. Am J Clin Pathol 2006;125:698-702.

155. Boyd LA, Earnhardt RC, Dunn JT, Frierson HG, Hanks JB. Preoperative evaluation and predictive value of fine-needle aspiration and frozen section of thyroid nodules. J Am Coll Surg 1998;187:494-502.

156. McHenry CR, Raeburn C, Strickland T, Marty JJ. The utility of routine frozen section for intra operative diagnosis of thyroid cancer. Am J Surg 1996;172:658-61.

157. Chen H, Zeiger MA, Clark DP, Westra WH, Udelsman R. Papillary carcinoma of the thyroid: can operative management be based solely on fine-needle aspiration? J Am Coll Surg 1997;184:605-10.

158. Gibb GK, Pasieka JL. Assessing the need for frozen sections: still a valuable tool in thyroid surgery. Surgery 1995;118:1005-9.

159. Aguilar-Diosdado M, Contreras A, Gavilan I, et al. Thyroid nodules. Role of fine needle aspiration and intra operative frozen section examination. Acta Cytol 1997;41:677-82.

160. Peng Y, Wang HH. A meta-analysis comparing fine-needle aspiration and frozen section for evaluating thyroid nodules. Diagn Cytopathol 2008;36:916-20.

161. Giard RW, Hermans J. Use and accuracy of fine-needle aspiration cytology in histologically proven thyroid carcinoma: an audit using a national pathology database. Cancer 2000;90:330-4.

162. Cramer H. Fine-needle aspiration cytology of the thyroid: an appraisal. Cancer 2000;90:325-9.

163. Richards ML, Bohnenblust E, Sirinek K, Bingener J. Nondiagnostic thyroid fine-needle aspiration biopsies are no longer a dilemma. Am J Surg 2008;196:398-402.

164. Banks ND, Kowalski J, Tsai HL, et al. A diagnostic predictor model for indeterminate or suspicious thyroid FNA samples. Thyroid 2008;18:933-41.

165. Raparia K, Min SK, Mody DR, Anton R, Amrikachi M. Clinical outcome for "suspicious" category in thyroid fine-needle aspiration biopsy: patient's sex and nodule size are possible predictors of malignancy. Arch Pathol Lab Med 2009;133:787-90.

166. Auger M, Nayar R, Khalbuss WE, et al. Implementation of the Bethesda System for Reporting thyroid Cytopatholgy: Observations from the 2011 thyroid supplemental questionnaire of the College of American Pathologists. Arch Pathol Lab Med 2013;137:1555-9.

167. Ohori NP, Schoedel KE. Variability in the atypia of undetermined significance/follicular lesion of undetermined significance diagnosis in the Bethesda System for Reporting Thyroid Cyto-

pathology: sources and recommendations. Acta Cytol, 2011;55:492-8.

168. Bongiovanni M, Spitale A, Faquin WC, Mazzucchelli L, Baloch ZW. The Bethesda System for Reporting Thyroid Cytopathology: a meta-analysis. Acta Cytol 2012;56:333-9.

169. Bose S, Walts AE. Thyroid fine needle aspirate: a post-Bethesda update. Adv Anat Pathol 2012;19:160-9.

170. Collins BT, Collins LE. Assessment of malignancy for atypia of undetermined significance in thyroid fine-needle aspiration biopsy evaluated by whole-slide image analysis. Am J Clin Pathol 2013;139:736-45.

171. Wong LQ, Baloch ZE. Analysis of the Bethesda system for reporting thyroid cytopathology and similar precursor thyroid cytopathology reporting schemes. Adv Anat Pathol 2012;19:313-9.

172. Onder S, Firat P, Ates D The Bethesda system for reporting thyroid cytopathology: an institutional experience of the outcome of indeterminate categories. Cytopathology 2013;Sept 2(Epub ahead of print).

173. VanderLann PA, Renshaw AA, Krane JF. Atypia of undetermined significance and nondiagnostic rates in The Bethesda System for Reporting Thyroid Cytopathology are inversely related. Am J Clin Pathol 2012;137:462-5.

174. Renshaw AA, Gould EW. Should "indeterminate" diagnoses be used for thyroid fine-needle aspirates of nodules smaller than 1 cm? Arch Pathol Lab Med 2013;137:1627-9.

175. Hosler GA, Clark I, Zakowski MF, Westra WH, Ali SZ. Cytopathologic analysis of thyroid lesions in the pediatric population. Diagn Cytopathol 2006;34:101-5.

176. Amrikachi M, Ponder TB, Wheeler TM, Smith D, Ramzy I. Thyroid fine-needle aspiration biopsy in children and adolescents: experience with 218 aspirates. Diagn Cytopathol 2005;32:189-92.

177. Caraway NP, Sneige N, Samaan NA. Diagnostic pitfalls in thyroid fine-needle aspiration biopsy: a review of 394 cases. Diagn Cytopathol 1993;9:345-50.

178. Heinmann A, Gritsman A. Diagnostic problems and pitfalls in aspiration cytology of thyroid nodules. In: Schmidt WA, ed. Cytopathology Annual 1993. Baltimore: Williams & Wilkins; 1993:207-237.

179. Betsill W. Thyroid fine needle aspiration in pregnant women. Diagn Cytopathol 1985;1:53-4.

180. Kini SR. Post-fine-needle biopsy infarction of thyroid neoplasms: a review of 28 cases. Diagn Cytopathol 1996;15:211-20.

181. LiVolsi VA, Merino MJ. Worrisome histologic alterations following fine-needle aspiration of the thyroid (WHAFFT). Pathol Annu 1994;29(Pt 2):99-120.

182. Vercelli-Retta J, Almeida E, Ardao G, et al. Capsular pseudoinvasion after fine-needle aspiration of follicular adenoma of the thyroid. Diagn Cytopathol 1997;17:295-7.

183. Axiotis CA, Merino MJ, Ain K, Norton JA. Papillary endothelial hyperplasia in the thyroid following fine-needle aspiration. Arch Pathol Lab Med 1991;115:240-2.

184. Tsang K, Duggan MA. Vascular proliferation of the thyroid. A complication of fine-needle aspiration. Arch Pathol Lab Med 1992;116:1040-2.

185. Haas SN. Acute thyroid swelling after needle biopsy of the thyroid. N Eng J Med 1982; 307:1349.

186. Dal Fabbro S, Barbazza R, Fabris C, Perelli R. Acute thyroid swelling after fine needle aspiration biopsy. J Endocrinol Invest 1987;10:105.

187. Van den Bruel A, Roelandt P, Drijkoningen M, Hudders JP, Decallonne B, Bouillon R. A thyroid thriller: acute transient and symmetric goiter after fine-needle aspiration of a solitary thyroid nodule. Thyroid 2008;18:81-4.

188. Velkeniers B, Noppen M, Vanhaelst L. Delayed swelling of prethyroid soft tissue after fine needle aspiration. J Endocrinol Invest 1988;11:225.

189. Kobayashi A, Kuma K, Matsuzuka F, Hirai K, Fukata S, Sugawara M. Thyrotoxicosis after needle aspiration of thyroid cyst. J Clin Endocrinol Metab 1992;75:21-4.

190. Shulkin BL. Hot nodule after fine needle aspiration. Clin Nucl Med 1988;13:131.

191. Powers CN. Fine needle aspiration biopsy: perspectives on complications—the reality behind the myth. In Schmidt WA (ed.), Cytopathology Annual 1995. Baltimore: Williams & Wilkins; 1996:69-96.

192. Hales MS, Hsu FS. Needle tract implantation of papillary carcinoma of the thyroid following aspiration biopsy. Acta Cytol 1990;34:801-4.

21 CLINICAL ASPECTS OF THYROID TUMORS

CLINICAL AND LABORATORY EVALUATION OF THYROID NODULES

Approximately 4 percent of the people in the United States between the ages of 30 and 60 years have one or more palpable thyroid nodules. Because most of these nodules are benign and not even neoplastic, the clinician evaluating them should be as selective as possible in the recommendation for surgical removal, while at the same time avoiding missing malignant tumors. The evaluation of the thyroid nodule includes the considerations listed below.

Demographics

Age (the incidence of malignancy is higher in children and the elderly), gender (the incidence of malignancy is higher in males), and geographic location (in reference to iodine-deficient areas) (1,2).

Family History

A strong family history unrelated to dietary iodine deficiency in a patient with thyroid nodule(s) suggests the diagnoses of dyshormonogenetic goiter (thyroid pathology: mainly nodular hyperplasia), multiple endocrine neoplasia (MEN) 2A, MEN 2B, and familial medullary thyroid carcinoma (FMTC) syndromes (thyroid pathology: medullary carcinoma), and Cowden syndrome (thyroid pathology: nodular hyperplasia, follicular adenoma, follicular carcinoma, papillary carcinoma (questionable), and other lesions) (3,4). Cowden syndrome is due to a germline mutation in *PTEN*, the loss of which is detected immunohistochemically in thyroidectomy specimens (5). Familial tumors account for about 5 percent of thyroid follicular and papillary carcinomas (6,7).

History of Hashimoto Thyroiditis

The association between Hashimoto thyroiditis and papillary thyroid carcinoma has been documented. The chances of a thyroid nodule being malignant, however, are similar among patients with and without Hashimoto thyroiditis (8,9).

Rate of Growth

Most adenomas are very slow growing, but this is also true for most well-differentiated follicular and papillary carcinomas. Rapid enlargement of a preexisting indolent nodule may signify the emergence of a high-grade malignant component or simply the spontaneous development of hemorrhage within the nodule.

Palpation

Solitary nodules are more likely to be malignant than multiple ones. However, approximately one third of clinically solitary nodules are shown to be multiple on scan and an even higher number on pathologic examination. Unusually prominent, hard, or irregular nodules that occur in a multinodular gland should be regarded as suspicious. Fixation of the thyroid gland, failure of the thyroid to move freely on swallowing, and vocal cord paralysis should heighten the suspicion of malignancy, although some of these signs are also seen in some forms of thyroiditis (10).

The presence of cervical adenopathy ipsilateral to a thyroid nodule is the strongest clinical indicator that the nodule is malignant, particularly if there is no evidence of an infection in the head and neck region.

Isotopic Imaging Study

This test, traditionally performed with ^{131}I, is now more commonly carried out with either ^{123}I or ^{99}Tc pertechnetate (Tc99m) in order to reduce the radiation exposure (11,12). Thyroid nodules are classified as hyperfunctional ("hot"), when trapping the isotope with greater avidity than (and sometimes to the exclusion of) the rest of the gland; functional ("cool" or "warm"), when trapping the isotope with the same avidity as the rest of the gland; and hypofunctional ("cold"), when failing to trap the isotope. A minimum diameter of 1 cm is necessary for a cold nodule to be detectable with this technique (13). Hyperfunctional nodules are almost always benign, and this is also true for most functional nodules. The incidence of carcinoma is higher for hypofunctional nodules, even though most of them (about 80 percent) are benign.

Ultrasonography (Ultrasound)

Solid nodules are more likely to be malignant than cystic ones, particularly if they have been found to be hypofunctioning by isotopic imaging study. Only 1 to 3 percent of the nodules found to be cystic by this technique prove to be malignant on pathologic examination. Ultrasonography is also useful for monitoring well-differentiated thyroid carcinomas, often done in combination with measurement of serum thyroglobulin levels (see below) (14).

Computerized Tomography (CT) and Magnetic Resonance Imaging (MRI)

The role of these two techniques in thyroid pathology is limited. MRI is said to be superior to CT for the evaluation of metastatic, retrotracheal, and mediastinal lesions (11).

Serum Thyroglobulin Levels

These levels are often elevated in patients with papillary and follicular carcinoma (particularly the latter), whereas they remain normal in patients with medullary or undifferentiated carcinoma. Since a similar elevation can also accompany follicular adenoma, this measurement does not allow benign tumors to be distinguished from malignant ones before surgery. The technique is more useful in monitoring patients after removal of a papillary or follicular carcinoma, especially if the excision was followed by radioactive iodine therapy (15). Repeated total-body scans may be omitted in patients with such tumors if the serum thyroglobulin levels are undetectable, unless a strong clinical indication exists (16–20).

Thyroglobulin mRNA transcripts have been successfully used to detect circulating tumor cells in the peripheral blood of patients with thyroid tumors (21).

Serum Calcitonin Levels

See chapters 1 and 12.

Frozen Section Examination

The role of frozen section in the management of thyroid nodules has greatly diminished after the widespread adoption of the fine-needle aspiration biopsy (FNAB) procedure (22,23) (see chapter 20). Lesions that are usually identifiable on frozen section are the conventional type of papillary carcinoma, widely invasive follicular carcinoma, poorly differentiated (including insular) carcinoma, undifferentiated (anaplastic) carcinoma, and medullary carcinoma. Cases of thyroiditis and of nodular hyperplasia (adenomatoid goiter) clinically simulating tumors are also recognizable without difficulty in most instances (24,25).

The main problem (and, unfortunately, a frequent one) is represented by the single encapsulated nodule with a follicular pattern of growth in which the differential diagnosis revolves around follicular adenoma, minimally invasive follicular carcinoma, and the encapsulated follicular variant of papillary carcinoma (26). This is by far the most significant factor responsible for the low sensitivity of frozen-section diagnosis of thyroid carcinomas (27,28). Factors contributing to the difficulty are the often focal nature of the capsular or vascular invasion in minimally invasive follicular carcinoma, and the fact that ground-glass nuclei, one of the most important hallmarks of papillary carcinoma and its follicular variant, are seen poorly or not at all in frozen-section material (29).

For this type of lesion, we believe that freezing of a maximum of three blocks, including the capsule, is adequate, regardless of the size of the nodule. If no capsular or vascular invasion is detected and if the cytoarchitectural features of the follicular variant of papillary carcinoma are not detectable, we think it is justifiable to make a diagnosis of "follicular lesion—diagnosis deferred to permanent sections." Because we believe that most cases of follicular adenoma, minimally invasive follicular carcinoma, and the encapsulated follicular variant of papillary carcinoma can be treated similarly (i.e., by the performance of either a lobectomy with isthmusectomy or a subtotal thyroidectomy), we do not regard the diagnostic deferral at the time of frozen section to be a significant drawback. This has also been the experience and conclusion of others (30–33). Of 359 patients with thyroid nodules studied by FNAB and intraoperative frozen sections that were analyzed by Hamburger and Hamburger (34), frozen-section diagnosis decisively influenced the surgical procedure in only 3 cases, i.e., less than 1 percent. A similar experience was recounted by Kopald et al. (35). Naturally, the role of frozen section will also largely depend on the preconceived notions of the surgeon. If he is of the belief that all thyroid nodules should be treated by a subtotal or total thyroidectomy, it follows that the frozen section result will hardly change his therapeutic choice (36).

Cytologic Evaluation

For a discussion of the role of cytopathology in the evaluation of thyroid tumors (including intraoperative cytology), see chapter 20.

PATHOLOGIC EVALUATION AND REPORTING

Described below is a set of guidelines for the handling, description, and microscopic sampling of surgical specimens from the thyroid gland. Only some general statements can be made in a section of this sort. The specific features of the individual specimen often call for a modification or even a substantial departure from these recommendations.

Handling

Weigh the specimen, and measure it in three dimensions.

Orient the specimen, if feasible (help from the surgeon may be necessary).

Search for parathyroid glands and lymph nodes in the surrounding fat.

Paint the outer aspect of the specimen with India ink or a similar dye.

Make parallel longitudinal cuts of the entire specimen, 3 to 5 mm apart, either in the fresh state or after formalin fixation.

If searching for papillary microcarcinoma (a lesion measuring less than 1 cm, by definition), we recommend slicing the specimen into 2- or 3-mm–thick sections and transilluminating them. Any sharply localized area with a fibrotic appearance should be regarded as suspicious, especially if it has a stellate shape.

Description

Indicate the type of specimen received: nodulectomy (an operation that has been largely abandoned), lobectomy, lobectomy with isthmusectomy, subtotal thyroidectomy, or total thyroidectomy. For specimens other than the last one, indicate the side from which most or all of the specimen was obtained.

State the weight, dimensions, shape, color, and consistency of the specimen.

Examine the cut surface for color and appearance. Note whether or not it is homogeneous and whether it is smooth or nodular.

When one or more nodules are present, note the number, size, shape, color; whether they are solid or cystic, calcified, hemorrhagic, or necrotic; and whether or not they are encapsulated. If a capsule is present, note whether it is thin or thick and regular or irregular. Note whether it is apparently intact or violated by tumor growth. Calculate the shortest distance from the edge of the nodule to the line of resection.

Sections for Histology

For diffuse and inflammatory lesions: take three sections from each lobe and one from the isthmus.

For solitary encapsulated nodules measuring up to 5 cm in diameter: make a 2- to 3-mm thick slice through the largest tumor circumference, divide into portions, being sure that the tumor capsule and surrounding non-neoplastic thyroid are included in all of them, and submit all tissue for microscopic examination. For a nodule measuring 5 cm in greatest diameter, 6 to 9 blocks are usually made (fig. 21-1).

For larger encapsulated nodules: submit one additional block for each centimeter over 5 cm (i.e., seven blocks for a 7-cm nodule, or 10 blocks for a 10-cm nodule).

For multinodular thyroid glands: submit a minimum of one section for each nodule (up to five nodules), including rim and adjacent gland. Submit additional sections for the nodules that are larger than or grossly different from the others.

For known papillary or medullary carcinoma: submit the entire gland and (separately) the line of resection, if the specimen is other than a total thyroidectomy.

For grossly invasive carcinoma other than papillary or medullary: submit a minimum of

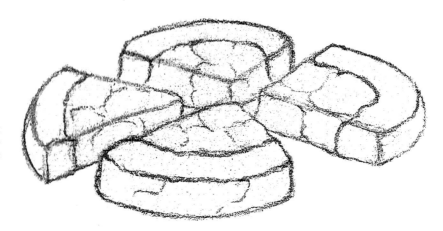

Figure 21-1

PROPER SAMPLING OF A THYROID NODULE

A slice of the nodule is cut in a pie-like fashion in order to sample the entire circumference of the capsule.

three blocks from the tumor, three of non-neoplastic gland (if present), and one from the line of resection (if other than total thyroidectomy).

For all cases: submit all parathyroid glands and lymph nodes that were found on gross inspection.

Example of Gross Description

"Received in the fresh state is a specimen identified as right lobectomy with isthmusectomy. A black suture is present at the isthmusectomy margin. The specimen weighs 30 g and measures 6.5 x 4.0 x 3.0 cm. The outer surface is smooth, and the consistency is homogeneously firm. An ill-defined bulging is noted in the lower pole of the right lobe. No parathyroid glands or lymph nodes are identified.

Parallel longitudinal sections of the specimen reveal a round nodule in the lower lobe measuring 2.5 cm in greatest diameter. It is entirely surrounded by a very thin fibrous capsule that shows no gross evidence of invasion. The cut surface of the nodule is solid, slightly bulging, and tan, with punctate areas of fresh hemorrhage. The capsule of the nodule is 0.5 cm distant from the thyroid capsule and 1.2 cm distant from the surgical margin at the isthmus. The rest of the thyroid shows no gross abnormalities.

Sections are submitted as follows:
A1, A2, A3: nodule
B1, B2: remainder of right lobe
C: surgical margin at the isthmus."

Standardized Reporting

In recent years, a trend has emerged for the standardized reporting of pathologic findings in tumor-containing surgical specimens spear-headed respectively by the Department of Pathology of Memorial Sloan Ketterin gCancer Center, and the Association of Directors of Anatomic and Surgical Pathology (ADASP). In the thyroid gland, this has resulted in the issuing of two protocols, one produced by ADASP, and the other by the College of American Pathologists (CAP) Both are in the synoptic style ("checklists"). It is up to the individual pathologist to decide which one to choose (if any) as long as the required information is contained in the final report.

ADASP Recommended Protocol/Checklist

See Table 21-1 for the ADASP recommended protocol, and Table 21-2 for the corresponding checklist (37).

CAP Recommended Protocol/Checklist

A detailed copy of this document, which is based on the American Joint Committee on Cancer/International Union Against Cancer (AJCC/UICC TNM), with list of authors, explanatory notes, and references has been posted in the CAP website (38) on November 2011 and updated (with a few minor changes) on August 12, 2014. In the few instances in which the terminology used was at variance with that of the rest of the Fascicle, no attempt at uniformity was made.

Microscopic Grading

The UICC recommends that all carcinomas of head and neck sites (including thyroid gland) be graded microscopically as follows:
GX   Grade cannot be assessed
G1   Well differentiated

Table 21-1

ADASP PROTOCOL FOR THE REPORTING OF CARCINOMA-CONTAINING THYROID SPECIMENS[a]

I. Carcinoma of the thyroid
  A. Features recommended to be included in the final report
    1. Organ—thyroid
    2. Type of specimen (surgical procedure)
    3. Tumor type (and subtype, when indicated)
    4. Tumor location
    5. Tumor largest diameter
    6. Presence of encapsulation
    7. Presence of capsular invasion
    8. Presence of blood vessel invasion
    9. Presence of extrathyroid extension
    10. Status of surgical margins
    11. Presence of tumor multicentricity
    12. Significant pathology in the gland away from the carcinoma—adenoma(s), nodular hyperplasia, lymphocytic/Hashimoto thyroiditis, C-cell hyperplasia (the latter for cases of medullary carcinoma)
    13. Number, appearance, and location of parathyroid glands, if any
    14. Number and status of lymph nodes, if any
    15. For metastatic lymph nodes—size of the largest involved node; presence of perinodal (extracapsular) tumor extension
  B. Optional features for the final report: These features may reflect institutional preferences and/or may be of inconclusive or controversial prognostic significance. The histologic grade can be listed as such (despite the fact that some tumor grading is implicit in the diagnosis of tumor type, i.e., poorly differentiated) or the features evaluated in a grading system (such as mitotic activity or necrosis) can be listed separately.

    1. Histologic grade
    2. Presence and degree of mitotic activity
    3. Presence and amount of tumor necrosis
    4. Presence of ancillary tumor features, such as squamous metaplasia, cytoplasmic clear cell change, mucinous features, psammoma bodies, other types of calcification, calcification, stromal (desmoplastic or "scirrhous") reactions, and amyloid deposition
  C. Features to be included in the gross description
    1. Type of specimen, how received fresh or fixed, intact or previously sectioned, etc.) and how identified
    2. Overall dimensions and weight
    3. Outer shape, color, symmetry, and consistency of entire specimen; presence and appearance of extrathyroid tissues
    4. Tumor description: number, location, size, shape, consistency, color, encapsulation, secondary changes (fibrosis, calcification, cystic degeneration, hemorrhage), and distance to surgical margins
    5. Appearance of thyroid gland away from tumor; presence of tumor multicentricity
    6. Number and appearance of parathyroid gland(s), if any
    7. Lymph node dissection, if included
      a. Type: extended radical, radical, modified radical, selective
      b. Presence of sternomastoid muscle/submandibular and/or parotid gland/jugular vein
      c. Presence of a palpable mass, and whether solitary or matted
      d. Size and location of gross tumor invasion of soft tissues, muscle, and jugular vein adjacent to involved lymph nodes
      e. Dimensions and appearance of sternomastoid muscle, major salivary glands, and internal jugular vein
      f. Size of lymph nodal masses (masses greater than 3 cm in diameter are to be regarded as confluent nodes or as an extension into soft tissue)

[a]ADASP = Association of Directors of Anatomic and Surgical Pathology; data from reference 37.

G2 Moderately differentiated
G3 Poorly differentiated
G4 Undifferentiated
Other (specify)

It should be understood that this grading system was proposed mainly for squamous cell carcinomas of the upper aerodigestive tract, for which it works well. In the thyroid gland, most tumors arising from follicular cells belong to either the well-differentiated or the undifferentiated types. The former includes nearly all of the minimally invasive follicular carcinomas (including those of oncocytic type) and the papillary carcinomas of either conventional or follicular variant types, whereas the undifferentiated grade is synonymous with the undifferentiated (anaplastic) type of carcinoma. We have proposed the term insular carcinoma for poorly differentiated tumors of either follicular or papillary type that exhibit an insular pattern of growth associated with mitotic activity and necrosis, and believe that this category can be expanded to include other poorly differentiated tumors of follicular cell origin that fit the insular pattern (see chapter 8). No grading system has been proposed for medullary carcinoma, even though the small cell variant of this tumor could be regarded as its poorly differentiated member.

Staging of Thyroid Carcinoma

The staging system most widely used for thyroid carcinoma is that recommended by the UICC in their Manual (currently in its seventh edition) and adopted by the AJCC (39-41). It is

Table 21-2

CHECKLIST TO BE USED WITH THE ADASP PROTOCOL OF TABLE 21-1

1. **Organ: Thyroid Gland**[a]
2. **Type of specimen**[b]
   Nodulectomy
   Lobectomy
   Subtotal thyroidectomy
   Total thyroidectomy
   Other : _____
3. **Tumor Type (and subtype)**
   Papillary carcinoma
      Classic type
      ____ type
   Follicular carcinoma
      Minimally invasive
      Widely invasive
   Hürthle cell carcinoma
      Minimally invasive
      Widely invasive
   Poorly differentiated carcinoma
      Insular type
      ____type
   Undifferentiated (anaplastic) carcinoma
      Without residual well-differentiated component
      With residual well-differentiated component, ___type
   Medullary carcinoma
      Classic type
      ____type
   Mixed medullary-follicular carcinoma
   Mixed medullary-papillary carcinoma
   Other ____
4. **Tumor Location**
   Right lobe (and isthmus)
   Left lobe (and isthmus)
   Both lobes (and isthmus)
   Isthmus
5. **Tumor Largest Diameter:** ____cm[c]
6. **Encapsulation**
   Absent
   Partial
   Complete
7. **Capsular Invasion**
   Absent
   Present (minimal)
   Present (extensive)
8. **Lymph Vessel Invasion**
   Absent
   Present (minimal)
   Present (extensive)

9. **Blood Vessel Invasion**
   Absent
   Present (minimal)
   Present (extensive
10. **Extrathyroid Extension**
    Absent
    Present (gross)
    Present (extensive)
11. **Surgical Margins**[d]
    Negative
    Positive
12. **Tumor Multicentricity**
    Absent
    Present[e]
13. **C-Cell Hyperplasia (for cases of medullary carcinoma only)**
    Absent
    Present
14. **Other Pathology**
    None
    Adenoma(s) (specify number, location, and size)
    Nodular hyperplasia
    Lymphocytic thyroiditis
    Hashimoto thyroiditis
    Atrophy
    Fibrosis
15. **Parathyroid Glands**[f]
    No
    Yes
    Number _____
    Location _____
       Normal
       Abnormal (specify)
16. **Lymph Nodes**
    No
    Yes
       Number
       Location (right, left, central) and level
       Negative
       Positive
17. **Positive (Metastatic) Lymph Nodes**
    Size of largest involved node: ____ cm
    Perinodal (extracapsular extension:
       Yes
       No

[a]If the thyroid gland is located ectopically (mediastinal, lingual, in a thyroglossal duct cyst, or in a teratoma), this should be indicated in the report.

[b]For nodulectomy or lobectomy specimens, the report should indicate whether the specimen is from the right or left side. (Nodulectomy is rarely, if ever, performed at present, but it is included in the checklist for the sake of completeness.) If the lobectomy specimen includes the isthmus (as is often the case), the report should make reference to this fact. For subtotal thyroidectomy specimens, the report should indicate which lobe was completely removed and which lobe was excised only partially.

[c]Provide a size estimate for tumor bulk if the tumor is multifocal. For cases of papillary microcarcinoma (less than 1 cm in diameter), indicate in the report the exact diameter of the tumor

[d]If positive, specify location (capsular or isthmic), number (single or multiple), and extent (minimal/microscopic or extensive), if feasible.

[e]Specify approximate number of tumor foci and whether these foci have the same or a different appearance. If the specimen is from a subtotal or total thyroidectomy, indicate whether the tumor foci involve one lobe or both lobes. In cases of papillary carcinoma, indicate whether psammoma bodies are present elsewhere in the gland or not, the former suggesting the presence of tumor multicentricity.

[f]Whenever possible, the location of the gland(s) should be specified; if this gland is intrathyroidal, this fact should be noted.

Table 21-3

UICC/AJCC STAGING SYSTEM FOR THYROID CARCINOMA (TNM)

Primary Tumor (T)

Note: All categories may be subdivided: (s) solitary tumor and (m) muliifocal tumor (the largest determines the classification).

TX   Primary tumor cannot be assessed
T0   No evidence of primary tumor
T1   Tumor 2 cm or less in greatest dimension limited to the thyroid
T1a   Tumor 1 cm or less, limited to the thyroid
T1b   Tumor more than 1 cm but not more than 2 cm in greatest dimension, limited to the thyroid
T2   Tumor more than 2 cm but not more than 4 cm in greatest dimension limited to the thyroid
T3   Tumor more than 4 cm in greatest dimension limited to the thyroid or any tumor with minimal extrathyroid extension (e.g., extension to sternothyroid muscle or perithyroid soft tissues)
T4a   Moderately advanced disease; tumor of any size extending beyond the thyroid capsule to invade subcutaneous soft tissues, larynx, trachea, esophagus, or recurrent laryngeal nerve
T4b   Very advanced disease; tumor invades prevertebral fascia or encases carotid artery or mediastinal vessels

All anaplastic carcinomas are considered T4 tumors
T4a   Intrathyroidal anaplastic carcinoma
T4b   Anaplastic carcinoma with gross extrathyroid extension

Regional Lymph Nodes (N)
Regional lymph nodes are the central compartment, lateral cervical, and upper mediastinal lymph nodes
NX   Regional lymph nodes cannot be assessed
N0   No regional lymph node metastasis
N1   Regional lymph node metastasis
N1a   Metastasis to Level VI (pretracheal, paratracheal, and prelaryngeal/Delphian lymph nodes)
N1b   Metastasis to unilateral, bilateral, or contralateral cervical (Level I, II, III, or IV) or retropharyngeal or superior mediastinal lymph nodes (Level VII)

Distant Metastasis (M)
M0   No distant metastasis
M1   Distant metastasis

---

based on the size and other morphologic features of the primary tumor: presence, absence, and level of regional lymph node metastases; and presence or absence of distant metastases (Table 21-3). This information is used to place the tumors into the various prognostic categories (Tables 21-4, 21-5).

ANCILLARY TESTING

A number of immunohistochemical markers have been proposed to confirm the diagnosis of papillary carcinoma, allowing for distinction from other lesions/tumors in the differential diagnosis. These markers include (but are not limited to) cytokeratin (CK) 19, galectin 3, and mesothelium-associated antibody, HBME-1. They are not totally specific for papillary carcinoma, however, and cannot relied on for the diagnosis of papillary carcinoma. At present, the morphologic criteria remain the "gold standard" in the diagnosis of papillary carcinoma.

Distinct genetic alterations that can be used as molecular markers have been identified in papil-lary carcinoma (PTC) (see chapter 19). The most important is the *BRAF* V600E mutation consisting of the substitution of valine (V) for glutamate (E) at residue 600 of *BRAF*, found in about 45 percent of cases. This mutation is common in classic PTC, and detected in almost all tall cell PTCs. In contrast, the follicular variant of PTC rarely presents the V600E mutation, but features instead less common *BRAF* variants, such as the *BRAF* K601E mutation in which glutamate (E) replaces lysine (K) at residue 601. The *RET/PTC* rearrangement is also found in PTC, typically in cases associated with radiation exposure.

RAS mutations are a molecular marker for follicular-patterned thyroid tumors, and as such are found in follicular adenoma, follicular carcinoma, and in the follicular variant of PTC (see chapter 19). The *PAX8/PPARγ* rearrangement is another marker for follicular-patterned lesions, found in a subset of follicular carcinomas, but also in some follicular adenomas and in the follicular variant PTCs (see chapter 19).

Table 21-4

UICC/AJCC ANATOMIC STAGE/PROGNOSTIC GROUPS

Separate stage groupings are recommended for papillary or follicular (differentiated), medullary, and anaplastic (undifferentiated) carcinoma.

Papillary or Follicular (differentiated)

Under 45 Years

Stage I	Any T	Any N	M0
Stage II	Any T	Any N	M1

45 Years and Older

Stage I	T1	N0	M0
Stage II	T2	N0	M0
Stage III	T3	N0	M0
	T1	N1a	M0
	T2	N1a	M0
	T3	N1a	M0
Stage IVA	T4a	N0	M0
	T4a	N1a	M0
	T1	N1a	M0
	T2	N1a	M0
	T3	N1b	M0
	T4a	N1b	M0
Stage IVB	T4b	Any N	M0
Stage IVC	Any T	Any N	M1

Medullary Carcinoma (all age groups)

Stage I	T1	N0	M0
Stage II	T2	N0	M0
	T3	N0	M0
Stage III	T1	N1a	M0
	T2	N1a	M0
	T3	N1a	M0
Stage IVA	T4a	N0	M0
	T4a	N1a	M0
	T1	N1b	M0
	T2	N1b	M0
	T3	N1b	M0
	T4a	N1b	M0
Stage IVB	T4b	Any N	M0
Stage IVC	Any T	Any N	M1

Anaplastic Carcinoma: all anaplastic carcinomas are considered Stage IV.

Stage IVA	T4a	Any N	M0
Stage IVB	T4b	Any N	M1
Stage IVC	Any T	Any N	M1

In spite of advances in the molecular categorization of thyroid follicular epithelial cell tumors, in general, and papillary carcinoma specifically, the use of molecular testing in the diagnosis and differential diagnosis of papillary carcinomas and follicular carcinomas is still evolving. In the United States, the Cancer Genome Atlas (TCGA) (http://cancergenome.nih.gov/), a National Institutes of Health project that began in 2006 to comprehensively study the molecular alterations of human cancers using high throughput molecular analysis, has selected papillary carcinoma as one of its targets. The results of this in-depth genomic analysis may contribute important insights and identify markers useful not only for the diagnosis, but also to define the prognosis and potentially treat thyroid tumors with specific, molecularly targeted therapies.

The molecular genetics of medullary carcinoma is well established, showing mutations in the *RET* proto-oncogene. Germline *RET* mutations are associated with hereditary medullary carcinomas, including familial medullary thyroid carcinoma and MEN 2A and 2B. In this setting, prophylactic total thyroidectomy is performed for family members based on the identification of *RET* oncogene mutations in DNA extracted from peripheral blood samples (42). Many of the thyroidectomy specimens appear grossly normal. In such cases, comprehensive examination of the entire thyroid gland is required to document the extent of C-cell hyperplasia and to assess for micromedullary carcinoma. Horizontal sections of each lobe should be taken serially in a superior to inferior direction, and the isthmus should be submitted separately. This serial sectioning of the thyroid is performed because C-cells are restricted to a zone deep within the middle to upper thirds of the lateral lobes. The extreme upper and lower poles of each lobe and the isthmic region are generally devoid of C-cells. Immunostains for calcitonin and carcinoembryonic antigen (CEA) are usually required to assess the extent of C-cell disease.

TREATMENT OF THYROID TUMORS

Some general statements regarding the therapy of thyroid tumors are made here. Specific considerations are discussed with the corresponding tumor types.

The initial therapeutic approach is usually surgical (43–45). The standard types of operation are lobectomy (often coupled with resection of the isthmus for cosmetic reasons), subtotal thyroidectomy, and total thyroidectomy (46–50). Nodulectomy (i.e., enucleation of a nodule) has been largely abandoned because of the definite risk of recurrence if the lesion is malignant. The morbidity associated with lobectomy and with subtotal thyroidectomy is comparable and of minimal magnitude (less than 1 percent). In contrast, significant morbidity in the form of permanent hypoparathyroidism or recurrent laryngeal nerve paralysis occurs in up to 10 percent of patients subjected to total thyroidectomy, even when performed by experienced surgeons. This operation should therefore be carried out only when strict criteria are met. Some authors, ourselves included, are skeptical about its indication for many well-differentiated follicular and papillary carcinomas, both in adults and children (46,51,52). Yet, this remains the most common procedure at present both in the United States and Europe (53,54), and the one recommended in the 2009 Updated American Thyroid Association Guidelines for Management of Thyroid Nodules and Differentiated Thyroid Cancer (except for small [under 1 cm] unifocal lesions) (44). As a matter of fact, it has been stated that the advantage of total thyroidectomy over lobectomy is clear and evidence-based, and that the debate has been closed (55–57). We remain unconvinced, and believe that only a properly conducted prospective randomized study will solve this issue (58,59). This issue is discussed in more detail in connection with the treatment of papillary carcinoma (see chapter 7).

The performance of a radical neck dissection in the presence of clinically negative nodes has been largely abandoned. A modified form of neck dissection is generally carried out if the nodes are thought to be involved, either clinically or at the time of thyroidectomy. This allows the preservation of the spinal accessory nerve, jugular vein, and sternocleidomastoid muscle, leading to a cosmetically superior result.

Postoperative oral administration of thyroid hormone on a long-term basis in a quantity sufficient to suppress thyroid-stimulating hormone activity is used routinely for follicular and papillary carcinomas, and with some frequency even for benign nodules, under the assumption that it results in a decrease in the incidence of clinical recurrence (60). However, a study by Cady et al. (61) showed no statistically significant improvement in survival with use of thyroid hormone in differentiated thyroid carcinoma when the patients were stratified by risk group and pathologic type.

Administration of radioactive iodine is another mainstay of thyroid cancer therapy (62,63). It is based on the principles that: 1) functioning thyroid tissue concentrates iodine; 2) most thyroid carcinomas are well differentiated enough to function; and 3) if a primary tumor takes up iodine, its metastases should be expected to behave similarly. We and others believe that use of radioactive iodine should be selective rather than routine, and that it should be generally restricted to nonresectable and metastatic well-differentiated carcinomas (64). In two very recent, carefully performed, randomized prospective studies carried out in patients with low-risk thyroid cancer, one in France and the other in the United Kingdom, it was shown that a low-dose (1.1 GBq) postoperative radioiodine ablation may be just as effective for the management of these patients as the doses currently employed (3.7 GBq) (65,66). These important studies have resulted in questioning whether postoperative radioiodine is needed at all, and will be addressed by another randomized trial in the United Kingdom (67,68).

External radiation therapy is reserved for tumors showing surgically uncontrollable local spread (69). In most series, its efficacy has been modest (70). The post-therapy monitoring includes (besides physical examination and chest X rays) radioactive scan and measurement of serum thyroglobulin levels for tumors of follicular cells and measurement of serum levels of calcitonin, CEA, and chromogranin A for tumors of C-cells.

Treatment of metastatic thyroid disease includes surgical excision (for local recurrence, lymph node metastases, or isolated distant metastases), radioactive iodine (highly effective for well-differentiated tumors), and external radiation therapy (64,71,72). In general, conventional cytotoxic chemotherapy, usually with doxorubicin, has proven of little benefit.

Molecular therapies with agents that target oncogenes and pathways activated in thyroid carcinoma are being evaluated in patients with tumors that do not respond to conventional treatment (73). In the United States, the Food and Drug Administration has approved the use of Vandetanib and Cabozantinib to treat advanced medullary carcinoma. Both are tyrosine kinase inhibitors with strong antiangiogenetic properties, active against RET as well as other tyrosine kinases. Although medullary carcinomas that harbor the *RET* M918T mutation may show a more favorable response, tumor genotyping is not currently required to administer the drug. The role for molecular therapy in the treatment

Table 21-5

PROPOSED PROGNOSTIC SCORING INDEXES

European Organization for Research and Treatment of Cancer (EORTC)	Total score = patient's age, +12 if male, +10 if poorly differentiated FTC,[a] +10 if invaded the thyroid capsule, +15 if 1 distant metastasis, +30 if 2 or more distant metastases
	Five risk groups:
	    Group 1 = a score <50
	    Group 2 = a score 50-65
	    Group 3 = a score 66-83
	    Group 4 = a score 84-108
	    Group 5 = a score >108

Mayo Clinic (Age, Grade, Extent, Size [AGES])	Total score = 0.05 x age in years (if aged ≥40) or +0 (if aged <40)
	+ 1 (if tumor grade 2) or + 3 (if tumor grade 3 or 4)
	+ 1 (if extrathyroidal invasion)
	+ 3 (if distant spread)
	+ 0.2 x tumor size (maximum diameter in cm)
	Four risk groups:
	    Group 1 = a score <4.00
	    Group 2 = a score 4.01-4.99
	    Group 3 = a score 5.00-5.99
	    Group 4 = a score ≥6

Lahey Clinic (Age, Metastases, Extent, Size [AMES])[b]	Two risk groups:
	Low-risk group =
	a. all younger patients without distant metastases (men <41 years, women <51 years)
	b. all older patients with:
	    1) intrathyroidal papillary cancer or minor tumor capsular involvement follicular carcinoma, and
	    2) tumor size < 5 cm, and
	    3) no distant metastases
	High-risk group =
	a. all patients with distant metastases
	b. all older patients with:
	    1) major capsular involvement papillary cancer or major capsular involvement follicular carcinoma and
	    2) tumor size ≥5cm

[a]FTC = follicular thyroid carcinoma.
[b]See Table 21-6.

of aggressive thyroid carcinomas of follicular cell derivation is less defined. Some results are encouraging, although bone metastases do not usually respond to tyrosine kinase inhibitors (73). Vemurafenib, a BRAF inhibitor approved for the treatment of malignant melanoma, is clinically active in some patients with aggressive *BRAF* V600E mutated tumors, including undifferentiated carcinomas, but definitive data on the efficacy of the drug is not yet available (74,75).

PROGNOSTIC FACTORS

Most of the clinical and pathologic factors related to prognosis are discussed with the specific tumor types. Overall, the most important prognostic indicators are age and gender of the patient, tumor microscopic type, presence and number of mitoses and necrosis, and tumor stage (76–81). These and other factors are combined in prognostic scoring indexes, of which no less than 17 have been generated, among which are those proposed by the European Organization for Research on Treatment of Cancer (EORTC), the Mayo Clinic (AGES score), and the Lahey Clinic (AMES system) (Table 21-5) (82–87).

Cady et al. (87) divided their patients with well-differentiated (papillary or follicular) carcinomas into two categories, with notably, different survival rates: 1) low risk (men under 40 years of age and women under 50 years of age) and 2) high risk (men over 40 years of age and women over 50 years of age). We have confirmed the great practical utility of this division for papillary carcinoma and found that, in

Table 21-6

MODIFIED LAHEY CLINIC RISK GROUP DEFINITION (CADY AND ROSS[a])

Low-Risk Group:
    All younger patients without distant metastases (men, <41 years; women, <51 years)
    All older patients with:
        intrathyroidal papillary cancer or minor tumor capsular involvement follicular carcinoma, and primary cancers
        <5 cm in diameter, and no distant metastases
    This group constituted 89 percent of all cases, and the death rate was 1.8 percent

High-Risk Group:[b]
    All patients with distant metastases
    All older patients with:
        extrathyroidal papillary cancer or major tumor capsular involvement follicular carcinoma, and primary cancers
        5 cm in diameter or larger regardless of extent of disease

[a]From reference 89.
[b]This group made up 11 percent of cases but carried a 46 percent mortality rate. Thus, a mortality ratio of 26:1 existed between the two groups.

our series, the prognostic difference was even more striking if the low-risk group was defined as including men under 40 years of age and women under 60 years of age (88).

Cady and Rossi (89) have proposed a modified version of their risk-group definition by incorporating some of the factors from the EORTC system (Table 21-6).

The genetic alterations found in thyroid carcinoma may have prognostic value (see chapters 2 and 19). *RET* M918T has been associated with unfavorable outcome in medullary carcinoma. In papillary carcinoma, a strong case has been made for the *BRAF* V600E mutation that, according to many studies, may identify a subset of patients with an increased risk for persistent disease, tumor recurrence, and even tumor-related death (73). TERT promoter mutations are emerging as an important marker of poor prognosis for papillary and follicular carcinomas (9, see chapter 2).

In terms of microscopic type, most deaths from thyroid epithelial malignancies result from undifferentiated, poorly differentiated, oncocytic, and medullary carcinomas, despite the fact that the sum of all of these types represents less than 25 percent of all thyroid carcinomas.

REFERENCES

1. Enewold L, Zhu K, Ron E, et al. Rising thyroid cancer incidence in the United States by demographic and tumor characteristics, 1980-2005. Cancer Epidemiol Biomarkers Prev 2009;18:784-91.
2. Aschebrook-Kilfoy B, Ward MH, Sabra MM, Devesa SS. Thyroid cancer incidence patterns in the United States by histologic type, 1992-2006. Thyroid 2011;21:125-34.
3. Nosé V. Familial follicular cell tumors: classification and morphological characteristics. Endocr Pathol 2010;21:219-26.
4. Harach HR, Soubeyran I, Brown A, Bonneau D, Longy M. Thyroid pathologic findings in patients with Cowden disease. Ann Diagn Pathol 1999;3:331-40.
5. Barletta JA, Bellizzi AM, Hornick JL. Immunohistochemical staining of thyroidectomy specimens for PTEN can aid in the identification of patients with Cowden syndrome. Am J Surg Pathol 2010;35:1505-11.
6. Nosé V. Familial thyroid cancer: a review. Mod Pathol 2011;24:S19-33.
7. Prazeres H, Torres J, Soares P, Sobrinho-Simões M. The familial counterparts of follicular cell—derived thyroid tumors. Int J Surg Pathol 2010;18:233-42.
8. Tamimi DM. The association between chronic lymphocytic thyroiditis and thyroid tumors. Int J Surg Pathol 2002;10:141-6.
9. Okayasu I. The relationship of lymphocytic thyroiditis to the development of thyroid carcinoma. Endocr Pathol 1997;8:225-30.
10. Hegedüs L. Clinical practice. The thyroid nodule. N Engl J Med 2004;351:1764-71.
11. Friedman M, Toriumi DM, Mafee MF. Diagnostic imaging techniques in thyroid cancer. Am J Surg 1988;155:215-23.
12. Shulkin BL, Shapiro B. The role of imaging tests in the diagnosis of thyroid carcinoma. Endocrinol Metab Clin North Am 1990;19:523-44.
13. Noyek AM, Greyson ND, Steinhardt MI, et al. Thyroid tumor imaging. Arch Otolaryngol 1983;109:205-24.
14. Pacini F, Molinaro E, Castagna MG, et al. Recombinant human thyrotropin-stimulated serum thyroglobulin combined with neck ultrasonography has the highest sensitivity in monitoring differentiated thyroid carcinoma. J Clin Endocrinol Metab 2003;88:3668-73.
15. Mazzaferri EL, Robbins RJ, Spencer CA, et al. A consensus report of the role of serum thyroglobulin as a monitoring method for low-risk patients with papillary thyroid carcinoma. J Clin Endocrinol Metab 2003;88:1433-41.
16. Ericsson UB, Tegler L, Lennquist S, Christensen SB, Stahl E, Thorell JI. Serum thyroglobulin in differentiated thyroid carcinoma. Acta Chir Scand 1984;150:367-75.
17. Ramanna L, Waxman AD, Brachman MB, et al. Correlation of thyroglobulin measurements and radioiodine scans in the follow-up of patients with differentiated thyroid cancer. Cancer 1985;55:1525-9.
18. Shlossberg AH, Jacobson JC, Ibbertson HK. Serum thyroglobulin in the diagnosis and management of thyroid carcinoma. Clin Endocrinol (Oxf) 1979;10:17-27.
19. Herle AJ, Uller RP. Elevated serum thyroglobulin. A marker of metastases in differentiated thyroid carcinomas. J Clin Invest 1975;56:272-7.
20. Pacini F, Capezzone M, Elisei R, Ceccarelli C, Taddei D, Pinchera A. Diagnostic 131-iodine whole-body scan may be avoided in thyroid cancer patients who have undetectable stimulated serum Tg levels after initial treatment. J Clin Endocrinol Metab 2002;87:1499-501.
21. Tallini G, Ghossein RA, Emanuel J, et al. Detection of thyroglobulin, thyroid peroxidase, and RET/PTC1 mRNA transcripts in the peripheral blood of patients with thyroid disease. Clin Oncol 1998;16:1158-66.
22. Hamburger JI, Husain M. Contribution of intraoperative pathology evaluation to surgical management of thyroid nodules. Endocrinol Metab Clin North Am 1990;19:509-22.
23. Osamura RY, Hunt JL. Current practices in performing frozen sections for thyroid and parathyroid pathology. Virchows Arch 2008;453:433-40.
24. Rigaud C. [The extemporaneous examination in thyroid pathology. Why and how?] Ann Pathol 1989;9:305-7. [French]
25. Anton RC, Wheeler TM. Frozen section of thyroid and parathyroid specimens. Arch Pathol Lab Med 2005;129:1575-84.
26. LiVolsi VA, Baloch ZW. Use and abuse of frozen section in the diagnosis of follicular thyroid lesions. Endocr Pathol 2005;16:285-93.
27. Rosen Y, Rosenblatt P, Saltzman E. Intraoperative pathologic diagnosis of thyroid neoplasms. Report on experience with 504 specimens. Cancer 1990;66:2001-6.

28. Leteurtre E, Leroy X, Pattou F, et al. Why do frozen sections have limited value in encapsulated or minimally invasive follicular carcinoma of the thyroid? Am J Clin Pathol. 2001;115:370-4.

29. Hapke MR, Dehner LP. The optically clear nucleus. A reliable sign of papillary carcinoma of the thyroid? Am J Surg Pathol 1979;3:31-8.

30. Bugis SP, Young JE, Archibald SD, Chen VS. Diagnostic accuracy of fine-needle aspiration biopsy versus frozen section in solitary thyroid nodules. Am J Surg 1986;152:411-6.

31. Keller MP, Crabbe MM, Norwood SH. Accuracy and significance of fine-needle aspiration and frozen section in determining the extent of thyroid resection. Surgery 1987;101:632-5.

32. Kraemer BB. Frozen section diagnosis and the thyroid. Semin Diagn Pathol 1987;4:169-89.

33. Pradeep PV, Vissa S. Follicular neoplasm involving one lobe of thyroid: is hemithyroidectomy the adequate initial procedure? Ir J Med Sci 2013;182:37-40.

34. Hamburger JI, Hamburger SW. Declining role of frozen section in surgical planning for thyroid nodules. Surgery 1985;98:307-12.

35. Kopald KH, Layfield LJ, Mohrmann R, Foshag LJ, Giuliano AE. Clarifying the role of fine-needle aspiration, cytologic evaluation and frozen section examination in the operative management of thyroid cancer. Arch Surg 1989;124:1201-5.

36. Antic T, Taxy JB. Thyroid frozen section. Supplementary or Unnecessary. Am J Surg Pathol 2013;37:282-6.

37. Association of Directors of Anatomic and Surgical Pathology: recommended reporting format for thyroid carcinoma. Virchows Arch 2000;437:351-3.

38. www.cap.org/apps/docs/committees/cancer/cancer_protocol/2014/Thyroid_14Protocol_3100.pdf.

39. Brierley JD, Panzarella T, Tsang RW, Gospodarowicz MK, O'Sullivan B. A comparison of different staging systems predictability of patient outcome. Thyroid carcinoma as an example. Cancer 1997;79:2414-23.

40. Sobin LH, Gospodarowicz MK, Wittekind C. TNM Classification of malignant tumours, 7th ed. Hoboken, NJ: Wiley-Blackwell; 2010.

41. Edge S, Byrd DR, compton CC, et al., eds. AJCC cancer staging manual, 7th ed. New York: Springer; 2010.

42. American Thyroid Association Guidelines Task Force, Kloos RT, Eng C, et al. Medullary thyroid cancer: management guidelines of the American Thyroid Association. Thyroid 2009;19:565-612.

43. McDougall R, Berry GJ. Management of thyroid cancer and related nodular disease. London: Springer; 2006.

44. American Thyroid Association (ATA) Guidelines Taskforce on Thyroid Nodules and Differentiated Thyroid Cancer, Cooper DS, Doherty GM, et al. Revised American Thyroid Association management guidelines for patients with thyroid nodules and differentiated thyroid cancer. Thyroid 2009:19:1167-214.

45. NCCN Clinical practice guidelines in oncology (NCCN GuidelinesTM). Thyroid carcinoma. Version 2.2012. NCCN.org.

46. Brooks JR, Starnes HF, Brooks DC, Pelkey JN. Surgical therapy for thyroid carcinoma: a review of 1249 solitary thyroid nodules. Surgery 1988;104:940-6.

47. Demeure MJ, Clark OH. Surgery in the treatment of thyroid cancer. Endocrinol Metab Clin North Am 1990;19:663-84.

48. Griffin JE. Management of thyroid nodules. Am J Med Sci 1988;296:336-47.

49. Mazzaferri EL. Treating differentiated thyroid carcinoma: where do we draw the line? Mayo Clin Proc 1991;66:105-11.

50. Hegedüs L. Clinical practice. The thyroid nodule. N Engl J Med 2004;351:1764-71.

51. Massimino M, Collini P, Leite SF, et al. Conservative surgical approach for thyroid and lymph-node involvement in papillary thyroid carcinoma of childhood and adolescence. Pediatr Blood Cancer 2006;46:307-13.

52. Mendelsohn AH, Elashoff DA, Abemayor E, St John MA. Surgery for papillary thyroid carcinoma: is lobectomy enough? Arch Otolaryngol Head Neck Surg 2010;136:1055-61.

53. Hundahl SA, Fleming ID, Fremgen AM, Menck HR. A National Cancer Data Base report on 53,856 cases of thyroid carcinoma treated in the U.S., 1985-1995. Cancer 1998;83:2638-48.

54. Hölzer S, Reiners C, Mann K, et al. Patterns of care for patients with primary differentiated carcinoma of the thyroid gland treated in Germany during 1996. U.S. and German Thyroid Cancer Group. Cancer 2000;89:192-201.

55. Hartl DM, Travagli JP. The updated American Thyroid Association Guidelines for management of thyroid nodules and differentiated thyroid cancer: a surgical perspective. Thyroid 2009;19:1149-51.

56. British Thyroid Association and Royal College of Physicians. Guidelines for the management of thyroid cancer in adults. London: Royal College of Physicians; 2002.

57. Bilimoria KY, Bentrem DJ, Ko CY, et al. Extent of surgery affects survival for papillary thyroid cancer. Ann Surg 2007;246:375-84.

58. Hundahl SA, Cady B, Cunningham MP, et al. Initial results from a prospective cohort study of 5583 cases of thyroid carcinoma treated in the United States during 1996. U.S. and German Thyroid Cancer Study Group. An American College of Surgeons Commission on Cancer Patient Care Evaluation study. Cancer 2000;89:202-17.

59. Shaha AR. The National Cancer Data Base Report on thyroid carcinoma: reflections of practice patterns. Cancer 1998;83:2434-6.

60. Clark OH. TSH suppression in the management of thyroid nodules and thyroid cancer. World J Surg 1981;5:39-47.

61. Cady B, Cohn K, Rossi RL, et al. The effect of thyroid hormone administration upon survival in patients with differentiated thyroid carcinoma. Surgery 1983;94:978-83.

62. Maxon HR 3rd, Smith HS. Radioiodine-131 in the diagnosis and treatment of metastatic well differentiated thyroid cancer. Endocrinol Metab Clin North Am 1990;19:685-718.

63. Haymart MR, Banerjee M, Stewart AK, Koenig RJ, Birkmeyer JD, Griggs JJ. Use of radioactive iodine for thyroid cancer. JAMA 2011;306:721-8.

64. Lee KY, Loré JM Jr. The treatment of metastatic thyroid disease. Otolaryngol Clin North Am 1990;23:475-93.

65. Schlumberger M, Catargi B, Borget I, et al. Strategies of radioiodine ablation in patients with low-risk thyroid cancer. N Engl J Med 2012;366:1663-73.

66. Mallick U, Harmer C, Yap B, et al. Ablation with low-dose radioiodine and thyrotropin alfa in thyroid cancer. N Engl J Med 2012;366:1674-85.

67. Alexander EK, Larsen PR. Radioiodine for thyroid cancer—is less more? N Engl J Med 2012;366:1732-3.

68. Mallick U, Harmer C, Hackshaw A, Moss L, IoN Trial Management Group. Iodine or Not (IoN) for low-risk differentiated thyroid cancer: the next UK National Cancer Research Network randomised trial following HiLo. Clin Oncol (R Coll Radiol) 2012;24:159-61.

69. Farahati J, Reiners C, Stuschke M, et al. Differentiated thyroid cancer. Impact of adjuvant external radiotherapy in patients with perithyroidal tumor infiltration (stage pT4). Cancer 1996;77:172-80.

70. Benker G, Olbricht T, Reinwein D, et al. Survival rates in patients with differentiated thyroid carcinoma. Influence of postoperative external radiotherapy. Cancer 1990;65:1517-20.

71. McWilliams RR, Giannini C, Hay ID, Atkinson JL, Stafford SL, Buckner JC. Management of brain metastases from thyroid carcinoma: a study of 16 pathologically confirmed cases over 25 years. Cancer 2003;98:356-62.

72. Sisson JC, Giordano TJ, Jamadar DA, et al. 131-I treatment of micronodular pulmonary metastases from papillary thyroid carcinoma. Cancer 1996;78:2184-92.

73. Xing M, Haugen BR, Schlumberger M. Progress in molecular-based management of differentiated thyroid cancer. Lancet 2013;381:1058-69.

74. Rosove MH, Peddi PF, Glaspy JA. BRAF V600E inhibition in anaplastic thyroid cancer. N Engl J Med 2013;368:684-5.

75. Kim KB, Cabanillas ME, Lazar AJ, et al. Clinical responses to vemurafenib in patients with metastatic papillary thyroid cancer harboring BRAF(V600E) mutation. Thyroid 2013;23:1277-83.

76. Lundgren CI, Hall P, Dickman PW, Zedenius J. Clinically significant prognostic factors for differentiated thyroid carcinoma: a population-based, nested case-control study. Cancer 2006;106:524-31.

77. Ghossein R. Problems and controversies in the histopathology of thyroid carcinomas of follicular cell origin. Arch Pathol Lab Med 2009;133:683-91.

78. Gilliland FD, Hunt WC, Morris DM, Key CR. Prognostic factors for thyroid carcinoma. A population-based study of 15,698 cases from the Surveillance, Epidemiology and End Results (SEER) program 1973-1991. Cancer 1997;79:564-73.

79. LiVolsi VA, Baloch ZW. Predicting prognosis in thyroid carcinoma: can histology do it? Am J Surg Pathol 2002;26:1064-5.

80. Wu HS, Young MT, Ituarte PH, et al. Death from thyroid cancer of follicular cell origin. J Am Coll Surg 2000;191:600-6.

81. Vini L, Hyer SL, Marshall J, A'Hern R, Harmer C. Long-term results in elderly patients with differentiated thyroid carcinoma. Cancer 2003;97:2736-42.

82. Lang BH, Lo CY, Chan WF, Lam KY, Wan KY. Staging system for papillary thyroid carcinoma: a review and comparison. Ann Surg 2007;245:366-78.

83. Byar DP, Green SB, Dor P, et al. A prognostic index for thyroid carcinoma. A study of the E.O.R.T.C. Thyroid Cancer Cooperative Group. Eur J Cancer 1979;15:1033-41.

84. Tennvall J, Biörklund A, Möller T, Ranstam J, Åkerman M. Is the EORTC prognostic index of thyroid cancer valid in differentiated thyroid carcinoma? Retrospective multivariate analysis of differentiated thyroid carcinoma with long term follow-up. Cancer 1986;57:1405-14.

85. Hay ID, Grant CS, Taylor WF, McConahey WM. Ipsilateral lobectomy versus bilateral lobar resection in papillary thyroid carcinoma: a retrospective analysis of surgical outcome using a novel prognostic scoring system. Surgery 1987;102:1088-95.
86. Hay ID. Papillary thyroid carcinoma. Endocrinol Metab Clin North Am 1990;19:545-76.
87. Cady B, Rossi R, Silverman M, Wool M. Further evidence of the validity of risk group definition in differentiated thyroid carcinoma. Surgery 1985;98:1171-8.
88. Carcangiu ML, Zampi G, Pupi A, Castagnoli A, Rosai J. Papillary carcinoma of the thyroid. A clinicopathologic study of 241 cases treated at the University of Florence, Italy. Cancer 1985;55:805-28.
89. Cady B, Rossi R. An expanded view of risk-group definition in differentiated thyroid carcinoma. Surgery 1988;104:947-53.

22 IMMUNOHISTOCHEMICAL MARKERS OF THE NORMAL AND NEOPLASTIC THYROID GLAND

As mentioned in chapter 1, a large number of molecules that are expressed in the normal follicular C-cells play a vital role in thyroid and bone metabolism. The most important of them, from a diagnostic or prognostic standpoint (such as thyroglobulin and calcitonin), have already been discussed in chapter 1 or mentioned with the various tumor types. In recent years, many other molecules have been evaluated at the immunohistochemical level in the normal, hyperplastic, and neoplastic thyroid gland. A listing of those molecules is given below, followed by a short description of their main features. A disclaimer is, however, in order. As a general rule, these molecules are not specific to the thyroid gland or to a special type of thyroid tumor. Allegedly, some of them show marked differences in the frequency and intensity of expression in the various conditions, differences that theoretically could be used for diagnostic purposes. This hope is tempered by the fact that there are often perplexing discrepancies in the results among the various series, and the equally frustrating realization that the differences found among benign and malignant thyroid conditions are almost always quantitative rather than qualitative, and therefore subject to wide variation of interpretation, depending on the degree of caution and enthusiasm exercised by the authors of the respective studies. The fact that many of these markers are not commercially available, thus preventing an independent confirmation of the literature claims, adds to the difficulty. In any event, here is the list, offered to the reader with the full realization that it will be already woefully incomplete by the time this Fascicle becomes available.

AgNOR. Although strictly speaking not an immunohistochemical technique, argyrophilic staining for the evaluation of the nucleolar organizer region (AgNOR) is listed here for convenience. It has been claimed that a significant difference in the expression of this marker exists between follicular adenoma and follicular carcinoma (but not between normal thyroid gland and follicular adenoma or between well-differentiated and undifferentiated [anaplastic] carcinoma) (1).

Apoptosis-Regulating Proteins. These are represented by the molecules BCL-2, BAX, MCL-1, and BCL-X. Normal thyroid tissues consistently express of BCL-2 and MCL-1 but not BAX or BCL-X. BAX is present in all papillary thyroid carcinomas and in most follicular carcinomas, whereas BCL-X is seen in all undifferentiated tumors (2).

Basement Membrane Components. Expression of basement membrane components (such as laminin, type IV collagen, and heparan sulphate proteoglycan) in the thyroid gland is related to follicle formation. These components are well-developed in follicular-patterned benign and malignant tumors, show an irregular and interrupted pattern in papillary carcinoma, and are absent in solid/trabecular neoplasms, including poorly differentiated and undifferentiated carcinomas (3).

Basic Fibroblastic Growth Factor. This molecule, which is barely detectable in normal follicular cells, is strongly expressed in papillary carcinoma, where it may stimulate the growth of vessels and other mesenchymal cells (4).

BAX. See Apoptosis-Regulating Proteins.
BCL-2. See Apoptosis-Regulating Proteins.
BCL-X. See Apoptosis-Regulating Proteins.
ß-Catenin. This is a widely expressed 90-kDa protein with a key role in cell adhesion and Wingless-type (Wnt) signaling. At the cell membrane site, β-catenin is complexed with E-cadherin (see below) to generate cell adhesion complexes that assure the structural integrity of many epithelial tissues. β-catenin increases in the nucleus when Wnt-driven carcinogenesis starts. In the thyroid gland, various alterations have been described, including decreased expression of β-catenin in widely invasive tumors; a shift from a membranous to a cytoplasmic/nuclear location; and presence in the nuclear pseudoinclusions of papillary carcinoma (5). It

has been claimed, however, that the key event in determining the degree of differentiation of thyroid carcinomas is E-cadherin loss rather than β-catenin alterations (6).

Blood Group Antigens. See Lewis-Type Antigens.

Calcitonin. See chapter 1.

Calcitonin Gene-Related Peptide. See chapter 1.

Carcinoembryonic Antigen (CEA). This is a glycoprotein of heterogeneous composition (molecular weight [MW], 200,000) that is normally detected in the glycocalix of fetal epithelial cells, particularly those of a mucin-secreting glandular nature. It is detectable only in small amounts in normal adult cells and benign tumors but is present in large quantities in carcinomas, particularly in adenocarcinomas of the digestive tract (including pancreas) and lung. In the thyroid gland, it is consistently expressed by thyroid medullary carcinoma.

Because CEA is primarily expressed by fetal tissues and malignant tumors, it is referred to as an oncofetal antigen. Monoclonal antibodies offer a greater degree of tumor specificity than conventional antisera. These are divided into five major groups according to the epitopes they recognize.

Cathepsins. Cathepsins B and D are endogenous proteinases that are linked to tumor progression at various sites. In the thyroid gland, there is greater staining intensity in follicular carcinomas than in follicular adenomas, especially when the former are widely invasive (7).

CD10. This molecule, originally described in lymphoid cells, is found in a wide variety of nonlymphoid tissues and tumors. In the thyroid gland, it characteristically stains the biotin-rich morules of optically clear nuclei (8).

CD15. This monocyte/granulocyte-related marker, typically present in the Reed-Sternberg cells of Hodgkin lymphoma, is detectable in most papillary carcinomas but only exceptionally in other malignant tumors and benign conditions of the thyroid gland (9).

CD26. This molecule, also known as dipeptidyl aminopeptidase IV, is a marker of proliferation. As such, it is barely detectable in the normal adult thyroid gland but present in both benign and malignant thyroid conditions accompanied by increased proliferation (10).

CD31. This antibody identifies the hematopoietic progenitor antigen ER-MP12, which is identical to the vascular endothelial adhesion molecule PECAM-1. It has emerged as one of the most useful markers of endothelial cells. As such, it is used for the detection of vascular invasion in thyroid tumors.

CD44. The variant isoform of CD44, known as CD44v6, has been detected more frequently in papillary than in follicular carcinomas and, among the former, in those associated with nodal metastases than in those without them (11).

CD98. CD98 is a component of the large neutral amino acid transporter (a cell surface amino acid transporter). Its expression is increased in a variety of carcinomas. In the thyroid gland, it is decreased in papillary carcinoma and Hashimoto thyroiditis (12).

Ceruloplasmin. Ceruloplasmin, a metal-binding serum glycoprotein, contains over 95 percent of the total serum copper in humans and acts as a copper transport protein. A study claiming that ceruloplasmin is not detectable immunohistochemically in the normal thyroid gland or in benign lesions but consistently expressed in follicular and papillary carcinomas (13) has not been independently confirmed (14). Similar negative conclusions have been expressed regarding the diagnostic value of two other metal-binding proteins, lactoferrin and transferrin (14).

Chromogranin. The chromogranin family is composed of acidic glycoproteins (MW, 20,000 to 100,000) located in the soluble fraction of neurosecretory granules. The most abundant is chromogranin A (MW, 75,000). Two others have been named chromogranin B (or secretogranin I) and chromogranin C (or secretogranin II). Nearly all types of neuroendocrine tumors are reactive, making the chromogranin stain the most widely used "panendocrine" marker.

Claudins. Claudins and occludins are integral components of tight junctions and are deregulated in a variety of malignant tumors. They are present in the normal thyroid gland and most thyroid neoplasms, and the differences among them are not particularly informative or useful. As expected, their expression is reduced in poorly differentiated and undifferentiated carcinomas (15).

Collagenase. The 72-kDa type IV collagenase (matrix metalloproteinase-2) is a neutral metalloproteinase that initiates the degradation of type IV collagen in the basement membranes. In the thyroid gland, it is virtually absent in normal thyroid tissue and nodular hyperplasia, while present in various types of carcinomas. Focal positivity has also been detected in Hashimoto thyroiditis and other conditions associated with inflammation, fibrosis, and distortion of the follicles (16).

Cyclooxigenase-2 (COX-2). This molecule, thought to play a role in carcinogenesis and carcinoma development, is almost absent in the normal thyroid gland but present to some extent in benign and malignant tumors, particularly papillary carcinoma (its amount correlating with increasing patient age) (17,18).

Cytokeratins. See Keratins.

E-Cadherin. E-cadherin is a calcium-dependent cell adhesion molecule that plays a major role in the maintenance of intercellular junctions in normal epithelial cells by forming a complex with β-catenin. The expression of this molecule is downregulated in thyroid tumors, especially in widely invasive ones (19). It has been claimed that the loss of E-cadherin is the key event in determining the degree of differentiation of thyroid carcinomas (6).

Emerin. Emerin is a nuclear membrane-associated protein. Its immunohistochemical detection allows a finer evaluation of the irregularities of the nuclear membrane that are associated with papillary carcinoma in both histologic and cytologic preparations (20,21).

Epidermal Growth Factor (EGF). EGF, one of the best known growth factors, is usually not evident at the immunohistochemical level in normal follicles, whereas both benign and malignant lesions contain a high percentage of positive cells, but apparently without significant differences among the two (22). *Epidermal growth factor receptor (EGFR)* shows a similar degree of expression among the various types of carcinoma, but with alterations of the functional polarization when compared with the normal gland (23). Some authors have found negativity in most adenomas (13).

Estrogen Receptors. See Hormone Receptors.

Fibrillin. Fibrillin is an extracellular matrix glycoprotein. It constitutes the main component of microfibrils, which are thought to support cell attachment and to influence cell differentiation and migration. It is expressed weakly and focally in the normal gland and in follicular tumors, but it is conspicuously present in all other types of carcinomas, particularly those of papillary type (24).

Galectin. The galectins constitute a family of lactose-binding soluble lectins sharing an affinity for β-galactoside residues and a significant sequence similarity in their carbohydrate-binding site. They have been implicated in cell growth and differentiation, intercellular recognition, and adhesion. They also appear to play a role in malignant transformation and metastases (25). The most extensively studied galectins are galectin-1 and galectin-3.

Increased galectin expression has been found in several carcinoma types, including those arising in the thyroid gland, endometrium, head and neck, kidney, bladder, large bowel, and pancreas. Galectin-3 has been studied in great detail in the thyroid gland, where it stains carcinomas (especially those of papillary type) in a stronger and more consistent fashion than adenomas (25,26). Alas, it is also often expressed (albeit focally) in the follicles of lymphocytic/Hashimoto thyroiditis, nodular hyperplasia, and follicular adenoma (27,28). Among the papillary carcinomas, it is said to be expressed in greater amounts in tumors associated with metastases than in those lacking them, a fact that does not fit well with the observation than the metastatic foci themselves tend to show lesser expression of galectin-3 than the corresponding primary tumors (28). Also perplexing is the fact that galectin-7 (another member of the galectins family) is more likely to be downregulated in follicular adenomas than in carcinomas (29). It has been argued that many of the reported differences observed with galectin-3 immunostaining among the various series are due to differences in methodology, and that a strict adherence to a set of technical requirements may be necessary to optimize the results (30).

Galectin-3 can be used alone or as part of a battery which may also include HBME-1, keratin 19, and thyroid peroxidase (31).

Ghrelin. Ghrelin is a growth hormone-releasing hormone produced by gastroenteropancreatic endocrine cells, hypothalamus, and pituitary gland. It is expressed in the fetal but not in the adult thyroid gland, and re-expressed in thyroid tumors, particularly medullary carcinoma, where it was first detected (32).

HBME-1. This monoclonal antibody recognizes an unknown antigen originally detected on the microvilli of mesothelial cells, and present in the majority of mesotheliomas. In the thyroid gland, it is said to be the most sensitive marker of malignancy. In the series of de Matos et al. (33), it was expressed in 94 percent of papillary carcinomas and 63 percent of follicular carcinomas. It is said to be particularly useful when used in conjunction with CK19 and galectin-3 (33,34). Its specificity is not absolute, however, since it sometimes also stains the abnormal follicles of Hashimoto thyroiditis or those entrapped in fibrous tissue.

Her-2Neu (c-erbB2). This proto-oncogene is expressed in nearly all medullary thyroid carcinomas, in about half of papillary carcinomas, and in 16 percent of undifferentiated carcinomas but not in follicular adenomas or follicular carcinomas (35,36).

Hormone Receptors. Several epidemiologic and experimental studies suggest a possible role of sex steroids in the pathogenesis or development of various human thyroid disorders (37). This impression is supported by the fact that labeling for both estrogen receptor (ER)-alpha and ER-beta is significantly higher in hyperplastic and neoplastic conditions than in the normal gland, which shows positivity in only a few follicular cells (38). In one study, ER expression was largely restricted to papillary carcinomas, whereas in another, there was a much wider distribution (39). Progesterone receptor (PR) is also present in many types of thyroid tumor (39).

Insulin-Like Growth Factor 1 (IGF-1). IGF-1 is hardly detectable in the normal thyroid gland but is commonly expressed in all types of benign and malignant proliferative processes of this organ (40,41)

Intermediate Filaments. This family of cytoplasmic filaments is so named because their diameter (8 to 10 nm) is intermediate between the diameters of actin (thin) and tubulin (thick). There are at least five biochemically and immunologically distinct types: cytokeratins, vimentin, desmin, glial fibrillary acidic protein, and neurofilaments (see individual headings).

Although originally these filaments were thought to be expressed in a stable, cell type-specific and differentiation-dependent fashion, it has been shown that their coexpression is a common phenomenon in fetal and neoplastic tissues.

Keratins. Keratins or cytokeratins (CKs) are a family of water-insoluble, intracellular fibrous proteins present in almost all epithelia. At least 20 well-defined subclasses of keratins have been identified on the basis of their molecular weight (ranging from 40,000 to 68,000) and isoelectric pH value (ranging from 5 to 8). This combination constitutes the so-called keratin catalog, which shows a tissue-specific distribution throughout the epithelia and which can be mapped using a battery of monoclonal antibodies. For scanning purposes, several of these antibodies are combined in the form of "cocktails" (such as AE1/AE3).

The normal thyroid gland strongly expresses simple epithelial-type CK7 and CK18 and, to a lesser degree, CK8 and CK19, but not stratified epithelial-type CKs (42). Papillary and follicular carcinomas share the expression of simple epithelial-type CK7, CK8, CK18, and CK19. CK19 is expressed particularly strongly by papillary carcinomas. The latter also usually express stratified-type CKs 5/6 and CK13. This reactivity pattern of papillary carcinoma is useful for identifying small tumor foci not easily found by conventional histologic examination and is maintained in the metastatic foci. Unfortunately, this rather distinct pattern of CK distribution in papillary carcinoma is often shared, at least focally, by the follicles of Hashimoto thyroiditis (43).

Ki-67. Ki-67 is an antigen that corresponds to a nuclear nonhistone protein expressed by cells in the proliferative phases G1, G2, M, and S. The original antibody against this marker worked only in fresh frozen sections, but monoclonal antibodies have subsequently been developed that detect formalin-resistant epitopes (MIB-1 and MIB-3). In the thyroid gland, the proliferative index, as measured with this marker, is higher in nodular and diffuse hyperplasia than in the normal gland. Among the neoplasms, the index is higher in follicular than in papillary carcinomas, and the highest index is found in undifferentiated carcinomas (44).

Lactoferrin. See Ceruloplasmin.

Laminin. This structural protein (MW, 900,000) is one of the two major components of the basement membrane, together with type IV collagen (see Basement Membrane Components). It is present in a linear fashion around normal thyroid follicles, and is preserved in benign lesions and well-differentiated carcinomas. Conversely, it is partially or completely lost in the solid areas of all types of thyroid carcinomas (45)

Leu-7. The antibody directed against this marker (initially described in a subset of lymphocytes) is expressed only weakly and focally in the normal thyroid gland and in follicular adenomas, but diffusely and with greater intensity in follicular and papillary carcinomas (46). The differences, however, are not large enough to be of diagnostic use (47). Interestingly, this marker is negative in medullary carcinoma (46).

Lewis-Type Antigens. Lewis type 1 (Lewis a, sialyl Lewis a, and Lewis B) and Lewis type 2 (precursor type 2, H type 2, Lexis x, sialyl Lewis x, and Lewis y) antigens are almost always absent from the normal thyroid gland and benign disorders, while often expressed in malignant tumors. In particular, expression of sialyl Lewis x is closely associated with papillary carcinoma (see also Simple Mucin-Type Antigens) (48).

MCl-1. See Apoptosis-Regulating proteins.

Metal-Binding Proteins. See Ceruloplasmin.

MIB-1. See Ki-67.

Mitochondrial Antigens. Two of the monoclonal antibodies currently available for the detection of mitochondrial antigens (and therefore useful for the identification of mitochondria-rich cells/oncocytes) are mES13, originally produced against bacterially expressed BACB *RAS* p21, and 113.1, obtained using Raji Burkitt lymphoma cells as the immunogen.

Mucin-Type Antigens. See Simple Mucin-Type Antigens.

Napsin A. Napsin A is an aspartic proteinase involved in the maturation of surfactant protein B. It is detected in the cytoplasm of type 2 pneumocytes and alveolar macrophages, and is a putative marker for pulmonary adenocarcinoma. Thyroid tumors are generally negative for this marker, although a minority of anaplastic, poorly differentiated, and papillary carcinomas do stain. Among the latter, a higher degree of positivity is said to be exhibited by papillary carcinomas with tall cell or micropapillary features (49,50).

Niban. Niban, a marker of renal carcinogenesis in experimental animals, is expressed in vari-

ous types of renal cell carcinoma in humans. It is not detected in the normal thyroid gland, but is found in oncocytic tumors and papillary carcinoma (less so in follicular carcinomas) (51).

Occludin. See Claudins.

p27kip1. This cell cycle inhibitory protein is expressed more strongly in the normal thyroid gland than in tumors, and in follicular adenomas or classic PTCs than in follicular carcinomas. It is present at very low levels in poorly differentiated and undifferentiated carcinomas (52,53).

p53. Mutations of the *p53* tumor-suppressor gene represent the most common genetic alteration in human tumors. The product of this gene is a nuclear protein thought to be involved in the control of the cell cycle and apoptosis, and the maintenance of genomic stability. The altered protein product of the mutant gene has an extended half-life and can be detected with immunohistochemical techniques. It should be noted, however, that accumulation of the protein can also occur as a result of epigenetic changes, and therefore, it is not an obligatory indicator of a gene mutation.

In the thyroid gland, as in most other sites, accumulation of p53 protein correlates with tumor differentiation (54). In one study, p53 was found to be always positive in undifferentiated carcinomas, less commonly positive in poorly differentiated or widely invasive follicular carcinomas, and consistently negative in the normal gland, benign tumors, follicular carcinomas, and papillary carcinomas (55). In another series, occult and intrathyroidal papillary carcinomas were usually negative, whereas their high-risk counterparts (extrathyroidal and tall cell papillary carcinoma) often overexpressed this product (55).

p63. This is a homolog of p53 that is consistently expressed by basal/stem cells of stratified epithelium, and myoepithelial cells of breast and salivary glands. Six isoforms exist, the functions of which are largely unknown.

PDCD4. Programmed cell death 4 (*PDCD4*) is a tumor suppressor gene whose expression is controlled by miR-21. Its downregulation is associated with undifferentiated cancer phenotypes and more advanced tumor stages, thus suggesting a role in thyroid carcinogenesis (56).

PPARγ. Peroxisomal proliferator-activated receptor gamma (PPARγ, also known as NR1C3) is a member of a nuclear hormone receptor superfamily that includes thyroid hormone, retinoic acid, and androgen and estrogen receptors. PPARγ is expressed at high levels in adipose tissue, where genes regulated by PPARγ control adipocyte function and differentiation. It is also expressed in muscle cells, vascular cells, macrophages, and various epithelial cells (e.g., mammary gland and colon). PPARγ is overexpressed in follicular adenomas and carcinomas carrying *PAX8/PPARγ* rearrangements. Strong nuclear immunoreactivity for PPARγ is considered a surrogate marker for the chromosomal rearrangement, but the correlation with immunohistochemistry is not perfect and should be confirmed by molecular methods (e.g., reverse transcriptase-polymerase chain reaction [RT-PCR]) (57,58).

P-Glycoprotein. This glycoprotein, which is associated with tumor multidrug resistance, is present in both benign and malignant thyroid tumors. The frequency of expression among these two groups is too small, however, to be of any diagnostic significance (59).

PAX8. See under Thyroid Transcription Factor-1 (TTF-1) and Other Transcription Factors.

Peroxidase. See Thyroid Peroxidase.

Progesterone Receptors. See Hormone Receptors.

Retinoblastoma. By immunohistochemistry, the protein product of this tumor-suppressor gene is expressed in the normal thyroid gland and in benign conditions, while absent in most malignant tumors, especially papillary carcinoma (60).

Retinoic Acid Receptor Betaprotein (RARß). This molecule, which has pleiotropic effects on epithelial cell growth and differentiation, is expressed in the nuclei of the follicular cells of normal thyroid gland and is markedly decreased in papillary carcinoma (61).

S-100 Protein. This is a family of acidic, dimeric calcium-binding proteins (MW, 21,000) composed of different combinations of alpha and beta subunits. It was first isolated in the central nervous system. A quantitative differentiation distribution has been found between the alpha and beta forms. It has both nuclear and cytoplasmic localization. An apparently positive stain for this marker showing only a cytoplasmic pattern should be questioned.

The wide expression of this antigen has substantially diminished its diagnostic utility.

In the thyroid gland, it is expressed in most papillary and follicular carcinomas, but not in insular or undifferentiated carcinomas (62). Interestingly, S-100A2, a member of the S-100 protein family, is expressed in most cases of undifferentiated carcinoma (63), whereas S-100A4, another family member, seems to be associated with the presence of metastases in papillary microcarcinoma (64).

Sialic Acid-Dependent Carbohydrate Epitope. Molecules containing this epitope, as recognized with the molecular antibody FB21, are seen in the cells of almost all follicular carcinomas, but also in about half of the papillary carcinomas and in a lesser number of follicular adenomas (65).

Syndecan-1. This proteoglycan, which regulates cell adhesion, is expressed in the stromal component of well-differentiated thyroid carcinomas (especially large papillary carcinomas) and in the epithelial tumor cells of poorly differentiated and undifferentiated thyroid carcinomas (66).

Simple Mucin-Type Antigens. This group of antigens, comprising T, Tn, and sialyl Tn, is almost always absent from the normal thyroid gland and benign disorders, while often expressed in malignant tumors, especially papillary carcinoma (see also Lewis-Type Antigens) (48).

Sodium Iodide Symporter (NIS). This protein mediates active iodide uptake across the basal membrane of thyroid follicles, resulting in a iodide concentration 20- to 40-fold higher than that in plasma. Levels of this molecule are higher in the normal thyroid gland and in benign conditions than in carcinomas (67).

T3 (Triiodothyronine) and T4 (Thyroxine). These are the two major thyroid hormones normally incorporated into thyroglobulin in the intraluminal colloid and released from it upon demand. Both of these hormones can be detected immunohistochemically, but this has been generally replaced by the search for thyroglobulin.

Thyroglobulin. Thyroglobulin is a large glycoprotein (MW, 670,000) formed by two identical subunits. It is produced by the thyroid follicular cells and serves as the substratum for iodination and hormonogenesis. It is a specific marker of thyroid differentiation and is widely used in the evaluation of thyroid neoplasms.

It has been suggested that the thyroglobulin produced by tumors is different from that manufactured by the normal gland, based on analysis of reactivity to various lectins (68,69). A pitfall associated with the interpretation of thyroglobulin immunostaining is the fact that this molecule tends to leak out from the follicle into the surrounding tissues, where it can be incorporated into the cytoplasm of other cell types that may be present (such as metastatic carcinoma or malignant lymphoma) and cause them to become spuriously positive (70).

Thyroid Peroxidase. Thyroid peroxidase (thyroperoxidase) is present in all normal follicular cells. In fetuses and infants, the staining is more intense on the apical side, whereas in the adult and elderly, it is often present in the form of a perinuclear ring (71). This marker is retained in adenomas but tends to be underexpressed in well-differentiated carcinomas and may be absent in lesser differentiated tumors (72–74).

Thyroid Transcription Factor-1 (TTF-1) and Other Transcription Factors. TTF-1 (also known as Nkx2-1) is a nuclear transcription factor which, together with TTF-2 (also known as Foxe-1), PAX8, and Hhex, is essential for thyroid organogenesis and differentiation (75,76). This DNA-binding protein was first identified in thyrocytes (hence its name) and later in lung pneumocytes. It is consistently expressed in all types of primary and metastatic thyroid carcinomas (including medullary carcinoma), except for the undifferentiated type (77). It is also present in most cases of lung carcinoma (including the small cell neuroendocrine type), and has become one of the most useful markers in the differentiation of lung carcinoma from carcinomas of other sites and from mesotheliomas, both in histologic sections and cytologic preparations. Unfortunately, staining for TTF-1 has also been documented in high-grade neuroendocrine carcinomas of nonpulmonary origin, and sporadically in Merkel cell carcinoma, ovarian epithelial neoplasms, and nephroblastomas (78–80). TTF-1

is not expressed in normal, hyperplastic, or adenomatous parathyroid tissue (81).

PAX8 may become of great potential diagnostic use if the claim that it stains almost 80 percent of undifferentiated thyroid carcinomas is confirmed (82).

Topoisomerase II. This enzyme affects replications, transcriptions, and chromosome segregation. In the thyroid gland, the presence of this marker correlates with tumor histology, since it is more frequently expressed in tumors associated with an aggressive clinical course (83).

Transferrin. See Ceruloplasmin.

Transforming Growth Factor-ß1 (TGFß1). This is a homodimeric protein present in virtually all cell types, of which three isoforms exist. They usually stimulate the growth of mesenchymal cells but inhibit epithelial cell proliferation. In the thyroid gland, there is a significantly higher expression of TGFβ1 in neoplasms than in the normal gland, and a higher prevalence in malignant tumors than in adenomatous lesions (84).

Type I Blood Group Antigen. Immunohistochemical expression of this antigen, which is dependent on the activity of alpha 2,3 sialyltransferase, is absent in the normal thyroid gland and in most follicular tumors, but usually expressed in papillary carcinoma (when using monoclonal antibodies against DU-PAN-2) (85).

Vascular Endothelial Growth Factor-D (VEGF-D). This molecule is known to promote lymphangiogenesis, which in turn is thought to promote lymph node metastases. In accordance with this theory, increased levels of VEGF-D have been correlated with nodal metastases in papillary carcinoma (86).

Vimentin. Vimentin, one of the major intermediate filaments, may be expressed in normal thyroid follicular cells, although not as intensely as in some tumors derived from them (42).

REFERENCES

1. Rüschoff J, Prasser C, Cortez T, Höhne HM, Hohenberger W, Hofstädter F. Diagnostic value of AgNOR staining in follicular cell neoplasms of the thyroid: comparison of evaluation methods and nucleolar features. Am J Surg Pathol 1993;17:1281-8.

2. Branet F, Brousset P, Krajewski S, et al. Expression of the cell death-inducing gene bax in carcinomas developed from the follicular cells of the thyroid gland. J Clin Endocrinol Metab 1996;81:2726-30.

3. Katoh R, Muramatsu A, Kawaoi A, et al. Alteration of the basement membrane in human thyroid diseases: an immunohistochemical study of type IV collagen, laminin and heparan sulphate proteoglycan. Virchows Arch A Pathol Anat Histopathol 1993;423:417-24.

4. Daa T, Kodama M, Kashima K, Yokoyama S, Nakayama I, Noguchi S. Identification of basic fibroblast growth factor in papillary carcinoma of the thyroid. Acta Pathol Jpn 1993;43:582-9.

5. Rezk S, Brynes RK, Nelson V, et al. Beta-catenin expression in thyroid follicular lesions: potential role in nuclear envelope changes in papillary carcinomas. Endocr Pathol 2004;15:329-37.

6. Rocha AS, Soares P, Fonseca E, Cameselle-Teijeiro J, Oliveira MC, Sobrinho-Simões M. E-cadherin loss rather than beta-catenin alterations is a common feature of poorly differentiated thyroid carcinomas. Histopathology 2003;42:580-7.

7. Ruhoy SM, Clarke MR. Cathepsin B and cathepsin D expression in follicular adenomas and carcinomas of the thyroid gland. Endocr Pathol 1997;8:49-57.

8. Cameselle-Teijeiro J, Alberte-Lista L, Chiarelli S, et al. CD10 is a characteristic marker of tumors forming morules with biotin-rich, optically clear nuclei that occur in different organs. Histopathology 2008;52:389-92.

9. Imamura Y, Fukuda M. CD15 (C3D-1) immunoreactivity in normal, benign and malignant thyroid lesions. Appl Immunohistochem Mol Morphol 1998;6:181-6.

10. Lima MA, Gontijo VA, Schmitt FC. CD26 (dipeptidyl aminopeptidase IV) expression in normal and diseased human thyroid glands. Endocr Pathol 1998;9:43-52.

11. Gu J, Daa T, Kashima K, Yokoyama S, Nakayama I, Noguchi S. Expression of splice variants of CD44 in thyroid neoplasms derived from follicular cells. Pathol Int 1998;48:184-90.

12. Anderson CE, Graham C, Herriot MM, Kamel HM, Salter DM. CD98 expression is decreased

in papillary carcinoma of the thyroid and Hashimoto's thyroiditis. Histopathology 2009;55:6836.

13. Song B. Immunohistochemical demonstration of epidermal growth factor receptor and ceruloplasmin in thyroid diseases. Acta Pathol Jpn 1991;41:336-43.

14. Raphael SJ, Asa SL. Immunohistochemical localization of metal binding proteins in thyroid tissues and tumors. Endocr Pathol 1992;3:182-7.

15. Tzelepi VN, Tsamandas AC, Vlotinou HD, Vagianos CE, Scopa CD. Tight junctions in thyroid carcinogenesis: diverse expression of claudin-1, claudin-4, claudin-7 and occludin in thyroid neoplasms. Mod Pathol 2008;21:22-30.

16. Campo E, Merino MJ, Liotta L, Neumann R, Stetler-Stevenson W. Distribution of the 72-kd typeIV collagenase in non-neoplastic thyroid tissue. Hum Pathol 1992;23:1395-401

17. Ito Y, Yoshida H, Nakano K, et al. Cyclooxygenase-2 expression in thyroid neoplasms. Histopathology 2003;42:492-7.

18. Siironen P, Ristimäki A, Nordling S, Louhimo J, Haapiainen R, Haglund C. Expression of COX-2 is increased with age in papillary thyroid cancer. Histopathology 2004;44:490-7.

19. Kato N, Tsuchiya T, Tamura G, Motoyama T. E-cadherin expression in follicular carcinoma of the thyroid. Pathol Int 2002;52:13-8.

20. Asioli S, Bussolati G. Emerin immunohistochemistry reveals diagnostic features of nuclear membrane arrangement in thyroid lesions. Histopathology 2009;54:571-9.

21. Asioli S, Maletta F, Pacchioni D, Lupo R, Bussolati G. Cytological detection of papillary thyroid carcinomas by nuclear membrane decoration with emerin staining. Virchows Arch 2010;457:43-51.

22. Mizukami Y, Nonomura A, Hashimoto T, et al. Immunohistochemical demonstration of epidermal growth factor and c-myc oncogene product in normal, benign and malignant thyroid tissues. Histopathology 1991;18:11-8.

23. Westermark K, Lundqvist M, Wallin G, et al. EGF-receptors in human normal and pathological thyroid tissue. Histopathology 1996;28:221-7.

24. Tseleni-Balafouta S, Gakiopoulou H, Fanourakis G, et al. Fibrillin expression and localization in various types of carcinomas of the thyroid gland. Mod Pathol 2006;19:695-700.

25. Xu XC, el-Naggar AK, Lotan R. Differential expression of galectin-1 and galectin-3 in thyroid tumors. Potential diagnostic implications. Am J Pathol 1995;147:815-22.

26. Volante M, Bozzalla-Cassione F, Orlandi F, Papotti M. Diagnostic role of galectin-3 in follicular thyroid tumors. Virchows Arch 2004;444:309-12.

27. Herrmann ME, LiVolsi VA, Pasha TL, Roberts SA, Wojcik EM, Baloch ZW. Immunohistochemical expression of galectin-3 in benign and malignant thyroid lesions. Arch Pathol Lab Med 2002;126:710-3.

28. Kawachi K, Matsushita Y, Yonezawa S, et al. Galectin-3 expression in various thyroid neoplasms and its possible role in metastasis formation. Hum Pathol 2000;31:428-33.

29. Rorive S, Eddafali B, Fernández S, et al. Changes in galectin-7 and cytokeratin-19 expression during the progression of malignancy in thyroid tumors: diagnostic and biological implications. Mod Pathol 2002;15:1294-301.

30. Bartolazzi A, Bellotti C, Sciacchitano S. Methodology and technical requirements of the galectin-3 test for the preoperative characterization of thyroid nodules. Appl Immunohistochem Mol Morphol 2012;20:2-7.

31. Weber KB, Shroyer KR, Heinz DE, Nawaz S, Said MS, Haugen BR. The use of a combination of galectin-3 and thyroid peroxidase for the diagnosis and prognosis of thyroid cancer. Am J Clin Pathol 2004;122:524-31.

32. Volante M, Allia E, Fulcheri E, et al. Ghrelin in fetal thyroid and follicular tumors and cell lines: expression and effects on tumor growth. Am J Pathol 2003;162:645-54.

33. de Matos PS, Ferreira AP, de Olivera Facuri F, Assumpção LV, Metze K, Ward LS. Usefulness of HBME-1, cytokeratin 19 and galectin-3 immunostaining in the diagnosis of thyroid malignancy. Histopathology 2005;47:391-401.

34. Rossi ED, Raffaelli M, Mule' A, et al. Simultaneous immunohistochemical expression of HBME-1 and galectin-3 differentiates papillary carcinomas from hyperfunctioning lesions of the thyroid. Histopathology 2006;48:795-800.

35. Utrilla JC, Martín-Lacave I, San Martín MV, Fernández-Santos JM, Galera-Davidson H. Expression of c-erbB-2 oncoprotein in human thyroid tumours. Histopathology 1999;34:60-5.

36. Elliott DD, Sherman SI, Busaidy NL, et al. Growth factor receptors expression in anaplastic thyroid carcinoma: potential markers for therapeutic stratification. Hum Pathol 2008;39:15-20.

37. van Hoeven KH, Menendez-Botet CJ, Strong EW, Huvos AG. Estrogen and progesterone receptor content in human thyroid disease. Am J Clin Pathol 1993;99:175-81.

38. Kawabata W, Suzuki T, Moriya T, et al. Estrogen receptors (alpha and beta) and 17beta-hydroxysteroid dehydrogenase type 1 and 2 in thyroid disorders: possible in situ estrogen synthesis and actions. Mod Pathol 2003;16:437-44.

39. Bur M, Shiraki W, Masood S. Estrogen and progesterone receptor detection in neoplastic and non-neoplastic thyroid tissues. Mod Pathol 1993;6:469-72.

40. Maiorano E, Ciampolillo A, Viale G, et al. Insulin-like growth factor 1 expression in thyroid tumors. Appl Immunohistochem Mol Morphol 2000;8:110-9.

41. Frittitta L, Sciacca L, Catalfamo R, et al. Functional insulin receptors are overexpressed in thyroid tumors: is this an early event in thyroid tumorigenesis? Cancer 1999;85:492-8.

42. Henzen-Longmans SC, Mullink H, Ramaekers FC, Tadema T, Meijer CJ. Expression of cytokeratins and vimentin in epithelial cells of normal and pathologic thyroid tissue. Virchows Arch 1987;410:347-54.

43. Fonseca E, Nesland JM, Höie J, Sobrinho-Simões M. Pattern of expression of intermediate cytokeratin filaments in the thyroid gland: an immunohistochemical study of simple and stratified epithelial-type cytokeratins. VIrchows Arch 1997;430:239-45.

44. Katoh R, Bray CE, Suzuki K, et al. Growth activity in hyperplastic and neoplastic human thyroid determined by an immunohistochemical staining procedure using monoclonal antibody MIB-1. Hum Pathol 1995;26:139-46.

45. Campo E. Pérez M, Charonis AA Axiotis CA, Merino MJ. Patterns of basement membrane lamin distribution in non-neoplastic thyroid tissue. Mod Pathol 1992;5:540-6.

46. Ghali VS, Jiménez EJ, Garciá RL. Distribution of Leu-7 antigen (HNK-1) in thyroid tumors: its usefulness as a diagnostic marker for follicular and papillary carcinomas. Hum Pathol 1992;23:21-5.

47. Loy TS, Darkow GV, Spollen LE, Diaz-Arias AA. Immunostaining for Leu-7 in the diagnosis of thyroid carcinoma. Arch Pathol Lab Med 1994;118:172-4.

48. Fonseca E, Castanhas S, Sobrinho-Simões M. Expression of simple mucin type antigens and lewis type 1 and type 2 chain antigens in the thyroid gland: an immunohistochemical study of normal thyroid tissues, benign lesions, and malignant tumors. Endocr Pathol 1996;7:291-301.

49. Bishop JA, Sharma R, Illei PB. Napsin A and thyroid transcription factor-1 expression in carcinomas of the lung, breast, pancreas, colon, kidney, thyroid, and malignant mesothelioma. Hum Pathol 2010;4:20-5.

50. Chernock RD, El-Mofty SK, Becker N, Lewis JS Jr. Napsin A expression in anaplastic, poorly differentiated, and micropapillary pattern thyroid carcinomas. Am J Surg Pathol 2013;37:1215-22.

489

51. Matsumoto F, Fujii H, Abe M, et al. A novel tumor marker, Niban, is expressed in subsets of thyroid tumors and Hashimoto's thyroiditis. Hum Pathol 2006;37:1592-600.

52. Erickson LA, Jin L, Wollan PC, Thompson GB, van Heerden J, Lloyd RV. Expression of p27kip1 and Ki-67 in benign and malignant thyroid tumors. Mod Pathol 1998;11:169-74.

53. Tallini G, Garciá-Rostán G, Herrero A, et al. Downregulation of p27Kip1 and Ki67/Mib1 labeling index support the classification of thyroid carcinoma into prognostically relevant categories. Am J Surg Pathol 1999;23:678-85.

54. Dobashi Y, Sakamoto A, Sugimura H, et al. Overexpression of p53 as a possible prognostic factor in human thyroid carcinoma. Am J Surg Pathol 1993;17:375-81.

55. Hosal SA, Apel RL, Freeman JL, et al. Immunohistochemical localization of p53 in human thyroid neoplasms: correlation with biological behavior. Endocr Pathol 1997;8:21-8.

56. Pennelli G, Fassan M, Mian C, et al. PDCD4 expression in thyroid neoplasia. Virchows Arch 2013;462:95-100.

57. Nikiforova MN, Biddinger PW, Caudill CM, Kroll TG, Nikiforov YE. PAX8-PPARgamma rearrangement in thyroid tumors: RT-PCR and immunohistochemical analyses. Am J Surg Pathol 2002;26:1016-23.

58. Sahin M, Allard BL, Yates M, et al. PPARgamma staining as a surrogate for PAX8/PPARgamma fusion oncogene expression in follicular neoplasms: clinicopathological correlation and histopathological diagnostic value. J Clin Endocrinol Metab 2005;90:463-8.

59. Loy TS, Gelven PL, Mullins D, Diaz-Arias AA. Immunostaining for P-glycoprotein in the diagnosis of thyroid carcinomas. Mod Pathol 1992;5:200-2.

60. Anwar F, Emond MJ, Schmidt RA, Hwang HC, Bronner MP. Retinoblastoma expression in thyroid neoplasms. Mod Pathol 2000;13:562-9.

61. Rochaix P, Monteil-Onteniente S, Rochette-Egly C, Caratero C, Voigt JJ, Jozan S. Reduced expression of retinoic acid receptor beta protein (RAR beta) in human papillary thyroid carcinoma: immunohistochemical and western blot study. Histopathology 1998;33:337-43.

62. Nishimura R, Yokose T, Mukai K. S-100 protein is a differentiation marker in thyroid carcinoma of follicular cell origin: an immunohistochemical study. Pathol Int 1997;47:673-9.

63. Ito Y, Yoshida H, Tomoda C, et al. Expression of S100A2 and S100A6 in thyroid carcinomas. Histopathology 2005;46:569-75.

64. Min HS, Choe G, Kim SW, et al. S100A4 expression is associated with lymph node metastasis in papillary microcarcinoma of the thyroid. Mod Pathol 2008;21:748-55.

65. Nozawa Y, Ami H, Suzuki S, Tuchiya A, Abe R, Abe M. Distribution of sialic acid-dependent carbohydrate epitope in thyroid tumors: immunoreactivity of FB21 in paraffin-embedded tissue sections. Pathol Int 1999;49:403-7.

66. Ito Y, Yoshida H, Nakano K, et al. Syndecan-1 expression in thyroid carcinoma: stromal expression followed by epithelial expression is significantly correlated with dedifferentiation. Histopathology 2003;43:157-64.

67. Lin JD, Hsueh C, Chao TC, Weng HF. Expression of sodium iodide symporter in benign and malignant human thyroid tissues. Endocr Pathol 2001;12:15-21.

68. Maruyama M, Kato R, Kobayashi S, Kasuga Y. A method to differentiate between thyroglobulin derived from normal thyroid tissue and from thyroid carcinoma based on analysis of reactivity to lectins. Arch Pathol Lab Med 1998;122:715-20.

69. Magro G, Perissinotto D, Schiappacassi M, et al. Proteomic and postproteomic characterization of keratan sulfate-glycanated isoforms of thyroglobulin and transferrin uniquely elaborated by papillary thyroid carcinomas. Am J Pathol 2003;163:183-96.

70. Rosai J, Carcangiu ML. Pitfalls in the diagnosis of thyroid neoplasms. Pathol Res Pract 1987;182:169-79.

71. Lima MA, Gontijo VA, Schmitt FC. Thyroid peroxidase and thyroglobulin expression in normal human thyroid glands. Endocr Pathol 1998;9:333-8.

72. Savin S, Cvejic D, Isic T, Paunovic I, Tatic S, Havelka M. Thyroid peroxidase and galectin-3 immunostaining in differentiated thyroid carcinoma with clinicopathologic correlation. Hum Pathol 2008;39:1656-63.

73. De Micco C, Ruf J, Chrestian MA, Gros N, Henry JF, Carayon P. Immunohistochemical study of thyroid peroxidase in normal, hyperplastic, and neoplastic human thyroid tissues. Cancer 1991;67:3036-41.

74. Yamashita H, Noguchi S, Murakami N, Adachi M, Maruta J. Immunohistological differentiation of benign thyroid follicular cell tumors from malignant ones: usefulness of anti-peroxidase and JT-95 antibodies. Acta Pathol Jpn 1993;43:670-3.

75. Lau SK, Luthringer DJ, Eisen RN. Thyroid transcription factor-1: a review. Appl Immunohistochem Mol Morphol 2002;10:97-102.

76. De Felice M, Di Lauro R. Thyroid development and its disorders: genetics and molecular mechanisms. Endocr Rev 2004;25:722-46.

77. Katoh R, Kawaoi A, Miyagi E, et al. Thyroid transcription factor-1 in normal, hyperplastic, and neoplastic follicular thyroid cells examined by immunohistochemistry and nonradioactive in situ hybridization. Mod Pathol 2000;13:570-6.

78. Bisceglia M, Ragazzi M, Galliani CA, Lastilla G, Rosai J. TTF-1 expression in neuroblastoma. Am J Surg Pathol 2009;33:454-61.

79. Kubba LA, McCluggage WG, Liu J, et al. Thyroid transcription factor-1 expression in ovarian epithelial neoplasms. Mod Pathol 2008;21:485-90.

80. Sierakowski A, Al-Janabi K, Dam H, Sood M. Metastatic Merkel cell carcinoma with positive expression of thyroid transcription factor-1—a case report. Am J Dermatopathol 2009;31:384-6.

81. Mantovani G, Corbetta S, Romoli R, Alberti L, Beck-Peccoz P, Spada A. Absence of thyroid transcription factor-1 expression in human parathyroid and pituitary glands. Mol Cell Endocrinol 2001;182:13-7.

82. Nonaka D, Tang Y, Chiriboga L, Rivera M, Ghossein R. Diagnostic utility of thyroid transcription factors Pax8 and TTF-2 (FoxE1) in thyroid epithelial neoplasms. Mod Pathol 2008;21:192-200.

83. Lee A, LiVolsi VA, Baloch ZW. Expression of DNA topoisomerase IIalpha in thyroid neoplasia. Mod Pathol 2000;13:396-400.

84. Maiorano E, Ciampolillo A, Gesualdo L, Ranieri E, Fanelli M, Viale G. Expression of transforming growth factor-ß1 in thyroid tumors. Appl Immunohistochem Mol Morphol 1999;7:135-41.

85. Kamoshida S, Ogane N, Yasuda M, et al. Immunohistochemical study of type-1 blood antigen expressions in thyroid tumors: the significance for papillary carcinomas. Mod Pathol 2000;13:736-41.

86. Yasuoka H, Nakamura Y, Zuo H, et al. VEGF-D expression and lymph vessels play an important role for lymph node metastasis in papillary thyroid carcinoma. Mod Pathol 2005;18:1127-33.

23 THE NORMAL PARATHYROID GLAND

Ivar Sandström (1) provided the first comprehensive description of the parathyroid glands in humans in 1880, although these glands had been recognized by Virchow 17 years earlier (2). Sandström chose the name *glandulae parathyroideae* to indicate the characteristic location of the four small glands next to the thyroid gland (2). The physiologic significance of the parathyroid glands, however, remained unknown until experimental studies revealed that their removal resulted in the tetany associated with hypocalcemia (3,4). The observation that the administration of parathyroid gland extract was capable of reversing hypocalcemia in parathyroidectomized animals led to the discovery and ultimate characterization of parathyroid hormone (PTH) (4).

EMBRYOLOGY

Detailed analyses of the development of the parathyroid glands are provided by Gilmour, Norris, and Weller (5–7). A brief review of the embryology of the glands, however, is necessary for an understanding of the topographic variations in their distribution in normal individuals.

The parathyroid glands are derived from branchial pouches III and IV. They are first recognizable in the 8- to 9-mm embryo (5 to 6 weeks of development) as localized thickenings of the anterodorsal pouch epithelium (5–7). The inferior parathyroid glands and the thymus are derived from branchial pouch III, and for that reason, they are also referred to as parathyroid III. The derivatives of pouch III have a complex pattern of migration and descent prior to attaining their final positions caudad to the derivatives of pouch IV.

Parathyroid III separates from the thymus at the 18-mm stage, when it is at the level of the lower pole of the thyroid gland. Failure of parathyroid III to separate from the thymus results in the appearance of the gland in the lower neck, within the thymic tongue, anterior mediastinum, or, less commonly, the posterior mediastinum. Early separation of parathyroid III from the thymus may result in the final position of the gland cephalad to the thyroid gland and parathyroid IV. Thus, parathyroid III or its remnants may be found along the entire course of migration of the third pouch derivatives from the angle of the jaw to the pericardium (5–7).

The superior glands (parathyroid IV) are derived from branchial pouch IV, together with the ultimobranchial bodies (5–7). Parathyroid IV separates from the ultimobranchial body and assumes its position as the upper gland. The location of parathyroid IV is close to the point where the inferior parathyroid artery crosses the recurrent laryngeal nerve at the cricothyroid junction. The final position of parathyroid IV is more constant than that of parathyroid III.

In the fetus, the parathyroid glands appear as well-vascularized collections of chief cells that are separated from the surrounding connective tissue by a thin connective tissue capsule (fig. 23-1).

Agenesis or hypoplasia of the parathyroid glands is rare in the absence of other anomalies. For example, parathyroid agenesis or hypoplasia is present in a high proportion of patients with the 22;1q2 syndrome (velocardiofacial/DiGeorge syndrome) (8,9). This syndrome is characterized by dysmorphic facies, conotruncal cardiac defects, hypocalcemic hypoparathyroidism, T cell–mediated immune deficiency, and absent or decreased numbers of C-cells. In one series, up to 61 percent of affected patients had complete hypoparathyroidism while 39 percent had partial hypoparathyroidism (10). Additional syndromes associated with parathyroid agenesis/hypoplasia include Smith-Lemli-Opitz syndrome (type II), X-linked recessive hypoparathyroidism, Kenny syndrome, Kearns-Sayre syndrome, and trisomy 18 (11).

Remnants of the third and fourth branchial pouches may persist in the neck postnatally as Kürsteiner canals. Small foci of heterotopic salivary glandular tissue associated with epithelium-lined cysts may be present close to or in

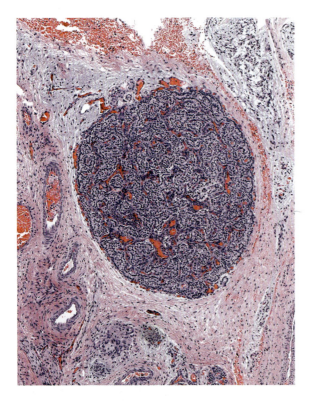

Figure 23-1

FETAL PARATHYROID GLAND (22 WEEKS' GESTATION)

The gland is separated from the surrounding connective tissue by a thin capsule. Chief cells appear clear. (Courtesy of Dr. M. DePaepe, Providence, RI.)

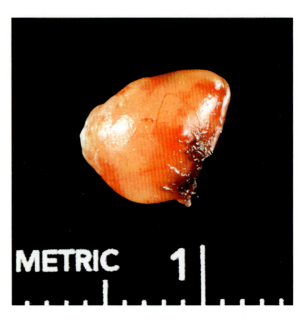

Figure 23-2

NORMAL ADULT PARATHYROID GLAND

The gland is encapsulated and pink-tan in color. (Courtesy of Drs. G. Randolph and P. Sadow, Boston, MA.)

direct contact with both normal and abnormal parathyroid glands (so-called heterotopic cyst units) (12). Most of these foci are present in relationship to the lower parathyroid glands.

ANATOMY

Gross and Microscopic Findings

Most individuals have four parathyroid glands that lie in close relationship to the posterior aspects of the thyroid lobes. The parathyroid glands are flattened, ovoid, or bean-shaped structures measuring 4 to 6 mm in length, 2 to 4 mm in width, and 1 to 2 mm in thickness (fig. 23-2). Occasional glands have an elongated, bilobated or multilobated shape. The glands are tan-brown when there is a high ratio of parenchymal cells to stromal fat, and yellow-brown when there is abundant stromal fat.

The average combined weight of the glands is 120 ± 5.2 mg for males and 142 +/– 5.2 mg for

females, with a maximum total glandular weight of 208 mg at the 95th percentile (13,14). In a large autopsy series, Grimelius et al. (14,15) found an individual mean glandular weight of 32 mg, with a maximum gland weight of 59 mg at the 95th percentile. Ghandur-Mnaymneh et al. (16) reported that glandular weights were greater in hospitalized patients (mean, 46.2 mg) than in patients who died suddenly (mean, 39.5 mg), with a 95 percent upper limit gland weight of 73.1 mg for healthy white subjects and 91.6 mg for healthy black subjects. Generally, individual gland weights in excess of 40 mg are considered abnormal.

The importance of determining parenchymal weight using planimetry or density gradients for the assessment of normal and abnormal functional states has been stressed by several groups (fig. 23-3) (see chapter 30) (15,17–19). The mean parenchymal weight of a single gland averages 22 mg, with a 95 percent upper limit of 39 mg (14). The mean parenchymal weight in adults is approximately 75 percent of the total glandular weight. There is an almost linear relationship between parenchymal cell volume and glandular density. These measurements can be used in conjunction with measurements of

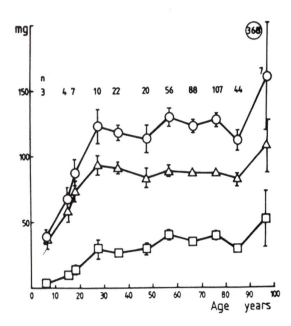

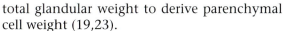

Figure 23-3

NORMAL PARATHYROID WEIGHTS

The total glandular weight (opened circles), total parenchymal cell weight (opened triangles), and total fat tissue weight (opened squares) are shown in relationship to patient age. Mean values +/- SEM. N=number of cases in each age group. The number in the right upper circle is the total number of cases. (Fig. 2 from Grimelius L, Akerstrom G, Johannson H, Bergstrom R. Anatomy and histopathology of human parathyroid glands. Pathol Annu 1981;16(Pt 2):6.)

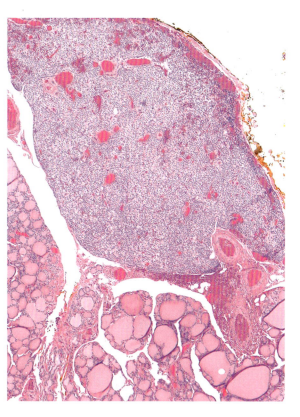

Figure 23-4

NORMAL PARATHYROID GLAND FROM 4-YEAR OLD MALE

There is essentially no stromal fat in the gland.

total glandular weight to derive parenchymal cell weight (19,23).

The amount of stromal fat is dependent on age and constitutional factors, particularly the amount of body fat. Parenchymal weights and total glandular weights are almost identical in individuals less than 18 years of age (fig. 23-4). After that age, the amount of stromal fat increases to 10 to 30 percent of the glandular volume, whereas the parenchymal weight remains more or less constant throughout life (figs. 23-5–23-7). Studies of normal adult parathyroid glands obtained at autopsy showed that two thirds had less than 20 percent stromal fat, while only 9 percent had more than 40 percent fat (20). Dufour et al. (21) reported that the average stromal fat content of normal adult glands was 17 percent. There may be considerable variation in the content of stromal fat in different glands in the

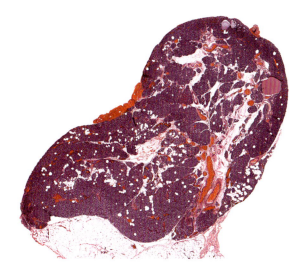

Figure 23-5

NORMAL PARATHYROID GLAND FROM NORMOCALCEMIC ADULT MALE

Stromal fat constitutes less than 10 percent of the gland area.

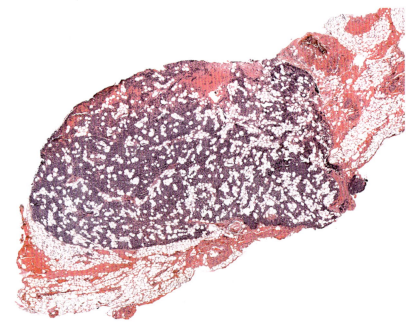

Figure 23-6

NORMAL PARATHYROID GLAND FROM NORMOCALCEMIC ADULT FEMALE

Stromal fat constitutes approximately 25 percent of the gland area.

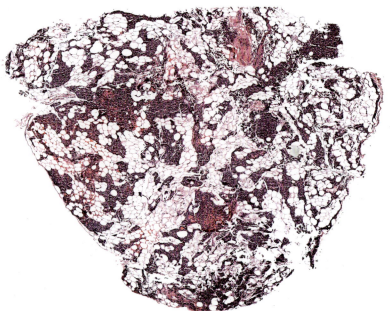

Figure 23-7

NORMAL PARATHYROID GLAND FROM NORMOCALCEMIC OBESE FEMALE

Stromal fat constitutes more than 50 percent of the gland area.

same individual (15). Moreover, stromal fat is distributed unequally within individual glands, with the polar regions richer in fat than the more central regions. Biopsies from the poles, therefore, may give spuriously high stromal fat to parenchymal cell ratios.

The superior parathyroid glands (parathyroid IV) are found most often within a circumscribed area at a distance of approximately 1 cm above the intersection of the recurrent laryngeal nerve and the inferior thyroid artery (fig. 23-8) (22). The glands are present in the connective tissue that binds the posterior edge of the thyroid gland to the pharynx. Occasional glands are present within the thyroid capsule, and in 0.2 percent of individuals, they are present within the thyroid parenchyma (22,23). Exceptionally, the superior parathyroid glands are found in the retropharyngeal or retroesophageal space (19).

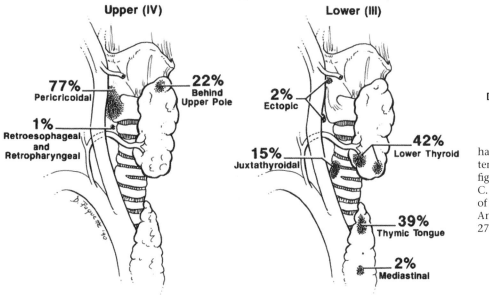

Upper (IV)

77% Pericricoidal

22% Behind Upper Pole

1% Retroesophageal and Retropharyngeal

Lower (III)

2% Ectopic

42% Lower Thyroid

15% Juxtathyroidal

39% Thymic Tongue

2% Mediastinal

Figure 23-8

ANATOMIC DISTRIBUTION OF PARATHYROID GLANDS

The thyroid lobes have been reflected anteriorly. (Adapted from figs. 1 and 2 from Wang C. The anatomic basis of parathyroid surgery. Ann Surg 1976;183: 271-5.)

The inferior parathyroids (parathyroid III), as noted in the in the discussion of embryologic development, are much more variable in their distribution than the superior glands. Akerström (19) reported that 61 percent of the inferior glands were present inferiorly, posteriorly, or laterally to the lower pole of the thyroid gland, and 17 percent were present high up on the anterior aspect of the thyroid lobe. In Akerström's series, other common sites of the inferior glands included the thyrothymic ligament and the cervical portion of the thymus. The inferior glands were located in the lower thymus in 2 percent of cases and in the anterior mediastinum below the thymus in 0.2 percent of cases. Of inferior glands, 2.8 percent were found in thymic tissue above the point of intersection of the recurrent laryngeal nerve and inferior thyroid artery. A small number of inferior glands were also found in the posterior mediastinum. Despite variations in their positions within the neck, the distribution of the glands tended to be bilaterally symmetrical.

The arterial supply of the glands is derived from branches of the superior thyroid artery (parathyroid IV) and the inferior thyroid artery (parathyroid III). As might be anticipated by the variability in their anatomic distribution, the vascular supply is equally variable (23,24). Venous drainage of parathyroid IV occurs via the superior or lateral thyroid vein, while drainage of the lower glands occurs via the lateral or inferior thyroid vein. Lymphatic drainage originates from a subcapsular plexus into the superior deep cervical, pretracheal, paratracheal, retropharyngeal, and deep cervical lymph nodes (22–24).

True supernumerary glands, defined as being located separate from the other four glands and weighing more than 5 mg, are present in up to 5 percent of normal individuals. Most individuals with true supernumerary glands have 5 glands, a few have 6 glands, and very few have 7 to 12 glands (19,24). In most patients with more than four parathyroid glands, the supernumerary glands are either rudimentary (less than 5 mg) or split (divided) (19,24). True supernumerary glands are found most commonly in the thymus or in relationship to the thyrothymic ligament (19,22,24). Supernumerary glands have also been found in the submucosa of the esophagus and hypopharynx. Lack et al. (25) demonstrated supernumerary or ectopic parathyroid tissue in 6 percent of vagus nerves of 32 children up to 1 year of age. Collections of parathyroid tissue in these cases ranged from 162 to 360 μm in diameter. Rarely, normal parathyroid tissue is present in extremely unusual anatomic sites, such as the vaginal wall in association with thyroid tissue (26). In approximately 3 percent of normal individuals, only three parathyroid

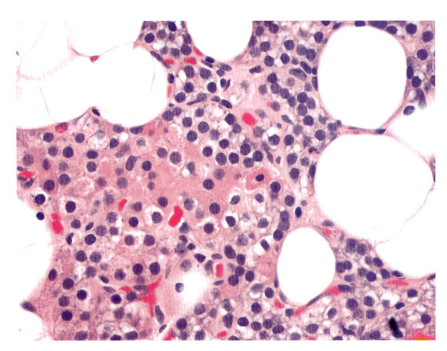

Figure 23-9

NORMOCELLULAR PARATHYROID GLAND

Chief cells have round, densely stained nuclei and clear cytoplasm. Oncocytes have abundant granular eosinophilic cytoplasm.

glands are found (19). The lower combined parathyroid weight in these individuals suggests that a fourth gland may have been missed during anatomic dissection.

The parathyroid glands are richly vascularized structures that are separated from the surrounding soft tissues of the neck by a thin connective tissue capsule (27). Occasional small clusters of parathyroid cells may be present external to the glandular capsule in the soft tissues of the neck. In patients with primary or secondary hyperplasia, these small cell clusters and nests may also become hyperplastic, a finding that has been referred to as *parathyromatosis* (see chapter 29) (28). Blood vessels enter and leave the gland through fibrous trabecula extending from the capsule. Although nerve bundles are present in proximity to the glandular cells, the role of neural control of physiologic function of the glands is unknown.

The parenchymal elements of the glands include chief cells, oncocytes, and transitional oncocytic cells (fig. 23-9) (23,27,29). In adults, the *chief cells* have a polyhedral shape and measure up to 10 μm in diameter (27). The nuclei are round and centrally placed, and have coarse chromatin with well-defined nuclear membranes. Because of the density of their chromatin, the nuclei appear pyknotic, particularly in thick sections. Mitotic figures are almost never seen in normal adult parathyroid glands. The cytoplasm of the chief cells in well-fixed samples is generally eosinophilic to amphophilic, while it sometimes has a clear or vacuolated appearance.

Chief cells are typically well glycogenated and contain variable amounts of neutral lipid in the form of 2 to 3 droplets per cell, as demonstrated with oil red O or azure A and Erie garnet B stains (fig. 23-10). Lipid droplets are present in up to 80 percent of chief cells in resting adult glands and in 30 to 40 percent of chief cells in children (27). Chief cells with clear cytoplasm should be distinguished from the water clear cells (Wasserhelle cells) which are found in water clear cell hyperplasias, and less commonly, in adenomas. Water clear cells contain multiple cytoplasmic vacuoles which are best demonstrated in 1-μm–thick plastic sections.

Chief cells in glands with little stromal fat are arranged in solid sheets. With increasing fat content, the chief cells tend to form branching and anastomosing cell cords (14,23). They also form small acinar or glandular structures, and occasional follicles containing an eosinophilic periodic acid–Schiff (PAS)-positive colloid-like material may be present (fig. 23-11). In some instances, the colloid-like material is congophilic and has the typical green birefringence of amyloid (30). Typically, the colloid in parathyroid glands does not contain calcium oxalate

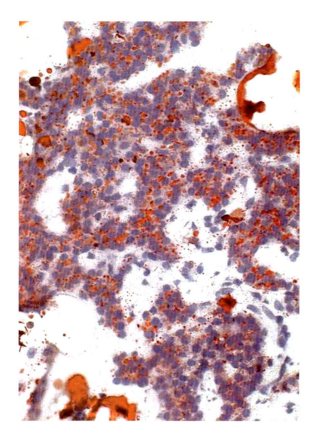

Figure 23-10

NORMOCELLULAR PARATHYROID GLAND

The chief cells contain oil red O-positive lipid deposits. Stromal fat cells are also stained.

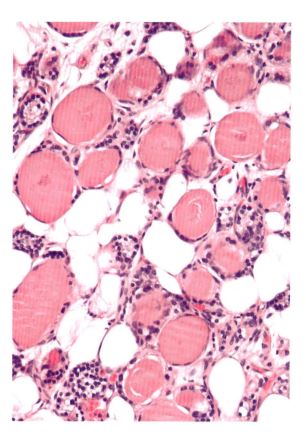

Figure 23-11

NORMOCELLULAR PARATHYROID GLAND

Small follicles contain eosinophilic colloid-like material.

crystals, in contrast to the colloid of the thyroid gland (31). Microcysts occur commonly in the parathyroid glands of older individuals.

Oncocytes (oxyphils) measure 12 to 20 μm in diameter and are characterized by the presence of deeply eosinophilic cytoplasmic granules. The nucleus is larger than that of the chief cells and nucleoli are prominent (14,23,27). Oncocytes are rich in oxidative enzymes and contain abundant mitochondria (32). These cells typically appear at puberty and increase in number with age, characteristically forming cell clusters and nodules (fig. 23-12). In some instances, large oncocytic nodules are impossible to distinguish from oncocytic adenomas. Transitional oncocytes are smaller and less eosinophilic than mature oncocytes.

In addition to mature fat cells, the stromal compartment of the parathyroid gland contains blood vessels, lymphatics, and variable amounts of fibrous tissue (24,25). The parathyroid glands of infants and children contain little stroma, while those of adults contain somewhat more abundant fibrous tissue which tends to accentuate the lobular appearance of the glands (29). Collections of lymphocytes may also be present in normal glands, and may be prominent in some cases (fig. 23-13).

Immunohistochemical Findings

Parathyroid chief cells contain cytokeratins (CK) 8, 18 and 19, while oncocytes contain identical cytokeratins although in lower concentrations (33). Vimentin is present in stromal cells and vascular endothelium, while the parenchymal cells of the gland are negative for this intermediate filament (33). Neurofilament proteins are present in occasional parenchymal cells of parathyroid adenomas, but normal glands are negative for this protein. In contrast

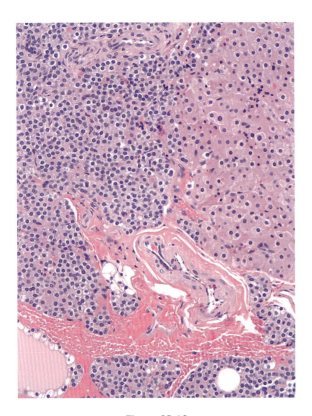

Figure 23-12

**ONCOCYTIC NODULE IN A
NORMOCALCEMIC ADULT FEMALE PATIENT**

The nodule is composed of cells with abundant eosinophilic cytoplasm.

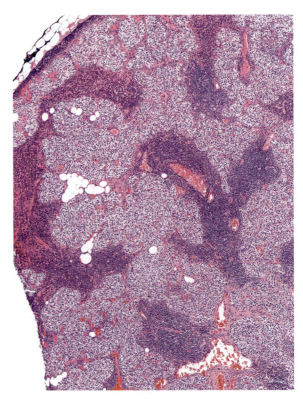

Figure 23-13

**LYMPHOCYTIC INFILTRATION
IN THE PARATHYROID GLAND**

In this parathyroid gland from a normocalcemic adult female patient there are prominent lymphoid infiltrates surrounding vascular spaces.

to thyroid follicular cells, parathyroid parenchymal cells are negative for thyroglobulin and thyroid transcription factor (TTF)-1.

Parathyroid hormone is present in most parenchymal cells, although staining is consistently stronger in chief cells than in oncocytes (figs. 23-14, 23-15) (34,35). Preproparathyroid hormone and PTH messenger RNA can be demonstrated by in situ hybridization methods (36,37). The glial cells missing 2 (Gcm2) transcription factor is also a sensitive marker for the identification of parathyroid cells (38). Chief cells are positive for chromogranin A (39). Vesicle-associated membrane protein (VAMP) and the synaptosomal protein of 23kDa (SNAP-23) are also expressed in normal chief cells (40). Normal parathyroid glands are negative for calcitonin; however, calcitonin and the calcitonin gene-related peptide have been reported to be present in a subset of PTH-producing hyperplastic and neoplastic

parathyroid glands (41,42). The calcitonin-positive cells also strongly express chromogranin B, which is not present in normal parathyroid glands. Monoclonal antibodies to a parathyroid receptor involved in the sensing of calcium react with the cell surface of normal and suppressed chief cells while adenomas and hyperplasias have lower levels of staining (43,44).

Parafibromin, a product of the *HRPT2/CDC73* gene, is expressed within the nuclei of normal chief cells (45). The protein gene product (PGP) 9.5 and galectin 3 are absent from normal parathyroid glands (46,47), while glycogen synthase 3β and the adenomatous polyposis coli (APC) gene product are present (48). PAX8 immunoreactivity is present in approximately one third of normal parathyroid glands (49).

CD4 immunoreactivity is present in chief cells, while oncocytes are nonreactive (50). Although the functional significance of CD4 in

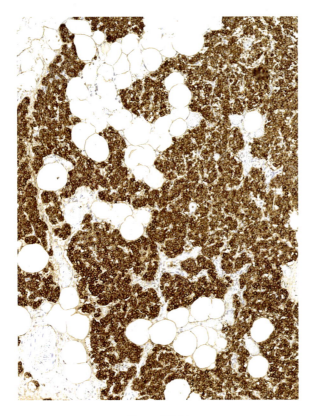

Figure 23-14

**NORMOCELLULAR PARATHYROID GLAND
STAINED FOR PARATHYROID HORMONE**

All of the parenchymal cells are positive for parathyroid hormone (PTH) (immunoperoxidase stain for PTH).

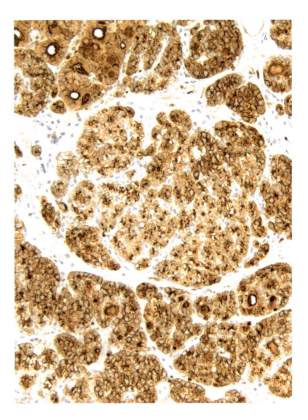

Figure 23-15

**NORMOCELLULAR PARATHYROID GLAND
STAINED FOR PARATHYROID HORMONE**

The oncocytic nodule (center) contains less PTH than the adjacent parenchymal cells (immunoperoxidase stain for PTH).

the parathyroid gland is unknown, this moiety may play a role in the calcium-regulated release of PTH. Cyclin D1 is expressed in less than 10 percent of normal parathyroid samples (51). The proliferative rate, as assessed with MIB-1, is in the range of 0.3 percent, while p27/Kip1, a cyclin-dependent kinase inhibitor, is highly expressed (52,53). The retinoblastoma gene product (RB protein) is present in normal chief cells (54).

Ultrastructural Findings

Chief cells in their resting phases have relatively straight plasma membranes, while increased functional activity is characterized by greater tortuosity of the plasma membranes (23,27,55,56). Resting chief cells contain few secretory granules, moderate numbers of mitochondria that are distributed randomly throughout the cytoplasm, and abundant glycogen deposits. The endoplasmic

reticulum is most often located in a perinuclear position, but occasional cisternae are present in the periphery of the cytoplasm (fig. 23-16). The Golgi regions have widened saccules and small empty appearing vesicles. Lipid droplets measuring 1 to 5 µm in diameter are also present.

The prosecretory granules in chief cells measure up to 0.2 µm and are generally round, with centrally located, moderately electron-dense cores that are separated from their limiting membranes by an electron-lucent space. Mature secretory granules are round, with an average diameter of 0.3 µm, and their contents are denser than those of prosecretory granules. Some mature secretory granules are ovoid or have a dumbbell configuration that makes their differentiation from lysosomes difficult.

Chief cells actively synthesizing PTH are usually smaller than resting chief cells and contain

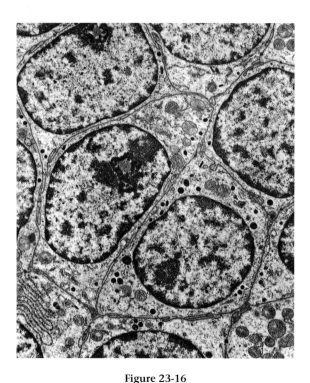

Figure 23-16

NORMAL PARATHYROID GLAND

Electron micrograph of normal parathyroid gland. The chief cells in the normal resting gland contain relatively few secretory granules.

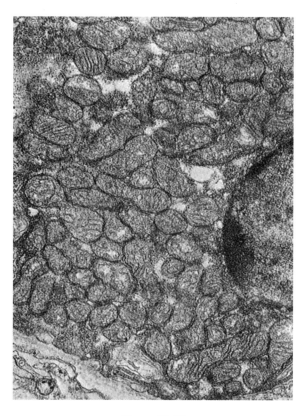

Figure 23-17

NORMAL PARATHYROID GLAND

Electron micrograph of normal parathyroid gland. The oncocyte is filled with mitochondria.

decreased amounts of glycogen and lipid (56). Granular endoplasmic reticulum is present in the form of multiple parallel stacks. In the packaging phase of the secretory cycle, the cells are small but the plasma membranes are highly tortuous. The Golgi region is well developed, with numerous vesicles and prosecretory granules. In the secretory phase, the cells become larger and secretory granules move toward the plasma membranes. With involution, the cells further enlarge with the accumulation of lipid and glycogen, while the plasma membranes become relatively straight.

Oncocytes are characterized by the presence of numerous mitochondria that fill the cytoplasm (fig. 23-17) (55,56). While most mitochondria are round, some are elongated or dumbbell shaped. The endoplasmic reticulum is less abundant than in chief cells, and Golgi regions tend to be considerably smaller. Prosecretory and secretory granules are present in smaller numbers than in chief cells and lipid droplets are smaller. Transitional oncocytes contain fewer mitochondria than oncocytes, but more mitochondria than chief cells.

REFERENCES

1. Sandström I. On a new gland in man and several mammals-glandulae parathyroideae. Uppsala Lakareforen Forh 1880;15:441-71.
2. Carney JA. The glandular parathyroideae of Ivar Sandström. Contributions from two continents. Am J. Surg Pathol 1996;20:1123-44.
3. Albright F. A page out of the history of hyperparathyroidism. J Clin Endocrinol Metab 1948;8:637-57.
4. Potts JT. Parathyroid hormone: past and present. J Endocrinol 2005;187:311-25.
5. Gilmour JR. The embryology of the parathyroid glands, the thymus and certain associated rudiments. J Pathol Bacteriol 1937;45:507-22.
6. Norris EH. The parathyroid glands and the lateral thyroid in man: their morphogenesis, histogenesis, topographic anatomy and prenatal growth. Contrib Embryol 1937;26:247-94.
7. Weller GL Jr. Development of the thyroid, parathyroid and thymus glands in man. Contrib Embryol 1933;141:93-139.
8. Burke BA, Johnson D, Gilbert EF, Drut RM, Ludwig J, Wick MR. Thyrocalcitonin-containing cells in the Di George anomaly. Hum Pathol 1987;18:355-60.
9. Cuneo BF. 22q11.2 deletion syndrome: DiGeorge, velocardiofacial, and conotruncal anomaly face syndrome. Curr Opin Pediatr 2001;13:465-72.
10. Al-Jenaidi F, Makitie O, Grunebaum E, Sochett E. Parathyroid hormone dysfunction in 22q11.2 deletion syndrome. Horm Res 2006;67:117-22.
11. Stocker JT, Dehner LP, Husain AN. Stocker & Dehner's pediatric pathology, 3rd ed. Philadelphia: Wolters Kluwer Health/Lippincott Williams & Williams; 2011:923.
12. Carney JA. Salivary heterotopia, cysts, and the parathyroid gland: branchial pouch derivatives and remnants. Am J Surg Pathol 2000;24:837-45.
13. Gilmour JR, Martin WJ. The weight of the parathyroid glands. J Pathol Bacteriol 1937;44:431-62.
14. Grimelius L, Akerström G, Johansson H, Juhlin C, Rastad J. The parathyroid glands. In: Kovacs K, Asa S, eds. Functional endocrine pathology, Vol. 1. Boston: Blackwell Scientific; 1991:375-95.
15. Grimelius, L, Akerström G, Johansson H, Bergström R. Anatomy and histopathology of human parathyroid glands. Pathol Annu 1981;16:1-24.
16. Ghandur-Mnaymneh L, Cassady J, Hajianpour MA, Paz J, Reiss E. The parathyroid gland in health and disease. Am J Pathol 1986;125:292-9.
17. Akerström G, Grimelius L, Johansson H, Lundqvist H, Pertoft H, Bergström R. The parenchymal cell mass in normal human parathyroid glands. Acta Pathol Microbiol Immunol Scand A 1981;89:367-75.
18. Akerström G, Grimelius L, Johnsson H, Pertroft H, Lundqvist H. Estimation of the parathyroid parenchymal cell mass by density gradients. Am J Pathol 1980;99:685-94.
19. Akerström G, Malmaeus J, Bergström R. Surgical anatomy of human parathyroid glands. Surgery 1984;95:14-21.
20. Dekker A, Dunsford HA, Geyer SJ. The normal parathyroid gland at autopsy: the significance of stromal fat in adult patients. J Pathol 1979;128:127-32.
21. Dufour DR, Wilkerson SY. The normal parathyroid revisited: percentage of stromal fat. Hum Pathol 1982;13;717-21.
22. Wang C. The anatomic basis of parathyroid surgery. Ann Surg 1976;183:271-5.
23. Castleman B, Roth SI. Tumors of the parathyroid glands. Atlas of Tumor Pathology, 2nd Series, Fascicle 14. Washington, DC: Armed Forces Institute of Pathology; 1978:1-94.
24. Gilmour JR. The gross anatomy of the parathyroid glands. J Pathol Bacteriol 1938;46:133-49.
25. Lack EE, Delay S, Linnoila RI. Ectopic parathyroid tissue within the vagus nerve: incidence and possible clinical significance. Arch Pathol Lab Med 1988;112:204-6.
26. Kurman RJ, Prabha AC. Thyroid and parathyroid glands in the vaginal wall: report of a case. Am J Clin Pathol 1973;59:503-7.
27. Roth SI, Sadow PM, Johnson NB, Abu-Jawdeh GM. Parathyroid. In: Mills SE, ed. Histology for pathologists, 4th ed. Philadelphia: Lippincott Williams & Wilkins; 2012:1209-30.
28. Reddick RL, Costa JC, Marx SJ. Parathyroid hyperplasia and parathyromatosis. Lancet 1977;1:549.
29. Gilmour JR. The normal histology of the parathyroid glands. J Pathol Bacteriol 1939;48:187-222.
30. Lieberman A, DeLellis RA. Intrafollicular amyloid in normal parathyroid glands. Arch Pathol 1973;95:422-3.
31. Isotalo PA, Lloyd RV. Presence of birefringent crystals is useful in distinguishing thyroid from parathyroid gland tissues. Am J Surg Pathol 2002;26:813-4.
32. Bedetti CD. Immunocytochemical demonstration of cytochrome C oxidase with an immunoperoxidase method: a specific stain for mitochondria in formalin-fixed and paraffin-embedded tissues. J Histochem Cytochem 1985;33:446-52.

33. Miettinen M, Clark R, Lehto VP, Virtanen I, Damjanov I. Intermediate-filament proteins in parathyroid glands and parathyroid adenomas. Arch Pathol Lab Med 1985;109:986-9.

34. Tomita, T. Immunocytochemical staining patterns for parathyroid hormone and chromogranin in parathyroid hyperplasia, adenoma and carcinoma. Endocr Pathol 1999;10:145-56.

35. Winkler B, Gooding GA, Montgomery CK, Clark OH, Arnaud C. Immunoperoxidase confirmation of parathyroid origin of ultrasound-guided fine needle aspirates of the parathyroid glands. Acta Cytol 1987;31:40-4.

36. Kendall CH, Roberts PA, Pringle JH, Lauder I. The expression of parathyroid hormone messenger RNA in normal and abnormal parathyroid tissue. J Pathol 1991;165:111-8.

37. Stork PJ, Herteaux C, Frazier R, Kronenberg H, Wolfe JH. Expression and distribution of parathyroid hormone and parathyroid hormone messenger RNA in pathological conditions of the parathyroid. Lab Invest 1989;60:92A (Abstract).

38. Nonaka D. Study of parathyroid transcription factor Gcm2 expression in parathyroid lesions. Am J Surg Pathol 2011;35:145-51.

39. Wilson BS, Lloyd RV. Detection of chromogranin in neuroendocrine cells with a monoclonal antibody. Am J Pathol 1984;115:458-68.

40. Lu M, Forsberg L, Hoog A, et al. Heterogeneous expression of SNARE proteins SNAP-23, SNAP-25, syntaxin-1 and VAMP in human parathyroid tissue. Mol Cell Endocrinol 2008;287:72-80.

41. Khan A, Tischler AS, Patwardhan NA, DeLellis RA. Calcitonin immunoreactivity in neoplastic and hyperplastic parathyroid glands: an immunohistochemical study. Endocr Pathol 2003;14:249-55.

42. Schmid KW, Morgan JM, Baumert M, Fischer-Colbrie R, Böcker W, Jasani B. Calcitonin and calcitonin gene-related peptide mRNA detection in a population of hyperplastic parathyroid cells also expressing chromogranin B. Lab Invest 1995;73:90-5.

43. Juhlin C, Akerström G, Klareskog L, et al. Monoclonal antiparathyroid antibodies revealing defect expression of calcium receptor mechanism in hyperparathyroidism. World J Surg 1988;12:552-8.

44. Juhlin C, Holmdahl R, Johansson H, Rastad J, Akerström G, Klareskog L. Monoclonal antibodies with exclusive reactivity against parathyroid cells and tubule cells of the kidney. Proc Natl Acad Sci U S A 1987;84:2990-4.

45. Tan MH, Morrison C, Wang P, et al. Loss of parafibromin immunoreactivity is a distinguishing feature of parathyroid carcinoma. Clin Cancer Res 2004;10:6629-37.

46. Bergero N, DePompa R, Sacerdote C, et al. Galectin-3 expresion in parathyroid carcinoma: immunohistochemical study of 26 cases. Hum Pathol 2005;36:908-14.

47. Howell VM, Gill A, Clarkson A, et al. Accuracy of combined protein gene product 9.5 and parafibromin markers for immunohistochemical diagnosis of parathyroid carcinoma. J Clin Endocrinol Metab 2009;94:434-41.

48. Juhlin CC, Haglund F, Villablanca A, et al. Loss of expression for the Wnt pathway components adenomatous polyposis coli and glycogen synthase kinase 3-beta in parathyroid carcinomas. Int J Oncol 2009;34:481-91.

49. Ozcan A, Shen SS, Hamilton C, et al. PAX-8 expression in non-neoplastic tissue, primary tumors and metastatic tumors: a comprehensive immunohistochemical study. Mod Pathol 2011;24:751-64.

50. Hellman P, Karlsson-Parra A, Klareskog L, et al. Expression and function of a CD4 like molecule in parathyroid tissue. Surgery 1996;120:985-92.

51. Vasef MA, Brynes RK, Sturm M, Bromley C, Robinson RA. Expression of cyclin D1 in parathyroid carcinomas, adenomas and hyperplasias: A paraffin immunohistochemical study. Mod Pathol 1999;12:412-6.

52. Abbona GC, Papotti M, Gasparri G, Bussolati G. Proliferative activity in parathyroid tumors as detected by Ki-67 immunostaining. Hum Pathol 1995:26:135-8.

53. Erickson LA, Jin L, Wollan P, Thompson GB, van Heerden JA. Parathyroid hyperplasia, adenomas and carcinomas: differential expression of p27Kip1 protein. Am J Surg Pathol 1999;23:288-95.

54. Cryns VL, Thor A, Xu J, et al. Loss of the retinoblastoma tumor suppressor gene in parathyroid carcinoma. New Engl J Med 1994;330:757-61.

55. Nilsson O. Studies on the ultrastructure of the human parathyroid glands in various pathological conditions. Acta Pathol Microbiol Scand Suppl 1977;263:1-88.

56. Roth SI, Capen CC. Ultrastructural and functional correlations of the parathyroid gland. Int Rev Exp Pathol 1974;13:161-221.

24 PHYSIOLOGY AND PATHOPHYSIOLOGY OF PARATHYROID GLANDS

CALCIUM HOMEOSTASIS

Calcium plays a key role in a wide variety of biologic processes and is distributed in three fractions in the blood (protein bound, ionized, and complexed). Approximately 50 percent of the total serum calcium is bound to proteins, primarily albumin and globulins (1). Under normal conditions, the total serum calcium ranges from 9.0 to 10.5 mg/dL (2.2 to 2.6 mmol/L), while ionized calcium levels range from 4.5 to 5.6 mg/dL (1.1 to 1.4 mmol/dL). Five to 10 percent of serum calcium is complexed to various anions, such as phosphate and citrate.

Ionized calcium is the most important regulator of the biosynthesis and secretion of parathyroid hormone (PTH) (1). Control of calcium homeostasis is mediated by PTH and 1,25-dihydroxy-vitamin D, their corresponding receptors, and the calcium sensing receptor (CaSR). CaSR is a member of the G-protein-coupled receptor family which senses the levels of ionized calcium in the blood. In addition to its presence in the parathyroid gland, CaSR is expressed in a wide variety of tissues, including kidney, intestine, bone, skin, and brain.

The CaSR determines the response of the parathyroid glands to ionized calcium through the regulation of PTH secretion and gene expression, and chief cell proliferative capacity (1). A decrease in ionized calcium leads to increased secretion of PTH. Serum calcium is subsequently increased as a result of activation of PTH receptor in bone, controlling resorption of calcium and its release into the circulation. Activation of PTH receptors in the kidneys leads to increased tubular resorption of calcium. In addition, renal secretion of 1,25-dihydroxy-vitamin D is increased, leading to activation of vitamin D receptors in the intestine with a resultant increase in calcium absorption. Calcium resorption in bone is also stimulated by the increased levels of 1,25-dihydroxy-vitamin D (2). The release of PTH is inhibited in response to increases in ionized calcium levels. While calcitonin has an important role in calcium homeostasis in fish and rodents, its biologic significance in humans is not clear.

PARATHYROID HORMONE AND PARATHYROID HORMONE-RELATED PROTEIN

PTH is an 84-amino acid peptide encoded by a gene on chromosome 11p15 (1,2). The hormone is synthesized within chief cells, and to lesser extent within oncocytes, as part of a large precursor protein, known as preproPTH (115 amino acids). The signal sequence ("pre") is cleaved from the amino terminus during the biosynthesis of the protein. As the signal sequence emerges from the ribosome, it binds to a signal recognition particle, which is an RNA protein complex that recognizes signal sequences on most secreted proteins. The signal recognition particle binds to a docking protein on the rough endoplasmic reticulum and directs preproPTH to a protein-lined channel. A signal peptidase then cleaves the signal sequence, resulting in the formation of proPTH within the endoplasmic reticulum. ProPTH is then transported to the Golgi apparatus, where the "pro" sequence is removed.

PTH is concentrated within dense-core secretory vesicles which ultimately fuse with the chief cell plasma membrane prior to its release into the circulation. The hormone is secreted predominantly as the intact 84-amino acid protein, although a variable proportion of carboxy terminal fragments are also secreted.

Most clinical laboratories currently use chemiluminescence assays for the evaluation of serum PTH levels. These assays are highly sensitive and specific for intact PTH, and they can be used intraoperatively because of their speed and the short half-life of the hormone. Normally, the levels of intact PTH range from 10 to 67 pg/mL (1.1 to 7.1 pmol/L).

PTH-related protein (PTHrP) is encoded by a single gene that is highly conserved among different species. Alternative RNA splicing yields transcripts that encode three proteins of 139, 141, and 173 residues (3). PTHrP was discovered as a result of efforts to identify the mediator of hypercalcemia of malignancy. The amino terminal portion of the molecule binds to the same receptors as PTH, but it also binds to other receptors. It is widely distributed throughout epithelial, mesenchymal, and neuronal cells where it controls proliferation, differentiation, and apoptosis (4,5). The actions of PTHrP are primarily local, and in all likelihood, it does not contribute to the control of calcium homeostasis under physiologic conditions.

HYPERCALCEMIA

Hypercalcemia is by far the most frequent manifestation of primary hyperparathyroidism and is also a common finding in patients with malignancies of various types (6). The clinical symptoms of hypercalcemia are protean and include disturbances in the central nervous system, gastrointestinal tract, kidney, and cardiovascular system. Central nervous system manifestations range from mild cognitive impairment to coma (hypercalcemic crisis). Gastrointestinal symptoms include anorexia, nausea, vomiting, constipation, and abdominal pain, which may be due to pancreatitis. Renal dysfunction is manifested by the presence of polyuria and polydipsia, while nephrolithiasis results in the development of renal colic. Cardiovascular manifestations include hypertension, a shortened QT interval, and increased sensitivity to digitalis.

While primary hyperparathyroidism is recognized most commonly in the outpatient setting, malignancy is the most common underlying cause of hypercalcemia in hospitalized patients (7). Still, the differential diagnosis of hypercalcemia is extensive, and includes vitamin D intoxication, sarcoidosis and other granulomatous diseases, hyperthyroidism, vitamin A intoxication, milk alkali syndrome, and administration of certain drugs such as thiazide diuretics (1). Lithium toxicity may be associated with increased levels of PTH and enlargement of the parathyroid glands (8). Following cessation of lithium therapy, PTH levels generally return to normal; however, a few patients develop clear-cut hyperparathyroidism secondary to parathyroid adenoma or hyperplasia. Hyperplasia appears to be more common in these patients than in those with sporadic hyperparathyroidism unassociated with lithium toxicity (8).

HYPERPARATHYROIDISM

General Considerations

Hyperparathyroidism is a metabolic disorder that is characterized by the increased production of PTH (9,10). In primary hyperparathyroidism, excess PTH originates from an adenoma, hyperplasia, or carcinoma of the parathyroid glands (11,12). The serum calcium and PTH levels are typically increased, although some patients have normocalcemic hyperparathyroidism characterized by normal serum calcium and increased PTH levels (6). Patients with normocalcemic primary hyperparathyroidism are usually identified on the basis of low bone densities.

Secondary hyperparathyroidism is an adaptive increase of PTH production induced most commonly by the hypocalcemia associated with chronic renal failure. Dietary insufficiency of calcium or vitamin D, malabsorption, administration of various drugs, and a variety of other mechanisms may also be responsible.

The term *tertiary hyperparathyroidism* refers to the development of apparent autonomous parathyroid hyperfunction in patients with secondary hyperparathyroidism. The latter designation is often used in the context of persistent secondary hyperparathyroidism after successful renal transplantation.

Primary Hyperparathyroidism

Primary hyperparathyroidism is now recognized as the third most common endocrine disorder. It is characterized by the excessive and unregulated secretion of PTH from one or more abnormal parathyroid glands (6,9,13). Increased circulating levels of PTH result in activation of PTH and calcitriol receptors in target organs, including the kidney, small intestine, and bone.

The diagnosis of primary hyperparathyroidism is confirmed by the demonstration of persistent hypercalcemia in the presence of inappropriately normal or elevated levels of intact PTH. The disorder is characterized by a shift of the set point and slope of the calcium-PTH response curve such that chief cells become less sensitive to the ability of calcium to suppress PTH synthesis and secretion. The 24-hour urinary calcium and creatinine levels should be measured to rule out familial hypocalciuric hypercalcemia (FHH) (6,14). Hypercalcemia in patients with primary hyperparathyroidism is most often associated with hypercalciuria rather than FHH.

Most cases of primary hyperparathyroidism occur sporadically, but increasing numbers of heritable hyperparathyroidism syndromes are recognized (15). Most of the syndromes have autosomal dominant patterns of inheritance. They may be associated with hyperplasia, adenomas, or carcinomas of the parathyroid glands (see chapter 27).

Prior to the mid 1970s, primary hyperparathyroidism was considered a rare disorder, with clinical manifestations dominated by renal and/or bone disease (13). The introduction of automated serum calcium measurements by multichannel analyzers profoundly altered the diagnosis of this disorder (10,16,17). Prior to the advent of routine serum calcium screening in June 1974, the age-adjusted incidence of primary hyperparathyroidism for males and females was 15.8 cases per 100,000 person years (1965 to June 1974) in Rochester, Minnesota (18). In the interval between July, 1975 and 1982, the combined incidence for males and females rose to 82.5 cases. The incidence for females climbed to 118.6 in this same interval as compared to 21.4 cases in 1965 to 1974. In the interval from 1983 to 1992, the incidence for males and females declined to 29.1 cases, with a further drop to 21.6 cases from 1993 to 2001. Data from 2001 demonstrate a combined incidence of 15.8 cases, which is roughly comparable to the incidence in the prescreening era.

The reasons for the continuing decline in the incidence of primary hyperparathyroidism since the mid 1980s are not entirely clear (18). The most likely possibility is that the decrease is the result of the "sweeping" effects of automated calcium screening that led to the identification of previously unrecognized cases of this disorder in the mid 1970s. An additional possibility is related to the long-term carcinogenic effects of therapeutic head and neck radiation for the treatment of benign childhood diseases in the

1930s and 1940s. It has also been suggested that women with mild underlying primary hyperparathyroidism may have their disease unmasked with the onset of estrogen deficiency at the time of the menopause since the administration of estrogen in women with mild primary hyperparathyroidism lowers serum calcium levels. Other factors that may have led to the declining incidence of primary hyperparathyroidism include the increased administration of calcium and vitamin D supplements.

Many patients with mild hypercalcemia associated with primary hyperparathyroidism do not have any clinical manifestations of the disease and only a small proportion develop a more severe form of hyperparathyroidism. There are no clinical or biochemical features that predict progression (6,19). The symptoms of hypercalcemia are a function of the rate of rise of serum calcium as well as its actual level. For patients with asymptomatic primary hyperparathyroidism, the most recently developed guidelines recommend that surgery should be performed when: 1) serum calcium is over 1 mg/dL (0.25 mmol/L) above normal; 2) creatinine clearance is reduced to less than 60 mL/min/1.73m2; 3) T-score is less than –2.5SD at the spine, hip (total or femoral neck), or distal third of the radius (which is composed primarily of cortical bone); and 4) patient age less than 50 years (20).

Bone Manifestations

While *osteitis fibrosa cystica* is decreasing in incidence in patients with hyperparathyroidism, the incidence of *diffuse osteopenia* is increasing (fig. 24-1) (6,10,11,21). This phenomenon is undoubtedly related to the earlier detection of hyperparathyroidism, particularly in postmenopausal women with osteoporosis (6). Less than 10 percent of patients have evidence of subperiosteal bone resorption at presentation based on X-ray examination of the hands. Patients with hyperparathyroidism have a statistically higher incidence of diffuse osteopenia of the spine, with associated fractures, as compared to age- and sex-matched controls. A significant proportion of patients have evidence of skeletal demineralization in cortical bone when studied by bone densitometry, with sparing of cancellous bone. In addition to osteopenia, patients with hyperparathyroidism manifest a variety of articular

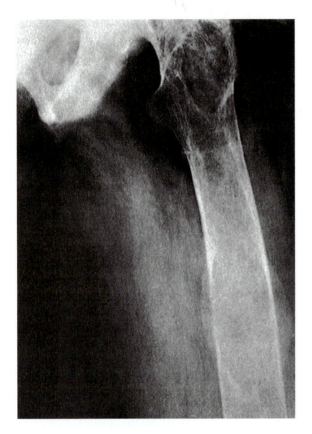

Figure 24-1

**OSTEITIS FIBROSA CYSTICA GENERALISITA
(VON RECKLINGHAUSEN DISEASE OF BONE)**

This radiograph of a femur demonstrates generalized osteopenia and multiple cysts.

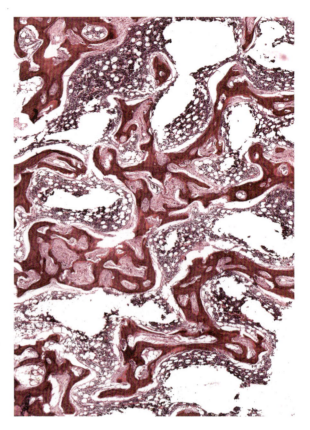

Figure 24-2

DISSECTING OSTEITIS

The bone trabeculae are invaded by fibrous tissue, with multiple areas of osteoclastic resorption.

disorders, including chondrocalcinosis with or without attacks of pseudogout, juxta-articular erosions, subchondral fractures, traumatic synovitis, calcific periarthritis, and true gout.

The earliest phases of bone disease are characterized by osteoclastic resorption of subperiosteal and endosteal bone surfaces and replacement of resorbed bone by fibrous tissue. A characteristic feature is dissecting osteitis in which bone trabeculae are hollowed out by osteoclasts and replaced with fibrous tissue (fig. 24-2). The latter finding is virtually diagnostic of hyperparathyroidism. The lytic lesions, which have a propensity to develop within the jaws, calvarium, and long tubular bones, are known as *"brown tumors,"* osteitis fibrosa cystica, or *von Recklinghausen disease* (fig. 24-3).

The development of brown tumors begins with resorption of bone trabeculae. The fibrous

response may develop as a consequence of microfractures within partially resorbed bone, followed by bleeding, hemosiderin deposition, and accumulation of giant cells. With further hemorrhage, cystic degeneration ultimately occurs. Giant cells, including osteoclasts and foreign body giant cells, are often aggregated in nodular foci around areas of hemosiderin deposition. Areas of osteoid and reactive bone are prominent in some brown tumors. So-called giant cell reparative granulomas frequently involve the jaws and the histologic distinction of this entity from brown tumors may be impossible. The giant cells found in true giant cell tumors tend to be more evenly spaced, the stromal cells tend to be plumper, and osteoblastic activity is less conspicuous than in brown tumors.

The giant cells of brown tumors have ultrastructural features similar to inactive osteoclasts,

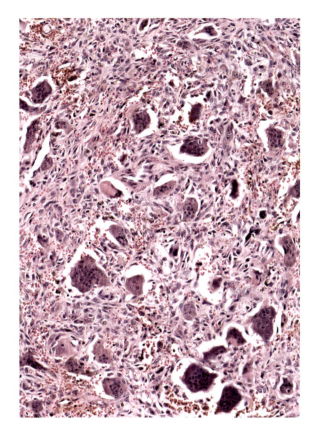

Figure 24-3

BROWN TUMOR

The central region of this brown tumor contains giant cells separated by plump stromal cells.

including numerous mitochondria, dilated endoplasmic reticulum, perinuclear Golgi regions, sparse lysosomes, and short filopodia (22). In contrast to active osteoclasts, the giant cells have prominent ruffled borders. The stromal compartment includes cells with the ultrastructural features of fibroblasts, myofibroblasts, and histiocytes.

Renal and Other Manifestations

Recurrent nephrolithiasis has been reported in 5 to 20 percent of patients with primary hyperparathyroidism in recent series, as compared to 70 percent in older series (6,10). In addition to the presence of calculi, renal disease is manifested by increased blood urea nitrogen and creatinine, decreased glomerular filtration rate, and a wide variety of tubular defects, including reduced net acid secretion, aminoaciduria, and glycosuria (23).

Neuromuscular manifestations include fatigue and muscle weakness, primarily affecting the proximal musculature (10). Histologically, the muscle weakness is manifested by atrophy of type II muscle fibers. Surgical treatment of hyperparathyroidism results in amelioration of muscle weakness in a significant proportion of patients.

Peptic ulcer disease had been regarded as a frequent complication of hyperparathyroidism in the past, but now is seen most commonly in those patients with type 1 multiple endocrine neoplasia (MEN) and gastrinomas. The association between pancreatitis, apart from that associated with the hypercalcemia per se, remains to be established.

Hypertension occurs in some patients with primary hyperparathyroidism, but it is not reversed by curative parathyroid surgery (6). The relationship of neuropsychiatric symptoms to primary hyperparathyroidism remains a subject of controversy.

HYPERCALCEMIA OF MALIGNANCY

Hypercalcemia occurs in approximately 10 percent of patients with advanced malignancies of various types (7,24–26). The development of hypercalcemia is often heralded by the onset of confusion, stupor, nausea, vomiting, or dehydration, and most affected patients die within 1 to 2 months of diagnosis (1). The pathogenesis of hypercalcemia is complex: it may result from the presence of circulating humoral factors (humoral hypercalcemia of malignancy) or by locally acting factors (localized osteolytic hypercalcemia). In some instances, mediators of hypercalcemia have both humoral and local effects.

Humoral hypercalcemia of malignancy is caused by the secretion of PTHrP, 1,25-dihydroxy-vitamin D, PTH, or prostaglandins by malignant tumors of various types (4,5,27–29). In most series, squamous cell carcinomas of the upper aerodigestive tract, lung, cervix, vulva, or skin are the most common tumor type associated with hypercalcemia secondary to the production of PTHrP. A wide variety of other tumors (breast, ovary, bladder, kidney), however, are also associated with hypercalcemia secondary to the production of PTHrP. For example, approximately one third of patients with small cell carcinoma of the ovary have evidence of hypercalcemia (30). Neuroendocrine tumors, including pheochromocytomas, pancreatic endocrine tumors, and carcinoid tumors, can also produce significant amounts of PTHrP (1). The aggressive T-cell lymphoma associated with human T-cell lymphotropic virus (HTLV-1) is also associated with the overproduction of PTHrP and hypercalcemia (31).

Since PTH and PTHrP share a common receptor, the biologic consequences of an excess of these products are similar. Humoral hypercalcemia secondary to the production of PTHrP and PTH results from enhanced resorption of calcium from bone and increased renal resorption of calcium. Both PTHrP and PTH are associated with hypophosphatemia secondary to a phosphaturic effect on the kidneys. Many tumors that produce excess PTHrP do so in the absence of skeletal metastases (4).

In addition to humoral hypercalcemia of malignancy, PTHrP is associated with localized osteolytic hypercalcemia secondary to the activation of osteoclasts immediately adjacent to tumor deposits. This phenomenon occurs most commonly in patients with widespread skeletal metastases of breast carcinoma.

Hypercalcemia in patients with lymphomas is most commonly due to the production of 1,25-dihydroxy-vitamin D (32,33). The hypercalcemic syndrome in these patients closely resembles the hypercalcemia associated with sarcoidosis.

Only a few examples of paraneoplastic production of PTH have been documented. These tumors are often small cell neuroendocrine or non-neuroendocrine carcinomas (24,34–36).

In addition, the production of PTH has been documented in carcinoma of the ovary (37,38), primitive neuroectodermal tumor (39), thymoma (40), squamous cell carcinoma of the lung (41,42), papillary thyroid carcinoma (43), and hepatocellular carcinoma (44). In one case of squamous cell carcinoma of the lung, the tumor cells produced both PTH and PTHrP (42).

Localized osteolytic hypercalcemia results from the production of osteoclast-stimulating cytokines by the tumor cells, including interleukin-1, tumor necrosis factor-α, interleukin-6, and transforming growth factor-α (45). Additionally, PTHrP may be responsible for localized osteolytic hypercalcemia. A critical osteoclastogenic pathway has been discovered that includes the osteoblast cell surface receptor RANK (receptor activator of nuclear factor κB); its ligand, RANKL; and a decoy receptor for RANKL, osteoprotegerin (46). RANKL has also been referred to as osteoclast differentiation factor, and by binding with the RANK receptor, promotes osteoclastic proliferation, differentiation, fusion, and activation. RANKL is secreted by tumor cells and the surrounding stroma in metastatic foci and results in osteolysis. Osteoprotegerin inhibits this pathway and represents a potential therapeutic agent in patients with hypercalcemia of malignancy (46).

Typically, patients with humoral hypercalcemia of malignancy due to the production of PTHrP or other mediators have suppressed levels of PTH, usually less than 2 ng/L (2 nmol/L). The parathyroid glands in these individuals are typically of normal size, with normal ratios of stromal fat to parenchymal cells (47).

REFERENCES

1. Bringhurst FR, Demay MD, Kronenberg HM. Hormones and disorders of mineral metabolism. In: Melmed S, Polonsky KS, Larsen PR, Kronenberg HM, eds. Williams Textbook of Endocrinology, 12th ed. Philadelphia: Elsevier/Saunders; 2011:1237-304.

2. Peacock, M. Calcium metabolism in health and diseases. Clin J Am Soc Nephrol 2010;5(Suppl 1):S23-30.

3. Philbrick WM. Parathyroid hormone-related protein: Gene structure, biosynthesis, metabolism and regulation. In: Bilezikian J, Marcus R, Levine MA, eds. The parathyroids: basic and clinical concepts, 2nd ed. San Diego: Academic Press; 2001:31-52.

4. Strewler GJ, Nissenson RA. Nonparathyroid hypercalcemia. Adv Intern Med 1987;32:235-58.

5. Strewler, GJ. Hypercalcemia of malignancy and parathyroid hormone-related protein. In: Clark OH, Duh QY, Kebebew E, eds. Textbook of endocrine surgery, 2nd ed. Philadelphia: Elsevier-Saunders; 2005:536-42.

6. Marcocci C, Cetani F. Clinical practice. Primary hyperparathyroidism. New Engl J Med 2011;365;2389-97.

7. Stewart AF. Clinical practice. Hypercalcemia associated with cancer. N Engl J Med 2005;352:373-9.

8. Saunders, BD, Saunders, F, Gauger, PG. Lithium therapy in hyperparathyroidism; an evidenced based assessment. World J Surg 2009;33:2314-23.

9. Fraser WD. Hyperparathyroidism. Lancet 2009;374:145-58.

10. Heath DA. Primary hyperparathyroidism. Clinical presentation and factors influencing clinical management. Endocrinol Metab Clin North Am 1989;18:631-46.

11. Castleman B, Roth SI. Tumors of the parathyroid glands. Atlas of Tumor Pathology, 2nd Series, Fascicle 14. Washington, DC: Armed Forces Institute of Pathology; 1978;1-94.

12. DeLellis RA. Tumors of the Parathyroid glands. AFIP Atlas of Tumor Pathology, 3rd Series, Fascicle 6. Washington, DC: American Registry of Pathology; 1993.

13. Melton LJ 3rd. The epidemiology of primary hyperparathyroidism in North America. J Bone Miner Res 2002;17(Suppl 2):N12-7.

14. Heath H 3rd. Familial benign (hypocalciuric) hypercalcemia. A troublesome mimic of mild primary hyperparathyroidism. Endocrinol Metab Clin North Am 1989;18:723-40.

15. Marx SJ. Hyperparathyroidism genes: sequences reveal answers and questions. Endocr Pract 2011;17(Suppl 3):18-27.

16. Palmër M, Jakobsson S, Akerström G, Ljunghall S. Prevalence of hypercalcemia in a health survey: a 14-year follow-up study of serum calcium values. Eur J Clin Invest 1988;18:39-46.

17. Palmër M, Ljunghall S, Akerström G, et al. Patients with primary hyperparathyroidism operated on over a 24-year period: temporal trends of clinical and laboratory findings. J Chronic Dis 1987;40:121-30.

18. Wermers RA, Khosla S, Atkinson EJ, et al. Incidence of primary hyperparathyroidism in Rochester Minnesota, 1993-2001: an update on the changing epidemiology of the disease. J Bone Miner Res 2006;21:171-7.

19. Scholz DA, Purnell DC. Asymptomatic primary hyperparathyroidism: 10-year prospective study. Mayo Clin Proc 1981;56:473-8.

20. Khan AA, Bilezikian JP, Potts JT Jr. Asymptomatic primary hyperparathyroidism: a commentary on the revised guidelines. Endocr Pract 2009;15:494-8.

21. Parisien M, Silverberg SJ, Shane E, Dempster DW, Bilezikian JP. Bone disease in primary hyperparathyroidism. Endocrinol Metab Clin North Am 1990;19:19-34.

22. Desai P, Steiner GC. Ultrastructure of brown tumor of hyperparathyroidism. Ultrastruct Pathol 1990;14:505-11.

23. Salusky IB, Colburn JW. The renal osteodystrophies. In: DeGroot LJ, ed. Endocrinology, Vol. 2, 2nd ed. Philadelphia: WB Saunders; 1989:1032-48.

24. Ohira S, Itoh K, Shiozawa T, et al. Ovarian non-small cell neuroendocrine carcinoma with paraneoplastic parathyroid hormone-related hypercalcemia. Int J Gynecol Pathol 2004;23:393-7.

25. Skrabanek P, McPartlin J, Powell D. Tumor hypercalcemia and "ectopic hyperparathyroidism." Medicine (Baltimore) 1980;59:262-82.

26. Stewart AF, Insogna K, Broadus AE. Malignancy associated hypercalcemia. In: DeGroot LJ, ed. Endocrinology, Vol. 2, 2nd ed. Philadelphia: WB Saunders; 1989:967-83.

27. DeLellis RA, Xia L. Paraneoplastic endocrine syndromes: a review. Endocr Pathol 2003;14:303-17.

28. Insogna KL. Humoral hypercalcemia of malignancy. The role of parathyroid hormone-related protein. Endocrinol Metab Clin North Am 1989;18:779-94.

29. Mundy GR. Hypercalcemic factors other than parathyroid hormone-related protein. Endocrinol Metab Clin North Am 1989;18:795-806.

30. Dickersin GR, Kline IW, Scully RE. Small cell carcinoma of the ovary with hypercalcemia: a report of eleven cases. Cancer 1982;49:188-97.
31. Shu, ST, Martin, CK, Thudi, NK, Dirksen WP, Rosol TJ. Osteolytic bone resorption in adult T-cell leukemia/lymphoma. Leuk Lymphoma 2010;51:702-14.
32. Davies M, Hayes ME, Yin JA, Berry JL, Mawer EB. Abnormal synthesis of 1,25-dihydroxyvitamin D in patients with malignant lymphoma. J Clin Endocrinol Metab 1994;78:1201-7.
33. Seymour JF, Gagel RF. Calcitriol: the major mediator of hypercalcemia in Hodgkin's disease and non-Hodgkin's lymphoma. Blood 1993;82:1383-4.
34. Chen L, Dinh TA, Haque A. Small cell carcinoma of the ovary with hypercalcemia and ectopic parathyroid hormone production. Arch Pathol Lab Med 2005;129:531-3.
35. Schmelzer HJ, Hesch RD, Mayer H. Parathyroid hormone and PTHmRNA in a human small cell lung cancer. Recent Results Cancer Res 1985;99:88-93.
36. Yoshimoto K, Yamasaki R, Sakai H, et al. Ectopic production of parathyroid hormone by small cell lung cancer in a patient with hypercalcemia. J Clin Endocrinol Metab 1989;68:976-81.
37. Nussbaum SR, Gaz RD, Arnold A. Hypercalcemia and ectopic secretion of parathyroid hormone by an ovarian carcinoma with rearrangement of the gene for parathyroid hormone. N Engl J Med 1990;323:1324-8.
38. Nussbaum SR, Zahradnik RJ, Lavigne JR, et al. Highly sensitive two-site immunoradiometric assay of parathyrin and its clinical utility in evaluating patients with hypercalcemia. Clin Chem 1987;33:1364-7.
39. Strewler GJ, Budayr AA, Clark OH, Nissenson RA. Production of parathyroid hormone by a malignant non-parathyroid tumor in a hypercalcemic patient. J Clin Endocrinol Metab 1993;76:1373-5.
40. Rizzoli R, Pache JC, Didierjean L, Bürger A, Bonjour JP. A thymoma as a cause of true ectopic hyperparathyroidism. J Clin Endocrinol Metab 1994;79:912-5.
41. Nielsen PK, Rasmussen AK, Feldt-Rasmussen U, Brandt M, Christensen L, Olgaard K. Ectopic production of intact parathyroid hormone by a squamous cell lung carcinoma in vivo and in vitro. J Clin Endocrinol Metab 1996;81:3793-6.
42. Uchimura K, Mokuno T, Nagasaka A, et al. Lung cancer associated with hypercalcemia induced by concurrently elevated parathyroid hormone and parathyroid hormone-relatedprotein levels. Metabolism 2002;51:871-5.
43. Iguchi H, Miyagi C, Tomita K, et al. Hypercalcemia caused by ectopic production of parathyroid hormone in a patient with papillary adenocarcinoma of the thyroid gland. J Clin Endocrinol Metab 1998;83:2653-7.
44. Koyama Y, Ishijima H, Ishitashi A, et al. Intact PTH-producing hepatocellular carcinoma treated by transcatheter arterial embolization. Abdom Imaging 1999;24:144-6.
45. Mundy GR, Edwards JR. PTH-related peptide (PTHrP) in hypercalcemia. J Am Soc Nephrol 2008;19:672-5.
46. Boyle WJ, Simonet WS, Lacey DL. Osteoclast differentiation and activation. Nature 2003;423:337-42.
47. Dufour DR, Marx SJ, Spiegel AM. Parathyroid gland morphology in non-parathyroid hormone-mediated hypercalcemia. Am J Surg Pathol 1985;9:43-51.

25 PARATHYROID ADENOMA AND VARIANTS

PARATHYROID ADENOMA

Definition. *Parathyroid adenoma* is a benign parathyroid neoplasm composed of chief cells, oncocytes, transitional oncocytes, or an admixture of these cell types (1,2).

General Features. Parathyroid adenoma is the single most common cause of primary hyperparathyroidism throughout the world. In most large series, 80 to 85 percent of all patients with primary hyperparathyroidism have a single adenoma (1,2). There is, however, considerable variation in the prevalence of adenomas in different published series that likely reflects the lack of uniformity of diagnostic criteria and variables in patterns of patient referrals.

There are few data relating to the etiology of parathyroid adenomas. These tumors are associated with type 1 or type 2 multiple endocrine neoplasia (MEN) syndromes in addition to other types of heritable hyperparathyroidism syndromes, as discussed in chapter 27 (3). Long-term lithium therapy is implicated in an increased prevalence of primary hyperparathyroidism, secondary to hyperplasia and adenoma, as discussed in chapter 24 (4).

External ionizing irradiation appears to have a role in the development of adenomas: up to 30 percent of patients with parathyroid adenomas in some series have had a history of radiation to the head and neck (5–7). Several studies have indicated that primary hyperparathyroidism and thyroid cancer occur together in those exposed to radiation more often than expected by chance alone (8,9). Survivors of the atomic blasts in Hiroshima had a fourfold increase in the incidence of parathyroid adenomas that appeared to be dose dependent (10). There is some evidence that the effects of radiation were greater for young individuals at the time of exposure (10). An increased risk of primary hyperparathyroidism has also been observed in a cohort of cleanup workers following the Chernobyl nuclear disaster (11). It has been sug-gested that exposure to strontium-90, which is a ligand for calcium-sensing receptor molecules, may be the cause of the primary hyperparathyroidism in this group (11).

Hyperparathyroidism occurs 15 to 20 years later than radiation-induced thyroid disease (52.6 ± 10 years versus 35.5 ± 13.8 years) (12). These observations suggest that patients with thyroid disease and a history of radiation exposure should be followed closely for the subsequent development of hyperparathyroidism. Interestingly, almost one third of the patients with hyperparathyroidism following radiation exposure have normal serum calcium levels despite elevated parathyroid hormone (PTH) levels and abnormal parathyroid glands (12).

The administration of diagnostic or therapeutic doses of radioactive iodine does not appear to be a significant risk factor for the development of parathyroid adenomas in humans (13,14). Triggs et al. (15), however, have reported that 61 percent of rats given radioactive iodine in the first 2 days of life develop parathyroid tumors. They suggest that this high frequency results from the fact that the parathyroid glands in rats are more deeply embedded in the thyroid gland than are the parathyroid glands in humans.

The histopathologic definition of parathyroid adenoma has remained controversial. In their seminal study of the pathology of hyperparathyroidism, Castleman and Mallory (16) stressed the localized character of the proliferative process in cases of adenoma, noting that it was limited not only to a single gland but was often confined to a portion of a single gland. Support for the concept of the neoplastic origin of adenomas was provided by the demonstration that an adjacent rim of parathyroid tissue was present in 40 percent of their cases and that there was no evidence of recurrent hyperparathyroidism after removal of the single enlarged gland (16).

Some studies, however, have suggested a relationship between hyperplasia and adenomas

(17,18). In a study of 172 cases of primary hyperparathyroidism, Ghandur-Mnaymneh and Kimura (19) concluded that hyperplasia with single gland involvement was responsible for 75 percent of cases of primary hyperparathyroidism. Akerström et al. (20) analyzed parathyroid glands obtained at autopsy from a large series of patients without evidence of advanced renal disease. Parathyroid hyperplasia was identified in 7 percent of cases while adenomas were found in 2.4 percent. The hyperplastic glands were frequently nodular and asymmetric, with increased numbers of oncocytes and chief cells, and some of the largest hyperplastic nodules were indistinguishable from adenomas. Serum calcium levels were increased in patients with adenomas and hyperplastic glands with large nodules. On the basis of these studies, Akerström et al. concluded that nodularity of parathyroid tissue is a sign of abnormality and that adenomas may arise from foci of nodular hyperplasia. This hypothesis has been supported by molecular studies that demonstrated clonality in some cases of primary and secondary chief cell hyperplasia (21).

The existence of double adenomas as a source of primary hyperparathyroidism has been a subject of controversy (22). Verdonk and Edis (23) reported double adenomas in approximately 2 percent of almost 2,000 patients with hyperparathyroidism. The criteria for inclusion in this study included: 1) the presence of two enlarged and hypercellular parathyroid glands and 2) the identification and preservation of two other normal-sized parathyroid glands.

One study has demonstrated that double adenomas occur in up to 15 percent of patients with primary hyperparathyroidism (24). Laboratory data, including serum calcium and PTH levels, were similar in patients with single and double parathyroid adenomas, as was the clinical symptomatology. Double adenomas occurred predominantly as bilateral superior parathyroid disease in 45 percent of cases (fourth pouch disease). The next most frequently involved sites were the lower glands (13 percent). The pattern of two-gland enlargement was characterized by a larger dominant gland combined with a considerably smaller second gland.

Clinical Features. Parathyroid adenomas occur predominantly in women (F:M, 3:1)

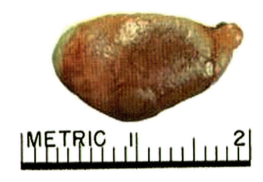

Figure 25-1

PARATHYROID ADENOMA

The adenoma in this case is relatively small.

with a peak incidence in the seventh decade; however, the incidence is similar in men and women before the age of 45 years (4). The clinical and laboratory findings are similar to those of primary hyperparathyroidism, as discussed in chapter 24. Most patients are asymptomatic and are identified on the basis of abnormal calcium levels.

Gross Findings. Parathyroid adenomas occur at any site in which normal parathyroid tissue is found (figs. 25-1–25-8) (1,16,25–27). Approximately 90 percent involve the upper or lower glands, with the lower glands involved more frequently. The remainder occur in a variety of other sites including the tracheoesophageal groove or paraesophagus (28 percent), mediastinum (26 percent), thymus (19 to 24 percent), thyroid gland (10 percent), carotid sheath (4 to 9 percent), base of skull (2 to 9 percent), and rarely, lateral to the carotid artery (28,29). Intrathyroidal adenomas tend to be smaller than those developing in extrathyroidal sites (30). Adenomas can also arise from ectopic or supernumerary parathyroid tissue present within the pericardium, soft tissue adjacent to the angle of the jaw, or the vagus and hypoglossal nerves (31–36).

The typical parathyroid adenoma is an encapsulated neoplasm. The capsule is generally thin, a feature that allows relatively easy surgical dissection of the tumor from the adjacent tissue. Adenomas vary considerably in size, ranging from less than 1 cm in diameter to more than 10 cm. *Microadenomas*, by definition, measure less than 0.6 cm in diameter (37). Microadenomas have also been defined on the basis of

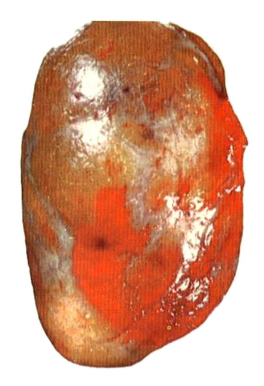

Figure 25-2

PARATHYROID ADENOMA

This tumor weighed 4.2 g.

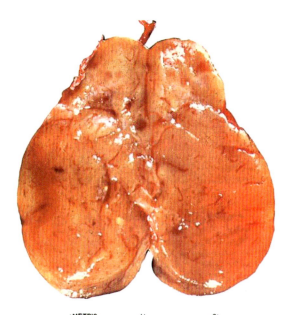

Figure 25-3

PARATHYROID ADENOMA

Cross section of 2.7-g adenoma.

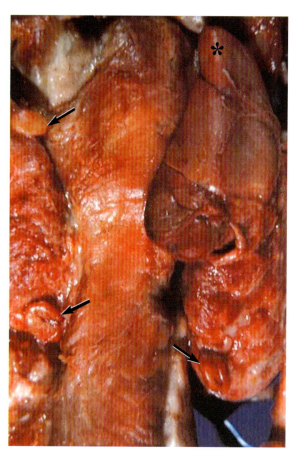

Figure 25-4

PARATHYROID ADENOMA

In situ postmortem dissection of the parathyroid glands in a patient with primary hyperparathyroidism. The lobes of the thyroid gland have been reflected anteriorly. The right upper parathyroid (asterisk) has been replaced by a large adenoma with a pyramidal shape and surface lobulations. The three remaining glands (arrows) are normal. (Courtesy of Dr. M. Stolte, Bayreuth, Germany.)

gland weight. Using an upper limit of 100 mg, Goasguen et al. (38) identified microadenomas in 6 percent of more than 1,000 patients with parathyroid adenomas. These lesions may be so small that they are missed on surgical exploration and frozen section examination (36). In several reported cases, microadenomas became evident only after serially sectioning the paraffin-embedded blocks (37,39).

There is some correlation between the clinical symptomatology and tumor weight, serum calcium level, and PTH level (1). In the cases reported from the Massachusetts General Hospital, adenomas associated with severe bone disease

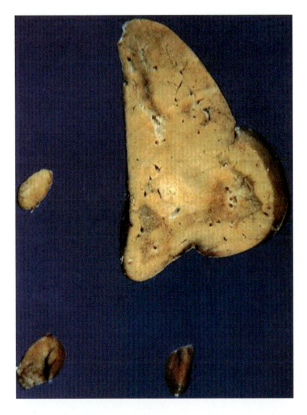

Figure 25-5

PARATHYROID ADENOMA

Following formalin fixation of the adenoma in figure 25-4, a solid appearance is seen on cross section. The remaining glands are normal. (Courtesy of Dr. M. Stolte, Bayreuth, Germany.)

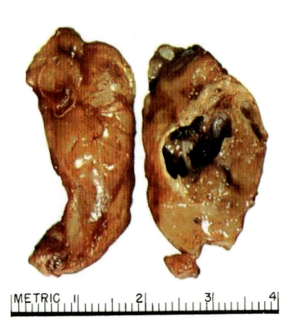

Figure 25-6

PARATHYROID ADENOMA

External (left) and cross section (right) of 3-g cystic adenoma.

Figure 25-7

MEDIASTINAL PARATHYROID ADENOMA

Thymus (left) and bisected adenoma (right). The adenoma has a few cystic foci.

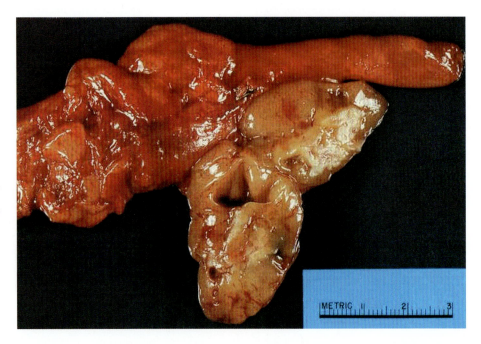

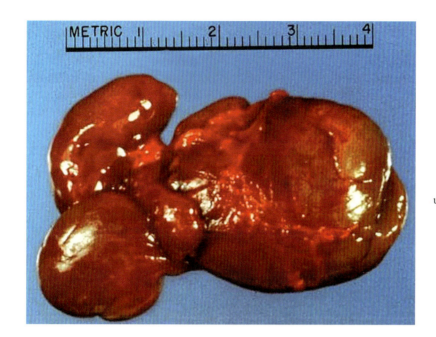

Figure 25-8

PARATHYROID ADENOMA

The tumor has a multilobated configuration.

had an average weight of 10 g while in individuals without bone disease the average weight was 1.3 g, with many weighing less than 0.5 g (1).

Large tumors are ovoid in configuration and sharply separated from the surrounding adipose tissue and thyroid gland. Some tumors are elongated and have a bilobated or multilobated configuration (fig. 25-8) (1,16). The risk of incomplete excision is higher in adenomas with a multilobated configuration than in ovoid tumors with smooth contours.

In most cases, the cut surface of the adenoma is tan to red brown, soft, and homogeneous (figs. 25-3, 25-5). Nodularity is evident in some cases. A rim of normal gland, commonly found in the hilar region, is generally light brown or yellow. The absence of a rim of residual parathyroid tissue does not exclude the diagnosis of an adenoma, while its presence does not confirm it.

Foci of cystic change are apparent in many cases, with individual cysts ranging from 0.1 to more than 1.0 cm in diameter (figs. 25-6, 25-7). The cysts are filled with clear straw-colored or brown fluid. Cystic degeneration may be extensive in some cases, with foci of fibrosis, calcification, and brown discoloration due to the presence of hemosiderin pigment (1,16). The walls of cystic adenomas may be markedly thickened, with adherence to the thyroid gland and adjacent soft tissues of the neck, raising the possibility of malignancy at the time of surgery.

Spontaneous infarction of parathyroid adenomas is a rare event that may be followed by resolution of the hyperparathyroidism (fig. 25-9) (40–42). Partial infarction may be followed by regeneration of the residual tumor and recurrence of hyperparathyroidism. Rarely, spontaneous rupture of a parathyroid adenoma presents as massive cervical hemorrhage (43).

Microscopic Findings. Most large parathyroid adenomas are encapsulated neoplasms that are composed of chief cells at varying stages of their secretory cycle (1,44–46). Microadenomas are impossible to distinguish from focally hyperplastic glands since the lesions are usually not encapsulated (fig. 25-10) (20). The cells are arranged in cords and nests, glandular formations, perivascular palisades, or diffuse sheets, with frequent admixtures of these patterns (figs. 25-11–25-13).

The dominant cell type in most adenomas is the chief cell (figs. 25-12, 25-13) (1,2,44–46). Typically, the adenoma cells are larger than those present in the adjacent normal parathyroid tissue. Most cells within adenomas measure 8 to 14 µm in diameter and have a polyhedral shape with an indistinct cell outline. Rarely, the tumor cells are spindle shaped (fig. 25-14).

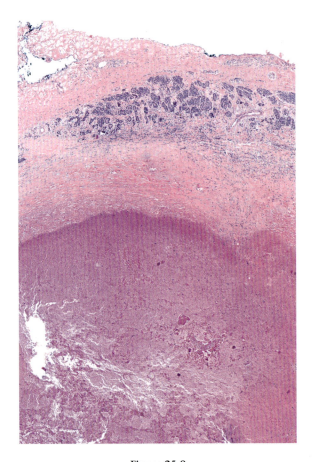

Figure 25-9

INFARCTED PARATHYROID ADENOMA

The tumor is almost completely necrotic (bottom). A small amount of residual adenoma is present in the fibrotic rim (top).

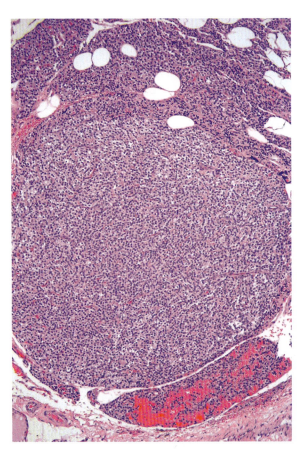

Figure 25-10

PARATHYROID CHIEF CELL MICROADENOMA

The tumor is nonencapsulated.

The cytoplasm is faintly eosinophilic but may appear clear (fig. 25-13). In some instances, the cytoplasm has a vacuolated appearance and some cells have perinuclear halos. Nodular aggregates of chief cells with more or less cytoplasm than the bulk of chief cells comprising the adenoma may be present (fig. 25-15). The larger cells often have abundant clear cytoplasm with sharply outlined plasma membranes and prominent glycogen deposits; the small chief cells have scanty eosinophilic cytoplasm.

The nuclei are generally round, regular, and centrally placed, with dense lymphocyte-like chromatin and occasional small nucleoli. Multinucleated adenoma cells are evident in some cases (fig. 25-16) (1,2,47,48). As in other endocrine tumors, enlarged hyperchromatic nuclei are present in up to 25 percent of all cases, with individual nuclei measuring up to 50 µm in diameter (fig. 25-17). Cells with enlarged hyperchromatic nuclei may be dispersed throughout the tumor or form small aggregates (1,2,47,48). In the absence of other features of malignancy, the presence of enlarged hyperchromatic nuclei should not be a criterion of malignancy. In fact, the presence of such bizarre nuclei may be used as a point in favor of the diagnosis of adenoma rather than hyperplasia or carcinoma.

The presence of mitoses has been considered in the past a feature highly suggestive of malignancy in parathyroid tumors. However, several studies have demonstrated that mitotic activity may be present in benign lesions, including adenomas and hyperplasias (fig. 25-18) (49,50). Snover and Foucar (50) found parenchymal mitoses in approximately 70 percent of adenomas: most cases contained less than 1 mitosis per

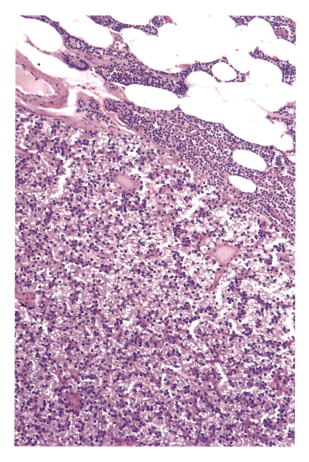

Figure 25-11

PARATHYROID CHIEF CELL ADENOMA

The tumor is separated from the adjacent parathyroid gland by a thin fibrous capsule.

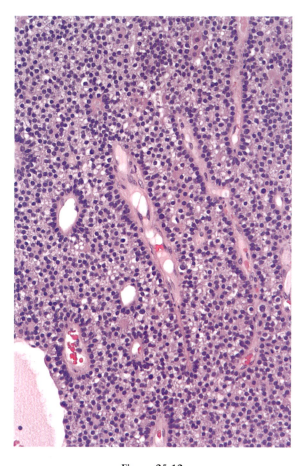

Figure 25-12

PARATHYROID CHIEF CELL ADENOMA

The tumor cells have a palisaded arrangement around blood vessels.

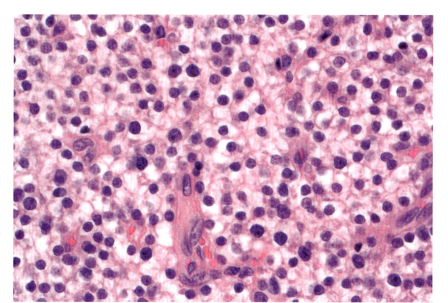

Figure 25-13

PARATHYROID CHIEF CELL ADENOMA

The tumor cell nuclei are small, round, and densely stained.

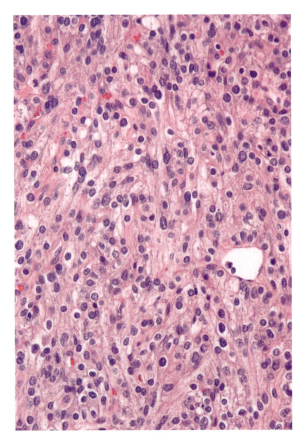

Figure 25-14

PARATHYROID CHIEF CELL ADENOMA

Many of the tumor cells have a spindle shape.

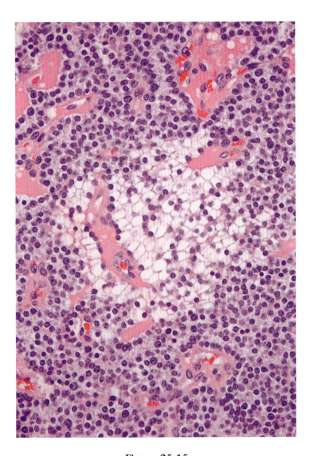

Figure 25-15

PARATHYROID CHIEF CELL ADENOMA

The nodule within the adenoma is composed of vacu-olated chief cells.

Figure 25-16

PARATHYROID CHIEF CELL ADENOMA

There are focal collections of multinucleated giant cells.

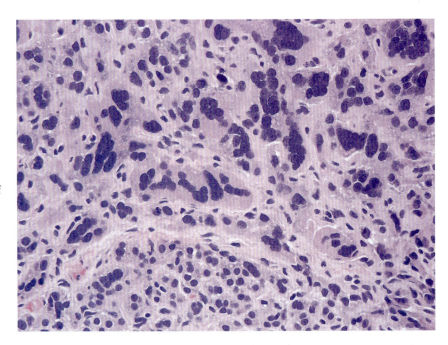

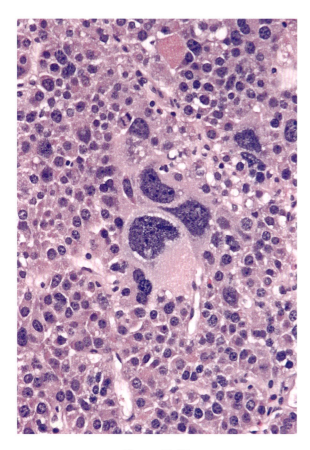

Figure 25-17

PARATHYROID CHIEF CELL ADENOMA

This tumor has scattered foci of cells with nuclear enlargement and hyperchromasia.

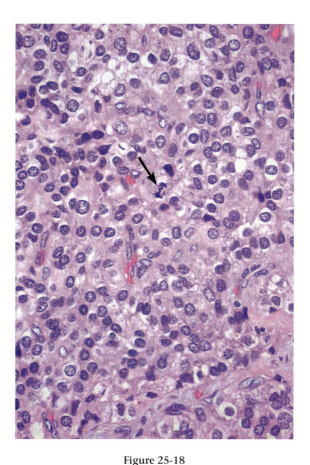

Figure 25-18

PARATHYROID CHIEF CELL ADENOMA

There is less than 1 mitosis (arrow) per 10 high-power microscopic fields in this tumor.

10 high-power microscopic fields, but approximately 10 percent had more than 1 mitosis per 10 high-power fields. None of the patients had evidence of recurrent or metastatic disease with a follow-up of 5.5 years. In the series of cases reviewed by San Juan et al. (49), 3 of 19 cases (16 percent) with mitoses and 1 of 7 cases (14 percent) without mitoses recurred. These data indicate that mitotic activity by itself should not be considered a criterion of malignancy. However, cases with more than 1 mitosis per 10 high-power fields should be evaluated carefully for the presence of other features suggestive of malignancy. Endothelial cells may be mitotically active in these tumors, and should be distinguished from mitoses occurring in parenchymal cells.

The proliferative activity of parathyroid adenomas has been assessed with antibodies to Ki-67 and proliferating cell nuclear antigen (PCNA), but more consistent results have been obtained with Ki-67 (51). The proliferative fractions of chief cell and oncocytic adenomas are generally less than 4 percent (52–55), while p27, a cyclin-dependent kinase inhibitor, is highly expressed (53,55).

Scattered follicle-like or glandular structures are present in many adenomas. Some adenomas, however, have a predominant follicular structure with accumulation of colloid-like material within the lumens (figs. 25-19, 25-20). The colloid is eosinophilic, and concentric laminations within the colloid may be calcified and may, therefore, resemble psammoma bodies. Cellular debris may be present within the follicles, and it has been suggested that the follicles arise as a result of cystic degeneration within the epithelium of hyperfunctioning parathyroid tissue (56). Congo red stains reveal that some of the intraluminal

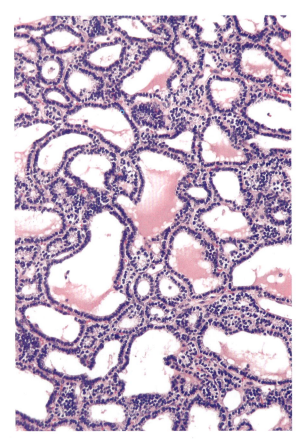

Figure 25-19

PARATHYROID CHIEF CELL ADENOMA

This tumor is composed of follicles containing a thin colloid-like material.

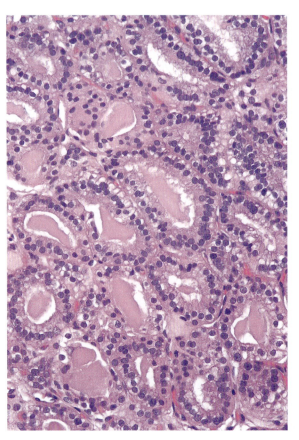

Figure 25-20

PARATHYROID CHIEF CELL ADENOMA

The follicles contain thick colloid-like material.

material shows the green birefringence typical of amyloid deposits (57).

The formation of papillae occurs rarely in parathyroid adenomas (fig. 25-21) (58). In a review of more than 100 adenomas, Sahin and Robinson (59) identified a single case in which the tumor had a partially papillary architecture. The papillae were composed of fibrovascular cores that were covered by cells with abundant eosinophilic cytoplasm and round nuclei with punctate chromatin. The presence of papillae in aspirated samples may lead to a mistaken diagnosis of papillary thyroid carcinoma.

The stroma contains numerous capillaries that can be demonstrated selectively with antibodies to factor VIII–related antigen, CD31, or CD34. Adenoma cells are typically arranged around the vessels in a palisade-like pattern (fig. 25-12). Occasional adenomas contain consider-

able amounts of fibrous connective tissue with extensive calcification and cyst formation (figs. 25-22–25-24). Fibrosis most likely develops as a result of degenerative changes within the adenoma, and the fibrotic areas frequently show evidence of hemosiderin deposition and chronic inflammation. Rarely, the stroma is extensively sclerotic in a pattern that has been referred to as *hyalinizing parathyroid adenoma* (60). Aggregates of lymphocytes are present in some cases, and on occasion, the degree of lymphocytic infiltration is extensive (fig. 25-25) (61). Stromal amyloid deposits may be present in patients with systemic amyloidosis (57).

Although most descriptions of parathyroid adenomas have stressed the absence of stromal fat as a major diagnostic criterion, adenomas may, in fact, contain mature adipose tissue (62). Adipocytes may be distributed uniformly

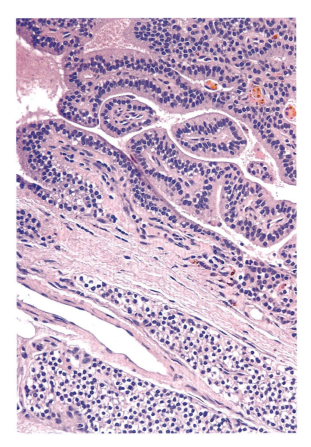

Figure 25-21

PARATHYROID CHIEF CELL ADENOMA

Focal papillary areas are seen.

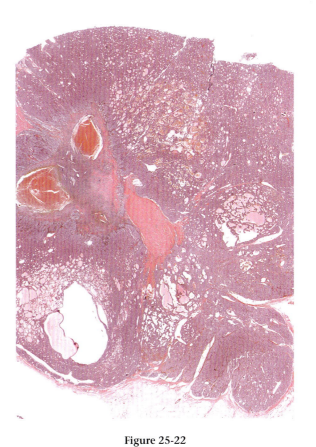

Figure 25-22

PARATHYROID CHIEF CELL ADENOMA

This degenerated adenoma has areas of fibrosis with hemorrhage and cystic change.

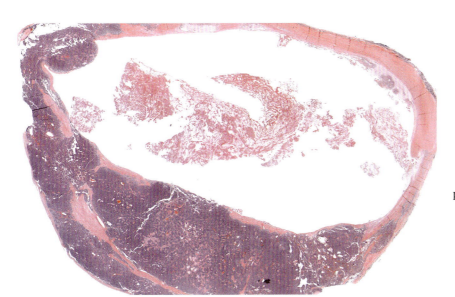

Figure 25-23

PARATHYROID CHIEF CELL ADENOMA

Extensive cystic change is present.

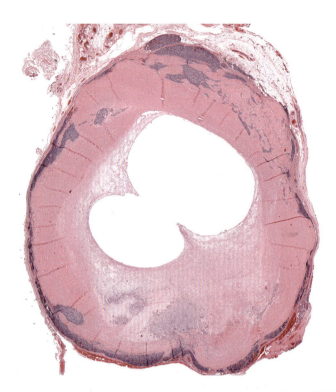
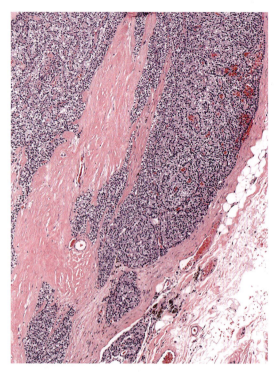

Figure 25-24

PARATHYROID CHIEF CELL ADENOMA

Left: The wall of this cystic adenoma is extensively fibrotic.
Right: Groups of residual adenoma cells are entrapped within the cyst wall.

Figure 25-25

**PARATHYROID
CHIEF CELL ADENOMA**

Infiltrates of lymphocytes are present in the periphery of the tumor. A rim of normal parathyroid is present at the upper right.

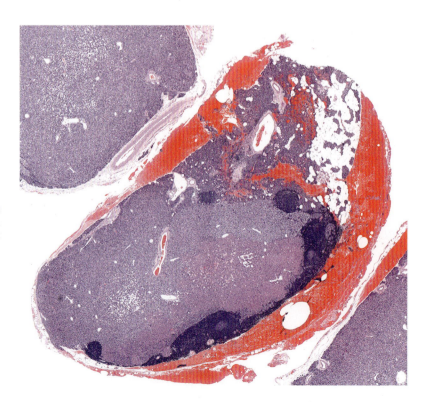

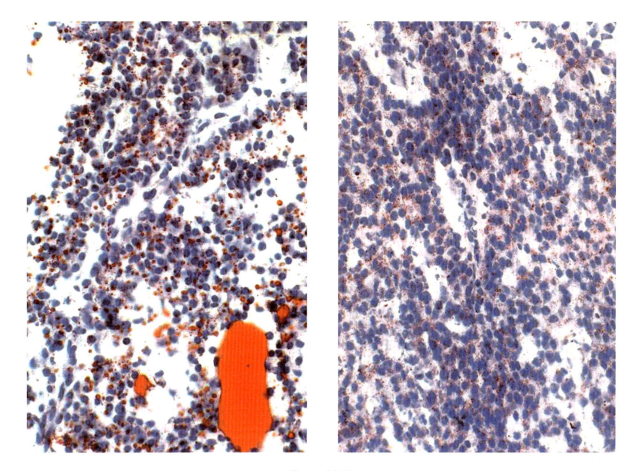

Figure 25-26

PARATHYROID CHIEF CELL ADENOMA

Left: Oil red O stains the rim surrounding the parathyroid chief cell adenoma. The cells contain prominent lipid droplets. The oil red O–positive area in the right lower corner is stromal fat.

Right: A small amount of finely dispersed lipid is present within the tumor cells.

throughout the tumor or be present in small aggregates. On occasion, stromal adipose tissue is so abundant that a small biopsy is interpreted as a normocellular gland.

The presence of a rim of normal or suppressed parathyroid tissue has been regarded as an important criterion to establish the diagnosis of adenoma. Approximately 30 to 50 percent of cases reported as adenoma have a rim of non-neoplastic chief cells. Generally, the probability of finding a rim is highest in small adenomas (16,25). Although the rim of parathyroid tissue is usually separated from the adenoma by a connective tissue capsule, the capsule may be indistinct or even absent. The parenchymal cells within the rim are typically smaller than those in the adenoma and contain more abundant

cytoplasmic lipid (fig. 25-26). The lipid droplets within the suppressed chief cells measure 0.5 to 1.5 µm in diameter (63,64). When lipid is present within adenoma cells, it tends to be more finely dispersed than in the suppressed rim (fig. 25-26).

Cytologic Findings. There are few studies on the use of fine-needle aspiration biopsy (FNAB) for the diagnosis of parathyroid proliferative lesions. Several groups have used needle aspirates in conjunction with noninvasive preoperative procedures, including ultrasonograph, thallium technetium scanning, magnetic resonance imaging (MRI), and computerized tomography (CT) scanning, particularly in patients with prior failed cervical explorations (65–69). In the series reported by Kendrick et al. (67), there were no instances of parathyromatosis following aspiration biopsy.

Aspirates of parathyroid adenomas are highly cellular, with numerous dissociated epithelial cells in addition to variably sized epithelial aggregates (figs. 25-27, 25-28) (69,70). The nuclei are variable in size, round to ovoid, and hyperchromatic. Numerous "naked" nuclei are often present, the chromatin is arranged in coarse granules, and occasional nucleoli may be evident. The cytoplasm is pale, amphophilic, and occasionally vacuolated, with ill-defined cell borders. Oncocytic cells are characterized by the presence of more abundant and granular cytoplasm. Occasional markedly enlarged and hyperchromatic nuclei are present in some cases (70). There are no cytologic criteria to distinguish cases of hyperplasia from adenoma; however, the presence of giant nuclei and morulas suggests that the lesion is an adenoma.

The differentiation of thyroid epithelium from parathyroid chief cells in aspirated material is particularly difficult. Cell groups in parathyroid aspirates are thick, cohesive, and branching, with frayed edges (figs. 25-27, 25-28) (70). Macrofollicular adenomas or adenomatous goiters have more evenly spaced "honeycomb" sheets. Aspirates from parathyroid adenomas may have a microfollicular pattern that is impossible to distinguish from thyroid microfollicular adenomas. The colloid-like material in parathyroid aspirates stains blue-green with the Papanicolaou stain, except for central regions which are more eosinophilic. Immunoperoxidase stains for PTH are the most specific approach for the identification of parathyroid tissue in aspirated material (fig. 25-27) (71). Concurrent assays for PTH also provide an invaluable approach for the identification of parathyroid tissue (68). When aspirating a lesion with the differential diagnosis of parathyroid adenoma versus thyroid adenoma, it is always wise to look for the most recent calcium level. Fine-needle aspiration biopsy of adenomas may, on occasion, lead to capsular disruption and other changes suspicious for malignancy (72). This subject is further discussed in chapter 26.

Immunohistochemical Findings. Adenoma cells are positive for cytokeratins (CK) 7, 8, 18, and 19. CK14 is expressed in most oncocytic adenomas and in approximately one third of chief cell adenomas (73). Occasional cells are positive for neurofilament proteins while vimentin is expressed predominantly in the stromal elements. The tumor cells are positive for PTH (fig. 25-29), chromogranin, and the glial cells missing 2 (Gcm2) transcription factor (74,75). Adenoma cells typically have less PTH and PTH messenger (m)RNA than the cells in the uninvolved rim of the gland (fig. 25-29) (76). The latter finding is consistent with the hypothesis that enhanced secretory function is largely a function of the increased total mass of the tumor cells. Stains for thyroglobulin and thyroid transcription factor (TTF)-1 are negative.

Most adenomas, with the exception of those associated with the hyperparathyroidism-jaw tumor syndrome, are positive for parafibromin, the product of the *HRPT2/CDC73* gene (fig. 25-30) (77,78). Parafibromin has a predominant nuclear localization, and is expressed in a wide variety of normal tissues (77,79). Adenomas are positive for the adenomatous polyposis coli (APC) gene product and glycogen synthases kinase 3-beta , while galectin-3 and PGP9.5 are expressed rarely (80–82). The latter proteins, in addition to parafibromin, have been suggested as potential markers to distinguish adenomas and carcinomas. This subject is discussed further in chapter 26.

The synaptosomal-associated protein of 25 kDa (SNAP-25) and syntaxin are present in 20 percent of adenomas while normal parathyroid tissue is negative for these markers (83). On the other hand, vesicle-associated membrane protein and SNAP-23, the cellular homologue of SNAP-25, are present both in normal and adenomatous parathyroid tissue (83).

Cyclin D1 immunoreactivity is present in 14 to 40 percent of adenomas, with nuclear staining present in 30 to 70 percent of the cells (84,85). PAX8 is expressed in approximately 40 percent of adenomas and hyperplasias (86) and occasional cases are positive for the renal cell carcinoma antigen, RCC (87). The retinoblastoma protein is present in most adenomas, although the extent of staining is variable among different cases (88). BCL-2 is present in 70 percent of cases (89), while most adenomas are negative for p53.

Calcium sensing receptor (CaSR) mRNA is significantly reduced in adenomas as compared

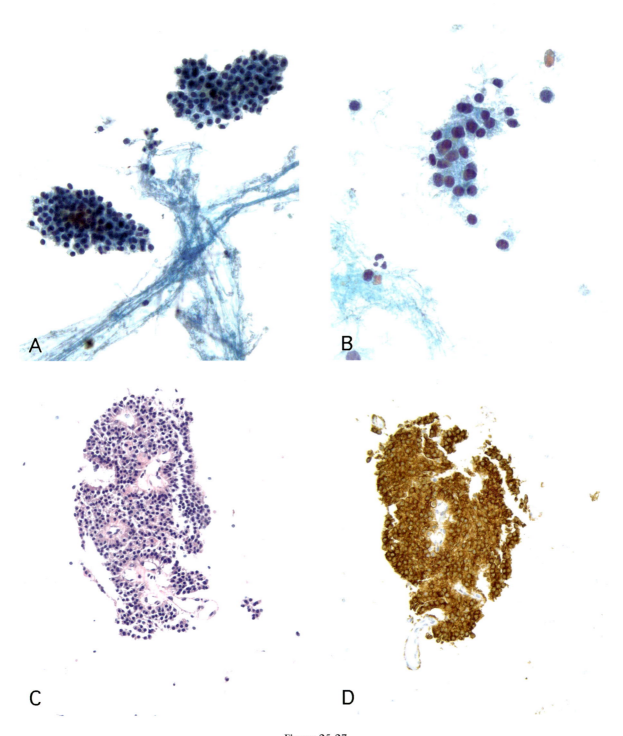

Figure 25-27

PARATHYROID CHIEF CELL ADENOMA

A: In this Thin Prep of a fine-needle aspiration biopsy (FNAB), there are variably sized groups of adenoma cells, in addition to isolated single cells and naked nuclei (Papanicolaou stain). (Courtesy of Dr. L. Pisharodi, Providence, RI.)

B: The cells have slightly irregular hyperchromatic nuclei (Papanicolaou stain; Thin Prep of FNAB).

C: Cell block of residual aspirated fluid. Small fragments of the adenoma are present (H&E stain).

D: Cell block of residual aspirated fluid. The adenoma cells are strongly and diffusely positive for parathyroid hormone (Immunoperoxidase stain).

Figure 25-28

PARATHYROID CHIEF-CELL ADENOMA

The tumor cells in this fine-needle aspirate are present as irregularly shaped aggregates admixed with red blood cells (Diff Quik stain).

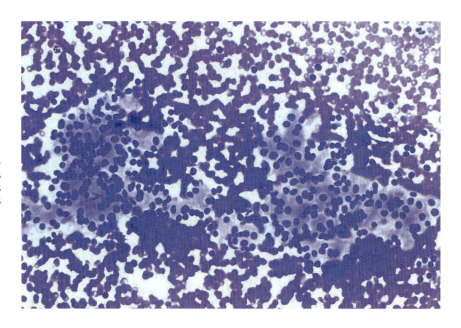

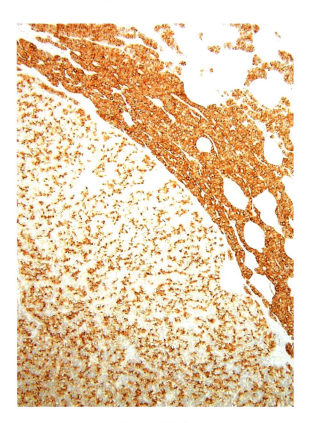

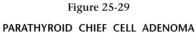

Figure 25-29

PARATHYROID CHIEF CELL ADENOMA STAINED FOR PARATHYROID HORMONE

The adenoma (lower left) contains less immunoreactive parathyroid hormone (PTH) than the cells in the adjacent rim (upper right) (Immunoperoxidase stain for PTH).

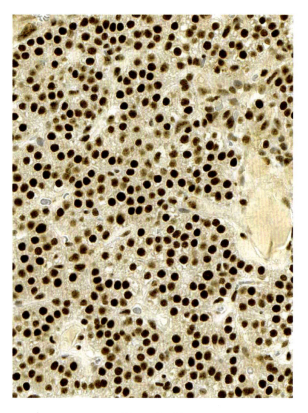

Figure 25-30

PARATHYROID CHIEF CELL ADENOMA STAINED FOR PARAFIBROMIN

The nuclei are uniformly and strongly stained (Immunoperoxidase stain for parafibromin). (Courtesy of Dr. A. Gill, Sydney, Australia.)

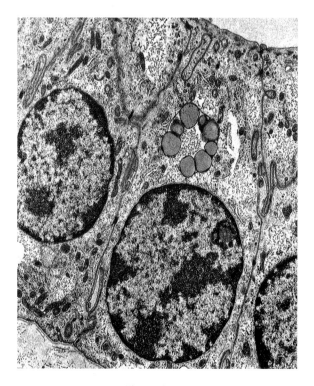

Figure 25-31

PARATHYROID CHIEF CELL ADENOMA

Electron micrograph of chief cell adenoma. The tumor cells are arranged in glandular formations. Plasma membranes have complex interdigitations. There are few secretory granules. Supranuclear lipid droplets are evident in some cells.

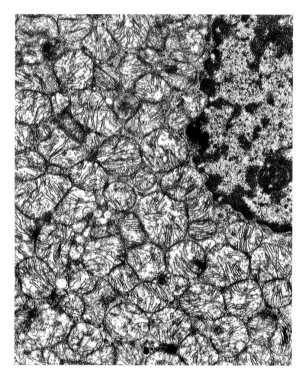

Figure 25-32

ONCOCYTIC PARATHYROID ADENOMA

Electron micrograph of oncocytic adenoma. The cytoplasm is filled with mitochondria.

to normal glands (90). This suggests that the lowered levels of CaSR mRNA in adenomas may contribute to the increased set point of PTH secretion. Reduction of CaSR has also been reported in adenomas from patients with secondary hyperparathyroidism (91).

Ultrastructural Findings. The cells of most parathyroid adenomas lack the normal integrated secretory and synthetic functions typical of normal chief cells (fig. 25-31) (44,45,92). It is often impossible to determine whether individual cells in these tumors are in the resting or synthetic phases of their cycles (93). Plasma membranes have more complex interdigitations than do normal chief cells. Generally, adenoma cells have a more extensive endoplasmic reticulum and a larger Golgi region with increased numbers of vesicles as compared to suppressed chief cells. There are no apparent increases in the numbers of prosecretory granules or mature secretory granules. There is some suggestion that the presence of extensive microvilli cor-

relates with the degree of synthetic activity in adenoma cells (94). Oncocytic adenoma cells (see Adenoma Variants below) are typically filled with mitochondria with few prosecretory and mature secretory granules (fig. 25-32). Water clear cell adenomas (see Adenoma Variants) are characterized by the presence of multiple cytoplasmic vesicles.

Molecular Genetic Findings. Early studies, based on glucose-6-phosphate dehydrogenase isoenzyme patterns, indicated that parathyroid adenomas were polyclonal proliferations (95). Subsequent analyses, however, have revealed that most are clonal lesions, as demonstrated by X-chromosome inactivation and DNA polymorphism studies (96,97).

The *PRAD1* (parathyroid adenoma)/(*CCND1*) cyclin D1 and *MEN1* genes have been implicated in the development of these tumors (98–101). Overexpression of the *CCND1* oncogene results from pericentric inversion of chromosome 11p with placement of the *CCND1* gene under the control of tissue-specific enhancer elements of the *PTH* gene promoter sequences (98–102). Translocations of this type are present in approximately 5 percent of adenomas; however, overexpression of cyclin D1 occurs in up to 40 percent of these tumors (103,104). These observations suggest that other mechanisms, in addition to translocations, are responsible for the overexpression of cyclin D1.

Mutations of the *MEN1* gene (11q13), which encodes menin, are responsible for the development of the multiple endocrine neoplasia 1 (MEN 1) syndrome (105,106). Loss of one *MEN 1* allele also occurs in up to 40 percent of sporadic adenomas, and an inactivating mutation in the other allele occurs in approximately 50 percent (21,107–109). There are no apparent mutations of the *MEN 1* gene in cases without loss of heterozygosity (LOH). The clinical and biochemical characteristics of patients are unrelated to the presence of LOH and *MEN 1* gene mutations (110). It has been suggested that the inactivation of the *MEN1* gene is an important genetic alteration in radiation-induced parathyroid adenomas (111).

The *HRPT2/CDC73* gene (1q25-q31), which encodes parafibromin, has been implicated in the development of adenomas and carcinomas in patients with the hyperparathyroidism-jaw tumor syndrome, but it does not play a significant role in the development of sporadic adenomas (112). Somatic mutations of the *CaSR*, *vitamin D receptor*, and *RET* genes have not been implicated in the development of sporadic parathyroid adenomas (95,113). Mutations of the *CDKI* genes occur in less than 5 percent of apparent sporadic adenomas (114–116).

Differential Diagnosis. Parathyroid adenomas must be distinguished from carcinomas and hyperplasias of the parathyroid glands (see chapters 26 and 27).

The distinction of parathyroid lesions from other neoplasms in this region is usually straightforward since most patients with primary hyperparathyroidism have evidence of hypercalcemia and increased serum levels of PTH. On occasion, however, it is difficult to distinguish primary thyroid neoplasms of both follicular and C-cell types from parathyroid adenomas. Since approximately 0.2 percent of normal parathyroid glands are within the thyroid parenchyma and a significant propor-

tion are contiguous with the thyroid capsule, parathyroid adenomas may have the gross appearance of a primary thyroid neoplasm.

Parathyroid adenomas with a completely follicular growth pattern are rare, but foci of follicle formation are common. In this situation, deeper sections often reveal areas more typical of parathyroid adenoma with solid cell sheets or cord-like growth patterns. Occasional thyroid adenomas contain abundant stromal fat and are classified as *adenolipomas* (117). Thyroid adenolipomas are particularly difficult to distinguish from parathyroid adenomas when there is a predominant microfollicular growth pattern and prominent stromal fat. Generally, the cells of parathyroid adenomas appear smaller and more vacuolated than the component cells of thyroid follicular neoplasms. Moreover, the nuclei of parathyroid cells are rounder, with a denser chromatin pattern than thyroid follicular cells.

The distinction of parathyroid adenomas from thyroid follicular cell neoplasms may be particularly challenging at the time of frozen section. Examination of sections in polarized light is helpful in this situation. The colloid of normal thyroid follicles and follicular neoplasms often contains birefringent calcium oxalate crystals, while the follicles in parathyroid adenoma do not (118,119).

Parathyroid adenomas contain more glycogen than do tumors of thyroid follicular cell origin, and the periodic acid–Schiff (PAS) stain helps make this distinction. Most thyroid follicular cell neoplasms contain little glycogen, except for the occasional clear cell type. Diastase-resistant PAS-positive material in thyroid follicular epithelium usually represents lipofuscin or colloid.

Immunohistochemistry is the most specific approach for the distinction of parathyroid and thyroid follicular cell neoplasms. Parathyroid neoplasms are positive for PTH, chromogranin, and Gcm2 transcription factor, but are negative for thyroglobulin and TTF-1 (74,75). Thyroid follicular cell neoplasms have the opposite immunophenotype.

Parathyroid adenomas rarely contain papillary structures (58). The presence of finely granular chromatin, nuclear grooves, and nuclear pseudoinclusions, together with positivity for thyroglobulin and TTF-1, distinguishes papillary thyroid carcinomas from papillary and pseudopapillary variants of parathyroid adenoma. Similarly, oncocytic parathyroid tumors (see Adenoma Variants below) are negative for thyroglobulin and TTF-1 but demonstrate positivity for parathyroid hormone and chromogranin.

Some parathyroid adenomas are difficult to distinguish from medullary thyroid carcinomas. The latter tumors have larger nuclei with coarsely clumped chromatin and finely granular or clear cytoplasm (see chapter 12). These tumors are typically positive for calcitonin, chromogranin, and carcinoembryonic antigen while parathyroid tumors are positive for chromogranin, PTH, and Gcm2. Occasional parathyroid adenomas, however, have been reported to be positive for calcitonin and the calcitonin gene-related peptide (120,121)

On occasion, the distinction of parathyroid adenoma from metastatic carcinoma, particularly of clear cell type, is a challenge. In this regard, it should be remembered that the RCC antigen may be expressed in parathyroid tumors (87). The demonstration of PTH or Gcm2 in such cases establishes the diagnosis of a parathyroid neoplasm.

Treatment and Prognosis. The optimal treatment of parathyroid adenoma is excision of the abnormal gland(s) with biopsy of a second (normal) gland or knowledge of intraoperative PTH levels (4,122), as discussed in chapter 30. The cure rate of the hyperparathyroidism is greater than 95 percent in the hands of experienced endocrine surgeons. In some series, however, the incidence of recurrent or persistent hyperparathyroidism is as high as 30 percent (28). Hyperparathyroidism diagnosed within 6 months of initial surgery is referred to as persistent disease, while hyperparathyroidism developing after 6 months is referred to as recurrent disease (28).

The causes of persistent/recurrent hyperparathyroidism include initial treatment failure due to the inability to locate a normally positioned gland, anatomic factors due to the presence of ectopic or supernumerary glands, and the biology of the underlying disease process (adenoma versus double adenoma versus hyperplasia) (28,29,123). In a small proportion of cases, recurrent/persistent disease results from an unrecognized carcinoma at the time of initial surgery (123). Capsular rupture with spillage of parathyroid cells or incomplete excision of a

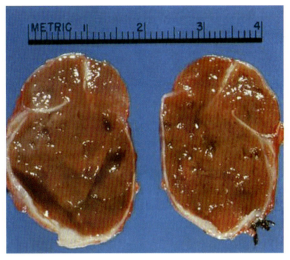

Figure 25-33

ONCOCYTIC PARATHYROID ADENOMA

The tumor is red-brown on cross section.

lobulated adenoma may also lead to the development of recurrent disease (4,124–126).

ADENOMA VARIANTS

Oncocytic Adenoma

Oncocytic adenomas are uncommon, accounting for 3 to 6 percent of all benign parathyroid tumors (127–131). Although earlier studies suggested that these tumors were nonfunctional, hyperparathyroidism has been documented in a substantial proportion of cases. The major criteria for the diagnosis of oncocytic adenoma, as summarized by Wolpert et al. (129), include: 1) at least 90 percent composition by oncocytic cells; 2) a second histologically normal parathyroid gland; and 3) postoperative alleviation of the hypercalcemia.

Grossly, oncocytic adenomas are soft and range in color from tan or dark brown to orange (fig. 25-33). The tumors are ellipsoidal or spherical in shape and are smooth or lobulated. Most weigh between 1 and 2 g (1,2,73).

The cells are typically arranged in broad sheets, anastomosing cords, or acini. They have abundant granular eosinophilic cytoplasm and round nuclei with dense chromatin and prominent nucleoli (fig. 25-34). Some of the tumors exhibit considerable variation in nuclear size and shape, with occasional bizarre hyperchromatic forms.

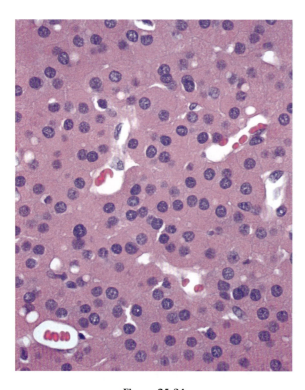

Figure 25-34

ONCOCYTIC PARATHYROID ADENOMA

The tumor is composed of large cells with abundant granular eosinophilic cytoplasm

Occasionally, groups of multinucleated cells, similar to those found in chief cell adenomas, are present. The cells of oncocytic adenoma have less intracellular lipid than the cells in the rims of the adjacent parathyroid gland.

Lipoadenoma

Lipoadenoma (hamartoma) is a rare benign tumor that is characterized by the proliferation of both stromal and parenchymal elements (132–136). These tumors may be functional or non-functional. The typical lipoadenoma presents as an encapsulated mass, which is soft, yellow-tan, and lobulated on cross section (fig. 25-35). Reported tumors have weighed between 0.5 and 420.0 g. While most lipoadenomas present as solitary lesions, rare examples of double lipoadenomas have been reported (137).

The stroma of lipoadenoma is characterized by an abundance of adipose tissue, with frequent areas of myxoid change and fibrosis (figs. 25-36, 25-37). Prominent collections of lymphoid cells are present in some cases. The parenchymal cells

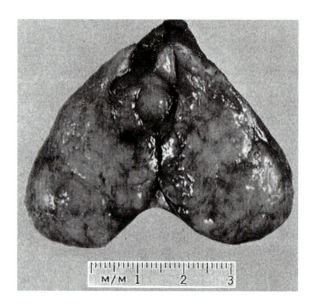

Figure 25-35

PARATHYROID LIPOADENOMA

On cross section, this encapsulated tumor has a lobular pattern.

include chief cells and small numbers of oncocytes arranged in a thin, branching, cord-like fashion. All reported cases have been benign. Otherwise typical chief cell adenomas may contain foci of lipoadenomatous change.

Water Clear Cell Adenoma

Water clear cell adenoma is a rare entity that is characterized by a solid or acinar growth pattern and the presence of large cells with finely vacuolated cytoplasm (figs. 25-38, 25-39) (138,139). Kuhel et al. (140) reported a case of synchronous water clear cell adenomas involving two glands. Since clear cell change occurs in a variety of thyroid follicular and C-cell tumors, immunohistochemical stains for thyroglobulin, calcitonin, and TTF-1 should be used to rule out a thyroid primary. Renal cell carcinomas, which on rare occasion metastasize to the parathyroid glands, should also be ruled out. The latter tumors typically demonstrate a sinusoidal pattern of blood vessels with frequent foci of intraluminal hemorrhage.

Atypical Adenoma

The term *atypical adenoma* describes a subset of parathyroid tumors that exhibit some of the features of parathyroid carcinoma but that lack

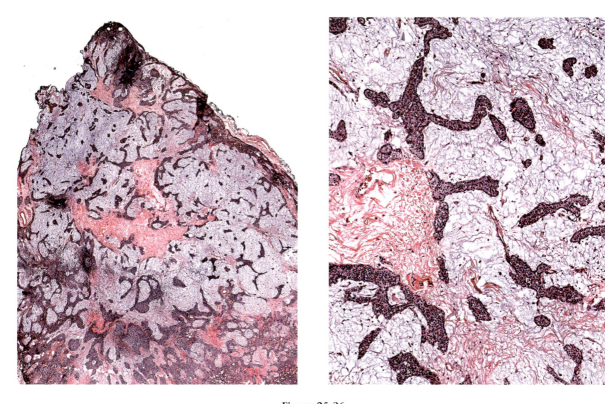

Figure 25-36

PARATHYROID LIPOADENOMA

Left: This tumor is composed of branching cords of chief cells embedded in a myxoid matrix.
Right: In addition to the myxoid matrix, there are focal areas of fibrosis.

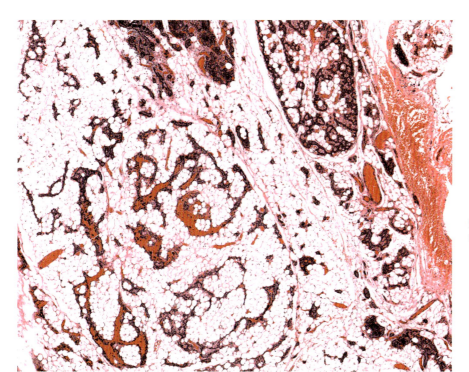

Figure 25-37

PARATHYROID LIPOADENOMA

The stroma of this tumor is composed almost entirely of mature fat cells.

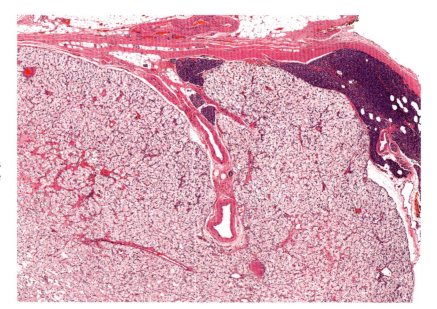

Figure 25-38

WATER CLEAR CELL ADENOMA

A rim of parathyroid tissue is present at the periphery of the tumor.

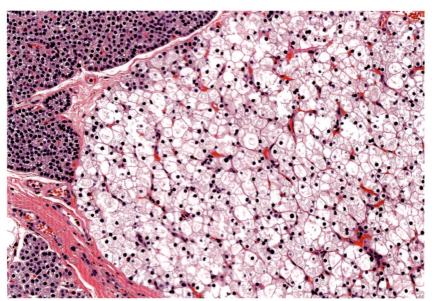

Figure 25-39

WATER CLEAR CELL ADENOMA

The component cells have abundant vacuolated cytoplasm.

unequivocal evidence of invasive growth (figs. 25-40–25-42) (2,141–147). As a group, atypical adenomas have also been described as parathyroid tumors of uncertain malignant potential. Gross and microscopic features may include the presence of banding fibrosis with or without associated hemosiderin deposition, adherence to, but not invasion of, contiguous structures, presence of tumor within the surrounding fibrous capsule, solid/trabecular growth patterns, and mitotic activity. However, none of these features, either individually or in combination, are diagnostic of malignancy.

Parathyroid adenomas may exhibit considerable fibrosis, often but not exclusively, in association with cystic change (figs. 25-22–25-24). In such instances, groups of neoplastic cells may be embedded or entrapped in the surrounding fibrous capsule, simulating invasion (fig. 25-24). However, there is no evidence of direct invasion of tumor into the surrounding soft tissues or contiguous structures. The presence of adherence of tumor to the surrounding structures often raises the possibility of malignancy to the surgeon. However, peri-tumoral adhesions, particularly if the tumor is large and cystic, may

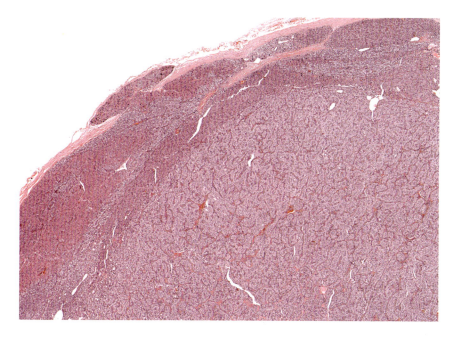

Figure 25-40

ATYPICAL PARATHYROID ADENOMA

There is a mild degree of pericapsular fibrosis. A nest of tumor cells is entrapped within the capsule.

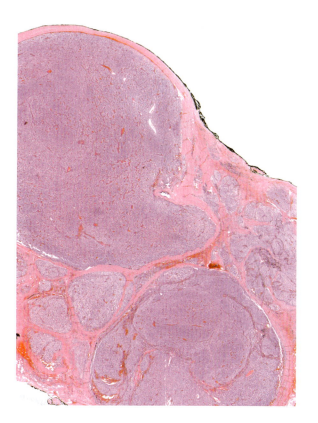

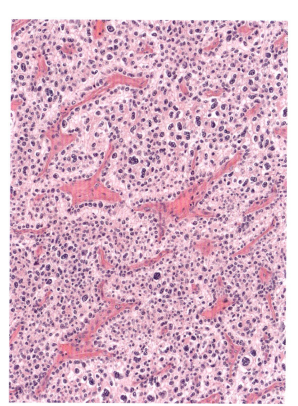

Figure 25-41

ATYPICAL PARATHYROID ADENOMA

Left: Extensive bands of fibrosis surround nodules of tumor. There is no evidence of extracapsular extension.

Right: The component cells have a palisaded arrangement around blood vessels. A few cells with enlarged hyperchromatic nuclei are scattered throughout the tumor.

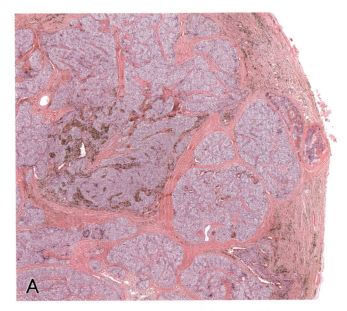

Figure 25-42

ATYPICAL PARATHYROID ADENOMA

A: Extensive areas of fibrosis dissect nodules and small groups of tumor cells. There is no evidence of extracapsular extension.

B: Dense collagenous bands separate nodules of tumor cells.

C: The tumor cells have round, densely stained nuclei.

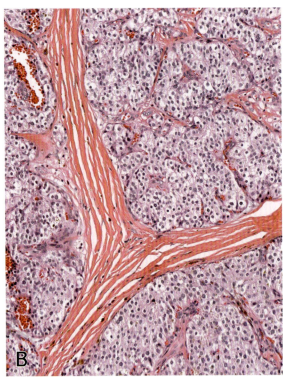

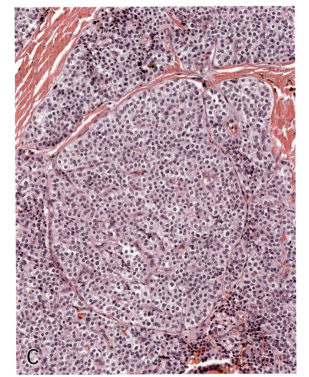

result from non-specific reactive changes associated with cystic degeneration. Finally, neither the presence of a solid/trabecular growth pattern nor mitotic activity is sufficient evidence for a diagnosis of malignancy.

Patients with atypical adenomas generally present with calcium levels intermediate between those of patients with typical adenomas and

carcinomas (143,144). On the basis of studies reported in the literature, most atypical adenomas (80 to 90 percent), as defined by the 2004 WHO criteria, pursue a benign clinical course (2).

There are relatively few studies on the immunohistochemical features of atypical adenomas. The immunophenotype of these tumors appears to be intermediate between that of typical adenomas and carcinomas with respect to the expression of p27, bcl-2, Ki-67, and mdm2 (147). Several studies have suggested that the use of parafibromin immunostaining, either alone or in combination with other markers, may be helpful in the distinction of atypical adenomas and parathyroid carcinomas (80,146,148,149). In general, parafibromin-positive atypical adenomas do not recur, while parafibromin negative tumors have a risk of recurrence of 10 to 20 percent and should be considered tumors of low malignant potential (149). It must be emphasized, however, that studies of parafibromin staining must be rigorously controlled and that reactivity of endothelial and stromal cells must be confirmed as an internal positive control for each case (149). A patient with a diagnosis of atypical adenoma should be monitored closely to rule out the possibility of recurrence (also see chapter 26).

Adenoma-Associated Parathyroid Glands

The classification of parathyroid lesions in the past as adenomas depended on the presence of an enlarged or abnormal gland together with the intraoperative identification of one or more normal parathyroid glands (4). The modern approach to these tumors in most practices now incorporates intraoperative decreases in serum PTH after tumor removal with subsequent prolonged normocalcemia (see chapter 30).

Nonadenomatous glands from patients with parathyroid adenomas traditionally are described as having a lower glandular and parenchymal weight and greater amounts of stromal fat than glands from normocalcemic individuals. In most instances, however, adenoma-associated parathyroid glands are indistinguishable from those of normocalcemic individuals, using standard histopathologic criteria (150). Parenchymal cells in adenoma-associated glands, however, contain prominent neutral lipid droplets which are independent of the stromal fat content (64).

The secretory set point of cells harvested from nonadenomatous glands is reduced below normal levels. The proliferative rate of nonadenomatous tissue is also reduced, based on analyses with Ki-67 labeling (151). A reduction in cell birth rate, combined with the persistence of apoptosis, could explain the small reduction in the weight of nonadenomatous glands in patients with parathyroid adenomas.

Ultrastructural analyses have revealed that adenoma-associated glands have reduced complexity and interdigitations of the plasma membranes, reduced amounts of granular endoplasmic reticulum and Golgi regions, small numbers of secretory granules and prosecretory granules, and increased amounts of cytoplasmic lipid (92). Based on the ultrastructural features, nonadenomatous parathyroid tissue is thought to be suppressed with respect to secretory function.

REFERENCES

1. Castleman B, Roth SI. Tumors of the parathyroid glands. Atlas of Tumor Pathology, 2nd Series, Fascicle 14. Washington, DC: Armed Forces Institute of Pathology; 1978:1-94.
2. Grimelius L, DeLellis RA, Bondeson L, et al. Parathyroid adenoma. In: DeLellis RA, Lloyd RV, Heitz PU, Eng C, eds. Pathology and genetics of tumours of endocrine organs (WHO Classification of Tumours). Lyons: IARC Press; 2004:128-32.
3. Marx SJ. Hyperparathyroidism genes: sequences reveal answers and questions. Endocrin Pract 2011;17(Suppl 3):18-27.
4. Marcocci C, Cetani F. Clinical practice. Primary hyperparathyroidism. N Engl J Med 2011; 365:2389-97.
5. Prinz RA, Barbato AL, Braithwaite SS, Brooks MH, Lawrence AM, Paloyan E. Prior irradiation and the development of coexistent differentiated thyroid cancer and hyperparathyroidism. Cancer 1982;49:874-7.
6. Russ JE, Scanlon EF, Sener SF. Parathyroid adenomas following irradiation. Cancer 1979;43:1078-83.
7. Tisell LE, Carlsson S, Lindberg S, Ragnhult I. Autonomous hyperparathyroidism: a possible late complication of neck radiotherapy. Acta Chir Scand 1976;142:367-73.

8. LiVolsi VA, LoGerfo P, Feind CR. Coexistent parathyroid adenomas anthyroid carcinomas. Can radiation be blamed? Arch Surg 1978;113:285-6.

9. Nishiyama R, Farhi D, Thompson NW. Radiation exposure and the simultaneous occurrence of primary hyperparathyroidism and thyroid nodules. In: DeGroot LJ, ed. Endocrinology. Philadelphia: WB Saunders; 1989:1013-31.

10. Fujiwara S, Sposto R, Ezaki H, et al. Hyperparathyroidism among atomic bomb survivors in Hiroshima. Radiat Res 1992;130:372-8.

11. Boehm BO, Rosinger S, Belyi D, Dietrich JW. The parathyroid as a target for radiation damage. N Engl J Med 2011;365;676-8.

12. Stephen AE, Chen KT, Milas M, Siperstein AE. The coming of age of radiation-induced hyperparathyroidism: evolving patterns of thyroid and parathyroid disease after head and neck irradiation. Surgery 2004;136:1143-53.

13. Cundiff JG, Portugal L, Sarne DH. Parathyroid adenoma after radioactive iodine therapy or multinodular goiter. Am J Otolaryngol 2001;22:374-5.

14. Rasmuson T, Tavelin B. Risk of parathyroid adenomas in patients with thyrotoxicosis exposed to radiaoactive iodine. Acta Oncol 2006;45:1059-61.

15. Triggs SM, Williams ED. Irradiation of thyroid as a cause of parathyroid adenoma. Lancet 1977;1:593-4.

16. Castleman B, Mallory TB. The pathology of the parathyroid gland in hyperparathyroidism: a study of 25 cases. Am J Pathol 1935;11:1-72.

17. Golden A, Canary JJ, Kerwin DM. Concurrence of hyperplasia and neoplasia of the parathyroid glands. Am J Med 1965;38:562-78.

18. Kramer WM. Association of parathyroid hyperplasia with neoplasia. Am J Clin Pathol 1970;53:275-83.

19. Ghandur-Mnaymneh L, Kimura N. The parathyroid adenoma. A histopathologic definition with a study of 172 cases of primary hyperparathyroidism. Am J Pathol 1984;115:70-83.

20. Akerström G, Rudberg C, Grimelius L, et al. Histologic parathyroid abnormalities in an autopsy series. Hum Pathol 1986;17:520-7.

21. Friedman E, Sakaguchi K, Bale AE, et al. Clonality of parathyroid tumors in familial multiple endocrine neoplasia type I. N Engl J Med 1989;321:213-8.

22. Harness JK, Ramsburg SR, Nishiyama RH, Thompson NW. Multiple adenomas of the parathyroids: do they exist? Arch Surg 1979;114:468-74.

23. Verdonk CA, Edis AJ. Parathyroid "double adenomas": fact or fiction? Surgery 1981;90:523-6.

24. Milas, M, Wagner K, Easley KA, Siperstein A, Weber CJ. Double adenoma revisited: Non-uniform distribution favors enlarged superior

parathyroids (fourth pouch disease). Surgery 2003;134:995-1004.

25. DeLellis RA. Tumors of the parathyroid gland. AFIP Atlas of Tumor Pathology, 3rd Series, Fascicle 6. Washington, DC: American Registry of Pathology; 1993.

26. Edis AJ. Surgical anatomy and techniques of neck exploration for primary hyperparathyroidism. Surg Clin North Am 1977;57:495-504.

27. Woolner LB, Keating FR Jr, Black BM. Tumors and hyperplasia of the parathyroid glands: a review of pathological findings in 140 cases of primary hyperparathyroidism. Cancer 1952;5:1069-88.

28. Caron NR, Sturgeon C, Clark OH. Persistent and recurrent hyperparathyroidism. Curr Treat Options Oncol 2004;5:335-45.

29. Cohn KH, Silen W. Lessons of parathyroid reoperations. Am J Surg 1982;144:511-7.

30. Mazeh H, Kouniavsky G, Schneider DF, et al. Intrathyroidal parathyroid glands: small, but mighty (a Napoleon phenomenon). Surgery 2012;152:1193-2000.

31. Karvounaris DC, Symeonidis N, Triantafyllou A, Flaris N, Sakadamis A. Ectopic parathyroid adenoma located inside the hypoglossal nerve. Head Neck 2010;32:1273-6.

32. Lack EE, Delay S, Linnoila RI. Ectopic parathyroid tissue within the vagus nerve. Incidence and possible clinical significance. Arch Pathol Lab Med 1988:112:304-6.

33. Pawlik TM, Richards M, Giordano TJ, Burney R, Thompson N. Identification and management of intravagal parathyroid adenoma. World J Surg 2001;25:419-23.

34. Reiling RB, Cady B, Clerkin EP. Aberrant parathyroid adenoma with a vagus nerve. Lahey Clin Bull 1972;21:158-62.

35. Saky MT, Hasinski S, Rose LI. Ectopic primary hyperparathyroidism. Endoc Pract 2001;7:272-4.

36. Devcic Z, Jeffrey RB, Kameya A, Desser TS. The elusive parathyroid adenoma: techniques for detection. Ultrasound Q 2013:29:179-87.

37. Rasbach DA, Monchik JM, Geelhoed GW, Harrison TS. Solitary parathyroid microadenoma. Surgery 1984;96:1092-8.

38. Goasguen N, Chirica M, Roger N, et al. Primary hyperparathyroidism from parathyroid microadenoma: specific features and implications for a surgical strategy in the era of minimally invasive parathyroidectomy. J Am Coll Surg 2010;210:456-62.

39. Liechty RD, Teter A, Suba EJ. The tiny parathyroid adenoma. Surgery 1986;100:1048-52.

40. Kovacs KA, Gay JD. Remission of primary hyperparathyroidism due to spontaneous infarction of a parathyroid adenoma. Case report and review of the literature. Medicine 1998;77:398-401.

41. Lucas DG, Lockett MA, Cole DJ. Spontaneous infarction of a parathyroid adenoma: two case reports and review of the literature. Am Surg 2002;68:1763-6.

42. Norris EH. Primary Hyperparathryoidism: a report of five cases that exemplify special features of this disease (infarction of a parathyroid adenoma; oxyphil adenoma). Arch Pathol (Chic) 1946;42:261-73.

43. Kihara M, Yokomuse H, Yamauchi A, Irie A, Matsusaka K, Miyauchi A. Spontaneous rupture of a parathyroid adenoma presenting as a massive cervical hemorrhage: report of a case. Surg Today 2001;31:222-4.

44. Altenähr E, Arps H, Montz R, Dorn G. Quantitative ultrastructural and radioimmunologic assessment of parathyroid gland activity in primary hyperparathyroidism. Lab Invest 1979;41:303-12.

45. Black WC 3rd. Correlative light and electron microscopy in primary hyperparathyroidism. Arch Pathol 1969;88:225-41

46. Black BK, Ackerman LV. Tumors of the parathyroid; a review of twenty-three cases. Cancer 1950;3:415-44.

47. Banerjee SS, Faragher B, Hasleton PS. Nuclear diameter in parathyroid disease. J Clin Pathol 1983;36:143-8.

48. Lloyd HM, Jacobi JM, Cooke RA. Nuclear diameter in parathyroid adenomas. J Clin Pathol 1979;32:1278-81.

49. San-Juan J, Monteagudo C, Fraker D, Norton J, Merino MJ. Significance of mitotic activity and other morphologic parameters in parathyroid adenomas and their correlation with clinical behavior Am J Clin Pathol 1989;92:523.

50. Snover DC, Foucar K. Mitotic activity in benign parathyroid disease. Am J Clin Pathol 1981;75:345-7.

51. Loda M, Lipman J, Cukor B, Bur M, Kwan P, DeLellis RA. Nodular foci in parathyroid adenomas and hyperplasia: an immunohistochemical analysis of proliferative activity. Hum Pathol 1994;25:1050-6.

52. Abbona GC, Papotti M, Gasparri P, Bussolati G. Proliferative activity on parathyroid tumors as detected by Ki-67 immunostaining. Hum Pathol 1995;26:135-8.

53. Erickson LA, Jin L, Wollan P, Thompson GB, van Heerden JA, Lloyd RV. Parathyroid hyperplasia, adenomas and carcinomas: differential expression of p27Kip1 protein. Am J Surg Pathol 1999;23:288-95.

54. Farnebo F, Auer G, Farnebo LO, et al. Evaluation of retinoblastoma and Ki-67 immunostaining as diagnostic markers of benigh and malignant parathyroid disease. World J Surg 1999;23:68-74.

55. Lloyd RV, Jin L, Qian X, Kulig E. Aberrant p27kip1 expression in endocrine and other tumors. Am J Pathol 1997;15:401-7.

56. Boquist L. Follicles in human parathyroid glands. Lab Invest 1973;28:313-20.

57. Anderson TJ, Ewen SW. Amyloid in normal and pathological parathyroid glands. J Clin Pathol 1974;27:656-63.

58. Friedman M, Shimaoka K, Lopez AC, Shedd DP. Parathyroid adenoma diagnosed as papillary carcinoma of the thyroid on needle aspiration smears. Acta Cytol 1983;27:337-40.

59. Sahin A, Robinson RA. Papillae formation in parathyroid adenoma. A source of possible diagnostic error. Arch Pathol Lab Med 1988;112:99-100.

60. Elgoweini M, Chetty R. Hyalinizing parathyroid adenoma and hyperplasia: report of 3 cases of an unusual histologic variant. Ann Diagn Pathol 2011;15:329-32.

61. Kovacs K, Bell CD, Juco J, Rotondo F, Anderson J. Parathyroid chief cell adenomas associated with massive chronic parathyroiditis in a woman with hyperparathyroidism. Endocr Pathol 2007:18:42-5.

62. Black WC 3rd, Utley JR. The differential diagnosis of parathyroid adenoma and chief cell hyperplasia. Am J Clin Pathol 1968;49:761-75.

63. Bondeson AG, Bondeson L, Ljungerg O, Tibblin S. Fat staining in parathyroid disease—diagnostic value and impact on surgical strategy: clinicopathologic analysis of 191 cases. Hum Pathol 1985;16:1255-63.

64. Roth SI, Gallagher MJ. The rapid identification of "normal" parathyroid glands by the presence of intracellular fat. Am J Pathol 1976;84:521-8.

65. Abati A, Skarulis MC, Shawker T, Solomon D. Ultrasound guided fine needle aspiration of parathyroid lesions: a morphologic and immunocytochemical approach. Hum Pathol 1995;26:338-43.

66. Agarwal AM, Bentz JS, Hungerford R, Abraham D. Parathyroid fine needle aspiration cytology in the evaluation of parathyroid adenoma: cytologic findings from 53 patients. Daign Cytopathol 2009;37:407-10.

67. Kendrick ML, Charboneau JW, Curlee KJ, van Heerden JA, Farley DR. Risk of parathyromatosis after fine-needle aspiration. Ann Surg 2001;67:290-3.

68. MacFarlane MP, Fraker DL, Shawker TH, et al. Use of fine-needle aspiration in patients undergoing reoperation for primary hyperparathyroidism. Surgery 1994;116:959-64.

69. Mincione GP, Borrelli D, Cicchi P, Ipponi PL, Fiorini A. Fine needle aspiration cytology of parathyroid adenoma. A review of seven cases. Acta Cytol 1986;30:65-9.

70. Davey DD, Glant MD, Berger EK, Parathyroid cytopathology. Diagn Cytopathol 1986;2:76-80.

71. Winkler B, Gooding GA, Montgomery CK, Clark OH, Arnaud C. Immunoperoxidase confirmation of parathyroid origin of ultrasound-guided fine needle aspirates of the parathyroid glands. Acta Cytol 1987;31:40-4.

72. Alwaheeb S, Rambaldini G, Boerner S, Coiré C, Fiser J, Asa SL. Worrisome histologic alterations following fine-needle aspiration of the parathyroid. J Clin Pathol 2006;59:1094-6.

73. Erickson L, Jin L, Papotti M, Lloyd RV. Oxyphil parathyroid carcinomas: a clinicopathologic and immunohistochemical study of 10 cases. Am J Surg Pathol 2002;26:344-9.

74. Nonaka D. Study of parathyroid transcription factor Gcm2 expression in parathyroid lesions. Am J Surg Pathol 2011;35:145-51.

75. Tomita T. Immunocytochemical staining patterns for parathyroid hormone and chromogranin in parathyroid hyperplasia, adenoma, and carcinoma. Endocr Pathol 1999;10:145-56.

76. Kendall CH, Roberts PA, Pringle JH, Lauder I. The expression of parathyroid hormone messenger RNA in normal and abnormal parathyroid tissue. J Pathol 1991;165:111-8.

77. Gill AJ, Clarkson A, Gimm O, Dralle H, Howell VM, Marsh DJ. Loss of nuclear expression of parafibromin distinguishes parathyroid carcinoma and hyperparathyroidism-jaw tumor (HPT-JT) syndrome-related adenomas from sporadic parathyroid adenomas and hyperplasias. Am J Surg Pathol 2006;30:1140-9.

78. Tan MH, Morrison C, Wang P, et al. Loss of parafibromin immunoreactivity is a distinguishing feature of parathyroid carcinoma. Clin Cancer Res 2004;10:6629-37.

79. Juhlin C, Larsson C, Yakoleva T, et al. Loss of parafibromin expression in a subset of parathyroid adenomas. Endocr Relat Cancer 2006;13:509-23.

80. Bergero N, De Pompa R, Sacerdote C, et al. Galectin-3 expression in parathyroid carcinoma: immunohistochemical study of 26 cases. Hum Pathol 2005;36:908-14.

81. Howell VM, Gill A, Clarkson A, et al. Accuracy of combined protein gene product 9.5 and parafibromin markers for immunohistochemical diagnosis of parathyroid carcinoma. J Clin Endocrinol Metab 2009;94:434-41.

82. Juhlin CC, Haglund F, Villablanca A, et al. Loss of expression for the Wnt pathway components adenomatous polyposis coli and glycogen synthase kinase 3-beta in parathyroid carcinomas. Int J Oncol 2009;34:481-92.

83. Lu M, Forsberg L, Höög A, et al. Heterogeneous expression of SNARE proteins SNAP-23, SNAP-25, Syntaxin-1 and VAMP in human parathyroid tissue. Mol Cell Endocriol 2008;287:72-80.

84. Haven CJ, van Pruijenbroek M, Karperien M, Fleuren GJ, Morreau H. Differential expression of the calcium sensing receptor and combined loss of chromosomes 1q and 11q in parathyroid carcinoma. J Pathol 2004;202:86-94.

85. Hsi ED, Zuckerberg LR, Yang WI, Arnold A. Cyclin D1/PRAD1 expression in parathyroid adenomas: an immunohistochemical study. J Clin Endocrinol Metab 1996;81:1736-9.

86. Ozcan A, Shen SS, Hamilton C, et al. PAX-8 expression in non-neoplastic tissues, primary tumors and metastatic tumors: a comprehensive immunohistochemical study. Mod Pathol 2011;24:751-64.

87. Bakshi N, Kunju LP, Giordano T, Shah RB. Expression of renal cell carcinoma antigen in nonrenal tumors: diagnostic implications. Appl Immunohistochem Mol Morphol 2007;15:310-5.

88. Cetani F, Pardi E, Viacava P, et al. A reappraisal of the Rb1 gene abnormalities in the diagnosis of parathyroid cancer. Clin Endocrinol (Oxf) 2004;60:99-106.

89. Vargas MP, Vargas HI, Kleiner DE, Medrino MJ. The role of prognostic markers (MIB-1, RB, bcl-2) in the diagnosis of parathyroid tumors. Mod Pathol 1997;10:12-7.

90. Farnebo F, Enberg U, Grimelius L, et al. Tumor-specific decreased expression of calcium sensing receptor messenger ribonucleic acid in sporadic hyperparathyroidism. J Clin Endocrinol Metab 1997;82:3481-6.

91. Kifor O, Moore FD Jr, Wang P, et al. Reduced staining for the extracellular Ca2+ sensing receptor in primary and uremic secondary hyperparathyroidism. J Clin Endocrinol Metab 1996;81:1598-606.

92. Roth SI, Munger BL. The cytology of the adenomatous, atrophic and hyperplastic parathyroid glands of man. A light- and electron-microscopic study. Virchows Arch Pathol Anat Physiol Klin Med 1962;335:389-410.

93. Cinti S, Colussi G, Minola E, Dickersin GR. Parathyroid glands in primary hyperparathyroidism: an ultrastructural study of 50 cases. Hum Pathol 1986;17:1036-46.

94. Aguilar-Parada E, González-Angulo A, del Peon L, Mravko E. Functioning microvillous adenoma of the parathyroid gland containing nuclear pores and annulate lamellae. Hum Pathol 1985;16:511-6.

95. Fialkow PJ, Jackson CE, Block MA, Greenawald KA. Multicellular origin of parathyroid adenomas. N Eng J Med 1977;297:696-8.

96. Arnold A, Kim HG, Gaz RD, et al Molecular cloning and chromosomal mapping of DNA rearranged with the parathyroid hormone gene in a parathyroid adenoma. J Clin Invest 1989;83:2034-40

97. Arnold A. Staunton CE, Kim HG, Gaz RD, Kronenberg HM. Monoclonality and abnormal parathyroid hormone genes in parathyroid adenomas. N Engl J Med 1988;318:658-62.

98. Arnold A, Shattuck TM, Mallya SM, et al. Molecular pathogenesis of primary hyperparathyroidism. J Bone Miner Res 2002;17:30-6.

99. Cetani F, Pardi E, Borsari S, Marcocci C. Molecular pathogenesis of primary hyperparathyroidism. J Endocrinol Invest 2011;34(Suppl 7):35-9.

100. Hendy GM. Molecular mechanisms of primary hyperparathyroidism. Rev Endocr Metab Disord 2000;1:297-305.

101. Westin G, Björklund P, Akerström G. Molecular genetics of parathyroid disease. World J Surg 2009;33:2224-33.

102. Yi Y, Nowak NJ, Pacchia AL, Morrison C. Chromosome 11 genomic changes in parathyroid adenoma and hyperplasia: array CGH, FISH, and tissue microarrays. Genes Chromosomes Cancer 2008;47:639-48.

103. Vasef MA, Brynes RK, Sturm M, Bromley C, Robinson RA. Expression of cyclin D1 in parathyroid carcinomas, adenomas, and hyperplasias: a paraffin immunohistochemical study. Mod Pathol 1999;12:412-6.

104. Hemmer S, Wasenius VM, Haglund C, et al. Deletion of 11q23 and cyclin D1 overexpression are frequent aberrations in parathyroid adenomas. Am J Pathol 2001;158:1355-62.

105. Chandrasekharappa SC, Guru SC, Manickam P, et al. Positional cloning of the gene for multiple endrocine neoplasia-type 1. Science 1997;276:404-7.

106. Lemmens I, Van de Ven WJ, Kas K, et al. Identification of the multiple endocrine neoplasia type 1 (MEN1) gene. The European Consortium on MEN1. Hum Mol Genet 1997;6:1177-83.

107. Dwight T, Twigg S, Delbridge L, et al. Loss of heterozygosity in sporadic parathyroid tumors: involvement of chromosome 1 and the MEN1 gene locus in 11q13. Clin Endocrinol (Oxf) 2000;53:85-92.

108. Farnebo F, Teh BT, Kytola S, et al. Alterations of the MEN1 gene in sporadic parathyroid tumors. J Clin Endocrinol Metab 1998;83:2627-30.

109. Heppner C, Kester MB, Agarwal K, et al. Somatic mutation of the MEN1 gene in parathyroid tumors. Nat Genet 1997;16:375-8.

110. Carling T, Correa P, Hessman O, et al. Parathyroid MEN1 mutations in relation to clinical characteristics of nonfamilial primary hyperparathyroidism. J Clin Endocrinol Metab 1998;82:2960-3.

111. Farnebo F, Kytölä S, Teh BT, et al. Alternative genetic pathways in parathyroid tumorigenesis. J Clin Endocrinol Metab 1999;84:3775-80.

112. Cetani F, Pardi E, Borsari S, et al. Genetic analyses of of the HRPT2 gene in primary hyperparathyroidism: germline and somatic mutations in familial and sporadic parathyroid tumors. J Clin Endocrinol Metab 2004;89:5583-91.

113. Padberg BC, Schröder S, Jochum W, et al. Absence of RET proto-oncogene point mutations in sporadic hyperplastic and neoplastic lesions of the parathyroid gland. Am J Pathol 1995;147:1600-7.

114. Costa-Guda J, Marinoni I, Molatore S, Pellegata NS, Arnold A. Somatic mutation and germline sequence abnormalities in CDKN1B, encoding p27Kip1, in sporadic parathyroid adenomas. J Clin Endocrinol Metab 2011;96:701-6.

115. Costa-Guda J, Arnold A. Genetic and epigenetic changes in sporadic endocrine tumors: parathyroid tumors. Mol Cell Endocrinol 2014;386:46-54.

116. Costa-Guda J, Soong CP, Parekh VI, Agarwal SK, Arnold A. Germline and somatic mutations in cyclin-dependent kinase inhibitor genes CDKN1A, CDKN2B, and CDKN2C in sporadic parathyroid adenomas. Horm Cancer 2013;4:301-7.

117. DeRienzo D, Truong L. Thyroid neoplasms containing mature fat: a report of two cases and review of the literature. Mod Pathol 1989;2:506-10.

118. Isotalo PA, Lloyd RV. Presence of birefringent crystals is useful in distinguishing thyroid from parathyroid gland tissues. Am J Surg Pathol 2002;26:813-4.

119. Wong KS, Lewis JS Jr, Gottipati S, Chernock RD. Utility of birefringent crystal identification by polarized light microscopy in distinguishing thyroid from parathyroid tissue on intraoperative frozen sections. Am J Surg Pathol 2014;38:1212-1219.

120. Schmid KW, Morgan JM, Baumert M, Fischer-Colbrie R, Böcker W, Jasani B. Calcitonin and calcitonin gene-related peptide mRNA detection in a population of hyperplastic parathyroid cells also expressing chromogranin B. Lab Invest 1995;73:90-5.

121. Khan A, Tischler AS, Patwardhan NA, DeLellis RA. Calcitonin immunoreactivity in neoplastic and hyperplastic parathyroid glands: an immunohistochemical study. Endocr Pathol 2003 ;14:249-55.

122. Greene AB, Butler RS, McIntyre S, et al. National trends in parathyroid surgery from 1998 to 2008: a decade of change. J Am Coll Surg 2009;209:332-43.

123. Rattner DW, Marrone GC, Kasdon E, Silen W. Recurrent hyperparathyroidism due to implantation of parathyroid tissue. Am J Surg 1985;149:745-8.

124. Fraker DL, Travis WD, Merendino JJ Jr, et al. Locally recurrent parathyroid neoplasms as a cause for recurrent and persistent primary hyperparathyroidism. Ann Surg 1991;213:58-65.

125. Fitko R, Roth SI, Hines JR, Roxe DM, Cahill E. Parathyromatosis in hyperparathyroidism. Hum Pathol 1990;21:234-7.

126. Reddick RL, Costa JC, Marx SJ. Parathyroid hyperplasia and parathyromatosis. Lancet 1997;1:549.

127. Bedetti CD, Dekker A, Watson CG. Functioning oxyphil cell adenoma of the parathyroid gland: a clinicopathologic study of ten patients with hyperparathyroidism. Hum Pathol 1984;15:1121-6.

128. Poole GV Jr, Albertson DA, Marshall RB, Myers RT. Oxyphil cell adenomas and hyperparathyroidism. Surgery 1982;92:799-805.

129. Wolpert HR, Vickery AL Jr, Wang CA. Functioning oxyphil cell adenomas of the parathyroid gland. A study of 15 cases. Am J Surg Pathol 1089;13:500-4.

130. McGregor DH, Lotuaco LG, Rao MS, Chu LL. Functioning oxyphil adenoma of parathyroid gland. An ultrastructural and biochemical study. Am J Pathol 1978;92:691-711.

131. Ordonez NG, Ibanez ML, Mackey B, Samaan NA, Hickey RC. Functioning oxyphil cell adenomas of parathyroid gland: immunoperoxidase evidence of hormonal activity in oxyphil cells. Am J Clin Pathol 1982;78:681-9.

132. Chow LS, Erickson LA, Abu-Lebdeh HS, Wermers RA. Parathyroid lipoadenomas: a rare cause of primary hyperparathyroidism. Endocr Pract 2006;12:131-6.

133. Fischer I, Wieczorek R, Sidhu GS, Pei Z, West B, Lee P. Myxoid lipoadenoma of the parathyroid gland: a case report and literature review. Ann Diagn Pathol 2006;10:294-6.

134. Geelhoed GW. Parathyroid adenolipoma: clinical and morphological features. Surgery 1982;92:806-10.

135. Ober WB, Kaiser GA. Hamartoma of the parathyroid. Cancer 1958;11:601-6.

136. Legolvan DP, Moore BP, Nishiyama RH. Parathyroid hamartoma: report of two cases and review of the literature. Am J Clin Pathol 1977;67:31-5.

137. Ogrin C. A rare case of double parathyroid lipoadenoma with hyperparathyroidism. Am J Med Sci 2013;346:432-4.

138. Dundar E, Grenko RT, Akalin A, Karahuseyinoglu E, Bildirici K. Intrathyroidal water-clear cell adenoma: a case report. Hum Pathol 2001;32:889-92.

139. Grenko RT, Anderson KM, Kauffman G, Abt AB. Water-clear cell adenoma of the parathyroid. A case report with immunohistochemistry and electron microscopy. Arch Pathol Lab Med 1995;119:1072-4.

140. Kuhel WI, Gonzales D, Hoda SA, et al. Synchronous water-clear cell double parathyroid adenomas a hitherto uncharacterized entity? Arch Pathol Lab Med 2001;125:256-9.

141. Levin KE, Galante M, Clark OH. Parathyroid carcinoma versus parathyroid adenoma in patients with profound hypercalcemia. Surgery 1987;101:649-60.

142. Levin KE, Chew KL, Ljung BM, Mayall BH, Siperstein AE, Clark OH. Deoxyribonucleic acid cytometry helps identify parathyroid carcinomas. J Clin Endocrinol Metab 1988;67:779-84.

143. Guiter GE, DeLellis RA. Risk of recurrence or metastasis in atypical parathyroid adenomas. Mod Pathol 2002;15:115A.

144. Fernandez-Ranvier GG, Khanafshar E, Jensen K, et al. Parathyroid carcinoma, atypical parathyroid adenoma or parathyromatosis? Cancer 2007;110:255-64.

145. Ippolito G, Palazzo FF, Sebag F, De Micco C, Henry JF. Intraoperative diagnosis and treatment of parathyroid cancer and atypical parathyroid adenoma. Br J Surg 2007;94:566-70.

146. Fernandez-Ranvier GG, Khanafshar E, Tacha D, et al. Defining a molecular phenotype for benign and malignant parathyroid tumors. Cancer 2009;115:334-44.

147. Stojadinovic A, Höös A, Nassar A, et al. Parathyroid neoplasms: clinical, histopathologic and tissue array-based molecular analysis. Hum Pathol 2003;34:54-64.

148. Kruijff S, Sidhu SB, Sywak MS, Gill AJ, Delbridge LW. Negative parafibromin staining predicts malignant behavior in atypical parathyroid adenomas. Ann Surg Oncol 2014;21:426-33.

149. Gill AJ. Understanding the genetic basis of parathyroid carcinoma. Endocr Pathol 2014;25:30-4.

150. Ejerblad S, Grimelius L, Johansson H, Werner I. Studies on the non-adenomatous glands in patients with a solitary parathyroid adenoma. Ups J Med Sci 1976;81:31-6.

151. Parfitt AM, Wang Q, Palnitkar S. Rates of cell proliferation in adenomatous, suppressed and normal parathyroid tissue: implications for pathogenesis. J Clin Endocrinol Metab 1998;83:863-9.

26 PARATHYROID CARCINOMA

Definition. *Parathyroid carcinoma* is a malignant tumor composed of parenchymal cells of the parathyroid gland.

GENERAL FEATURES

Parathyroid carcinomas are rare neoplasms that account for less than 1 percent of cases of primary hyperparathyroidism in North America (1,2). They have a high probability of local recurrence and the potential to metastasize to regional nodes and distant sites late in their course (3). The incidence rate is less than 1 per million population per year in the United States, based on the Surveillance, Epidemiology, and End Results (SEER) database; however, the incidence increased from 3.58 to 5.73 cases per 10^7 population between 1988 to 1991 and 2000 to 2003, resepctively (4). A similar trend has been noted in studies from Australia (4,5). Possible reasons for this change include increased screening, evolving diagnostic criteria based on the use of biomarkers, and a true increased incidence of the disease.

There is some apparent geographic variation in the prevalence of the disease in different parts of the world. Studies from Italy (6) and Japan (7) have shown that 5 to 6 percent of cases of primary hyperparathyroidism are due to parathyroid carcinoma, and these rates are substantially higher than those observed in North America (1,2). Although some of the reported variation is likely due to differing criteria for the diagnosis of this malignancy, there may be true geographic differences in the incidence of the disease.

Little is known about the etiology and pathogenesis of parathyroid carcinoma. Based on an analysis of 286 cases treated in the United States between 1985 and 1995, there was no disproportionate clustering by ethnicity, race, income group, or geographic location (8). In contrast to adenoma, parathyroid carcinoma has been reported rarely following neck irradiation (9).

The incidence of parathyroid carcinoma is increased in patients with the hyperparathy-roidism-jaw tumor syndrome (HPT-JT) (10). Parathyroid carcinoma has been reported in association with familial (isolated) hyperparathyroidism (11) and occurs very rarely in patients with multiple endocrine neoplasia (MEN)1 (12,13) and MEN 2A (14).

Parathyroid carcinoma occurs in patients with chronic renal failure but is rare. Berland et al. (15) reported the first such case in 1982. Since that time, approximately 20 patients with chronic renal failure on maintenance hemodialysis have been reported with parathyroid carcinoma (16,17). One reported patient also had a history of prior neck irradiation (18). Five of the patients had local tumor invasion, while two had evidence of distant metastases. In all cases, the remaining parathyroid glands had evidence of hyperplasia. Parathyroid carcinoma has also been reported in a patient with celiac disease (16).

To date, there are no morphologic or molecular data to support an adenoma to carcinoma progression for parathyroid tumorigenesis, other than in the HPT-JT syndrome (19).

CLINICAL FEATURES

The mean age of patients with parathyroid carcinoma in the series reported by Wang and Gaz (3) was 45 years, with a range of 28 to 72 years. In a series of 286 cases reported from the National Cancer Data Base (NCDB) (8), the mean and median ages were 54.5 and 55.1 years, respectively. In contrast to adenomas, which occur most commonly in women, the sex ratio of patients with carcinomas is roughly equal (20,21).

Most patients with parathyroid carcinoma have evidence of metabolic complications at presentation, with marked symptomatic hypercalcemia (1,20–23). The serum calcium levels are usually in excess of 14 mg/dL (or approximately 3 to 4 mg/dL above the upper limit of normal) with concomitant marked elevations of serum parathyroid hormone (PTH). Occasional patients present in hypercalcemic crisis. In most

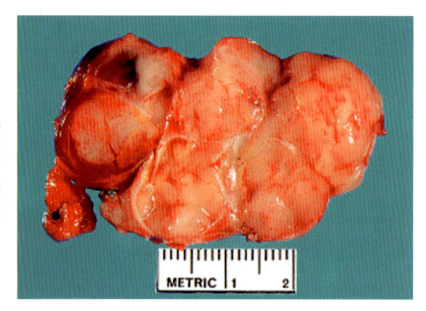

Figure 26-1

PARATHYROID CARCINOMA

The cut surface of this tumor is distinctly nodular due to the formation of fibrous bands. (Fig. 57-32 from Roth SI. The parathyroid gland. In: Silverberg SA, DeLellis RA, Frable WJ, eds. Principles and practice of surgical pathology and cytopathology, 3rd ed. New York: Churchill Livingstone; 1997:2732.)

cases, the degree of hypercalcemia is greater in patients with parathyroid carcinoma than in those with adenoma. It should be noted, however, that some carcinomas are nonfunctional and may simulate thyroid carcinoma both clinically and pathologically (24–26).

Many patients have symptoms attributable to renal disease, with more than two thirds having nephrolithiasis. In some series, more than half of the patients had diminished renal function with azotemia and creatinine clearances of less than 50 mL/min (20). A similar proportion had evidence of bone disease, including osteitis fibrosa cystica, subperiosteal bone resorption, diffuse osteoporosis, "salt and pepper" skull, and absence of lamina dura. Additional common signs and symptoms include fatigue, weakness, weight loss, anorexia, nausea, vomiting, polyuria, and polydipsia (20,21). A palpable neck mass occurs in 30 to 75 percent of patients. This clinical finding is strikingly different from the very low frequency of palpable neck masses in patients with parathyroid adenomas. The presence of recurrent laryngeal nerve paralysis in a patient with primary hyperparathyroidism is also suggestive of parathyroid carcinoma.

GROSS FINDINGS

Parathyroid carcinoma most often appears as a poorly circumscribed mass which is densely adherent to the surrounding soft tissues of the neck or thyroid gland (fig. 26-1) (27–29). Oc-

casional tumors, however, may be grossly encapsulated and otherwise resemble parathyroid adenomas. Carcinomas range in weight from 1.5 to 27.0 g (mean, 6.7 g) (3), but occasional tumors are considerably larger. On cross section, parathyroid carcinomas are firm and pink-tan. Foci of necrosis may be apparent as small yellow areas.

MICROSCOPIC FINDINGS

The histopathologic diagnosis of parathyroid carcinoma is challenging, with considerable interobserver diagnostic variability. In some series, a significant proportion of cases that recurred or metastasized were classified as adenomas at initial presentation (30). On the other hand, only a small proportion of cases classified initially as carcinomas behaved as true malignancies (31). Whether the latter cases represent carcinomas cured by simple excision or atypical adenomas is unknown.

Parathyroid carcinomas are often surrounded by a thick fibrous capsule which extends into the central region of the neoplasm (fig. 26-2) (28,32). Thus, many carcinomas have a nodular appearance due to the presence of thick fibrous bands. Most carcinomas have a predominantly solid growth pattern with a variable trabecular architecture (28,32). Nesting patterns may also be evident, and occasional tumors have follicular or spindle cell growth patterns. Rare tumors have a carcinosarcomatous pattern (33,34).

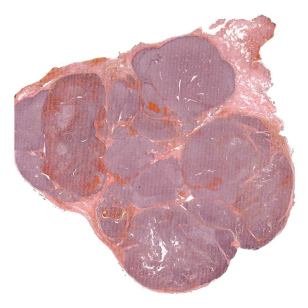

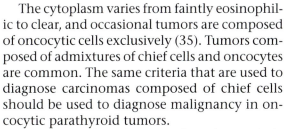

Figure 26-2

PARATHYROID CARCINOMA

The tumor has a thick fibrous capsule, prominent fibrous bands, and a nodular growth pattern.

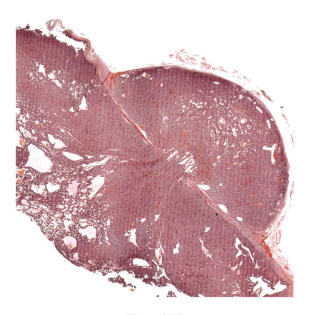

Figure 26-3

PARATHYROID CARCINOMA

The tumor invades through the capsule in a mushroom-like pattern.

The cytoplasm varies from faintly eosinophilic to clear, and occasional tumors are composed of oncocytic cells exclusively (35). Tumors composed of admixtures of chief cells and oncocytes are common. The same criteria that are used to diagnose carcinomas composed of chief cells should be used to diagnose malignancy in oncocytic parathyroid tumors.

As described by Schantz and Castleman (36), the important features of carcinomas include the presence of thick fibrous bands, capsular invasion, vascular invasion, and mitotic activity. Fibrous band formation, which occurs in 90 percent of cases, is characterized by the presence of relatively acellular collagenous tissue which subdivides the tumor into irregularly shaped compartments (fig. 26-2). Fibrous bands, however, are not specific for carcinomas and are also seen in large adenomas that have undergone retrogressive changes and in atypical adenomas (31,37,38). While hemosiderin is present frequently in degenerated adenomas, it also occurs in carcinomas. Extensive areas of fibrosis and hemosiderin deposition may also be present in glands from patients with secondary hyperparathyroidism.

Capsular invasion has been reported in approximately two thirds of carcinomas (36). This feature is characterized by the extension of tongue-like protrusions of the tumor into the collagenous network of the capsule, with variable extension into contiguous soft tissue, perineural spaces, thyroid gland, and esophagus (figs. 26-3–26-7). Often, foci of invasion are accompanied by a fibrous tissue response (fig. 26-4). Capsular invasion should be distinguished from entrapment of tumor cells within the capsules of adenomas. The latter change may be particularly prominent in the thickened capsules of adenomas that have undergone cystic degeneration.

Mitotic activity occurs in approximately 80 percent of carcinomas (28,36); however, mitoses are also common in adenomas and hyperplasias of primary and secondary types (38,39). In some studies, the frequency of mitoses in carcinomas did not exceed that in adenomas (32,40). In Bondeson's series (32), however, a substantial proportion of carcinomas had a markedly higher mitotic rate, which was prognostically significant with respect to tumor aggressiveness. When assessing mitotic activity, mitoses in endothelial

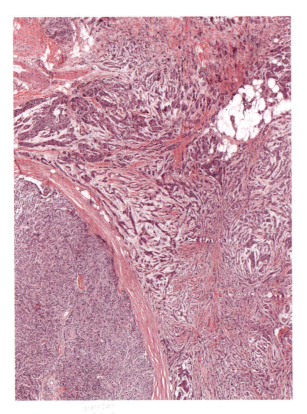 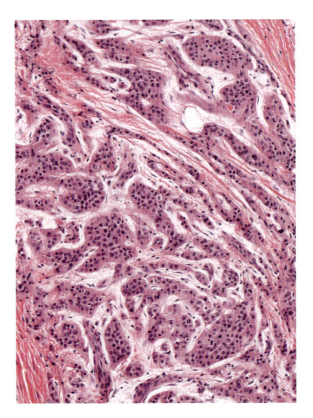

Figure 26-4

PARATHYROID CARCINOMA

Left: This tumor (upper right) has extensively invaded the surrounding soft tissues.
Right: The invasive tumor is accompanied by a fibrous stroma.

cells and other stromal elements should be distinguished from those occurring in tumor cells.

Studies using Ki-67 have revealed higher values in carcinomas (6.0 to 8.4 percent) than in adenomas (less than 3 to 4 percent); however, the overlap of values in equivocal cases has limited the usefulness of this approach (41). As compared with adenomas, carcinomas have a 3- to 4-fold decrease in p27 expression (42). These findings have suggested that p27 and Ki-67 labeling indices may be helpful in the distinction of parathyroid adenomas (decreased Ki-67, increased p27) and carcinomas (increased Ki-67, decreased p27) (42,43).

Schantz and Castleman (35) noted that cellular atypia and variation were not useful criteria for the diagnosis of carcinoma and that most of the tumors in their series had a fairly uniform and bland cell pattern (figs. 26-6, 26-8, 26-10). In the series reported by Bondeson et al. (32), on the other hand, most unequivo-

cal carcinomas, as defined by the presence of invasion or recurrence, had significant nuclear atypia and occasional foci of necrosis (figs. 26-11–26-14). They also defined a number of partially interrelated cytologic features, including macronucleoli, marked mitotic activity, and an aberrant nuclear DNA pattern (aneuploidy), that were associated with a high risk of malignancy. Certain patterns of fibrosis and necrosis (fig. 26-14) were common in carcinomas but were not pathognomonic of malignancy.

Vascular invasion was present in up to 15 percent of the parathyroid carcinomas reported by Schantz and Castleman (36), although other authors (44) have reported higher frequencies of this finding (figs. 26-15–26-17). To qualify as true vascular invasion, the following criteria must be met: 1) the tumor should be located in capsular vessels or in vessels in the surrounding soft tissue; 2) the tumor should be attached to the vessel wall, at least partially; 3) fibrin may be

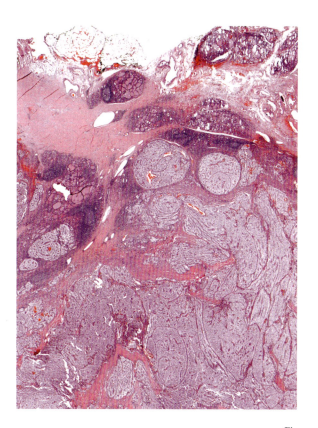 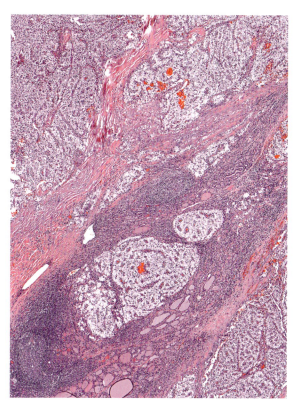

Figure 26-5

PARATHYROID CARCINOMA

Left: This tumor has extensively invaded the thyroid gland (top).
Right: Thyroid tissue is present in the lower portion of the figure. The nodules of the tumor have clear cell features.

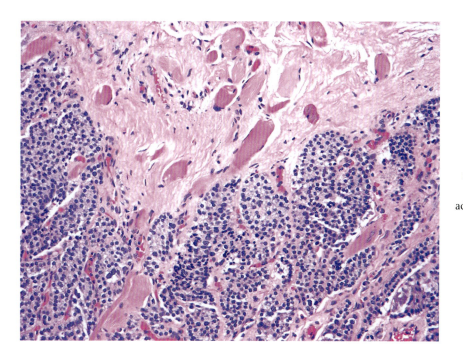

Figure 26-6

PARATHYROID CARCINOMA

This tumor has invaded the adjacent skeletal muscle.

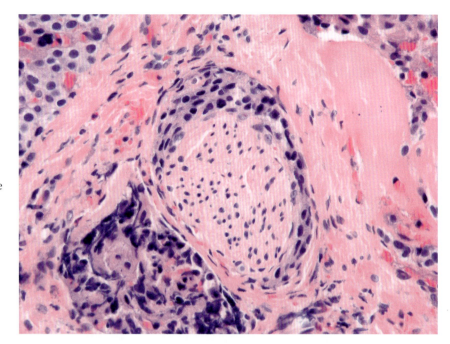

Figure 26-7

PARATHYROID CARCINOMA

This tumor has invaded the perineural space.

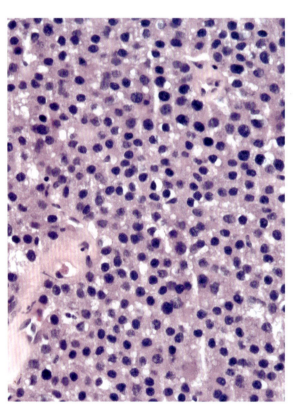

Figure 26-8

PARATHYROID CARCINOMA

This recurrent tumor has relatively bland cytologic features.

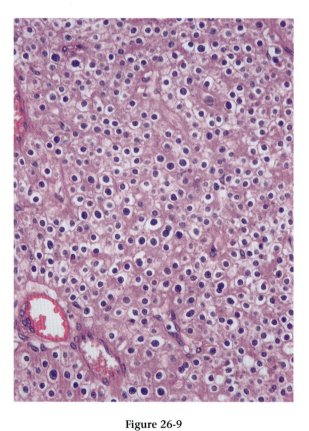

Figure 26-9

PARATHYROID CARCINOMA

Parathyroid carcinoma from a patient with the hyperparathyroidism-jaw tumor syndrome. There is mild variation in nuclear size.

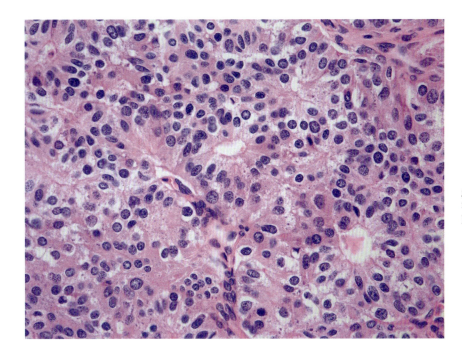

Figure 26-10

PARATHYROID CARCINOMA

This tumor forms ill-defined gland structures. There is a mild degree of nuclear pleomorphism.

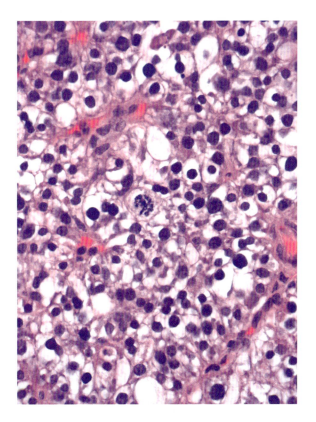

Figure 26-11

PARATHYROID CARCINOMA

An abnormal mitotic figure is present in the center of the image.

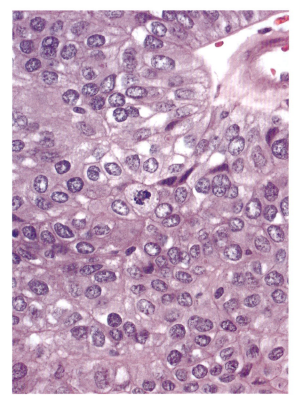

Figure 26-12

PARATHYROID CARCINOMA

The nuclei in this mitotically active tumor are markedly atypical.

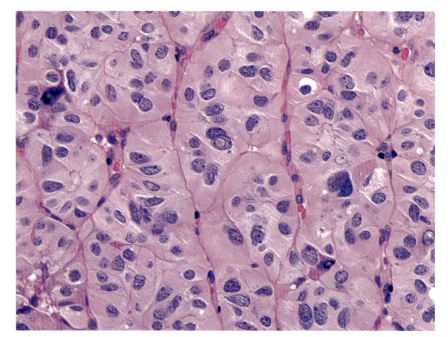

Figure 26-13

PARATHYROID CARCINOMA

This tumor has a trabecular growth pattern. The nuclei are markedly atypical and contain nuclear pseudoinclusions.

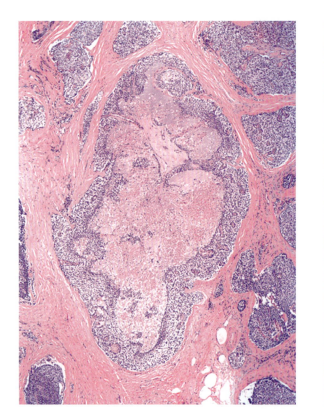

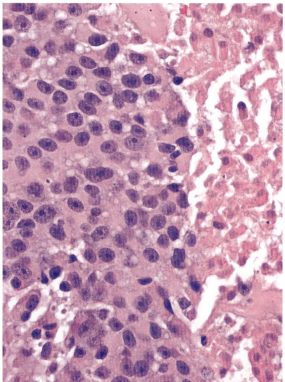

Figure 26-14

PARATHYROID CARCINOMA

Left: This case demonstrates central areas of necrosis (comedonecrosis) in tumor cell nests.
Right: The tumor cells in this case have macronucleoli. Zonal necrosis is present.

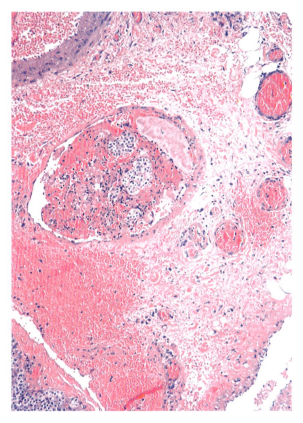

Figure 26-15

PARATHYROID CARCINOMA

Intravascular tumor cells are associated with fibrin thrombi.

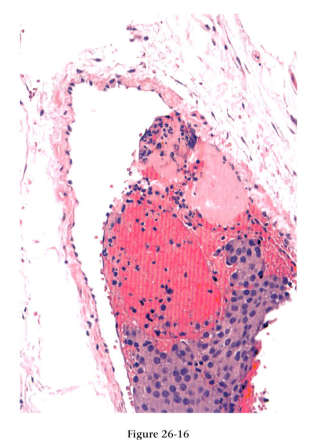

Figure 26-16

PARATHYROID CARCINOMA

A tumor thrombus is present in a vessel within the soft tissue surrounding a parathyroid carcinoma.

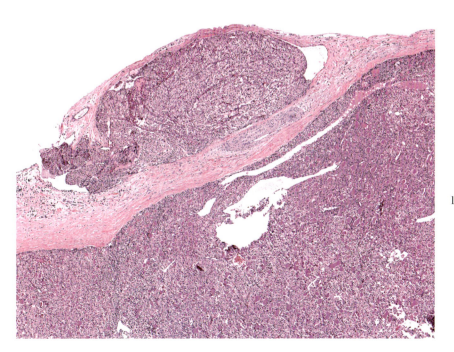

Figure 26-17

PARATHYROID CARCINOMA

A capsular vessel contains a large tumor thrombus.

present in association with the tumor; and 4) an endothelial covering may or may not be present. Artifactually dislodged tumor deposits in vascular channels are usually irregularly shaped and are not endothelialized or associated with fibrin. While vascular invasion is uncommon in parathyroid carcinomas, its presence is diagnostic of malignancy. Invasion of perineural spaces is also diagnostic of malignancy, but this feature is less common than vascular invasion.

Several studies have established that, in the absence of unequivocal evidence of invasion or metastasis, histopathologic features are unable to establish the diagnosis of malignancy (32,40). This view is also supported by the World Health Organization (45). The diagnosis of malignancy, therefore, should be restricted to those cases that have evidence of invasion of adjacent soft tissues and associated structures, vascular channels, or perineural spaces or to tumors with documented metastases (29,45).

Both flow cytometry and static DNA imaging have been used to assess ploidy status in parathyroid neoplasms. Although aneuploidy is more frequent in carcinomas, a significant proportion of adenomas contains aneuploid populations, particularly when assessed by flow cytometry. Accordingly, there is uncertainty about the extent to which nuclear DNA cytometry should be considered an important modality for the assessment of malignancy in these tumors. This subject is further discussed in chapter 30.

CYTOLOGIC FINDINGS

There are few studies of parathyroid carcinoma in aspirated material (46–49), and there are no consistent cytologic criteria that permit the distinction of adenoma and carcinoma with this type of sample. Concurrent assays of PTH in aspirated material have been used to identify sites of recurrent or persistent disease in patients undergoing re-operation for primary hyperparathyroidism, including those with parathyroid carcinoma (22,49). A case of tumor seeding along a needle track has been reported 5 years following aspiration biopsy of a parathyroid carcinoma (46). It should be noted that fine-needle aspiration biopsy of adenomas may be followed by a variety of atypical changes simulating carcinoma, including fibrosis, exten-

sion of tumor into the surrounding soft tissues, nuclear atypia, and mitotic activity (50).

IMMUNOHISTOCHEMICAL FINDINGS

Parathyroid carcinomas are usually positive for chromogranin and PTH, although the staining pattern may be more irregular than that seen in adenomas. The cytokeratin profile is similar to that of adenomas (see chapter 25). Thus, the tumors are typically positive for cytokeratins (CK) 7, 8, 18, and 19 while CK20 is negative. Cyclin D1 is expressed in 90 percent of carcinomas, as compared to 40 percent of adenomas and 60 percent of hyperplasias (51); however, these differences are not diagnostically useful.

Studies of cell cycle regulatory proteins and proteins that play important roles in the p53 pathway have shown that parathyroid carcinomas tend to have higher levels of expression of Ki-67 and lower levels of expression of p27, bcl-2, and mdm2 than adenomas (43). Staining for the RB protein is generally negative in parathyroid carcinomas, while adenomas are variably positive (52,53). However, other groups have concluded that RB staining is not useful for the distinction of parathyroid adenomas and carcinomas (54).

There is extensive literature on the use of immunohistochemical stains for parafibromin, a product of the *HRPT2/CDC73* gene, for the distinction of parathyroid adenomas and carcinomas (55–66). Early studies reported an absence of nuclear staining in parathyroid carcinomas and in adenomas associated with the HPT-JT syndrome, while sporadic adenomas were positive in more than 99 percent of cases (56,57,60). In well-controlled studies complete loss of staining occurs in 60 to 70 percent of carcinomas, with positive staining of stromal and endothelial cells as internal positive controls (fig. 26-18) (56,60). Some investigators have suggested that absent parafibromin staining could replace *HRPT2/CDC73* gene analysis for the diagnosis of parathyroid carcinoma (65). Other studies, however, have revealed partial or complete loss of nuclear or nucleolar staining in 30 to 80 percent of cases of carcinoma (55,58,59,62,63,66). Interestingly, parathyroid carcinomas developing in some patients with chronic renal failure are positive for parafibromin (65), suggesting an alternative genetic pathway for the development of these tumors.

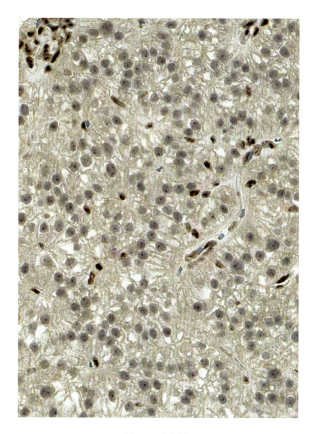

Figure 26-18

PARATHYROID CARCINOMA: PARAFIBROMIN STAIN

The tumor cell nuclei are unreactive, while endothelial and stromal cell nuclei (internal control) are positive. (Courtesy of Dr. A. Gill, Sydney, Australia.)

Some of the observed variability in parafibromin reactivity is undoubtedly related to case selection criteria, with respect to the inclusion of unequivocal (invasive) and equivocal (noninvasive) tumors. Other factors that may be responsible for the staining variability include differences in tissue fixation, primary antibodies and retrieval methods, and differing criteria for the assessment of staining patterns (partial versus complete loss) (62,63). The results of parafibromin staining should, therefore, be interpreted with caution and in the context of the histopathologic features (57). Absent or patchy nuclear staining for parafibromin should raise the possibility of carcinoma; however, the final diagnosis should be based on the conventional criteria for invasive growth.

Additional markers that have been used, either alone or in combination with parafibromin, for the distinction of parathyroid carcinoma and adenoma include galectin-3, the adenomatous polyposis coli (APC) protein, glycogen synthase 3β, and protein gene product 9.5 (PGP 9.5). Galectin-3 is present in the majority of carcinomas but is negative in most adenomas (55,67). However, the potential value of galectin-3 in distinguishing benign and malignant lesions appears to be reduced in patients with multiglandular disease (68).

The APC protein is uniformly expressed in adenomas but is absent from the majority of carcinomas, while glycogen synthase is not helpful in the distinction of these tumors (69). PGP 9.5 has been reported to have a sensitivity of 78 percent for the detection of parathyroid carcinoma or the *HRPT2/CDC73* mutation and a specificity of 100 percent (66). While alterations in parafibromin and other markers may heighten the suspicion of carcinoma, the diagnosis of malignancy should depend on the demonstration of invasive growth.

ULTRASTRUCTURAL FINDINGS

There are few ultrastructural studies of parathyroid carcinomas (25,35,70–72). Some cells have extensively developed Golgi regions with numerous prosecretory granules and mature secretory granules while others have prominent stacks of granular endoplasmic reticulum. In one case from an unpublished observation, the plasma membranes were extensively tortuous and there were occasional intracytoplasmic lumens. Oncocytic carcinomas, similar to their benign counterparts, are filled with mitochondria (35).

MOLECULAR GENETIC FINDINGS

The molecular genetic features of parathyroid malignancies are reviewed in several publications (21,23,73,74). Germline mutations of the *HRPT2/CDC73* gene, which encodes parafibromin, are responsible for the development of parathyroid carcinoma in the HPT-JT syndrome (75). Somatic mutations of this gene also occur in approximately 70 percent of sporadic parathyroid carcinomas (10,76,77). Most of the mutations are of the nonsense type and are predicted to result in a loss of parafibromin expression, but mutations in noncoding regulatory sequences or gene inactivation by methylation have also been implicated (78). Sporadic adenomas rarely harbor *HRPT2/*

CDC73 mutations (76). Parafibromin inhibits cell proliferation and promotes apoptosis (79).

The *RB* and *BRCA2* genes have also been implicated in the development of parathyroid carcinoma (52,80,81). Early studies reported that most of these tumors lacked an *RB* allele (52). The *RB* and *BRCA2* genes are located in the same region of chromosome 13 (80). In one study, loss of heterozygosity (LOH) for at least one marker of the *RB* allele was found in all parathyroid carcinomas while LOH for *BRCA2* was present in 60 percent of cases (53). In the same series, LOH for *RB* and *BRCA2* was present in 28 percent and 17 percent, respectively, of adenomas. Direct sequencing of parathyroid carcinoma with losses of *RB* and *BRCA2*, however, was negative for microdeletions, insertions, or point mutations in either gene (81). These findings demonstrate that neither *RB* nor *BRCA2* are likely to act as classic tumor suppressor genes. These observations, however, do not exclude the possibility that the decreased functions of *RB* in carcinomas, whether secondary or due to epigenetic effects, may have a role in tumor development (81).

DIFFERENTIAL DIAGNOSIS

Parathyroid carcinomas must be distinguished from both thyroid follicular and C-cell neoplasms, as well as metastatic tumors in this region, as discussed in previous chapters.

The distinction of classic parathyroid carcinoma from typical parathyroid adenoma is generally straightforward. Atypical adenomas, on the other hand, present considerable differential diagnostic difficulties (31,37,82–86). By definition, atypical adenomas lack evidence of invasion, as discussed in chapter 25. Atypical adenomas may be positive or negative for parafibromin (55,57,59,87), while carcinomas are more consistently negative. In well controlled studies, the risk for recurrence of parafibromin negative cases is approximately 10 to 20 percent, while the risk is essentially nil in parafibromin positive cases (57,87). In contrast to carcinomas, galectin-3 positivity and loss of APC have been reported in a few cases of atypical adenoma (24).

Occasional patients who have had previous surgery for parathyroid adenoma or hyperplasia may develop recurrent hyperparathyroidism, suggesting the possibility of malignancy. Benign parathyroid tissue that has been spilled in the operative field may regrow and simulate carcinoma both grossly and microscopically (88–90). This phenomenon has been referred to as parathyromatosis (91). Rattner et al. (89) reported their experience with inadvertently implanted parathyroid tissue at the time of surgery in 4 of 23 cases of recurrent hyperparathyroidism. Two of the 4 patients had multiple parathyroid implants in the previous operative field and 1 of these patients had documented spillage of a cystic adenoma during the original surgery. The remaining 2 patients had recurrent adenomas containing fragments of suture material.

The distinction of parathyroid carcinoma and parathyromatosis (see chapter 29) is challenging. In a series of 13 cases of parathyromatosis reported by Fernandez-Ranvier et al. (82), 12 patients had recurrent or persistent hyperparathyroidism following prior parathyroid surgery, while 1 patient had de novo parathyromatosis. The diagnosis was established by finding multiple small fragments of parathyroid tissue scattered in the neck and upper mediastinum. Fibrosis and scarring are present in most cases of secondary (post-surgical) parathyromatosis. In addition, invasion of the soft issues of the neck and mitotic activity occur in 15 percent of the cases, but no patients have had evidence of vascular invasion, lymph node involvement, or distant metastases with an average follow-up of 58 months. The immunophenotype of parathyromatosis is reported to be similar to that of parathyroid reported to be adenoma (55).

TREATMENT AND PROGNOSIS

The optimal treatment for patients with parathyroid carcinoma is en bloc resection of the tumor at the time of initial surgery (1,7,92). Failure to remove the adjacent tissue together with the tumor leads to local recurrence in a high proportion of patients (figs. 26-19–26-21). En bloc resection generally includes removal of the adjacent thyroid lobe and paratracheal soft tissues and lymph nodes. Tracheoesophageal, paratracheal, and upper mediastinal nodes may be removed at initial surgery, but a neck dissection is performed only when there is evidence of nodal involvement.

If a diagnosis of carcinoma is made postoperatively on the basis of microscopic features, immediate reoperation may not be necessary

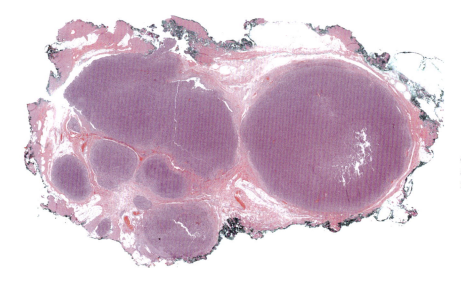

Figure 26-19

RECURRENT PARATHYROID CARCINOMA

This tumor, in the soft tissue of the neck, has a multinodular appearance with intervening fibrous bands.

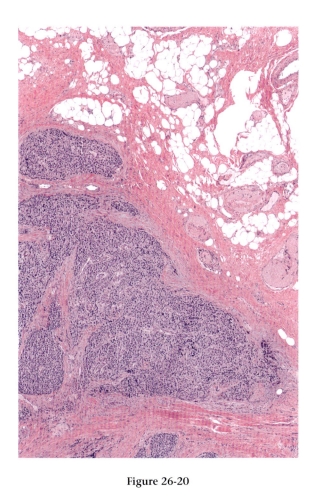

Figure 26-20

RECURRENT PARATHYROID CARCINOMA

There is extensive fibrosis surrounding the areas of tumor.

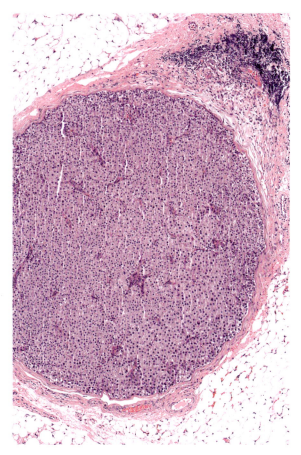

Figure 26-21

RECURRENT PARATHYROID CARCINOMA

This tumor implant, in a patient with the hyperparathyroidism-jaw tumor syndrome, is surrounded by a fibrous capsule.

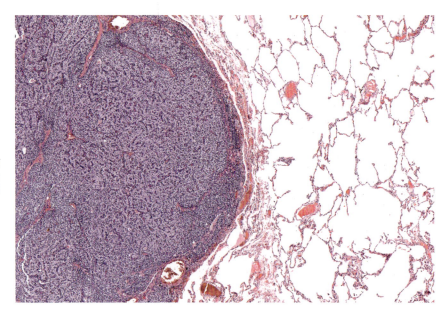

Figure 26-22

METASTATIC PARATHYROID CARCINOMA (LUNG)

The patient had a history of secondary hyperparathyroidism associated with chronic renal failure.

since the initial resection of the tumor may be curative. A decision to reoperate should be based on regular monitoring of PTH and calcium levels. Recurrent disease in the neck should be treated by wide local excision of the involved area, including regional nodes. External beam radiation may reduce recurrence rates, although this modality has not been evaluated extensively. There is no effective chemotherapy. Palliative surgery with excision of sites of recurrence and metastases may be effective in prolonging survival in selected patients (93). The administration of calcimimetics is effective in treating the metabolic complications of recurrent and metastatic disease (1).

Most parathyroid carcinomas are indolent tumors with a low malignant potential (22). The tumors characteristically recur locally and spread to contiguous structures in the neck (figs. 26-19–26-21). In the series reported by Koea and Shaw (94), the most common sites of local involvement included the ipsilateral thyroid gland (89 percent), strap muscles (71 percent), ipsilateral recurrent laryngeal nerve (66 percent), esophagus (18 percent), and trachea (17 percent). Metastatic spread tends to occur late in the course of the disease. The most common sites of metastases include cervical lymph nodes (30 percent) and lung (40 percent), followed by liver (10 percent) (fig. 26-22). Other sites that may be involved include bone, pleura, and pericardium. Rarely, metastases to the brain have

been documented (95,96). Downregulation of CaSR, global loss of parafibromin reactivity, and the presence of an *HRPT2/CDC73* mutation have been proposed as determinants of increased malignant potential (61).

STAGING OF PARATHYROID CARCINOMA

The American Joint Committee of Cancer/International Union Against Cancer has not as yet developed a staging system for parathyroid carcinoma. However, Shaha and Shah (97) have proposed a staging system that divides the tumors into four categories. In their proposal, the T1 category includes tumors measuring less than 3 cm; T2 refers to tumors greater than 3 cm; the T3 refers to tumors of any size with invasion of the surrounding soft tissue, thyroid gland, or strap muscles; and T4 refers to tumors with massive central compartment involvement with invasion of the trachea and esophagus or recurrent parathyroid carcinoma. Talat and Schultz (44) have proposed a system that divides tumors into those with capsular invasion alone (T1) or invasion of surrounding soft tissue, excluding the trachea, larynx, or esophagus (T2). The T3 category in their system refers to tumors with vascular invasion while the T4 category includes cases in which there is invasion of hypopharynx, trachea, esophagus, larynx, recurrent laryngeal nerve, or carotid artery. They further propose a system that divides tumors into low risk (capsular invasion or invasion of soft tissue, i.e., T1 or T2) and high risk (vascular invasion [T3] and/or invasion of vital organs [T4] and/or nodal metastases [N1] and/or distant metastases [M1]) categories. They report that this system identifies a 3.5- to 7.0-fold higher risk of recurrence and death in those patients with high-risk tumors.

Kameyama and Takami (98) in 2005 also proposed a classification of parathyroid carcinoma based on the extent of invasion. This classification divides tumors into those showing minimal or widespread capsular and vascular invasion. In their series, all 5 patients with widespread invasion had evidence of remote metastases while the 12 patients with minimally invasive tumors had no evidence of recurrence or metastasis.

REFERENCES

1. Fang SH, Lal G. Parathyroid cancer. Endocr Pract 2011;17(Suppl 1):36-43.
2. McKeown PP, McGarity WC, Sewell CW. Carcinoma of the parathyroid gland: is it over diagnosed? A report of three cases. Am J Surg 1984;147:292-8.
3. Wang CA, Gaz RD. Natural history of parathyroid carcinoma. Diagnosis, treatment and results. Am J Surg 1985;149:522-7.
4. Lee PK, Jarosek SL, Virnig BA, Evasovich M, Tuttle TM. Trends in the incidence and treatment of parathyroid cancer in the United States. Cancer 2007;109:1736-41.
5. Brown S, O'Neill CO, Suliburk J, et al. Parathyroid carcinoma: increasing incidence and changing presentation. ANZ J Surg 2011;81:428-532.
6. Favia G, Lumachi F, Polistina F, D'Amico DF. Parathyroid carcinoma: sixteen new cases and suggestions for contact management. World J Surg 1998;22:1225-30.
7. Obara T. [Diagnosis and treatment of primary hyperparathyroidism.] Nihon Naibunpi Gakkai Zassli 1992;68:1167-76. [Japanese]
8. Hundahl SA, Fleming ID, Fremgen AM, Menck HR. Two hundred eighty-six cases of parathyroid carcinoma treated in the US between 1985-1995: a National Cancer Data Base Report. The American College of Surgeons Commission on Cancer and the American Cancer Society. Cancer 1999;86:538-44.
9. Christmas TJ, Chapple CR, Noble JG, Milroy EJ, Cowie AG. Hyperparathyroidism after neck irradiation. Br J Surg 1988;75:873-4.
10. Shattuck TM, Välimäki S, Obara T, et al. Somatic and germ-line mutations of the HRPT2 gene in sporadic parathyroid carcinoma. N Engl J Med 2003;349:1722-9.
11. Wassif WS, Moniz CF, Friedman C, et al. Familial isolated hyperparathyroidism: a distinct genetic entity with an increased risk of parathyroid carcinoma. J Clin Endocrinol Metab 1993;77:1485-9.
12. Agha A, Carpenter R, Bhattacharya S, Edmonson SJ, Carlsen E, Monson JP. Parathyroid carcinoma in multiple endocrine neoplasia type 1 (MEN1) syndrome: two case reports of an unrecognized entity. J Endocrinol Invest 2007;30:145-9.
13. Shih RY, Fackler S, Matuso S, True MW, Brennan J, Wells D. Parathyroid carcinoma in multiple endocrine neoplasia type 1 with a classic germline mutation. Endocr Pract 2009;15:567-72.
14. Jenkins PJ, Satta MA, Simmergen M, et al. Metastatic parathyroid carcinoma in the MEN2A syndrome. Clin Endocrinol (Oxf) 1977;47:747-51.
15. Berland Y, Olmer M, Labreuil G, Grisoli J. Parathyroid carcinoma, adenoma and hyperplasia in a case of chronic renal insufficiency on dialysis. Clin Nephrol 1982;18:154-8.
16. Boyle NH, Ogg CS, Hartley RB, Owen WJ. Parathyroid carcinoma secondary to prolonged hyperplasia in chronic renal failure and celiac disease. Eur J Clin Oncol 1999;25:100-3.
17. Miki H, Sumitomo M, Inoue H, Kita S, Monden Y. Parathyroid carcinoma in patients with chronic renal failure on maintenance hemodialysis. Surgery 1996;120:897-901.
18. Ireland J, Fleming S, Levison D, Cattell WR, Baker LR. Parathyroid carcinoma associated with chronic renal failure and previous radiotherapy to the neck. J Clin Pathol 1985;38:1114-8.
19. Haven CJ, Howell VM, Eilers PH, et al. Gene expression of parathyroid tumors: molecular subclassification and identification of the potential malignant phenotype. Cancer Res 2004;64:7405-11.
20. Shane E. Clinical review 122: Parathyroid carcinoma. J. Clin Endocrinol Metab 2001;86:485-93.
21. Sharretts JM, Kebebew E, Simonds WF. Parathyroid carcinoma. Semin Oncol 2010;37:580-90.
22. Harari A, Waring A, Fernandez-Ranvier G, et al Parathyroid carcinoma: a 43-year outcome and survival analysis. J Clin Endocrinol Metab 2011;96:3679-86.

23. Marcocci C, Cetani F, Rubin MR, Silverberg SJ, Pinchera A, Bilezikian JP. Parathyroid carcinoma. J Bone Miner Res 2008;23:1869-80.
24. Fernandez-Ranvier GG, Jensen K, Khanafshar E, et al. Non-functioning parathyroid carcinoma: a case report and review of the literature. Endocr Pract 2007;13:750-7.
25. Murphy MN, Glennon PG, Diocee MS, Wick MR, Cavers DJ. Nonsecretory parathyroid carcinoma of the mediastinum. Light microscopic, immunocytochemical and ultrastructural features of a case, and a review of the literature. Cancer 1986;58:2468-76.
26. Ordonez NG, Ibánez ML, Samaan NA, Hickey RC. Immunoperoxidase study of uncommon parathyroid tumors. Report of two cases of nonfunctioning parathyroid carcinoma and one intrathyroid parathyroid tumor-producing amyloid. Am J Surg Pathol 1983;7:535-42.
27. Black BK. Carcinoma of the parathyroid. Ann Surg 1954;139:355-63.
28. Castleman B, Roth SI. Tumors of the parathyroid glands. Atlas of Tumor Pathology, 2nd Series, Fascicle 14, Washington DC: Armed Forces Institute of Pathology; 1978:1-94.
29. DeLellis RA. Parathyroid tumors and related disorders. Mod Pathol 2011;24(Suppl 2):S578-93.
30. Sandelin K, Tullgren O, Farnebo O. Clinical course of parathyroid cancer. World J Surg 1994;18:594-8.
31. Ippolito G, Palazzo FF, Sebag F, De Micco C, Henry JF. Intraoperative diagnosis and treatment of parathyroid cancer and atypical parathyroid adenoma. Br J Surg 2007;94:566-70.
32. Bondeson L, Sandelin K, Grimelius L. Histopathological variables and DNA cytometry in parathyroid carcinomas. Am J Surg Pathol 1993;17:820-9.
33. Nacamuli R, Rumore GJ, Clark G. Parathyroid carcinosarcoma: a previously unreported entity. Am Surg 2002;68:900-3.
34. Taggart JL, Summerlin DJ, Moore MG. Parathyroid carcinosarcoma: a rare form of parathyroid carcinoma with normal parathyroid hormone levels. Int J Surg Pathol 2013;21:394-8.
35. Obara T, Fujimoto Y, Yamaguchi K, Takanashi R, Kino I, Sasaki Y. Parathyroid carcinoma of the oxyphil cell type. A report of two cases, light and electron microscopic study. Cancer 1985;55:1482-9.
36. Schantz A, Castleman B. Parathyroid carcinoma. A study of 70 cases. Cancer 1973;31:600-5.
37. Levin KE, Galante M, Clark OH. Parathyroid carcinoma versus parathyroid adenoma in patients with profound hypercalcemia. Surgery 1987;101:649-60.
38. San Juan J, Monteagudo C, Fraker D, Norton J, Merino M. Significance of mitotic activity and other morphologic parameters in parathyroid adenomas and their correlation with clinical behavior [Abstract]. Am J Clin Pathol 1989;92:523.
39. Snover DC, Foucar K. Mitotic activity in benign parathyroid disease. Am J Clin Pathol 1981;75:345-7.
40. Sandelin K, Auer G, Bondeson L, Grimelius L, Farnebo LO. Prognostic factors in parathyroid carcinoma: a review of 95 cases. World J Surg 1992;16:724-31.
41. Abbona GC, Papotti M, Gasparri G, Bussolati G. Proliferative activity in parathyroid tumors as detected by Ki-67 immunostaining. Hum Pathol 1995;26:135-8.
42. Erickson LA, Jin L, Wollan P, Thompson GB, van Heerden LA, Lloyd RV. Parathyroid hyperplasia, adenomas and carcinoma: differential expression of p27kip protein. Am J Surg Pathol 1999;23:288-5.
43. Stojadinovic A, Hoos A, Nissan A, et al. Parathyroid neoplasms: clinical, histopathologic and tissue microarray-based molecular analysis. Hum Pathol 2003;34:54-4.
44. Talat N, Schulte KM. Clinical presentation, staging and long term evolution of parathyroid cancer. Ann Surg Oncol 2010;17:2156-74.
45. Bondeson L, Grimelius L, DeLellis RA, et al. Parathyroid carcinoma. In: DeLellis RA, Lloyd RV, Heitz PU, Eng C, eds. Pathology and genetics of tumours of endocrine organs. WHO Classification of Endocrine Tumours. Lyon: IARC Press; 2004:124-7.
46. Agarwal G, Dhingra S, Mishra SK, Krishnani N. Implantation of parathyroid carcinoma along fine needle aspiration track. Langerbecks Arch Surg 2006;391:623-6.
47. Hara H, Oyama T, Kimura M, et al. Cytologic characteristics of parathyroid carcinoma: a case report. Diagn Cytopathol 1998;18:192-8.
48. Ikeda K, Tate G, Suzuki T, Mitsuya T. Cytologic comparison of a primary parathyroid cancer and its metastatic lesions: a case report. Diagn Cytopathol 2006;34:50-5.
49. MacFarlane MP, Fraker DL, Shawker TH, et al. Use of preoperative fine-needle aspiration in patients undergoing reoperation for primary hyperparathyroidism. Surgery 1994;116:959-64.
50. Alwaheeb S, Rambaldini G, Boerner S, Coiré C, Fiser J, Asa SL. Worrisome histologic alterations following fine needle aspiration of the parathyroid. J Clin Pathol 2006;59:1094-6.
51. Vasef MA, Brynes RK, Sturm M, Bromley C, Robinson RA. Expression of cyclin D1 in parathyroid carcinomas, adenomas and hyperplasia: a paraffin immunohistochemical study. Mod Pathol 1999;12:412-6.

52. Cryns VL, Thor A, Xu HJ, et al. Loss of the retinoblastoma tumor-suppressor gene in parathyroid carcinoma. N Engl J Med 1994;330:757-61.

53. Cetani F, Pardi E, Vlacava P, et al. A reappraisal of the Rb1 gene abnormalities in the diagnoses of parathyroid carcinoma. Clin Endocrinol (Oxf) 2004;60:99-106.

54. Farnebo F, Auer G, Farnebo LO, et al. Evaluation of retinoblastoma and Ki-67 immunostaining as diagnostic markers of benign and malignant parathyroid disease. World J Surg 1999;23:68-74.

55. Fernandez-Ranvier GG, Khanafshar E, Tacha D, et al. Defining a molecular phenotype for benign and malignant parathyroid tumors. Cancer 2009;115:334-44.

56. Gill AJ, Clarkson A, Gimm O, et al. Loss of nuclear expression of parafibromin distinguishes parathyroid carcinoma and hyperparathyroidism-jaw tumor (HPT-JT) syndrome-related adenomas from sporadic parathyroid adenomas and hyperplasias. Am J Surg Pathol 2006;30:1140-9.

57. Gill AJ. Understanding the genetic basis of parathyroid carcinoma. Endocr Pathol 2014;25:30-4.

58. Juhlin CC, Haglund F, Obara T, Arnold A, Larsson C, Höög A. Absence of nucleolar parafibromin immunoreactivity in subsets of parathyroid malignant tumors. Virchows Arch 2011;459:47-53.

59. Juhlin CC, Villablanca A, Sandelin K, et al. Parafibromin immunoreactivity; its use as an additional diagnostic marker for parathyroid tumor classification. Endocr Relat Cancer 2007;24:501-2.

60. Tan MH, Morrison C, Wang P, et al. Loss of parafibromin immunoreactivity is a distinguishing feature of parathyroid carcinoma. Clin Cancer Res 2004;10:6629-37.

61. Witteveen JE, Hamdy NA, Dekkers OM, et al. Downregulation of CASR expression and global loss of parafibromin staining are strong negative determinants of progress in parathyroid carcinoma. Mod Pathol 2011;24:688-97.

62. Mangray S, DeLellis RA. Parafibromin as a tool for the diagnosis of parathyroid tumors. Adv Anat Pathol 2008;15:179.

63. Mangray S, Kurek KC, Sabo E, DeLellis RA. Immunohistochemical expression of parafibromin is of limited value in distinguishing parathyroid carcinoma from adenoma. Mod Pathol 2008; 21: 108A. (Abstract).

64. Tominaga Y, Tsuzuki T, Matsuoka A, et al. Expression of parafibromin in distant metastatic parathyroid tumors in patients with advanced secondary hyperparathyroidism due to chronic kidney disease. World J Surg 2008;32:815-1.

65. Cetani F, Ambrogini E, Viacava P, et al. Should parafibromin staining replace HRPT2 gene analysis as an additional tool for histologic diagnosis of parathyroid carcinoma? Eur J Endocrinol 2007;156:547-54.

66. Howell VM, Gill A, Clarkson A, et al. Accuracy of combined protein gene product 9.5 and parafibromin markers for immunohistochemical diagnosis of parathyroid carcinoma. J Clin Endocrinol Metab 2009;94:434-41.

67. Bergero N, DePompa R, Sacerdote C, et al. Galectin-3 expression in parathyroid carcinoma: immunohistochemical study of 26 cases. Hum Pathol 2005;36:908-14.

68. Saggiorato E, Bergero N, Volante M, et al. Galectin-3 and Ki-67 expression in multiglandular parathyroid lesions. Am J Clin Pathol 2006;126:59-66.

69. Juhlin CC, Haglund F, Villablanca A, et al. Loss of expression for the Wnt pathway components adenomatous polyposis coli and glycogen synthase kinase 3-β in parathyroid carcinomas. Int J Oncol 2009;34:481-92.

70. Altenähr E, Saeger W. Light and electron microscopy of parathyroid carcinoma. Report of three cases. Virchows Arch A Pathol Pathol Anat 1973;360:107-22.

71. de la Garza S, Flores de la Garza E, Hernandez-Batres F. Functional parathyroid carcinoma. Cytology, histology and ultrastructure of a case. Diagn Cytopathol 1985;1:232-5.

72. Faccini JM. The ultrastructure of parathyroid glands removed from patients with primary hyperparathyroidism: a report of 40 cases, including four carcinomata. J Pathol 1970;102:189-99.

73. Cetani F, Pardi E, Borsari S Marcocci C. Molecular pathogenesis of primary hyperparathyroidism. J Endocrinol Invest 2011;34(Suppl 7):35-9.

74. Weinstein LS, Simonds WF. HRPT2, a marker of parathyroid cancer. N Engl J Med 2003;349:1691-2.

75. Carpten JD, Robbins CM, Villablanca A, et al. HRPT2 encoding parafibromin is mutated in hyperparathyroidism-jaw tumor syndrome. Nat Genet 2002;32:676-80.

76. Cetani F, Pardi E, Borsari S, et al. Genetic analyses of the HRPT2 gene in primary hyperparathyroidism: Germline and sporadic mutations in familial and sporadic parathyroid tumors. J Clin Endocrinol Metab 2004;89:5583-91.

77. Howell VM, Haven CJ, Kahnoski K, et al. HRPT2 mutations are associated with malignancy in sporadic parathyroid tumors. J Med Genet 2003;40:657-63.

78. Hewitt KM, Sharma PK, Samowitz W, Hobbs M. Aberrant methylation of the HRPT2 gene in parathyroid carcinoma. Ann Otol Rhinol Laryngol 2007;116:928-33.

79. Zhang C, Kong D, Tan MH, et al. Parafibromin inhibits cancer cell growth and causes G1 phase arrest. Biochem Biophys Res Commun 2006;350:17-24.

80. Pearce SH, Trump D, Wooding C, Sheppard MN, Clayton RN, Thakker RV. Loss of heterozygosity studies at the retinoblastoma and breast cancer susceptibility (BRCA2) loci in pituitary, parathyroid, pancreatic and carcinoid tumours. Clin Endocrinol (Oxf) 1996;45:195-200.

81. Shattuck TM1, Kim TS, Costa J, et al. Mutational analyses of RB and BRCA2 as candidate tumour suppressor genes in parathyroid carcinoma. Clin Endocrinol (Oxf) 2003;59:180-9.

82. Fernandez-Ranvier GG, Khanafshar E, Jensen K, et al. Parathyroid carcinoma, atypical parathyroid adenoma or parathyromatosis? Cancer 2007;110:255-64.

83. Guiter GE, DeLellis RA. Risk of recurrence or metastasis in atypical parathyroid adenomas. Mod Pathol 2002;15:115A (Abstract).

84. Levin KE Chew KL Ljung BM, Mayall BH, Siperstein AE, Clark OH. Deoxyribonucleic acid cytometry helps identify parathyroid carcinomas. J Clin Endocrinol Metab 1988;67:779-84.

85. Farnebo F, Svensson A, Thompson NW, et al. Expression of matrix metalloproteinase gelatinase A messenger ribonucleic acid in parathyroid carcinomas. Surgery 1999;126:1183-7.

86. Juhlin CC, Nilsson IL, Johansson K, et al. Parafibromin and APC as screening markers for malignant potential in atypical parathyroid adenomas. Endocr Pathol 2010;21:166-77.

87. Kruijff S, Sidhu SB, Sywak MS, Gill AJ, Delbridge LW. Negative parafibromin staining predicts malignant behavior in atypical parathyroid adenomas. Ann Surg Oncol 2014;21:426-33.

88. Fitko R, Roth SI, Hines JR, Roxe DM, Cahill E. Parathyromatosis in hyperparathyroidism. Hum Pathol 1990;21:234-7.

89. Rattner DW, Marrone GC, Kasdon E, Silen W. Recurrent hyperparathyroidism. Am J Surg 1985;149:745-8.

90. Fraker DL, Travis WD, Merendino JJ Jr, et al. Locally recurrent parathyroid neoplasms as a cause for recurrent and persistent primary hyperparathyroidism. Ann Surg 1991;213:58-65.

91. Reddick RL, Costa J, Marx SJ. Parathyroid hyperplasia and parathyromatosis. Lancet 1997;1:549.

92. Wei CH, Harari A. Parathyroid carcinoma: update and guidelines for management. Curr Treat Options Oncol 2012;13:11-23.

93. Fujimoto Y, Obara T, Ito Y, Kodama T, Nobori M, Ebihara S. Localization and surgical resection of metastatic parathyroid carcinoma. World J Surg 1986;10:539-47.

94. Koea JB, Shaw JH. Parathyroid cancer: biology and management. Surg Oncol 1999;8:155-65.

95. Tyler D, Mandybur G, Dhillon G, Fratkin L. Intracranial metastatic parathyroid carcinoma: case Report. Neurosurgery 2001;48:937-40.

96. Yamamoto T, Matsumura A, Fujita K, Kawakami Y, Yamashita K, Nose T. Cerebral metastases of parathyroid carcinoma. Neurol Med Chir (Tokyo) 1996;36:96-8.

97. Shaha AR, Shah JP. Parathyroid carcinoma: a diagnostic and therapeutic challenge. Cancer 1999;86:378-80.

98. Kameyama K, Takami H. Proposal for the histological classification of parathyroid carcinoma. Endocr Pathol 2005;16:49-52.

27 PRIMARY CHIEF CELL HYPERPLASIA, CLEAR CELL HYPERPLASIA, AND HERITABLE HYPERPARATHYROIDISM SYNDROMES

PRIMARY CHIEF CELL HYPERPLASIA

Definition. *Primary chief cell hyperplasia* of the parathyroid glands is characterized by an absolute increase in the parathyroid parenchymal mass resulting from a proliferation of chief cells, oncocytes, and transitional oncocytes in multiple parathyroid glands in the absence of a known stimulus for parathyroid hormone (PTH) hypersecretion.

General Features. Primary chief cell hyperplasia was first reported as a cause of primary hyperparathyroidism by Cope et al. in 1958 (1). These authors recognized that it was difficult, if not impossible, to distinguish chief cell hyperplasia from adenoma by examining a single gland. In most series, primary chief cell hyperplasia accounts for approximately 15 percent of all cases of primary hyperparathyroidism (2).

This disorder occurs sporadically (75 percent) or as a component of one of the heritable hyperparathyroidism syndromes (25 percent). The prevalence of sporadic hyperplasia increases with age. Akerström et al. (3) found evidence of parathyroid hyperplasia in 7 percent of routinely examined glands at autopsy. None of the patients had evidence of chronic renal disease, thereby ruling out secondary parathyroid hyperplasia.

Clinical Features. The clinical features of sporadic primary chief cell hyperplasia do not differ significantly from those of adenomas (4,5). Affected patients have excessive and inappropriate secretion of PTH with attendant hypercalcemia and hypophosphatemia. The stimulus for the chief cell hyperplasia and PTH secretion is unknown although some studies have implicated a circulating parathyroid mitogenic factor in the genesis of this disease (6).

Gross Findings. Black and Haff (7) recognized three major patterns of gland involvement in patients with primary chief cell hyperplasia: classic, pseudoadenomatous, and occult. In

the usual or classic type, all of the glands are enlarged to some extent. In the pseudoadenomatous variant, there is considerable variation in the extent of gland enlargement, with some glands markedly enlarged and other glands minimally enlarged or even normal in size (fig. 27-1). The occult cases are characterized by glands that are only minimally enlarged with only subtle microscopic changes of hyperplasia.

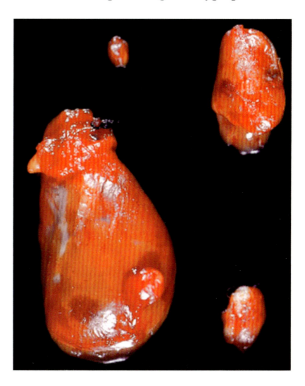

Figure 27-1

PRIMARY CHIEF CELL HYPERPLASIA

There is a marked disparity in the gland sizes. The left lower gland weighs more than the combined weight of the other three glands. The left upper gland is indistinguishable from normal. (Fig. 57-23 from Roth SI. The parathyroid gland. In: Silverberg SA, DeLellis RA, Frable WJ, eds. Principles and practice of surgical pathology and cytopathology, 3rd ed. New York: Churchill Livingstone; 1997:2727.)

Akerström et al. (8) reported that only two parathyroid glands were enlarged in approximately two thirds of their cases of primary chief cell hyperplasia. In a series reported from the Massachusetts General Hospital (2), approximately 50 percent of the cases had glands of approximately equal size while in the remaining cases, one gland was significantly larger than the other three. In the same series, total gland weight was less than 1 g in 54 percent of the patients and 1 to 5 g in 28 percent; only 18 percent had gland weights between 5 and 10 g and none had a weight in excess of 10 g.

Minimally enlarged glands may be difficult to distinguish from normal-sized glands. With increasing size, the parathyroid glands often assume irregular configurations, with pseudopodal projections from their surfaces. On cut section, the glands vary from yellow-brown to red. In most cases, the cut surface appears homogeneous, but distinct nodularity is evident in some instances. Cystic changes may occur, particularly in larger glands (9).

Microscopic Findings. Chief cell hyperplasia is characterized by increased parenchymal cell mass (fig. 27-2). The predominant cell type in this form of hyperplasia is the chief cell, although variable numbers of oncocytes and transitional oncocytes may be present (2). Stromal fat cells are markedly decreased. Because of the regional variation in the distribution of stromal fat cells, however, small biopsies of hyperplastic glands may show a normal chief cell to stromal fat ratio (2,10).

Primary chief cell hyperplasia may have a predominant diffuse (fig. 27-2) or nodular growth pattern (figs. 27-3–27-7). The nodular foci contain few or no stromal fat cells while the internodular and perinodular regions contain more numerous stromal fat cells (fig. 27-7). In some cases, fibrous septa surround the nodules.

Occasional cases of primary chief cell hyperplasia have abundant stromal fat cells, and small biopsies of such glands may lead to an erroneous diagnosis of a normocellular gland (fig. 27-2). If the pathologist has not examined the intact gland grossly, it may not be evident that it is enlarged. Straus et al. (10) introduced the term *lipohyperplasia* to describe hyperplastic glands with abundant stromal fat. Most of the resected glands in their series weighed between

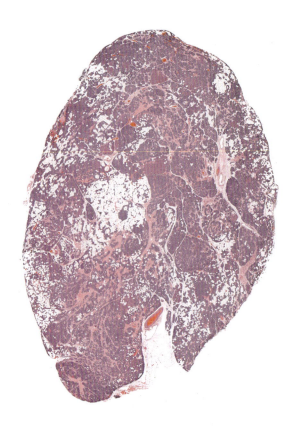

Figure 27-2

DIFFUSE CHIEF CELL HYPERPLASIA

There is considerable regional variation in the distribution of stromal fat in this enlarged gland.

100 and 200 mg, with the largest gland weighing 820 mg.

Aggregates of hyperplastic chief cells may also be evident in the soft tissues of the neck in patients with primary chief cell hyperplasia (chapter 29). In a study reported by Reddick et al. (11), 3 of 40 patients with primary chief cell hyperplasia had multiple parathyroid nests in the soft tissues of the neck or mediastinum. These lesions are referred to as *parathyromatosis* and may be responsible for persistent or recurrent hyperparathyroidism in patients treated by subtotal parathyroidectomy for chief cell hyperplasia. Supernumerary parathyroid glands also may become hyperplastic in patients with primary chief cell hyperplasia.

Hyperplastic chief cells are arranged in solid nests, cords, sheets, or follicles (figs. 27-3,

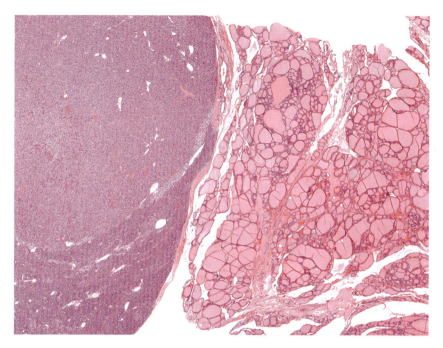

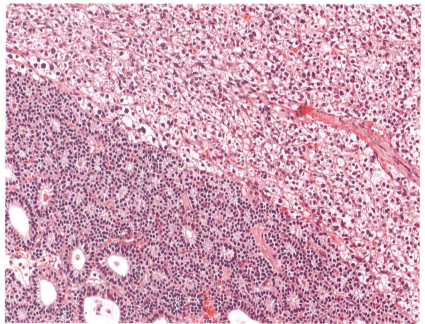

Figure 27-3

NODULAR CHIEF CELL HYPERPLASIA

Top: Nodular chief cell hyperplasia in a patient with multiple endocrine neoplasia type 1 (MEN 1).

Bottom: The nodule in the lower portion of the field has a partially follicular growth pattern.

bottom; 27-5). Proliferating chief cells, which are slightly larger than normal chief cells, predominate, but increased numbers of oncocytes and transitional oncocytic cells may also be evident. Nodules may be composed of fairly pure populations of one or another of these cell types. The parathyroid tissue adjacent to the nodules may contain stromal fat cells (fig. 27-7). It is often impossible to distinguish mild forms of diffuse hyperplasia adjacent to a hyperplastic nodule from a rim of normal parathyroid tissue adjacent to an adenoma. Fat stains are useful in making this distinction since hyperplastic chief cells generally contain decreased amounts of intracellular lipid as compared to normal or suppressed chief cells. It should be remembered, however, that occasional hyperplastic chief cells may contain abundant intracellular lipid.

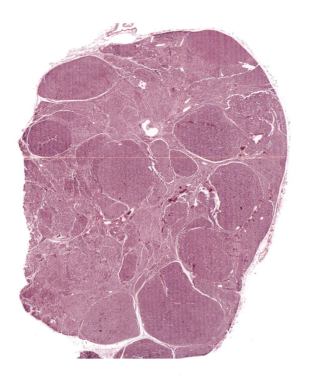

Figure 27-4

NODULAR CHIEF CELL HYPERPLASIA

Nodules are present throughout this enlarged gland of a patient with MEN 1.

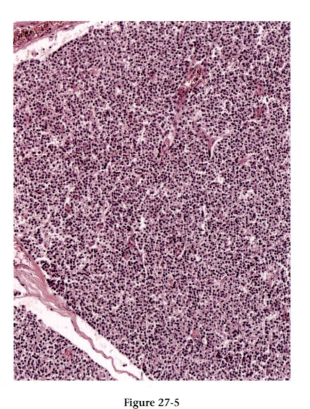

Figure 27-5

NODULAR CHIEF CELL HYPERPLASIA

Nodular chief cell hyperplasia in a patient with MEN 1 consists of nodules composed of diffuse proliferations of chief cells.

Figure 27-6

NODULAR CHIEFF CELL HYPERPLASIA

Multiple nodules are present throughout this enlarged gland in a patient with MEN 2A.

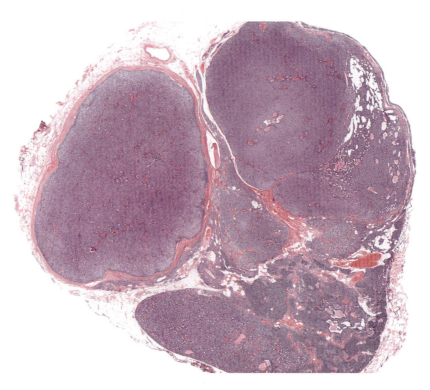

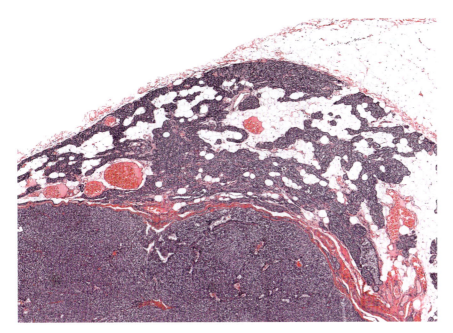

Figure 27-7

NODULAR CHIEF CELL HYPERPLASIA

A rim of parathyroid tissue (top), similar to that seen in an adenoma, is present adjacent to one of the nodules in a patient with MEN 2A.

Mitotic activity may be present in cases of hyperplasia (12,13). Snover and Foucar (13) reported mitoses in 80 percent of cases, with 60 percent having less than 1 mitotic figure per 10 high-power fields and 20 percent having greater than 1 mitosis per 10 high-power fields.

Hyperplastic chief cells may exhibit slight variation in nuclear size and shape, with enlarged and hyperchromatic nuclear forms in some cases. Pronounced nuclear enlargement and hyperchromasia, however, are more typical of adenomas. Hyperplastic glands, particularly if they are markedly enlarged, may show evidence of fibrosis and hemosiderin deposition.

Chronic parathyroiditis is associated with primary chief cell hyperplasia in occasional cases (14,15). In two cases reported by Bondeson et al. (14), dense collections of lymphocytes were noted in the stroma of the glands. In some areas, the stroma was densely fibrotic while other areas had a loose and edematous texture. Foci of lymphoid follicle formation, plasmacytic infiltration, and areas of parenchymal destruction were also noted. The lymphoid infiltration was considerably more extensive in these cases than the focal perivascular lymphoid infiltrates noted in occasional normal parathyroid glands. Although the origin of the lymphoid infiltrates in cases of parathyroiditis is unknown, it has been suggested that this disorder may have an

autoimmune basis. A similar change has been observed in rabbits exposed to ozone (16).

Cystic change in primary chief cell hyperplasia is uncommon (9). When present, cyst formation is most likely to occur in large hyperplastic glands. Mallette et al. (17) described an unusual familial variant of primary chief cell hyperplasia in 1987. It is now recognized, however, that this disorder represents the hyperparathyroidism-jaw tumor syndrome.

Immunohistochemical and Ultrastructural Findings. The immunohistochemical and ultrastructural features of primary chief cell hyperplasia are generally similar to those of chief cell adenoma (4,18–21).

Molecular Genetic Findings. Most cases of primary chief cell hyperplasia represent clonal proliferations. There are few molecular studies of nonfamilial chief cell hyperplasia, but the multiple endocrine neoplasia (MEN) 1 gene appears to be involved in the genesis of some cases. Molecular genetic features of MEN 1 and other heritable hyperparathyroidism syndromes are discussed below.

Differential Diagnosis. Parathyroid hyperplasia must be distinguished from parathyroid adenoma, and knowledge of the intraoperative findings or the results of intraoperative PTH levels is essential for this distinction. In patients with primary chief cell hyperplasia, enlargement of at least two glands is apparent grossly in cases in which the bilateral surgical approach has been used. The use of intraoperative PTH assays for single gland disease is well accepted (see chapter 30). Generally, a 50 percent decrease from baseline at 5 and 10 minutes is predictive of cure in 95 percent of patients. The value of this assay for cases of hyperplasia, however, is less clear (22). In the series of hyperplasia cases reported by Weber et al. (21), the 50 percent rule would have missed 20 percent of the patients with hyperplasia. The authors concluded that a 90 percent drop in PTH levels from baseline may be required to confirm complete excision of hyperfunctioning parathyroid tissue in patients with parathyroid hyperplasia of primary and secondary types (see chapter 30).

The presence of a rim of normal parathyroid tissue is considered an important criterion to distinguish adenoma from hyperplasia. However, cases of chief cell hyperplasia, particularly of the nodular type, may exhibit portions of compressed, mildly hyperplastic or normal parathyroid tissue at the periphery, referred to as a "pseudorim." Such areas are often impossible to distinguish from a compressed rim of parathyroid tissue adjacent to an adenoma. Although the pseudorims of hyperplastic glands should have a relatively low intracellular lipid content, abundant lipid is observed in some cases.

Biopsy of a second gland in a patient with chief cell hyperplasia should also show evidence of hyperplasia. Some hyperplastic glands, however, are normal or only slightly enlarged. Although intraoperative fat stains are expected to show decreased intracellular lipid in hyperplastic glands, this is not always the case. Bondeson (23) has shown that hyperplastic parathyroid tissue, in contrast to normal or suppressed glands, is likely to have divergent areas of intracellular lipid staining. Thus, some areas of hyperplastic glands may contain prominent intracellular lipid, while other areas are devoid of lipid.

Bondeson et al. (23) have shown that access to two complete glands and the use of fat stains allow for the highly reproducible and reliable distinction of adenoma and hyperplasia. Equivocal findings were seen in only 8 percent of cases. As with other special procedures, fat stains should not be used alone for the evaluation of parathyroid hyperplasia. The combined use of fat stains, careful morphologic assessment, and knowledge of the intraoperative PTH levels provides an optimal approach to the analysis of parathyroid disease (see chapter 30).

Treatment and Prognosis. The treatment of choice for patients with primary chief cell hyperplasia is subtotal parathyroidectomy (24,25). Generally, three entire glands and a portion of a fourth gland are removed, leaving a well-vascularized remnant of 50 to 80 mg. Each thymic tongue is also removed in order to ensure that all parathyroid tissue has been excised. Alternatively, some surgeons advocate total parathyroidectomy with autotransplantation of approximately 50 mg of parathyroid tissue into the forearm.

In patients treated by subtotal parathyroidectomy, recurrent hypercalcemia occurred in 16 percent at 1 to 16 years after surgery (26). Many of these patients were subsequently cured at reoperation by the removal of glands that had been left behind during the first procedure. A rare cause of recurrent hypercalcemia in patients treated surgically for chief cell hyperplasia is implantation of parathyroid tissue throughout the soft tissue of the neck and mediastinum, resulting in parathyromatosis (27,28) (see chapter 29).

CLEAR CELL HYPERPLASIA

Definition. *Clear cell hyperplasia* is characterized by an absolute increase in parathyroid parenchymal mass resulting from the proliferation of vacuolated water-clear (Wasserhelle) cells in multiple parathyroid glands in the absence of a known stimulus for PTH hypersecretion.

General Features. Clear cell hyperplasia is a rare disorder: only 19 patients were seen at the Massachusetts General Hospital between 1930 and 1975 (2,29). Since that time, few additional cases have been documented (30,31). Similar to primary hyperparathyroidism diagnosed prior to 1975, most patients with clear cell hyperplasia have evidence of renal calculi or bone disease. There are no apparent familial associations (32).

Clinical Features. The clinical presentation is similar to that of other primary hyperparathyroidism diseases.

Gross Findings. All parathyroid glands are enlarged in most patients with primary clear cell hyperplasia, but on occasion, only three glands are involved. There may be considerable variation in glandular size in individual cases, but the upper glands are usually larger than the lower (fig. 27-8). In the series from the Massachusetts General Hospital, almost half of the cases had total gland weights ranging from 10 to 60 g (2,29); the remaining cases had total glandular weights of less than 10 g.

The shape of the glands is irregular, with pseudopodal extensions into the surrounding adipose tissue of the neck. The glands vary in color from red-brown to brown, and more severe cases may have foci of cystic change, fibrosis, and hemosiderin deposition.

Microscopic Findings. The cells most often grow in a diffuse pattern, but follicular arrangements may be evident. The individual cells are generally polyhedral, with sharply defined plasma membranes (figs. 27-9, 27-10) (2). They have an average diameter of 15 to 20 µm, but range up to 40 µm in size. The nuclei have an average diameter of 8 µm, are frequently multiple, and tend to be round to slightly ovoid and moderately hyperchromatic, with an eccentrically placed nucleolus. The nuclei are aligned toward the vascular pole of the cells, which results in a characteristic "bunch of berries" appearance (2,29). Occasional nuclei are markedly enlarged and hyperchromatic. The cytoplasm has a strikingly clear appearance due to the presence of multiple small vacuoles measuring up to 0.8 µm in diameter. The cells

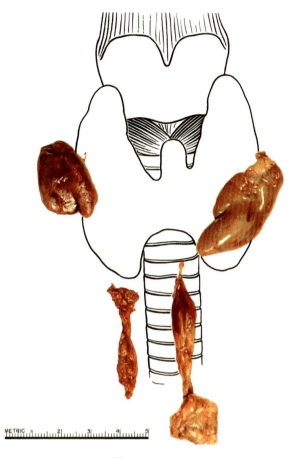

Figure 27-8

PRIMARY CLEAR CELL HYPERPLASIA

The upper glands are considerably larger than the lower glands.

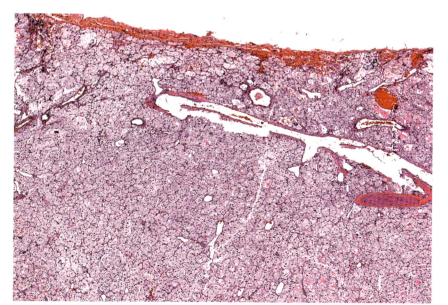

Figure 27-9

PRIMARY CLEAR CELL HYPERPLASIA

The clear cells have a diffuse pattern of growth.

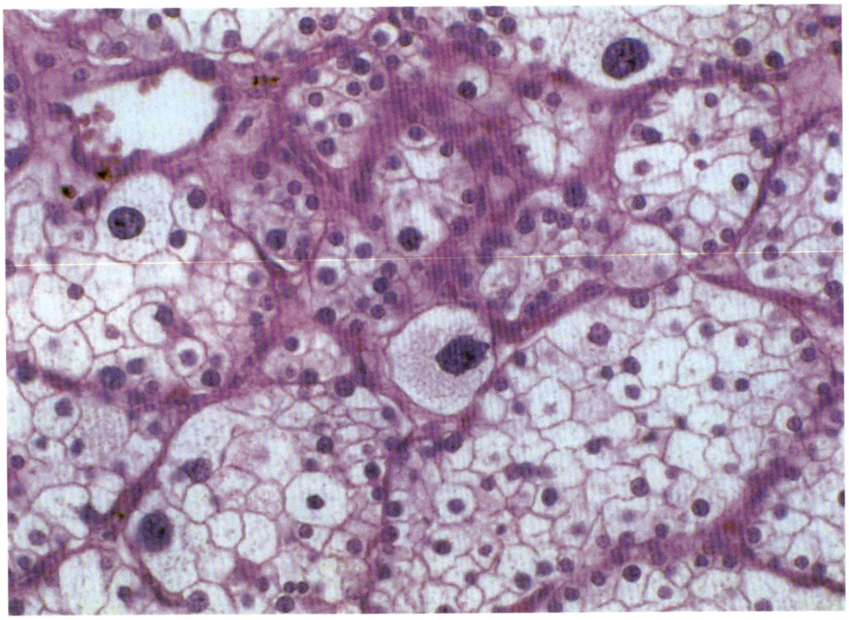

Figure 27-10

PRIMARY CLEAR CELL HYPERPLASIA

Scattered cells have enlarged and hyperchromatic nuclei.

contain moderate amounts of glycogen but are typically negative for neutral lipids.

Ultrastructurally, the cells contain multiple vacuoles which appear to arise from the Golgi vesicles (fig. 27-11) (33). Some of the vacuoles contain dense secretory material which most likely represents stored PTH. The lesional cells contain scant endoplasmic reticulum and there are few secretory and presecretory granules. Dawkins et al. (34) have demonstrated that the concentration of PTH is approximately 1,000 times lower than in normal glands or chief cell adenomas.

Foci of cystic change may occur, with individual cysts lined by a layer of clear cells. The cyst lumen often contains eosinophilic proteinaceous material.

Treatment. The treatment is similar to that of primary chief cell hyperplasia.

HERITABLE HYPERPARATHYROIDISM SYNDROMES

Although occasional kindreds with dominantly inherited parathyroid adenomas and carcinomas have been reported, most patients with *familial hyperparathyroidism* have chief cell hyperplasia associated with MEN 1 or MEN 2 (Table 27-1) (5,35,36). Less common causes of familial hyperparathyroidism include cystic parathyroid adenomatosis with fibro-osseous jaw tumors (hyperparathyroidism-jaw tumor [HPT-JT] syndrome) or apparently isolated parathyroid hyperplasia, adenoma, or carcinoma. Familial benign hypocalciuric hypercalcemia is a syndrome characterized by glands that appear histologically normal although some degree of glandular enlargement may occur.

The possibility of a familial hyperparathyroidism syndrome should be considered in patients presenting with hypercalcemia at less than 30 years of age. A family history of hypercalcemia, with or without neuroendocrine tumors, should suggest a heritable hyperparathyroidism syndrome. The presence of MEN 1-associated skin lesions, including facial angiofibromas, collagenomas, lipomas, and mucosal neuromas, should lead to calcium screening studies of first-degree relatives (5).

Multiple Endocrine Neoplasia Type 1

Multiple endocrine neoplasia type 1 is a complex endocrinopathy. Most cases are familial, with an autosomal dominant pattern of inheritance, while a subset is apparently sporadic (37,38). Most of the clinical manifestation of MEN 1 result from hypersecretion of PTH, gastrin, and prolactin.

By far, hyperparathyroidism is the most common manifestation of MEN 1, with prevalence rates ranging from 80 to 100 percent (36–38). Hyperparathyroidism may occur as early as 5 to 8 years of age; the penetrance increases to 50 percent between the ages of 20 and 30 and 95 percent between the ages of 40 and 50. In contrast

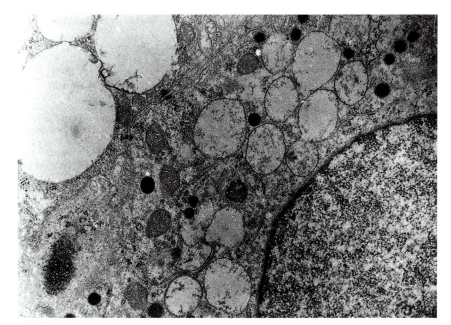

Figure 27-11

**PRIMARY CLEAR
CELL HYPERPLASIA**

In this electron micrograph, the cells contain membrane limited vacuoles and scattered secretory granules.

Table 27-1

FAMILIAL HYPERPARATHYROIDISM SYNDROMES

Syndrome	OMIM No.[a]	Inheritance[b]	Gene	Chromosomal location	Parathyroid Pathology
Multiple endocrine neoplasia, type 1 (MEN 1)	131100	AD	*MEN1*	11q13 (CDK1 gene family [p27, p18, p21])[d]	Hyperplasia[c]
Multiple endocrine neoplasia, type 2A (MEN 2A)	171400	AD	*RET*	10q21	Hyperplasia
Multiple endocrine neoplasia, type 4 (MEN 4)	610755	AD	*CDKN1*	12p13.1	Hyperplasia; adenoma
Hyperparathyroidism-jaw tumor syndrome (HPT-JT)	145001	AD	*HRPT2/ CDC73*	1q24-32	Adenomas with cystic changes; carcinoma; hyperplasia
Familial isolated hyperparathyroidism (FIHP)	145000	AD	?[e] *MEN1* *HRPT2/CDC73* *CaSR*	11q13 19p13.3 1q24-32	Hyperplasia; adenoma; carcinoma
Familial hypocalciuric hypercalcemia (FHH)	145980	AD	*CaSR*	3q21-24[f] 19p13.3 19q13	Normocellular to mildly hypercellular glands
Neonatal severe primary hyperparathyroidism (NSHPT)	239200	AR	*CaSR*	3q21-24	Severe hyperplasia

[a]OMIM = Online mendelian inheritance in man.
[b]AD = autosomal dominant; AR = autosomal recessive.
[c]Although the parathyroid lesions in MEN 1 are classified traditionally as hyperplasia, molecular studies indicate that they are clonal proliferations.
[d]A small proportion of patients lacking *MEN 1* gene mutations have *CDK1* mutations, and some of these patients are classified as having MEN 4. The designation MEN 4 was chosen to describe the latter syndrome, since the term MEN 3 has been used by some investigators to describe patients with MEN 2B.
[e]After causes for a weakly expressed syndrome (MEN 1, FHH, HPT-JT) have been eliminated, approximately 70% of kindreds with FIH do not have an identifiable mutation in a major hyperparathyroid syndromal gene (35).
[f]Most cases of FHH map to the *CaSR* gene (calcium sensing receptor) on 3q21-24, but a few show linkage to 19p13.3 or 19q13.

to patients with sporadic hyperparathyroidism who have an average onset of disease at 55 years of age, the average age at onset in patients with MEN 1 is 25 years. The female:male ratio of hyperparathyroidism in patients with sporadic disease is 3:1 while the ratio is 1:1 in those with MEN 1. While most patients with sporadic primary hyperparathyroidism have uniglandular parathyroid disease, the disease in patients with MEN 1 is typically multiglandular (37).

Gastrin-producing enteropancreatic tumors occur in approximately 40 percent of MEN 1 patients, and they are typically multicentric (37). The clinical features of the associated Zollinger-Ellison syndrome include multiple peptic ulcers with abdominal pain, reflux symptoms, and diarrhea. Most gastrinomas are less than 1 cm in diameter and occur primarily within the duodenum. In some patients, evidence of gastrinoma may precede the hyperparathyroidism. Insulinomas occur in 10 to 30 percent of patients while nonfunctional tumors synthesizing pancreatic polypeptide (PPomas) occur in up to 20 percent. Other products produced by enteropancreatic tumors include glucagon, vasoactive intestinal peptide (VIP), somatostatin, growth hormone-releasing hormone, and adrenocorticotropic hormone (ACTH).

Symptoms of hyperpituitarism occur in 10 to 30 percent of MEN 1 patients and most secrete prolactin. Nonfunctional tumors synthesizing subunits of glycoprotein hormones are also common, while tumors producing prolactin and growth hormone, growth hormone alone, ACTH, or thyroid-stimulating hormone (TSH) are rare.

Gastrointestinal neuroendocrine (carcinoid) tumors in MEN 1 patients are primarily of foregut origin, developing in the thymus, bronchus, stomach, duodenum, and pancreas. The thymic tumors occur predominately in males while bronchial carcinoids predominate in females. Other endocrine tumors occurring in patients with MEN 1 include adrenal cortical adenomas and thyroid follicular adenomas. Nonendocrine tumors include multiple lipomas, facial angiofibromas, and collagenomas.

The inherited mutation of the *MEN 1* gene is unmasked by inactivation (deletion) of the second allele (39–43). More than 1,000 mutations spread over the entire coding region have been detected without apparent hotspots, and there

is no apparent correlation between the genotype and the *MEN 1* phenotype (44). Presymptomatic testing can identify the carrier status up to 20 years before clinical symptomatology is evident. However, the use of genetic screening in individuals at risk for the development of MEN 1 is controversial, since prophylactic surgery is not indicated for any of the components of this disorder.

Approximately 30 percent of patients with MEN 1 have no evidence of a mutation of the *MEN 1* gene (35). Possible causes for unidentified mutations include a mutation outside the zone amplified by the polymerase chain reaction (PCR) and the presence of a large heterozygous deletion of more than a complex copy of the syndromal gene (35). One group of candidate genes that may harbor a mutation is the cyclin-dependent kinase inhibitor (*CDKI*) gene family (45,46). Mutations of *CDKIB/p27(KIP1)* have been demonstrated in a small subset of MEN 1 patients that were negative for *MEN 1* mutations (44). Other *CDKI* genes that have been found in *MEN 1* mutation-negative patients include p15, p18, and p21 (47,48). Because of the rarity of *CDKI* mutations, it is likely that other genes will be implicated in MEN 1 mutation-negative individuals.

Multiple Endocrine Neoplasia Type 2

Multiple endocrine neoplasia type 2A is an autosomal dominant disorder characterized by medullary thyroid carcinoma, pheochromocytoma, and parathyroid abnormalities (see chapter 12) (49). The hyperparathyroidism associated with MEN 2A is generally mild, with 15 to 20 percent of affected individuals developing clinical signs and symptoms of their disease (44). The median age at diagnosis of the hyperparathyroidism is 38 years. Patients with a codon 634 mutation are likely to have hyperparathyroidism and should be monitored annually with measurements of serum calcium and PTH. In most patients, evidence of hyperparathyroidism develops 10 to 12 years following the diagnosis of medullary thyroid carcinoma; however, the hyperparathyroidism precedes the development of the thyroid tumors in a few patients.

Patients with multiple endocrine neoplasia type 2B (MEN 2B) rarely develop hyperparathyroidism. Studies reported by Carney et al. (50) demonstrated that the microscopic appearance of the glands is normal in MEN 2B patients less than 17 years of age. With increasing age, the glands show mildly increased cellularity unassociated with clinical or laboratory evidence of hyperparathyroidism. By definition, hyperparathyroidism does not occur in patients with familial medullary thyroid carcinoma (FMTC).

Multiple Endocrine Neoplasia Type 4

A syndrome combining features of MEN 1 and MEN 2 was discovered in a colony of Sprague-Dawley rats in 2006 (45). Affected animals developed multiple endocrine tumors involving the pituitary gland, adrenal medulla, C-cells, parathyroid glands, and pancreatic islets (45), and this association was referred to as MEN X. The gene responsible for the syndrome in the rat was identified as *Cdkn1b*. Mutations in the human homolog of the gene, *CDKN1B*, were subsequently identified as a subset of MEN 1-like cases without mutations in the *MEN1* gene (38,45,47,48). Affected patients had evidence of parathyroid hyperplasia or adenoma, pituitary adenomas, and occasional other endocrine and nonendocrine tumors, including renal angiomyolipomas. The designation MEN 4 was chosen for the latter syndrome since the term MEN 3 has been used by some to describe patients with MEN 2B (38,47). In contrast to the autosomal recessive pattern of inheritance of MEN X in the rat, MEN 4 appears to be an autosomal dominant trait in humans.

Hyperparathyroidism-Jaw Tumor Syndrome

Hyperparathyroidism-jaw tumor (HPT-JT) *syndrome* is a complex autosomal dominant disorder characterized by the presence of multiple cystic parathyroid tumors and fibro-osseous tumors of the maxilla or mandible (51,52). Additional features include the presence of renal cysts, hamartomas, and Wilms tumor. Pancreatic adenocarcinoma, renal cell carcinoma, testicular germ cell tumors, uterine tumors, and Hürthle cell thyroid adenomas have also been reported (52).

Most patients present with a single (cystic) parathyroid adenoma, but multiple adenomas may occur synchronously or metachronously (52). Parathyroid carcinomas have been found in approximately 15 percent of patients and some examples of parathyroid hyperplasia have also been reported.

The HPT-JT syndrome develops as a result of mutations of the *HRPT2/CDC73* gene on chromosome 1q34-32. The parathyroid tumors show loss of the wild-type allele, consistent with the concept that *HRPT2/CDC73* is a tumor suppressor gene (53,54). The product of the gene is parafibromin, and parathyroid lesions in this syndrome are negative for parafibromin (53,54). It has been suggested that genetic testing be performed 5 to 10 years prior to the earliest diagnosis of hyperparathyroidism and possibly at birth in families with a known mutation of the *HRPT2/CDC73* gene (55).

Familial Hypocalciuric Hypercalcemia and Neonatal Severe Primary Hyperparathyroidism

Familial hypocalciuric hypercalcemia (FHH), also termed *benign familial hypercalcemia*, is an autosomal dominant disorder that is distinct from other syndromes associated with hyperparathyroid states (56,57). The prevalence of FHH has been reported to be as high as 1 in 16,000 (56).

Most affected patients are asymptomatic. FHH is characterized by lifelong and generally mild hypercalcemia with inappropriately normal or mildly elevated PTH levels. In addition to the hypercalcemia, affected individuals typically manifest normal or low urinary calcium levels. Parathyroidectomy has no effect on the hypercalcemia. Genetic testing for FHH-associated mutations (*CaSR* gene) can help to prevent unnecessary and inappropriate parathyroidectomy, although approximately 40 percent of FHH patients do not have *CaSR* mutations (58).

This disorder is caused by heterozygous loss of function germline mutations of the calcium sensing receptor (*CaSR*) gene, resulting in insensitivity of the parathyroid glands and other target sites (e.g., kidney) to inhibition by serum calcium (57). As a result, higher than normal levels of calcium are required to suppress the biosynthesis and secretion of PTH. In the kidney, abnormal function of the receptor leads to increased calcium reabsorption. The responsible gene was first mapped to chromosome 3q21-24 and was ultimately identified as the *CaSR* gene (59). A few cases have shown linkage to 19p or 19q (35). Most mutations associated with the syndrome are present within the first 300 amino acids of the extracellular domain of the protein. Less commonly, mutations occur proximal to the first transmembrane segment or within the transmembrane segments and intracellular or extracellular loops.

In most patients with FHH, the parathyroid glands are histologically normal or slightly enlarged. In a study of 18 patients from eight kindreds, the average parathyroid parenchymal area was increased as compared to normal controls, but less than that seen in patients with primary parathyroid hyperplasia (60). Rarely, examples of parathyroid hyperplasia or adenoma are reported in association with this syndrome. In a report by Carling et al. (61) of a kindred with a novel mutation in the cytoplasmic tail of the *CaSR* gene, the clinical and laboratory features of FHH and primary hyperparathyroidism overlapped. Seven of nine patients had chief cell hyperplasia, one had an adenoma, and one had equivocal findings on examination of the parathyroid glands.

Neonatal severe primary hyperparathyroidism (NSHPT) is due to the homozygous loss of function of *CaSR* mutations and is usually diagnosed within a week of birth (35,36). Typically, serum PTH levels are markedly elevated. The clinical features include anorexia, constipation, failure to thrive, myotonia, and respiratory distress. Skeletal X rays show severe bone demineralization, widening of metaphyses, fractures, and osteitis fibrosa cystica. Hypercalcemia is usually severe and relative hypocalciuria may be present. Additional phenotypic features include dysmorphic facies and anorectal or anovaginal fistulas, the latter findings suggesting that the *CaSR* gene may have a role in morphogenesis.

Resected parathyroid glands of patients with NSHPT typically demonstrate chief cell hyperplasia, although examples of water clear cell hyperplasia have also been reported. Patients are typically treated on an emergent basis by total parathyroidectomy with implantation of a small amount of parathyroid tissue (62).

Familial Isolated Hyperparathyroidism

Familial isolated hyperparathyroidism (FIHPT) is a rare autosomal dominant disorder characterized by hyperparathyroidism without evidence of other endocrinopathies. A variety of mutations have been reported in patients with FIHPT, including those affecting *MEN 1* (0 to 23 percent), *CaSR* (14 percent), and *HRPT2* (rare) (63,64). Up to 70 percent of patients have no identifiable mutations in these genes. Cases with known mutations are probably best reclassified as weakly expressed MEN 1, HPT-JT, or FHH (35).

In most cases, the resected parathyroid glands show evidence of single or multiple parathyroid adenomas or chief cell hyperplasia. The increased incidence of parathyroid carcinoma in some kindreds with FIHPT most likely reflects the inclusion of those patients with *HRPT2/CDC73* mutations.

REFERENCES

1. Cope O, Keynes WM, Roth SI, Castleman B. Primary chief-cell hyperplasia of the parathyroid glands: a new entity in the surgery of hyperparathyroidism. Ann Surg 1958;148:375-88.
2. Castleman B, Roth SI. Tumors of the parathyroid glands. Atlas of Tumor Pathology, 2nd Series. Fascicle 14. Washington, DC: Armed Forces Institute of Pathology; 1978:1-94.
3. Akerström G, Rudberg C, Grimelius L, et al. Histological parathyroid abnormalities in an autopsy series. Hum Pathol 1986;17:520-27.
4. Bringhurst FR, Demay MD, Kronenberg HM. Hormones and disorders of mineral metabolism. In: Melmed S, Polonsky KS, Larsen PR, Kronenberg HM, eds. Williams textbook of endocrinology, 12th ed. Philadelphia: Elsevier/Saunders; 2011:1237-304.
5. Marcocci C, Cetani F. Clinical practice. Primary hyperparathyroidism. N Engl J Med 2011;365:2389-97.
6. Brandi ML. Multiple endocrine neoplasia type I: general features and new insights into etiology. J Endocrinol Invest 1991;14:61-72.
7. Black WC, Haff RC. The surgical pathology of parathyroid chief cell hyperplasia. Am J Clin Pathol 1970;53:565-79.
8. Akerström G, Bergström R, Grimelius L, et al. Relation between changes in clinical and histopathological features of primary hyperparathyroidism. World J Surg 1986;10:696-702.

9. Clark OH. Hyperparathyroidism due to primary cystic parathyroid hyperplasia. Arch Surg 1978;113:748-50.

10. Straus FH 2nd, Kaplan EL, Nishiyama RH, Bigos ST. Five cases of parathyroid lipohyperplasia. Surgery 1983;94:901-5.

11. Reddick RL, Costa JC, Marx SJ. Parathyroid hyperplasia and parathyromatosis. Lancet 1977;1:549.

12. San Juan J, Monteagudo C, Fraker D, Norton J, Merino M. Significance of mitotic activity and other morphologic parameters in clinical behavior [Abstract]. Am J Clin Pathol 1989;92:523.

13. Snover DC, Foucar K. Mitotic activity in benign parathyroid disease. Am J Clin Pathol 1981;75:345-7.

14. Bondeson AG, Bondeson L, Ljungberg O. Chronic parathyroiditis associated with parathyroid hyperplasia and hyperparathyroidism. Am J Surg Pathol 1984;8:211-5.

15. Boyce BF, Doherty VR, Mortimer G. Hyperplastic parathyroiditis—a new autoimmune disease? J Clin Pathol 1982;35:812-4.

16. Atwal OS, Samagh BS, Bhatnagar MK. A possible autoimmune parathyroiditis following ozone inhalation. II. A histopathologic, ultrastructural, and immunofluorescent study. Am J Pathol 1975;80:53-68.

17. Mallette LE, Malini S, Rappaport MP, Kirkland JL. Familial cystic parathyroid adenomatosis. Ann Intern Med 1987;107:54-60.

18. Alternähr E, Arps H, Montz R, Dorn G. Quantitative ultrastructural and radioimmunologic assessment of parathyroid gland activity in primary hyperparathyroidism. Lab Invest 1979;41:303-12.

19. Cinti S, Colussi G, Minola E, Dickersin GR. Parathyroid glands in primary hyperparathyroidism: an ultrastructural study of 50 cases. Hum Pathol 1986;17:1036-46.

20. Nilsson O. Studies on the ultrastructure of the human parathyroid glands in various pathological conditions. Acta Pathol Microbiol Immunol Scand Suppl 1977;263:1-88.

21. Roth SI, Munger BL. The cytology of adenomatous, atrophic and hyperplastic parathyroid glands of man. A light and electron-microscopic study. Virchows Arch Pathol Anat Physiol Klin Med 1962;335:389-410.

22. Weber KJ, Misra S, Lee JK, Wilhelm SW, DeCresce R, Prinz RA. Intraoperative monitoring in parathyroid hyperplasia requires stricter criteria for success. Surgery 2004;134:1154-9.

23. Bondeson AG, Bondeson L, Ljungberg O, Tibblin S. Fat staining in parathyroid disease—diagnostic value and impact on surgical strategy: clinicopathological analysis of 191 cases. Hum Pathol 1985;16:1255-63.

24. Malmaeus J, Benson L, Johansson H, et al. Parathyroid surgery in the multiple endocrine neoplasia type 1 syndrome: choice of surgical procedure. World J Surg 1986;10:668-72.

25. Palmer JA, Brown WA, Kerr WH, Rosen IB, Watters NA. The surgical aspects of hyperparathyroidism. Arch Surg 1975;110:1004-7.

26. Rudberg C, Akerström G, Palmér M, et al. Late results of operation for primary hyperparathyroidism in 441 patients. Surgery 1986;99:643-51.

27. Rattner DW, Marrone GC, Kadson E, Silen W. Recurrent hyperparathyroidism due to implantation of parathyroid tissue. Am J Surg 1985;149:745-8.

28. Fitko R, Roth SI, Hines JR, Roxe DM, Cahill E. Parathyromatosis in hyperparathyroidism. Hum Pathol 1990;21:234-7.

29. Albright F, Bloomberg E, Castleman B, Churchill ED. Hyperparathyroidism due to diffuse hyperplasia of all parathyroid glands rather than adenoma of one. Clinical studies on three such cases. Arch Intern Med 1934;54:315-29.

30. Dorado AE, Hensley G, Castleman B. Water clear cell hyperplasia of parathyroid: autopsy report of a case with supernumerary glands. Cancer 1976;38:1676-83.

31. Ezzat T, Maclean GM, Parameswaran R, et al. Primary hyperparathyroidism with water clear cell content: the impact of histological diagnosis on clinical management and outcome. Ann R Coll Surg Engl 2013;95:e60-2.

32. Tisell LE, Hedman I, Hansson G. Clinical characteristics and surgical results in hyperparathyroidism caused by water-clear cell hyperplasia. World J Surg 1981;5:565-71.

33. Roth SI. The ultrastructure of primary water-clear cell hyperplasia of the parathyroid glands. Am J Pathol 1970;61:233-40.

34. Dawkins RL, Tashjian AH Jr, Castleman B, Moore EW. Hyperparathyroidism due to clear cell hyperplasia. Serial determinations of serum ionized calcium, parathyroid hormone and calcitonin. Am J Med 1973;54:119-26.

35. Marx SJ. Hyperparathyroidism genes: sequences reveal answers and questions. Endocr Pract 2011;17(Suppl 3):18-27.

36. Marx SJ, Simonds WF, Agarwal SK, et al. Hyperparathyroidism in hereditary syndromes: special expressions and special managements. J Bone Miner Res 2002;17(Suppl 2):N37-43.

37. Calender A, Morrison CD, Kommioth P, Scoazec JY, Sweet KM, Teh BR. Multiple endocrine neoplasia type1. In: DeLellis R, Lloyd RV, Heitz PU, Eng C, eds. Pathology and genetics of tumours of endocrine organs. WHO Classification of Endocrine Tumours. Lyon: IARC Press; 2004:218-27.

38. Thakker RV. Multiple endocrine neoplasia type 1 (MEN1) and type 4 (MEN4). Mol Cell Endocrinol 2014;386:2-15.

39. Agarwal SK, Guru SC, Heppner C, et al. Menin interacts with the AP1 transcription factor JunD and represses JunD activated transcription. Cell 1999;96:143-52.

40. Agarwal SK, Lee Burns A, Sukhodolets KE, et al. Molecular pathology of the MEN1 gene. Ann N Y Acad Sci 2004;1014:189-98.

41. Chandrasekharappa SC, Guru SC, Manickam P, et al. Postional cloning of the gene for multiple endocrine neoplasia-type 1. Science 1997;276:3404-7.

42. Larsson C, Skogseid, B, Oberg K, Nakamura Y, Nordenskjold M. Multiple endocrine neoplasia type 1 gene maps to chromosome 11 and is lost in insulinoma. Nature 1988;332:85-7.

43. Lemmens I, Van de Ven WJ, Kas K, et al. Identification of the multiple endocrine neoplasia type1 (MEN1) gene. The European Consortium on MEN1. Hum Mol Genet 1997;6:1177-83.

44. Cetani F, Pardi E, Borsari S, Marcocci C. Molecular pathogenesis of primary hyperparathyroidism. J Endocrinol Invest 2011;34(Suppl 7):35-9.

45. Pellegata NS, Quintanilla-Martinez L, Siggelkow H, et al. Germ-line mutations in p27 Kip1 cause a multiple endocrine neoplasia syndrome in rats and humans. Proc Nat Acad Sci 2006;103:15558-63.

46. Agarwal SK, Mateo CM, Marx SJ. Rare germline mutations in cyclin dependent kinase inhibitor genes in multiple endocrine neoplasia type 1 and related states. J Clin Endocrinal Metab 2009;94:1826-34.

47. Georgitsi M. MEN-4 and other multiple endocrine neoplasias due to cyclin-dependent kinase inhibitors (p27(Kip1) and p18(INK4C)) mutations. Best Pract Res Clin Endocrinol Metab 2010;24:425-37.

48. Costa-Guda J, Arnold A. Genetic and epigenetic changes in sporadic endocrine tumors: Parathyroid tumors. Mol Cell Endocrinol 2014;386:46-54.

49. Gimm O, Morrison CD, Suster S, et al. Multiple endocrine neoplasia type2. In: DeLellis RA, Lloyd RV, Heitz PU, Eng C. MEN2 Pathology of genetics of tumours of endocrine organs. WHO Classification of Endocrine Tumours. Lyon: IARC Press; 2004;211-7.

50. Carney JA, Roth SI, Heath H 3rd, Sizemore GW, Hayles AB. The parathyroid glands in multiple endocrine neoplasia type 2b. Am J Pathol 1980;99:387-98.

51. Chen JD, Morrison C, Zhang C, Kahnoski K, Carpten JD, Teh BT. Hyperparathyroidism-jaw tumor syndrome. J Int Med 2003;253:634-42.

52. Teh BT, Sweet KM, Morrison CD. Hyperparathyroidism-jaw tumour syndrome. In: DeLellis RA, Lloyd RV, Heitz PU, Eng C, eds. Pathology of genetics of tumours of endocrine organs. WHO Classification of Endocrine Tumours. Lyon: IARC Press; 2004:228-9.

53. Newey PJ, Bowl MR, Thakker RV. Parafibromin-functional insights. J Int Med 2009;266:84-98.

54. Carpten JD, Robbins CM, Villablanca A, et al. HRPT2 encoding parafibromin is mutated in hyperparathyroidism-jaw tumor syndrome. Nat Genet 2002;32:676-80.

55. Pichardo-Lowden AR, Manni A, Saunders BD, Baker MJ. Familial hyperparathyroidism due to a germline mutation of the CDC73 gene: Implications for management and age appropriate testing of relatives at risk. Endocr Pract 2011;17:602-9.

56. Gunn IR, Gaffney D. Clinical and laboratory features of calcium sensing receptor disorders: a systematic review. Ann Clin Biochem 2004;41:441-58.

57. Thakker RV. Diseases associated with the extra-cellular calcium-sensing receptor. Cell Calcium 2004;35:275-82.

58. Mizusawa N, Uchino S, Tsuyuguchi M, et al. Genetic analyses in patients with familial isolated hyperparathyroidism and hyperparathyroidism-jaw tumor syndrome. Clin Endocrinol 2006;65:9-16.

59. Chou YH, Pollak MR, Brandi ML, et al. Mutations in the human Ca(2+)-sensing-receptor gene that cause familial hypocalciuric hypercalcemia. Am J Hum Genet 1995;56:1075-9.

60. Thorgeirsson U, Costa J, Marx SF. The parathyroid glands in familial hypocalciuric hypercalcemia. Hum Pathol 1981;12:229-37.

61. Carling T, Szabo E, Bai M, et al. Familial hypercalcemia and hypercalciuria caused by a novel mutation in the cytoplasmic tail of the calcium receptor. J Clin Endocrinol Metab 2000;85:2042-7.

62. Al-Shanafey S, Al-Hoisani R, Al-Ashwad A, Al-Rebeeah A. Surgical management of severe neonatal hyperparathyroidism: one center's experience. J Pediatr Surg 2010;45:714-7.

63. Simonds WF, James-Newton O, Agarwal SK, et al. Familial isolated hyperparathyroidism: clinical and genetic characterizations of 36 kindreds. Medicine (Baltimore) 2002;81:1-26.

64. Warner J, Epstein M, Sweet A, et al. Genetic testing in familial isolated hyperparathyroidism: unexpected results and their implications. J Med Genet 2004;41:155-60.

28 SECONDARY AND TERTIARY HYPERPARATHYROIDISM, AND PARATHYROID GRAFTS

SECONDARY HYPERPARATHYROIDISM

Definition. *Secondary hyperparathyroidism* is an adaptive increase in parathyroid parenchymal mass resulting from a proliferation of chief cells, oncocytic cells, and transitional oncocytic cells in multiple parathyroid glands in the presence of a known stimulus for parathyroid hormone (PTH) hypersecretion.

General Features. The relationship between chronic renal failure and enlargement of multiple parathyroid glands has been known for many years (1,2). Papenheimer and Wilens in 1935 (3) reported that parathyroid glands from patients with chronic renal disease were 50 to 100 percent larger than glands from normal individuals. Overproduction of PTH and parathyroid proliferation in this setting result from hyperphosphatemia, low levels of ionized calcium in the blood, and impaired 1,25-dihydroxy-vitamin D synthesis by the diseased kidneys. When plasma levels of calcium decrease, the calcium sensing receptor (CaSR) responds by increasing the secretion of PTH, resulting in a compensatory mechanism to restore normal function (4).

Secondary hyperparathyroidism also occurs in patients with deficiency of vitamin D, abnormal vitamin D metabolism, malabsorptive states, resistance of peripheral tissues to the effects of PTH (pseudohypoparathyroidism), or following the administration of certain drugs. Once the process of parathyroid hyperplasia begins, the set point for the control of PTH secretion by ionized calcium rises and this leads to further hyperplasia of the glands and hypersecretion of PTH (5,6).

Clinical Features. The clinical features of secondary hyperparathyroidism are dominated by skeletal pain and deformities resulting from the increased secretion of PTH and the decreased synthesis of 1, 25-dihydroxy-vitamin D (6). In patients with chronic renal failure, extensive visceral, soft tissue, and periarticular calcifications also occur (6).

Gross Findings. The appearance of the parathyroid glands in patients with secondary hyperparathyroidism is generally similar to that seen in patients with primary chief cell hyperplasia (7–9). The size of the glands, however, tends to be more uniform early in the course of secondary hyperplasia (fig. 28-1). The extent of the hyperplasia generally parallels the severity of the underlying condition that predisposes the patient to secondary hyperparathyroidism. In advanced secondary hyperplasia, variations in gland size may be considerable (fig. 28-2), and the glands may exhibit considerable fibrosis, cyst formation, and calcification.

Microscopic Findings. The earliest change in the parathyroid glands is a decrease in the number of stromal fat cells and their partial replacement by widened cords and nests of chief cells (9). Typically, the proliferating chief cells are present in diffuse sheets, but some areas have cord-like, acinar, or trabecular growth patterns. Advanced stages of secondary hyperplasia are characterized by nodular proliferations of chief cells and oncocytes (figs. 28-3–28-6). The nodules in these areas may be surrounded by fibrosis and some are entirely encapsulated. Irregular areas of fibrosis, hemorrhage, and cyst formation may also be evident. In some cases, the presence of fibrous bands may suggest atypical adenoma or parathyroid carcinoma; however, there is no evidence of invasion in most cases of secondary hyperplasia.

The characteristic cell in cases of secondary hyperplasia is the vacuolated chief cell (9). The nucleus is small and dense, and occupies an eccentric position within the cytoplasm (10). Vacuolated chief cells are typically rich in glycogen, with little neutral lipid. In some cases, the chief cells assume a distinctive organoid or adenomatoid growth pattern (9). In addition to

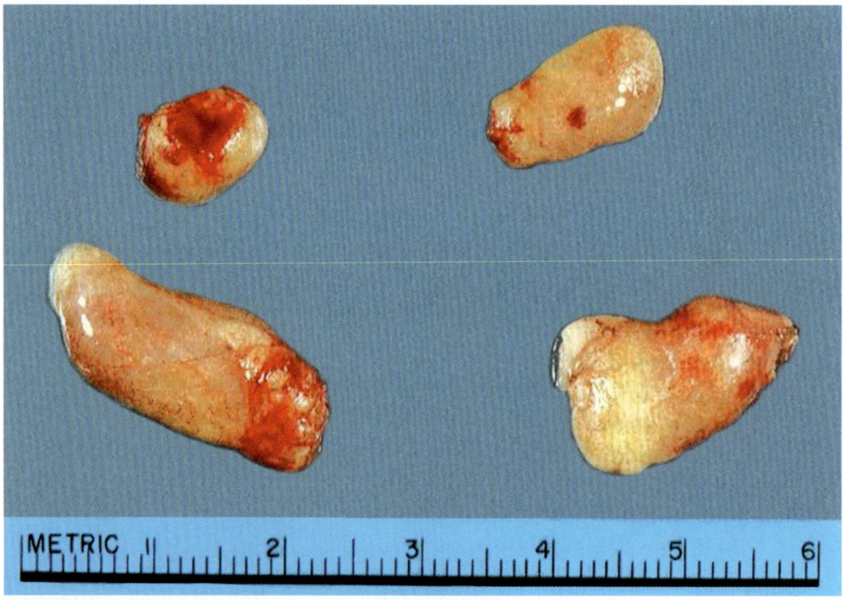

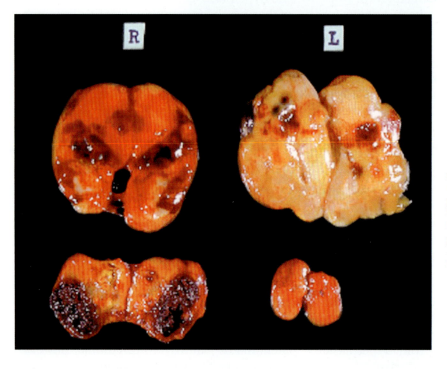

Figure 28-1

SECONDARY HYPERPARATHYROIDISM: CHRONIC RENAL FAILURE

All four glands are enlarged with mild variation in size.

Figure 28-2

SECONDARY HYPERPARATHYROIDISM: CHRONIC RENAL FAILURE

Cross sections reveal variations in sizes and color of glands. (Fig. 57-38 from Roth SI. The parathyroid gland. In: Silverberg SA, DeLellis RA, Frable WJ, eds. Principles and practice of surgical pathology and cytopathology, 3rd ed. New York: Churchill Livingstone; 1997:2737.)

chief cells, the glands contain increased numbers of oncocytes and transitional oncocytes.

Immunohistochemical Findings. The immunohistochemical features of secondary hyperplasia are generally similar to those of adenomas and primary hyperplasia.

Ultrastructural Findings. Ultrastructural studies have demonstrated that the chief cells in secondary hyperparathyroidism have fairly straight plasma membranes with few desmosomal attachment sites (11). The cytoplasm is electron transparent and contains occasional cisternae of granular endoplasmic reticulum. Numerous secretory granules may be present, adjacent to Golgi regions or plasma membranes (9). Oncocytes and transitional oncocytes are increased in proportion to the extent of functional renal impairment.

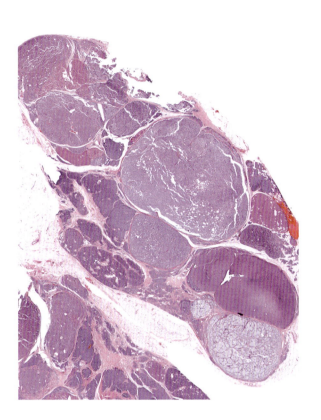 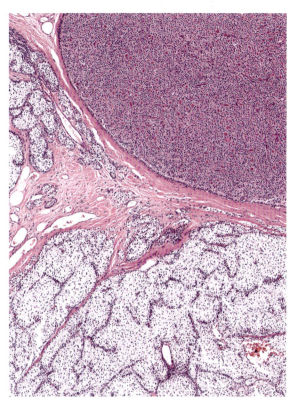

Figure 28-3

SECONDARY HYPERPARATHYROIDISM: CHRONIC RENAL FAILURE

Left: In secondary hyperparathyroidism associated with chronic renal failure, multiple nodules are composed of varying cell types.

Right: The nodule in the lower portion of the image is composed of vacuolated chief cells.

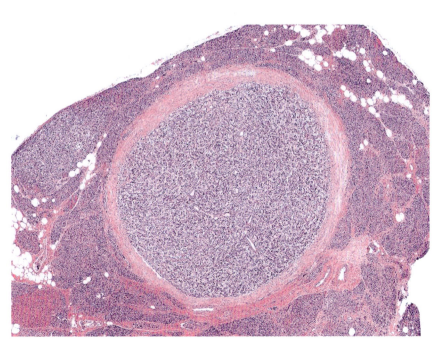

Figure 28-4

SECONDARY HYPERPARATHYROIDISM: CHRONIC RENAL FAILURE

The chief cell nodule in the center is surrounded by a complete fibrous capsule. The adjacent parathyroid tissue is diffusely hyperplastic.

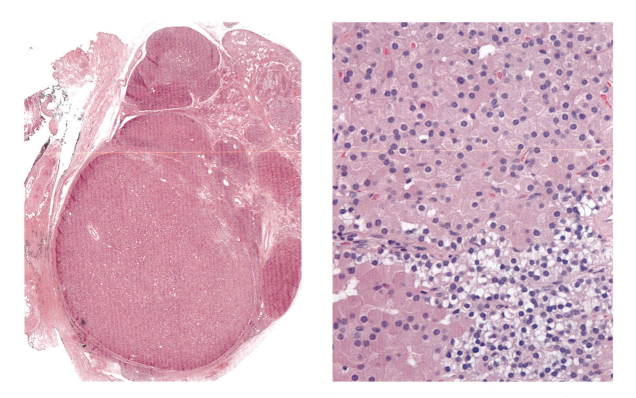

Figure 28-5

SECONDARY HYPERPARATHYROIDISM: CHRONIC RENAL FAILURE

Left: The nodules are composed predominantly of oncocytes.
Right: Oncocytes are admixed with scattered groups of vacuolated chief cells.

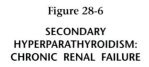

Figure 28-6

SECONDARY HYPERPARATHYROIDISM: CHRONIC RENAL FAILURE

This intrathymic parathyroid gland shows predominant diffuse chief cell hyperplasia with areas of fibrosis at the periphery.

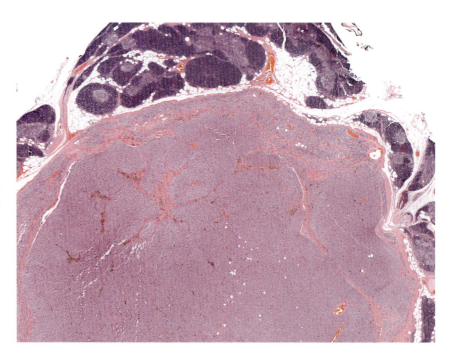

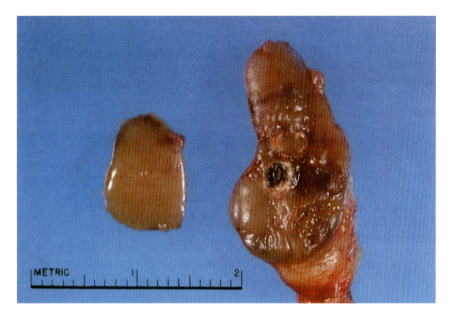

Figure 28-7

TERTIARY HYPERPARATHYROIDISM: CHRONIC RENAL FAILURE

This bisected gland shows nodular hyperplasia with foci of calcification and hemorrhage.

Molecular Genetic Findings. A significant proportion of cases of secondary hyperplasia represents clonal proliferations.

Treatment and Prognosis. Calcimimetics bind to the CaSR and increase its sensitivity to extracellular calcium, with a significant reduction in levels of PTH (4). The rationale for parathyroidectomy in patients with secondary hyperparathyroidism is to halt the often disabling bone disease. Treatment includes subtotal parathyroidectomy with approximately 50 mg of parathyroid tissue left in situ or transplanted to the forearm (5,12–14). Since the stimulus for the parathyroid hyperplasia (most often chronic renal failure) is still present, the residual parathyroid tissue in the neck or forearm may eventually become hyperplastic and the patient may require surgical re-exploration (15).

TERTIARY HYPERPARATHYROIDISM

Definition. *Tertiary hyperparathyroidism (uremic refractory secondary hyperparathyroidism)* refers to the development of autonomous parathyroid hyperfunction in patients with previously documented secondary hyperparathyroidism (16). This disorder occurs in less than 10 percent of patients with secondary hyperparathyroidism following successful renal transplantation and is characterized by significant metabolic complications.

General Features. The mechanisms for the development of tertiary hyperparathyroidism are unknown, although it most likely results from an increased calcium set point and a depletion of vitamin D receptors (4,6). According to this hypothesis, the cellular response function is shifted away from normal toward higher calcium concentrations (6). Parathyroid chief cells, which have higher set points of suppression, increase their biosynthetic and secretory activities and are stimulated to divide even at normal calcium concentrations. This chain of events leads to an increased parenchymal parathyroid mass.

Microscopic Findings. Krause and Hedinger (17) reviewed the pathologic findings in 128 resected parathyroid glands from 41 patients with tertiary hyperparathyroidism. Only 5 percent of the patients had adenomas; the remainder had evidence of hyperplasia. Similar results have been reported by Kebebew et al. (18). The hyperplasia is predominantly diffuse in 40 percent, and nodular in the remainder (figs. 28-7, 28-8). The glandular weight in diffuse hyperplasia is significantly less than that of nodular hyperplasia. Moreover, gland enlargement in diffuse hyperplasia tends to be symmetric, while resected glands with nodular hyperplasia often have an asymmetric appearance.

The predominant cell type in diffuse hyperplasia is the chief cell, although oncocytes and transitional oncocytic cells are also present. In patients with nodular hyperplasia, individual nodules are composed of chief cells, although nodules of oncocytic cells are also present.

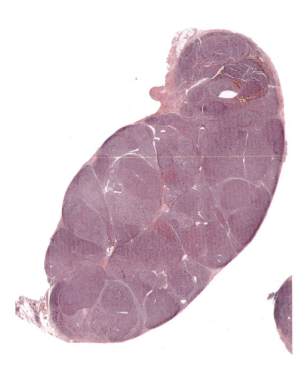

Figure 28-8

TERTIARY HYPERPARATHYROIDISM: CHRONIC RENAL FAILURE

The enlarged gland contains multiple nodules of chief cells and small numbers of oncocytes.

Overall mitotic activity is low and nuclear pleomorphism slight, except in oncocytic areas (19). Foci of fibrosis, cyst formation, iron deposition, and calcification are common The parenchymal cells between the nodules are diffusely hyperplastic. Compression of the internodular areas sometimes results in the appearance of small atrophic cells in a rim of tissue similar to that of patients with adenoma.

Ultrastructural Findings. The ultrastructural features of glands with tertiary hyperparathyroidism have been described in detail (9,20). The chief cell cytoplasm is typically rich in granular endoplasmic reticulum with variable numbers of secretory granules and prominent Golgi regions.

Molecular Genetic Findings. The majority of patients who develop tertiary hyperparathyroidism have clonal parathyroid lesions as documented by X-chromosome inactivation studies (21). Genome wide molecular allelotyping and comparative genomic hybridization studies have identified recurrent clonal DNA abnormalities that suggest the existence and localization of genes that are important in the development of tertiary hyperparathyroidism. These studies also indicate that there are markedly different molecular pathogenetic processes for clonal outgrowth in severe tertiary hyperparathyroidism as compared to common parathyroid adenomas (21)

Treatment and Prognosis. Subtotal or total parathyroidectomy with autotransplantation is recommended for patients with asymptomatic disease with calcium levels in excess of 12.0 mg/dL for more than 1 year, for those with acute hypercalcemia, and for patients with symptomatic hypercalcemia. Kebebew et al. (18) have concluded that localizing studies and intraoperative PTH assays are insufficiently accurate to predict which patients would benefit from a focused neck exploration without the direct examination of other glands.

PARATHYROID GRAFTS

Total parathyroidectomy with autotransplantation of parathyroid tissue into the muscles of the forearm is a useful technique for the treatment of primary and secondary hyperparathyroidism (13,14). However, graft failure or graft hypofunction may occur, resulting in hypoparathyroidism. Occasional patients develop recurrent hyperparathyroidism, with serum PTH concentrations highest in the forearm bearing the graft (figs. 28-9, 28-10).

Klempa et al. (22) noted recurrent hyperparathyroidism in 6 of 42 uremic patients who had forearm autotransplants. Although only 20 to 40 mg of parathyroid tissue had been implanted originally, the removed grafts weighed between 0.9 to 3.1 g. Compared to the originally excised parathyroid tissue, the nuclei of the transplanted cells were often larger and more pleomorphic. In 2 cases, mitotic activity was apparent. A striking finding was the presence of small nests of parathyroid tissue next to and at some distance from the autograft within skeletal muscle and connective tissue. On occasion, these abnormalities were extreme enough to simulate malignancy. In addition, the grafts may exhibit extensive areas of banding fibrosis reminiscent of the changes seen in atypical adenomas and carcinomas (figs. 28-9, 28-10).

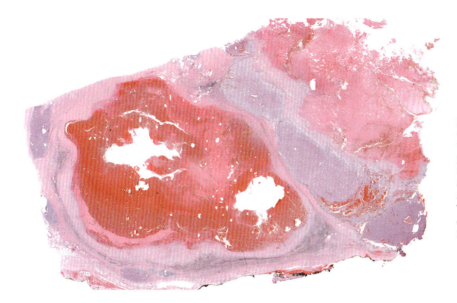

Figure 28-9

PARATHYROID GRAFT

Parathyroid tissue was implanted into the forearm of a uremic patient treated by total parathyroidectomy. The patient subsequently developed recurrent hyperparathyroidism, and the graft was injected with alcohol prior to its excision. There is extensive necrosis of chief cell nodules. (Courtesy of Dr. J. Monchik, Providence, RI.)

Figure 28-10

PARATHYROID GRAFT

Autotransplanted parathyroid tissue in the forearm of a patient with secondary hyperparathyroidism treated by total parathyroidectomy and subsequent recurrent hyperparathyroidism. Nodules of hyperplastic chief cells and oncocytes surrounded by broad bands of fibrous connective tissue are present in the soft tissue.

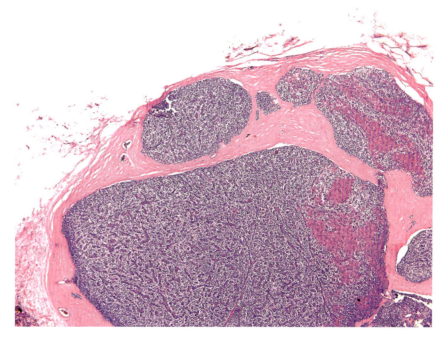

REFERENCES

1. Castleman B, Mallory TB. Parathyroid hyperplasia in chronic renal insufficiency. Am J Pathol 1937;13:553-74.

2. Sitges-Serra A, Caralps-Riera A. Hyperparathyroidism associated with renal disease. Pathogenesis, natural history, and surgical treatment. Surg Clin North Am 1987;67:359-77.

3. Pappenheimer AM, Wilens SL. Enlargement of the parathyroid glands in renal disease. Am J Pathol 1935;11:73-91.

4. Fraser WD. Hyperparathyroidism. Lancet 2009; 374:145-58.

5. Breslau NA. Update on secondary forms of hyperparathyroidism. Am J Med Sci 1987;294:120-31.

6. Salusky IB, Colburn JW. The renal osteodystrophies. In: DeGroot LJ, ed. Endocrinology, Vol. 2, 2nd ed. Philadelphia: WB Saunders; 1989:1032.

7. Akerström G, Malmaeus J, Grimelius L, Ljunghall S, Bergström R. Histological changes in parathyroid glands in subclinical and clinical renal disease. An autopsy investigation. Scand J Urol Nephrol 1984;18:75-84.

8. Castleman B, Roth SI. Tumors of the parathyroid glands. Atlas of Tumor Pathology, 2nd Series, Fascicle 14. Washington, DC: Armed Forces Institute of Pathology; 1978:1-94.

9. Roth SI, Marshall RB. Pathology and ultrastructure of the human parathyroid glands in chronic renal failure. Arch Intern Med 1969;124:397-407.

10. Banerjee SS, Faragher B, Haslton PS. Nuclear diameter in parathyroid disease. J Clin Pathol 1983;36:143-8.

11. Hasleton PS, Ali HH. The parathyroid in cronic renal failure—a light and electron microscopic study. J Pathol 1980;132:307-23.

12. Wallfelt C, Larsson R, Gylfe E, Ljunghall S, Rastad J, Alderström G. Secretory disturbance in hyperplastic parathyroid nodules of uremic hyperparathyroid-ism: implication for parathyroid autotransplantation. World J Surg 1988;12:431-8.

13. Wells SA Jr, Ellis GJ, Gunnels JC, Schneider AB, Sherwood LM. Parathyroid autotransplantation in primary parathyroid hyperplasia. N Engl J Med 1976;295:57-62.

14. Wells SA, Jr, Gunnells JC, Shelburne JD, Schneider AB, Sherwood LM. Transplantation of the parathyroid glands in man: clinical indications and results. Surgery 1975;78:34-44.

15. Fitko R, Roth SI, Hines JR, Roxe DM, Cahill E. Parathyromatosis in hyperparathyroidism. Hum Pathol 1990;21:234-7.

16. Nichols G Jr, Roth SJ. Case 29-1963—chronic renal disease and hypercalcemia. N Engl J Med 1963;268:943-53.

17. Krause MW, Hedinger CE. Pathologic study of parathyroid glands in tertiary hyperparathyroidism. Hum Pathol 1985;16:772-84.

18. Kebebew E, Duh QY, Clark OH. Tertiary hyperparathyroidism: histological patterns of disease and results of parathyroidectomy. Arch Surg 2004;139:974-7.

19. Snover DC, Foucar K. Mitotic activity in benign parathyroid disease. Am J Clin Pathol 1981; 75:345-7.

20. Altenähr E, Arps H, Montz R, Dorn G. Quantitative ultrastructural and radioimmunologic assessment of parathyroid gland activity in primary hyperparathyroidism. Lab Invest 1979;41:303-12.

21. Imanishi Y, Tahara H, Palanisamym N, et al. Clonal chromosomal defects in the molecular pathogenesis of refractory hyperparathyroidism of uremia. J Am Soc Nephrol 2002;13:1490-8.

22. Klempa I, Frei U, Röttger P, Schneider M, Koch KM. Parathyroid autografts—morphology and function: six years' experience with parathyroid autotransplantation in uremic patients. World J Surg 1984;8:540-6.

29 MISCELLANEOUS PARATHYROID LESIONS

PARATHYROID CYSTS

Parathyroid cysts are rare lesions that present most commonly in the fourth and fifth decades of life (1–4). They develop most often in the neck in proximity to the lower parathyroid glands, but they also occur in the mediastinum (5).

Most parathyroid cysts are nonfunctional remnants of the third and fourth branchial pouches. They also develop as a result of coalescence of the microcysts commonly present in the parathyroid glands of older individuals. Rarely, parathyroid cysts are found within the thyroid gland (6). Heterotopic salivary glandular tissue may be present in association with the cysts (7). Mediastinal parathyroid cysts may contain small fragments of thymic tissue and are sometimes referred to as *third pharyngeal pouch cysts* (8).

Most patients present with a neck mass, with or without compressive symptoms, raising the possibility of a thyroid lesion (4). The cysts vary in size, up to 10 cm in diameter (fig. 29-1). They are usually unilocular and their walls are gray-white and paper thin (5).

Microscopically, the cyst wall is composed of fibrous tissue with occasional smooth muscle cells. Groups of chief cells and oncocytes may be present within the wall. A flattened layer of chief cells may line portions of the cyst (fig. 29-2). The cyst fluid is usually thin, water-clear or straw-colored but may appear opalescent or bloody, especially following aspiration of the fluid. Water-clear fluid aspirated from a neck cyst in the area of the parathyroid glands is virtually diagnostic of a parathyroid cyst. The fluid is typically positive for parathyroid hormone (PTH), with levels higher than those present in the serum (9).

Some parathyroid cysts may develop as a result of degeneration of a parathyroid neoplasm or hyperplasia (see chapters 25 and 27) (1,10,11). These cysts are more accurately characterized as *pseudocysts*. In such cases, portions of abnormal parathyroid tissue may be present in the cyst wall. However, if extensive scarring has occurred, residual parathyroid tissue may be impossible to identify.

PARATHYROMATOSIS

The term *parathyromatosis* refers to the presence of multiple nodules of hyperfunctioning parathyroid tissue beyond the confines of the normal parathyroid glands (12). Developmental rests of parathyroid tissue are common in the soft tissues of the neck and mediastinum, often in proximity to normal glands. In patients with primary or secondary hyperplasia, the rests may become hyperplastic, a phenomenon that has been termed *developmental* or *ontogenous parathyromatosis*, in view of the developmental origin of the rests. Ontogenous parathyromatosis may be responsible for persistent or recurrent

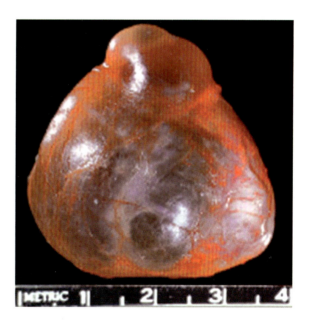

Figure 29-1

PARATHYROID CYST

The cyst contains colorless clear fluid. (Fig. 57-47 from Roth SI. The parathyroid gland. In: Silverberg SA, DeLellis RA, Frable WJ, eds. Principles and practice of surgical pathology and cytopathology, 3rd ed. New York: Churchill Livingstone; 1997:2740.)

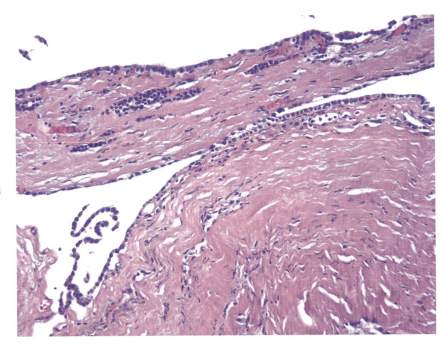

Figure 29-2

PARATHYROID CYST

The cyst is lined by a flattened layer of chief cells.

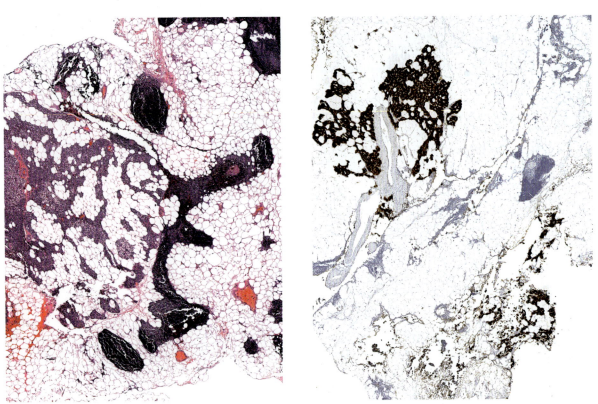

Figure 29-3

DEVELOPMENTAL/PRIMARY (ONTOGENOUS) PARATHYROMATOSIS

Left: The thymus gland in a patient with primary chief cell hyperplasia without a history of prior surgery contains multiple, scattered collections of chief cells.

Right: The chief cells are positive for parathyroid hormone (PTH) (immunoperoxidase stain for PTH).

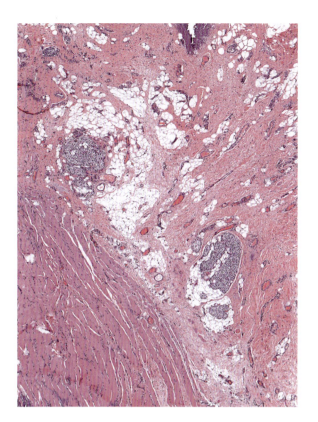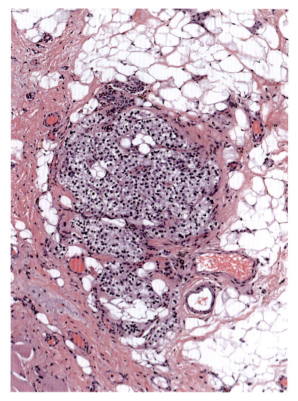

Figure 29-4

SECONDARY (POSTSURGICAL) PARATHYROMATOSIS

Left: This patient with primary chief cell hyperplasia developed recurrent hyperparathyroidism after subtotal parathyroidectomy. Multiple foci of hyperplastic chief cells surrounded by areas of fibrosis were present in the cervical soft tissue on exploration for recurrent hyperparathyroidism.

Right: In contrast to recurrent parathyroid carcinoma, the nests of chief cells lack an expansile pattern of growth and are not associated with vascular invasion.

hyperparathyroidism following incomplete parathyroidectomy (fig. 29-3) (13–16). A second mechanism for the development of parathyromatosis is seeding of the operative field during parathyroidectomy or incomplete excision of hyperplastic or neoplastic parathyroid lesions (*secondary* or *postsurgical parathyromatosis*) (fig. 29-4).

Distinguishing parathyromatosis from parathyroid carcinoma is challenging. In patients with previously untreated primary or secondary hyperplasia, foci of parathyromatosis are unassociated with desmoplasia. In patients with previous surgery, however, parathyromatosis may be associated with considerable fibrosis, invasion of skeletal muscle and soft tissues, and mitotic activity, features that are similar to parathyroid autotransplants. Vascular invasion is absent (17). Some studies have indicated that

the molecular profiles of parathyromatosis are more similar to those of adenomas than carcinomas (18).

SECONDARY TUMORS

Secondary involvement of the parathyroid glands by tumor occurs through extension from adjacent structures (thyroid, larynx) (fig. 29-5) or by metastatic spread (fig. 29-6) (19). In a prospective series of 160 autopsies of patients with cancer, Horwitz et al. (20) found metastasis to at least one parathyroid gland in 19 cases (11.9 percent). The most common sites of origin, in order of decreasing frequency, were breast, blood (leukemia), skin (melanoma), lung, and soft tissue. De la Monte et al. (21) described parathyroid metastases in 6 percent of patients with widely disseminated breast cancer.

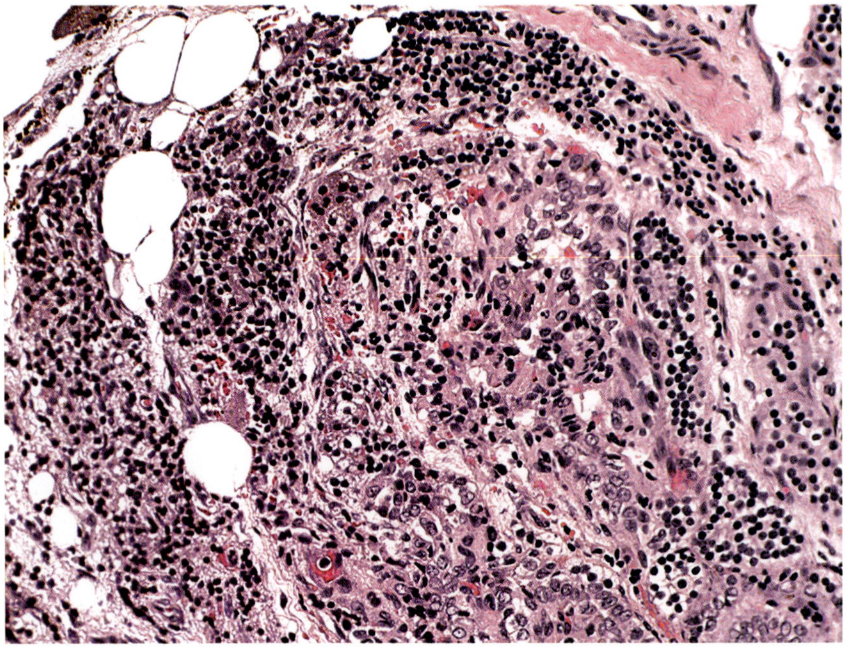

Figure 29-5

**EXTENSION OF
PAPILLARY THYROID
CARCINOMA INTO
PARATHYROID GLAND**

Tumor is present in the center
of this parathyroid gland.

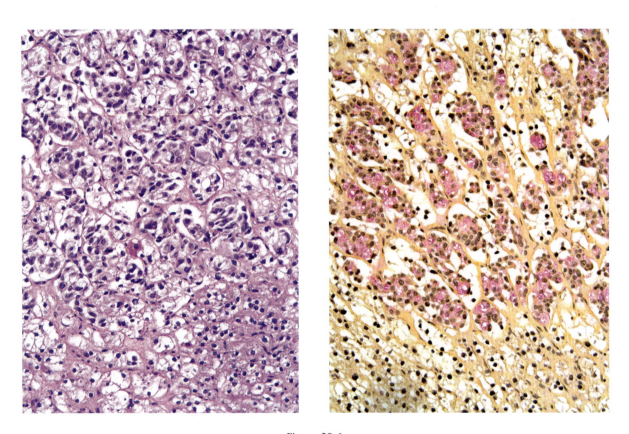

Figure 29-6

METASTATIC BREAST CARCINOMA INVOLVING PARATHYROID ADENOMA

Left: A small amount of residual adenoma is present at the bottom.
Right: The mucicarmine stain is positive in the tumor cells.

Hypoparathyroidism, occurring as a result of tumorous destruction of the parathyroid glands, however, is rare (20). Hypocalcemia and hyperphosphatemia were recorded in only 2 of 19 patients from the series of Horowitz et al. (20). In both instances, more than 70 percent of the parathyroid parenchyma was replaced by tumor.

REFERENCES

1. Castleman B, Roth SI. Tumors of the parathyroid glands. Atlas of Tumor Pathology, 2nd Series, Fascicle 14. Washington, DC: Armed Forces Institute of Pathology; 1978:1-94.
2. Haid SP, Method HL, Beal JM. Parathyroid cysts. Report of two cases and review of the literature. Arch Surg 1967;94:421-6.
3. Hoehn JG, Beahrs OH, Woolner LB. Unusual surgical lesions of the parathyroid gland. Am J Surg 1969;118:770-8.
4. Wang C, Vickery AL Jr, Maloof F. Large parathyroid cysts mimicking thyroid nodules. Ann Surg 1972;175:448-53.
5. Fortson JK, Patel VG, Henderson VJ. Parathyroid cysts: a case report and review of the literature. Largngoscope 2001;111:1726-8.
6. Atwan M, Chetty R. An unusual "thyroid cyst": intrathyroidal parathyroid cyst. Endocr Pathol 2011;22:108-11.
7. Carney JA. Salivary heterotopia, cysts and the parathyroid land: branchial pouch derivatives and remnants. Am J Surg Pathol 2000;24:837-45.
8. Wick MR. Mediastinal cysts and intrathoracic thyroid tumors. Semin Diagn Pathol 1990;7:285-94.
9. Silverman JF, Khazanie PG, Norris HT, Fore WW. Parathyroid hormone (PTH) assay of parathyroid cysts examined by fine needle aspiration biopsy. Am J Clin Pathol 1986;86:776-80.
10. Calandra DB, Shah KH, Prinz RA, et al. Parathyroid cysts: a report of eleven cases including two associated with hyperparathyroid crisis. Surgery 1983;94:887-92.
11. Shields TW, Staley CJ. Functioning parathyroid cysts. Arch Surg 1961;82:937-42.
12. Reddick RL, Costa J, Marx SJ. Parathyroid hyperplasia and parathyromatosis. Lancet 1997;1:549.
13. Rattner DW, Marrone GC, Kasdon E, Silen W. Recurrent hyperparathyroidism due to implantation of parathyroid tissue. Am J Surg 1985;149:745-8.
14. Fitko R, Roth SI, Hines JR, Roxe DM, Cahill E. Parathyromatosis in hyperparathyroidism. Hum Pathol 1990;21:234-7.
15. Fraker DL, Travis WD, Merendino JJ Jr, et al. Locally recurrent parathyroid neoplasms as a cause for recurrent and persistent primary hyperparathyroidism. Ann Surg 1991;213:58-65.
16. Lee P, Mateo RB, Clarke MR, Brown ML, Carty SE. Parathyromatosis: a cause for recurrent hyperparathyroidism. Endocr Pract 2001;7:189-92.
17. Fernandez-Ranvier GG, Khanafshar E, Jensen K, et al. Parathyroid carcinoma, atypical parathyroid adenoma or parathyromatosis? Cancer 2007;110:255-64.
18. Fernandez-Ranvier GG, Khanafshar E, Tacha D, et al. Defining a molecular phenotype for benign and malignant parathyroid tumors. Cancer 2009;115:334-44.
19. DeLellis, RA. Secondary tumours of the thyroid. In: DeLellis RA, Lloyd RV, Heita PU, Eng C, eds. Pathology and genetics of tumours of endocrine organs (World Health Organization Classification of Tumours). Lyon: IARC Press; 2004:122.
20. Horwitz CA, Myers WP, Foote FW Jr. Secondary malignant tumors of the parathyroid glands. Report of two cases with associated hypoparathyroidism. Am J Med 1972;52:797-808.
21. de la Monte SM, Hutchins GM, Moore GW. Endocrine organ metastases from breast carcinoma. Am J Pathol 1984;114:131-6.

30 DIAGNOSTIC APPROACHES TO PARATHYROID LESIONS

According to current clinical practice in most centers, surgery for parathyroid adenoma is performed following preoperative localization studies together with intraoperative assays of parathyroid hormone (minimal access parathyroidectomy). Conventional open parathyroidectomy is now more commonly performed for patients suspected of having parathyroid hyperplasia. Pathologic examination of the glands obtained by the conventional approach, including the use of fat stains, density gradient measurements, and DNA cytometry, is discussed first. Immunohistochemical and molecular approaches for the analysis of specific parathyroid disorders have been discussed in previous chapters of this volume.

INTRAOPERATIVE DIAGNOSIS

The optimal treatment of patients with hyperparathyroidism requires a close working relationship between the endocrinologist, radiologist, pathologist, and surgeon (1–3). The pathologist should be apprised of any pertinent history relating to previous endocrine disorders, including the family history. The major task of the pathologist at the time of the frozen section is to determine whether a biopsy or excision of a neck nodule represents parathyroid tissue (2,4,5). Based on a series of more than 1,500 frozen sections from the Johns Hopkins Hospital, the correct identification of parathyroid tissue was achieved in more than 99 percent of cases, excluding cases (0.4 percent) in which the diagnosis was deferred (6). Deferred or incorrect diagnoses in this study were the result of frozen section artifact, sampling problems, and interpretative errors.

Parathyroid tissue may be difficult to distinguish grossly from a variety of other tissues in the neck including fat, lymph node, thyroid, and ectopic thymus. The surgeon, depending on experience, may request frozen sections on a number of such samples to confirm the presence or absence of parathyroid tissue. On occasion, the distinction between thyroid and parathyroid tissue is difficult, particularly if the parathyroid biopsy contains follicular structures. Generally, the follicles in parathyroid tissue are smaller than those in normal thyroid tissue and the cells have clear or vacuolated cytoplasm. Thyroid tissue may contain a predominance of oncocytic cells, similar to those found in the parathyroid gland. Deeper sections of equivocal cases may reveal areas more typical of parathyroid tissue. The presence of birefringent oxalate crystals within follicles is helpful in identifying thyroid tissue (7,8). Fragments of ectopic thymus may be composed almost exclusively of epithelial elements that may be difficult to differentiate from parathyroid tissue. The presence of Hassal corpuscles clearly establishes a thymic origin in such instances.

The distinction of normal versus hyperplastic tissue in biopsy material is problematic. In the era of intraoperative parathyroid hormone (PTH) assays, however, the challenges of distinguishing hyperplasia from normal and adenomatous glands has become less acute both for surgeons and pathologists (see section, Preoperative Localization and Intraoperative Parathyroid Hormone Assays).

Depending on variations in the distribution of chief cells in a parathyroid gland and on constitutional factors, a biopsy of a normal-sized gland may appear hypercellular and the pathologist may erroneously render a diagnosis of hyperplasia. On the other hand, a biopsy of a hyperplastic gland or adenoma containing stromal fat may be misinterpreted as a normal gland if knowledge of the gland size is not known (9).

Upon receipt by the pathologist, each intact gland or biopsy specimen should be labeled as to anatomic site, and should be measured and weighed after removing the surrounding fat. The gross description should include information on the external appearance, color, and consistency of each gland. Representative samples, if sufficient tissue is available, should be frozen at -70° for possible molecular studies.

The critical issue in distinguishing hyperplasia from adenoma at surgery is the determination of the number of enlarged parathyroid glands. Most patients with parathyroid adenoma have involvement of one gland, and the remaining glands are of normal size. In most instances, the surgeon will remove the largest gland first. The gland should be carefully weighed and a representative section, which includes the capsule, should be selected for frozen section examination. Since a rim of adjacent parathyroid tissue is seen in only a subset of cases at the time of frozen section, the pathologist cannot rely on this criterion alone to render a diagnosis of adenoma (2).

The presence of stromal fat cannot be used to exclude the diagnosis of adenoma, since adenomas may contain at least some stromal fat, and occasional adenomas may contain an abundance of stromal fat (9). In many instances, the pathologist can only report that the resected gland is hypercellular and that it may represent adenoma or hyperplasia. The surgeon must then sample another gland. If this gland is of normal size and cellularity, both the surgeon and pathologist can be satisfied that the diagnosis is most likely adenoma (1).

The diagnosis of hyperplasia is likely when multiple glands are involved. It should be remembered, however, that hyperplasia may not involve all glands equally and that one dominant gland may be present. A biopsy of a second gland in this situation, particularly if the biopsy is from one of the poles, may reveal a high proportion of stromal fat. In such instances, it is imperative to know the size of the gland. If the second gland is enlarged, the likelihood of hyperplasia is high.

Geelhoed and Silverberg (10) advocate the use of intraoperative imprints for the rapid identification of parathyroid tissue. The procedure permits cytologic evaluation in less than 1 minute per specimen, with accurate and reproducible determination of the presence or absence of parathyroid tissue. Pathologic diagnoses are possible on abnormal parathyroid glands when the imprint is used as a screening procedure to select specimens for subsequent frozen section examination.

FAT STAINS

The use of fat stains, including oil red O and Sudan IV, for the evaluation of the parathyroid gland is based on the observation that the intracellular or lipid content is decreased or absent in hyperfunctioning chief cells as compared to normal or suppressed chief cells. Roth and Gallagher (11), using Sudan IV stains to evaluate frozen sections of parathyroid tissue, demonstrated prominent intracellular sudanophilic deposits in up to 80 percent of chief cells of suppressed parathyroid glands; the cases of chief cell hyperplasia and adenoma, on the other hand, contained little or no stainable lipid.

Some authors, however, have noted considerable variation in the intracellular lipid content of hyperplasia and adenoma cases (12–16). Dufour and Durkowski (12) reported positive intracellular lipid staining in at least one gland from patients with hyperplasia, and in 5 of 6 cases the staining was intense. Moreover, variation in intracellular lipid content was seen within individual glands. Bondeson et al. (17) also studied the lipid content of hyperplastic glands and reported considerable variation in staining in the same gland and in different glands from the same patient. All the hyperplastic glands showed distinctly divergent areas of parenchymal fat in different areas. In 73 patients with normal glands obtained at autopsy, 15 percent had reduced intracellular lipid staining, suggesting the presence of hyperfunctioning parathyroid tissue.

Using the oil red O technique, Bondeson et al. (17) examined the parathyroid glands from almost 200 cases of surgically treated hyperparathyroidism. On the basis of careful histologic examination and clinical follow-up, they concluded that access to two complete glands and the use of fat stains allowed the highly reproducible and reliable distinction between adenoma and hyperplasia. The rate of equivocal findings for cases in which two glands were available was 8 percent.

As with other special procedures, fat stains should not be used in isolation for the evaluation of parathyroid disease. The combination of fat stains and careful morphologic assessment provides an optimal approach.

DENSITY GRADIENTS

Density measurements, based on the differences in density between the parenchymal cells and stromal fat cells, provide an objective evaluation of the ratio of these two cell types (18,19). The medium used for density gradient measurements is Percoll equilibrated with sodium chloride to iso-osmotic conditions. Akerström et al. (18) found that the density of parathyroid glands is related linearly to the parenchymal cell content. The density of the parathyroid gland indirectly allows an estimate of the parenchymal content, and with knowledge of the total glandular weight, it is possible to calculate the parenchymal weight.

DNA CYTOMETRY

Both static and flow cytometric methods have been used for the assessment of the DNA content of proliferative lesions of the parathyroid glands (20). Most of the data now available are based on studies using formalin-fixed, paraffin-embedded samples processed according to the method of Hedley et al. (21). Using this approach, most normal parathyroid glands have a diploid DNA pattern, although some normal glands exhibit small tetraploid peaks. The considerable variation in the frequency of tetraploidy in parathyroid adenomas ranges from 8 to 80 percent (22–25). It has been suggested that the high frequency of tetraploidy reported in some of these studies may have resulted from the contamination of the samples by cell aggregates.

The frequency of aneuploidy in adenomas ranges from 3 to nearly 50 percent in different series using flow cytometry of formalin-fixed and paraffin-embedded samples (20,23,26–28). A comparable frequency of aneuploidy has been noted in parathyroid carcinomas using similar technical approaches. Moreover, 25 to 50 percent of glands from patients with primary or secondary hyperplasia may exhibit aneuploidy (21,26,29). These findings indicate that flow cytometry is generally not a useful approach in distinguishing parathyroid adenoma from carcinoma.

Obara et al. (28) reported that the analysis of DNA content by flow cytometry may be useful for the prediction of clinical outcome of patients with parathyroid carcinoma. In their study,

patients with aneuploid carcinomas were more likely to have an aggressive form of the disease than those with diploid carcinomas.

Examination of Feulgen-stained sections by image cytometry appears to provide more consistent results than flow cytometry of formalin-fixed paraffin-embedded samples. Image cytometry has demonstrated a significantly greater mean DNA content in carcinomas as compared to typical adenomas, adenomas associated with marked hypercalcemia, and atypical adenomas (30,31). In the series reported by Levin et al. (30,31), aneuploidy was restricted to 4 of 9 carcinomas, including 2 cases originally classified as atypical adenomas. Other studies have demonstrated that most specimens with definite criteria of malignancy are aneuploid, while specimens lacking these criteria are euploid (32). Studies using image cytometry have suggested that aneuploid carcinomas are likely to pursue a more aggressive course than diploid carcinomas (33).

Kinetic analyses of normal parathyroid glands show mean S-phase fractions of 1.2 percent, while mean S-phase fractions of adenomas and secondary hyperplasias are 1.5 percent and 0.8 percent, respectively (23). Carcinomas have a mean S-phase fraction of 6.0 percent. On the basis of these studies, Harlow et al. (23) concluded that a diagnosis of carcinoma should be considered in the presence of an S-phase fraction of greater than 4.0 percent and a DNA index greater than 1.2.

PREOPERATIVE LOCALIZATION AND INTRAOPERATIVE PARATHYROID HORMONE ASSAYS

Parathyroid surgery has evolved from conventional open parathyroidectomy with exploration of all four glands to minimal access (focused) open or endoscopic parathyroidectomy (34–41). This evolution was made possible by the development of high resolution radiologic techniques together with the development of the rapid intraoperative parathyroid hormone (IOPTH) assay (figs. 30-1, 30-2) (42).

Sonography and technetium-99-m-sestamibi (99mTc-sestamibi) scintigraphy are the most commonly used imaging techniques for the demonstration of parathyroid lesions. Comparative studies have revealed similar sensitivities

591

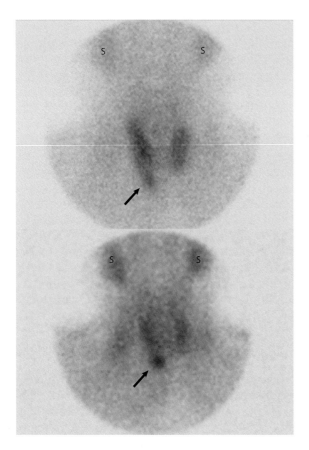

Figure 30-1

TECHNETIUM-SESTAMIBI SCAN

The immediate image shows a suggestion of an abnormality (arrow) at the lower right thyroid pole (upper panel). The 2-hour delayed scan (lower panel) shows a clear-cut nodule, which proved to be a parathyroid adenoma at the same site (arrow). S, submandibular gland. (Courtesy of Drs. M. Beland and P. Mazzaglia, Providence, RI.)

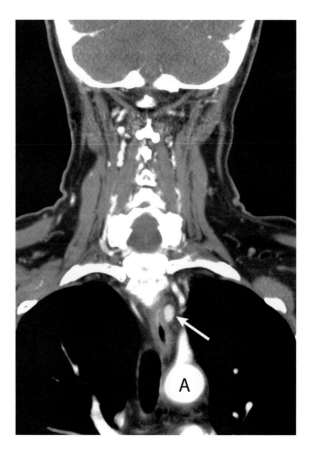

Figure 30-2

4D COMPUTERIZED TOMOGRAPHY

A paraesophageal adenoma is present at the arrow. A, aorta. (Courtesy of Dr. M. Beland, Providence, RI.)

and specificities for the detection of adenomas using these approaches. Adenomas are usually hypoechoic to the overlying thyroid gland on grayscale imaging (43). Color and power Doppler imaging frequently show a characteristic extrathyroidal feeding vessel that enters the gland at one of the poles and frequently branches around the tumor, producing a rimlike effect (44). The sensitivity of sonography for the detection of single adenomas ranges from 72 to 89 percent while the sensitivity for multiglandular disease is considerably less (45).

99mTc-sestamibi is concentrated both by the thyroid and parathyroid glands, but hyperactive parathyroid glands typically have more avid uptake of the tracer and retain it for longer inter-

vals than the thyroid gland (fig. 30-1) (46). On delayed imaging at 2 hours, the tracer is retained by abnormal parathyroid tissue but washes out from the thyroid gland. Single photon emission tomography (SPECT) with a pinhole collimator can further help to discriminate thyroid and parathyroid tissue (47). The sensitivity of 99mTc-sestamibi using SPECT ranges from 68 to 95 percent for the identification of single gland disease, but this approach is considerably less successful for the detection of multiglandular disease (48). Modifications of the original sestamibi scan protocol include the use of radioactive iodine to subtract the thyroid image.

The development of the rapid IOPTH assay was a major advance in the treatment of hyperparathyroidism, since this approach can accurately confirm or refute the preoperative localization studies (49–51). Laboratory turnaround time for this assay averages 13 to 15 minutes. Multiple studies have confirmed the ability of IOPTH to guide intraoperative decision making. This is accomplished by estimating whether additional hypersecreting glands remain after removal of the gland identified by preoperative localization studies. The success of this approach is based on the fact that PTH has a half-life of less than 5 minutes. A drop in PTH levels of 50 percent or greater from the baseline or pre-excision value is the criterion by which most surgeons conclude that all abnormal glands have been removed, without having to identify all remaining glands (52). In a series of more than 600 cases, the rates for double adenomas and hyperplasia were 11 percent and 7 percent, respectively, for the traditional four-gland approach and 5.1 percent and 1.6 percent, respectively, for a minimally invasive procedure (53). These findings underscore the fact that a subset of patients had enlarged glands that were not identified by ultrasonography,

sestamibi, or IOPTH, but which might have been discovered using the traditional four-gland approach. The question remains as to whether enlarged glands that were not hypersecreting at the time of initial surgery will cause recurrence of hyperparathyroidism in the future. Follow-up studies from the University of Miami have demonstrated a cure rate of 98 percent with a focused surgical approach (54).

In some series, a false positive intraoperative excess of PTH of 50 percent has been noted in 2 to 3 percent of patients. A similar proportion of patients have had a false negative drop (55,56).

Occasional normocalcemic patients have increased levels of PTH at 1 to 5 years after apparent curative surgery (57). At present, there is no evidence that the postoperative PTH increases are indicative of surgical failure. Potential mechanisms for PTH elevation in the setting of normocalcemia include vitamin D deficiency, hungry bone syndrome, and PTH resistance.

REFERENCES

1. Norton JA, Aurbach GD, Marx SJ, Doppman JL. Surgical management of hyperparathyroidism. In: DeGroot LJ, ed. Endocrinology, Vol 2, 2nd ed. Philadelphia: WB Saunders; 1989:1013-31.
2. Roth SI. The parathyroid gland. In: Silverberg SG, DeLellis RA, Frable, WJ, eds. Principles and practice of surgical pathology and cytopathology, 3rd ed. New York: Churchill & Livingstone; 1997:2709-50.
3. Roth SI, Wang CA, Potts JT Jr. The team approach to primary hyperparathyroidism. Hum Pathol 1975;6:645-8.
4. Akerström G, Bergström R, Grimelius L, et al. Relation between changes in clinical and histopathological features of primary hyperparathyroidism. World J Surg 1986;10:696-702.
5. Castleman R, Roth SI. Tumors of the parathyroid glands. Atlas of Tumor Pathology, 2nd Series, Fascicle 14. Washington, DC: Armed Forces Institute of Pathology; 1978:1-94.
6. Westra WH, Pritchett DD, Udelsman R. Intraoperative confirmation of parathyroid tissue during parathyroid exploration; a retrospective

evaluation of the frozen section. Am J Surg Pathol 1998;22:538-44.
7. Isotalo PA, Lloyd RV. Presence of birefringent crystals is useful in distinguishing thyroid from parathyroid gland tissue. Am J Surg Pathol 1999;23:288-95.
8. Wong KS, Lewis JS Jr, Gottipati S, Chernock RD. Utility of birefringent crystal identification by polarized light microscopy in distinguishing thyroid from parathyroid tissue on intraoperative frozen sections. Am J Surg Pathol 2014;38:1212-1219.
9. Abul-Haj SK, Conklin H, Hewitt WC. Functioning lipoadenoma of the parathyroid gland. Report of a unique case. N Engl J Med 1962;266:121-3.
10. Geelhoed GW, Silverberg SG. Intraoperative imprints for the identification of parathyroid tissue. Surgery 1984;96:1124-31.
11. Roth SI, Gallagher MJ. The rapid identification of "normal" parathyroid glands by the presence of intracellular fat. Am J Pathol 1976;84:521-8.
12. Dufour DR, Durkowski C. Sudan IV stain. Its limitations in evaluating parathyroid functional status. Arch Pathol Lab Med 1982;106:224-7.

13. Kasdon EJ, Rosen S, Cohen RB, Silen W. Surgical pathology of hyperparathyroidism. Usefulness of fat stain and problems in interpretation. Am J Surg Pathol 1981;5:381-4.

14. King DT, Hirose FM. Chief cell intracytoplasmic fat used to evaluate parathyroid disease in frozen section. Arch Pathol Lab Med 1979;103:609-12.

15. Ljungberg O, Tibblin S. Preoperative fat staining of frozen sections in primary hyperparathyroidism. Am J Pathol 1979;95:633-41.

16. Monchik JM, Farrugia R, Teplitz C, Teplitz J, Brown S. Parathyroid surgery: the role of chief cell intracellular fat staining with osmium carmine in the intraoperative management of patients with primary hyperparathyroidism. Surgery 1983:94:877-86.

17. Bondeson AG, Bondeson L, Ljungberg O, Tibblin S. Fat staining in parathyroid disease—diagnostic value and impact on surgical strategy: clinico-pathologic analysis of 191 cases. Hum Pathol 1985;16:1255-63.

18. Akerström G, Grimelius L, Johansson H, Pertoft H, Lundqvist H. Estimation of the parathyroid parenchymal cell mass by density gradients. Am J Pathol 1980;99:685-94.

19. Wang C, Rieder SV. A density test for the intraoperative differentiation of parathyroid hyperplasia from neoplasia. Ann Surg 1978;187:63-7.

20. Mallette LE. DNA quantitation in the study of parathyroid lesions. A review. Am J Clin Pathol 1992;98:305-11.

21. Hedley DW, Friedlander ML, Taylor IW, Rugg CA, Musgrove EA. Method for analysis of cellular DNA content of paraffin-embedded pathological material using flow cytometry. J Histochem Cytochem 1983;31:1333-5.

22. Bowlby L, DeBault LE, Abraham S. Flow cytometric DNA analysis of parathyroid glands. Relationship between nuclear DNA and pathologic classifications. Am J Pathol 1987;128:338-44.

23. Harlow S. Roth SI, Bauer K, Marshall RB. Flow cytometric DNA analysis of normal and pathologic parathyroid glands. Mod Pathol 1991;4:310-5.

24. Irvin GL 3rd, Bagwell CB. Identification of histologically undetectable parathyroid hyperplasia by flow cytometry. Am J Surg 1979;138:567-71.

25. Irvin GL 3rd, Taupier MA, Block NL, Reiss E. DNA patterns in parathyroid disease predict postoperative hormone secretion. Surgery 1988;104:1115-20.

26. Berczi C, Bocsi J, Balazs G, Lukacs G. Flow cytometric DNA analysis of benign hyperfunctioning parathyroid glands: significant difference in the S phase fraction and proliferative index between adenomas and hyperplasias. Pathology 2002;34:442-5.

27. Joensuu H, Klemi PJ. DNA aneuploidy in adenomas of endocrine organs. Am J Pathol 1988;132:145-51.

28. Obara T, Fujimoto Y, Hirayama A, et al. Flow cytometric DNA analysis of parathyroid tumors with special reference to its diagnostic and prognostic value in parathyroid carcinoma. Cancer 1990;65:1789-93.

29. Obara T, Fujimoto Y, Kanaji Y, et al. Flow cytometric DNA analysis of parathyroid tumors. Implication of aneuploidy for pathologic and biologic classification. Cancer 1990;66:1555-62.

30. Levin KE, Chew KL, Ljung BM, Mayall BH, Siperstein AE, Clark OH. Deoxyribonucleic acid cytometry helps identify parathyroid carcinomas. J Clin Endocrinol Metab 1988;67:779-84.

31. Levin KE, Galante M, Clark OH. Parathyroid carcinoma versus parathyroid adenoma in patients with profound hypercalcemia. Surgery 1987;101:649-60.

32. Sandelin K, Auer G, Bondeson L, Grimelius L, Farnebo LO. Prognostic factors in parathyroid cancer: a review of 95 cases. World J Surg 1992;16:724-31.

33. Bondeson L, Sandelin K, Grimelius L. Histopathological variables and DNA cytometry in parathyroid carcinoma. Am J Surg Pathol 1993;17:820-9.

34. Duh QY. Surgical approach to primary hyperparathyroidism (bilateral approach). In: Clark OH, Duh QY, eds. Textbook of endocrine surgery. Philadelphia: WB Saunders; 1997:357-63.

35. Greene AB, Butler RS, McIntyre S, et al. National trends in parathyroid surgery from 1998-2008: a decade of change. J Am Coll Surg 2009;209:332-43.

36. Marcocci C, Cetani F. Clinical practice. Primary hyperparathyroidism. N Engl J Med 2011;365:2389-97.

37. Miccoli P, Bendinelli C, Berti P, Vignali E, Pinchera A, Marcocci C. Video-assisted versus conventional parathyroidectomy in primary hyperparathyroidism: a prospective randomized study. Surgery 1999;126:1117-21.

38. Monchik JM, Barellini L, Langer P, Kahya A. Minimally invasive parathyroid surgery in 103 patients with local/regional anesthesia, without exclusion criteria. Surgery 2002;131:502-8.

39. Sosa JA, Udelsman R. Minimally invasive parathyroidectomy. Surg Oncol 2003;12:125-34.

40. Tibblin SA, Bergenfelz AO. Surgical approach to primary hyperparathyroidism (unilateral approach). In: Clark OH, Duh QY, eds. Textbook of endocrine surgery. Philadelphia: WB Saunders; 1997;365-71.

41. Wang CA. Surgical management of primary hyperparathyroidism. Curr Probl Surg 1985;22:1-50.

42. Lumachi F, Ermani M, Basso S, Zucchetta P, Borsato N, Favia G. Localization of parathyroid tumors in the minimally invasive era: which technique should be chosen? Population based analysis of 253 patients undergoing parathyroidectomy and factors affecting parathyroid glands detection. Endocr Relat Cancer 2001;8:63-9.

43. Johnson NA, Tublin ME, Ogilve JB. Parathyroid imaging: technique and role in the prospective evaluation of primary hyperparathyroidism. AJR Am J Roentgenol 2007;188:1706-15.

44. Scheiner JD, Dupuy DE, Monchik JM, Noto RB, Cronan JJ. Pre-operative localization of parathyroid adenomas: a comparison of power and color Doppler ultrasonography with nuclear medicine scintography. Clin Radiol 2001;56:984-8.

45. Solarzano CC, Carneiro-Pla DM, Irvin GL 3rd. Surgeon-performed ultrasonography as the initial and only localizing study in sporadic primary hyperparathyroidism. J Am Coll Surg 2006;202:18-24.

46. Taillefer R, Boucher Y, Potvin C, Lambert R. Detection and localization of parathyroid adenomas in patients with hypoparathyroidism using a single radionuclide imaging procedure with technetiuym-99m-sestamibi (double phase study). J Nucl Med 1992;33:1801-7.

47. Sharma J, Mazzaglia P, Milas M, et al. Radionuclide imaging for hyperparathyroidism (HPT): which is the best technetium-99m sestamibi modality? Surgery 2006;140:856-63.

48. Light VL, McHenry CR, Jarjoura D, Sodee DB, Miron SD. Prospective comparison of dual phase technetium-99 sestamibi scintigraphy and high resolution ultrasonography in the evaluation of abnormal parathyroid glands. Am Surg 1996;62:563-7.

49. Irvin GL 3rd, Dembrow VD, Prudhomime DL. Clinical usefulness of an intraoperative quick parathyroid hormone assay. Surgery 1993;114:1019-23.

50. Irvin III 3rd, Dembrow, VD, Prudhomme DL. Operative monitoring of parathyroid gland hyperfunction. Am J Surg 1991;162:299-302.

51. Nussbaum SR, Zahradnik RJ, Lavigne JR, et al. Highly sensitive two-site immunoradiometric assay of parathyrin, and its clinical utility in evaluating patients with hypercalcemia. Clin Chem 1987;33:1364-7.

52. Carneiro D, Solarzano CC, Nader MC, Ramirez M, Irvin GL 3rd. Comparison of intraoperative iPTH assay (QPTH) criteria in guiding parathyroidectomy: which criterion is the most accurate? Surgery 2003;134:973-81.

53. Udelsman R. Six hundred fifty-six consecutive explorations for primary hyperparathyroidism. Ann Surg 2002:235:665-70.

54. Carneiro D, Solarzano CC, Irvin GL 3rd. Recurrent disease after limited parathyroidectomy for sporadic primary hyperparathyroidism. J Am Coll Surg 2004;199:849-53.

55. Garner SC, Leight GS Jr. Initial experience with intraoperative PTH determinations in the surgical management of 130 consecutive cases of primary hyperparathyroidism. Surgery 1999;126:1132-7.

56. Vignali E, Picone A, Materazzi G, et al. A quick intraoperative parathyroid hormone assay in the surgical management of patients with primary hyperparathyroidism: a study of 206 consecutive cases. Eur J Endocrinol 2002;146:783-8.

57. Biskobing DM. Significance of elevated parathyroid hormone after parathyroidectomy. Endocr Pract 2009;16:112-7.

Index*

A

ADASP (Association of Directors of Anatomic and Surgical Pathology) reporting protocol, 468
Adenochondroma, 78
Adenoid cystic carcinoma, 320
Adenoid cystic variant of papillary carcinoma, 431
Adenolipoma, 78
Adenoma-associated parathyroid glands, 537
Adenoma, parathyroid gland, *see* Parathyroid adenoma
Adenoma, thyroid gland, *see* Thyroid adenoma
Adenoma, thyroid gland, with bizarre nuclei, follicular, 73
Adenoma, thyroid gland, with papillary features, follicular, 79
Adenomatoid/adenomatous goiter, 331
Adenomatous hyperplasia, 331
AKT gene, 39
ALK, 374
American Joint Committee on Cancer (AJCC) protocol, 468
Amphicrine cell medullary carcinoma, 264
Amyloid goiter, 349
Anaplastic carcinoma, *see* Undifferentiated carcinoma
Anatomy, 3, 494
	normal parathyroid gland, 494
	normal thyroid gland, 3
Angioinvasive oncocytic carcinoma, 211
Angiolipoma, 315
Angiosarcoma, 291
Angiosarcoma-like medullary carcinoma, 265
Askanazy cells, 200
Association of Directors of Anatomic and Surgical Pathology (ADASP) report protocol, 468
Atypia of undetermined significance/follicular lesion of undetermined significance (AUS/FLUS), 450
Atypical adenoma, 78, 532
	parathyroid gland, 532
	thyroid gland, 78

B

B-catenin/APC/wnt pathway, 42
Benign follicular nodule, 73
Benign familial hypercalcemia, 571
Benign oncocytoma, 203
Benign thyroid nodule, 400
Bethesda system for reporting thyroid cytopathology, 396, 453
Biphasic carcinoma, 267
Black thyroid, 104
BRAF genes, 37
BRAF mutations, in papillary carcinoma, 371

C

C-cell, normal, 11
	calcitonin, 12, **14**
	calcitonin gene-related peptide, 13
	embryology, 3
	gastrin-releasing peptide, 13
	somatostatin, 13
C-cell carcinoma, 241
C-cell hyperplasia, 272
	association with MEN 2, 272
	peritumoral C-cell hyperplasia, 273
	primary (neoplastic) C-cell hyperplasia, 273
	secondary (physiologic) C-cell hyperplasia, 273
Calcitonin, 12, **14**
Calcitonin gene-related peptide, 13, **14**
Calcium homeostasis, parathyroid gland, 505
CAP reporting protocol, 468
Carcinoma, thyroid gland, *see* Thyroid carcinoma
Carcinoma showing thymus-like differentiation, 232, 319
Carcinosarcoma, 177
Cellular follicular lesion, 403
Chernobyl-related thyroid carcinoma, 58
Chief cell adenoma, parathyroid gland, 517
Chief cell hyperplasia, primary, parathyroid gland, *see* Primary chief cell hyperplasia, parathyroid gland

*In a series of numbers, those in boldface indicate the main discussion of the entity. All entities refer to the thyroid gland unless specified otherwise.

Chromosomal DNA alterations, 369, 375
  in follicular carcinoma, 369
  in papillary carcinoma, 375
Chronic lymphocytic hyperplasia, 404
Classification of thyroid tumors, 61
Clear cell carcinoma, **221**, 262, 439
  cytopathology, 439
  follicular, 222
  lipid-rich follicular, 226
  medullary, 227, 262
  oncocytic, 222
  papillary, 226
  signet ring follicular, 225
  undifferentiated, 227
Clear cell hyperplasia, parathyroid gland, 566
Clear cell medullary carcinoma, 227, **262**
Clear cell tumors, **221**, 439
  cytology, 439
  follicular, 222
  lipid-rich follicular, 226
  medullary, 227
  oncocytic, 222
  papillary, 226
  signet ring follicular, 225
  undifferentiated, 227
Clinical features of thyroid tumors, 465
College of American Pathologists (CAP) reporting
  protocol, 468
Colloid goiter, 331
Colloid nodule, 402
Columnar cell papillary carcinoma, **146**, 378, 429
  cytopathology, 429
  molecular genetic alterations, 378
Composite/compound carcinoma, 267
Cribriform/morular papillary carcinoma, **149**, 378
  molecular genetic alterations, 382
CTNNB1 gene, 42
Cysts, parathyroid gland, 583
Cytopathology of thyroid tumors, 395
  Bethesda system for reporting thyroid cyto-
    pathology, 396
  clear cell neoplasms, 439
  diffuse hyperplasia, 404
  fine-needle aspiration biopsy, 395, *see also*
    Fine-needle aspiration biopsy
  follicular neoplasms, 406
  Hashimoto thyroiditis, 404
  insular carcinoma, 431
  lymphoma, 445

  medullary carcinoma, 441
  nodular hyperplasia, 400
  normal gland, 397
  oncocytic neoplasms, 433
  papillary carcinoma, 416
  papillary carcinoma variants, 427
  secondary tumors, 447
  specimen adequacy, 397
  squamous cell neoplasms, 440
  undifferentiated carcinoma, 433

D

Density gradient measurement, parathyroid gland,
  591
DeQuervain thyroiditis, 342
Differentiated carcinoma, 267
Diffuse hyperplasia, **335**, 404
  cytopathology, 404
Diffuse lipomatosis, 315
Diffuse sclerosing variant of papillary carcinoma,
  141, 377, 429
  cytopathology, 429
DNA cytometry, parathyroid gland, 591
Dyshormonogenetic goiter, 336

E

Ectopic cervical thymoma, 315
Ectopic hamartomatous thymoma, 316
Ectopic thyroid tissue, 355
Embryology, 1, 493
  normal parathyroid gland, 493
  normal thyroid gland, 1
Encapsulated follicular variant of papillary car-
  cinoma, **135**, 377
Encapsulated medullary carcinoma, 265
Encapsulated oncocytic carcinoma, 211
Encapsulated papillary carcinoma, 130
Encapsulated oncocytic papillary neoplasm, 216

F

Familial hyperparathyroidism syndromes, 568
  familial hypocalciuric hypercalcemia, 571
  familial isolated hyperparathyroidism, 572
  hyperparathyroidism-jaw tumor syndrome, 571
  multiple endocrine neoplasia, type 1, 568
  multiple endocrine neoplasia, type 2, 570
  multiple endocrine neoplasia, type 4, 571
  neonatal severe primary hyperparathyroidism, 571

Familial hypocalciuric hypercalcemia, 571
Familial isolated hyperparathyroidism, 572
Familial medullary thyroid carcinoma, 242
Fat stains, parathyroid gland, 590
Fibrosing thyroiditis, 342
Fine-needle aspiration biopsy, thyroid gland, 395,
    see also Cytopathology, thyroid gland
  accuracy of, 452
  Bethesda classification, 396
  classification scheme, 396
  complications, 456
  histologic alterations following FNAB, 456
  indications for, 395
  molecular pathology, 450
  normal gland, 397
  pitfalls of, 455
  specimen adequacy, 397
Follicular adenoma, 65, 95, 203, 226, **365**, 367, 407
  cytopathology, 407
  differentiation from carcinoma, 72; from nod-
    ular hyperplasia, 73; from oncocytic carci-
    noma, 214
  hereditary syndromes, 367
  general and clinical features, 65
  gross findings, 65
  immunohistochemical findings, 71
  microscopic findings, 66
  molecular genetic alterations, 365
  treatment, 73
  ultrastructural findings, 72
  variants, 73
    adenochondroma, 78
    adenolipoma, 78
    adenoma with bizarre nuclei, 73
    adenoma with papillary features, 79
    atypical adenoma, 78
    hyalinizing trabecular adenoma, 73, 367
    lipid rich, 226
    of oxyphilic cell type, 203
    toxic adenoma, 81, 367
  with focal atypical features, 95
Follicular adenoma of oxyphilic cell type, 203
Follicular carcinoma, 72, **85**, 233, 367, 370, 406
  clear cell type, 222
  cytopathology, 407
  differentiation from follicular adenoma, 72;
    from parathyroid adenoma, 530
  follicular variant of papillary carcinoma, 85, *see*
    also Papillary thyroid carcinoma

hereditary syndromes, 370
lipid rich, 226
medullary carcinoma, follicular, 261
minimally invasive (encapsulated) type, 86
  capsular invasion, 87
  differentiation from adenoma, papillary car-
    cinoma, medullary carcinoma, 94
  pseudoinvasion, 89
  vascular invasion, 90
noninvasive follicular carcinoma, 94
oncocytic variant, 85, 209
poorly differentiated, 85, 172
squamous cell, 232
widely invasive type, 97
Follicular cells, normal, 8
  hormones, 10
Follicular lesion of undetermined significance, 406,
  450, 453
Follicular lymphoma, cytopathology, 452
Follicular tumor of uncertain malignant potential,
  95, 135
Follicular variant of papillary carcinoma (FVPTC),
  85, **131**, 135, 376, 416, 427
  cytopathology, 416, 427
  differentiation from medullary carcinoma, 257
  microfollicular variant, 135
Frozen section evaluation, thyroid gland, 466

G

Gastrin-releasing peptide, 13
Genes in tumorigenesis, thyroid gland, **23**
  AKT gene, 40
  B-catenin/APC/wnt pathway, 42
  BRAF genes, 37
  CTNNB1 gene, 42
  GNAS gene, 30
  MAPK gene pathway, 31
  MET gene, 36
  NTRK1 gene, 34, 374
  NTRK3 gene, 374
  PAX gene, 41
  PAX/PPRG rearrangement, 41
  PI3K/PTEN/AKT pathway, 39
  PPARγ rearrangement, 41
  PRKAR1A gene, 31
  PTEN gene, 40
  RAS genes, 36
  RET gene, 32
  RET/PTC oncogene, 33

TERT, 41, 375

TP53 gene, 45

TSH (thyroid-stimulating hormone) receptor/ cAMP (cyclic adenosine monophosphate) gene pathway, 25

TSHR gene, 29

tyrosine kinase receptors (RET, NTRK1, MET), 31

Genetic alterations, *see* Molecular genetic alterations

Giant cell medullary carcinoma, 261

GNAS gene, 30

Grading thyroid tumors, 468

Granular cell tumor, 315

Graves disease, **335**, 404

    cytopathology, 404

H

Hashimoto thyroiditis, **339**, 404, 465

    association with thyroid carcinoma, 465

    cytopathology, 404

    hashitoxicosis, 340

    nodular Hashimoto thyroiditis, 340

Hemangioma, 314

Hemangiopericytoma, 314

Histology, normal thyroid gland, 4

Hodgkin lymphoma, 305

Hormones, thyroid gland, 10

Hürthle cells, 199

Hürthle cell adenoma, *see* Oncocytic adenoma

Hürthle cell carcinoma, *see* Oncocytic tumors

Hürthle cell tumors, *see* Oncocytic tumors

Hyalinizing parathyroid adenoma, 522

Hyalinizing trabecular adenoma, **73**, 367, 412

    cytopathology, 416

    molecular genetic alterations, 367

Hyalinizing trabecular tumor, differentiation from medullary carcinoma, 258

Hypercalcemia, 506

Hypercalcemia of malignancy, 509

Hyperfunctioning adenoma, 81, 367

Hypernephroid tumor, 223

Hyperparathyroidism, 245, **506**, 513

    and medullary thyroid carcinoma, 245

    and parathyroid adenoma, 513

    bone manifestations, 507

    general considerations, 506

    primary hyperparathyroidism, 506

    renal manifestations, 509

    secondary hyperparathyroidism, 506, 575

tertiary hyperparathyroidism, 506, 579

Hyperparathyroidism-jaw tumor syndrome, 571

Hyperplastic papillary adenoma, 81

I

Implanted thyroid tissue, 358

Immunohistochemical markers, 481

Inclusion in lymph node, 360

Inflammatory pseudotumor, 307

Insular carcinoma, 85, **165,** 431

    cytopathology, 431

International union against cancer (UICC) grading scheme, 468

Intraoperative parathyroid hormone assay, 591

Intraoperative parathyroid tumor diagnosis, 589

Intrathyroidal epithelial thymoma, 319

Intrathyroidal glands, 311

Iodine deficiency and thyroid carcinogenesis, 57

L

Langerhans cell histiocytosis, 347

Large B-cell lymphoma, cytopathology, 445

Large cells, 200

Leiomyoma, 315

Leiomyosarcoma, 289

Lingual thyroid tissue, 355

Lipid-rich follicular adenoma/carcinoma, 226

Lipoadenoma, parathyroid gland, 532

Lipohyperplasia, parathyroid gland, 562

Lymphangioma, 314

Lymphoepithelioma-like carcinoma, 189

Lymphoma, 191, 258, **299**, 445

    Burkitt lymphoma, cytology, 447

    cytopathology, 445

    differentiation from undifferentiated carcinoma, 191; from medullary carcinoma, 258

    diffuse large B-cell lymphomas, 300

    follicular type lymphoma, cytopathology, 447

    Hodgkin lymphoma, 305

    large B-cell lymphoma, cytopathology, 445

    marginal zone B-cell lymphomas, 300

    mucosa-associated lymphoid tissue (MALT) lymphoma, 300, 445

    cytopathology, 445

    plasma cell granuloma, 307

    plasmacytoma, 307

Lymph nodes, thyroid inclusions in, 360

M

Macrofollicular variant of papillary carcinoma, 430
Malakoplakia, 347
Malignant hemangioendothelioma, 291
Malignant lymphoma, *see* Lymphoma
Malignant teratoma, 318
MAPK gene pathway, 30
Marginal zone B-cell lymphoma, 300
Mechanical implantation of thyroid tissue, 357
Medullary carcinoma, 190, 227, **241**, 266, 441, 531
    association with MEN 2, 242
    clear cell, 227
    clinical features, 244
    cytopathology, 441
    definition and general features, 241
    differential diagnosis, 257; differentiation from
        undifferentiated carcinoma, 189; from mixed
        medullary and follicular carcinoma, 271;
        from paraganglioma, 313; from parathyroid
        adenoma, 531
    familial medullary thyroid carcinoma, 242
    gross findings, 246
    heritable forms, 266
    histochemical and immunohistochemical find-
        ings, 251
    hyperparathyroidism, 242
    laboratory diagnosis, 245
    microscopic findings, 246
    mixed medullary and follicular cell carcinoma, 266
    molecular pathogenesis, 243
    mucinous type, 234
    spread and metastases, 259
    treatment and prognosis, 259
    ultrastructural findings, 256
    variants, 261
        amphicrine cell, 264
        angiosarcoma-like, 265
        clear cell, 262
        encapsulated, 265
        follicular, 261
        giant cell, 261
        medullary microcarcinoma, 265
        melanotic, 262
        oncocytic, 262
        papillary, 261
        paraganglioma-like, 264
        small cell, 261
        squamous cell, 264
Medullary microcarcinoma, 265
Melanotic medullary carcinoma, 262
MET gene, 36
Metaplastic carcinoma, 177
Metastatic tumors, *see* Secondary tumors
Mixed follicular and C-cell carcinoma, 267
Mixed medullary and follicular cell carcinoma, 266
    clinical features, 271
    definition and general features, 266
    differentiation from medullary carcinoma, 271
    gross and microscopic findings, 271
    treatment and prognosis, 272
Molecular genetic alterations, **365**, 450
    fine-needle aspiration biopsy alterations, 450
    follicular adenomas, 365
        hereditary syndromes, 367
        hyalinizing trabecular adenoma, 367
        toxic adenoma, 367
    follicular carcinoma, 367
        chromosomal alterations, 369
        hereditary syndromes, 367
        PI3K/PTEN/AKT pathway dysregulation, 369
        PPARγ rearrangement, 368
        RAS mutation, 367
    papillary carcinoma, 371
        BRAF mutations, 371
        chromosomal alterations, 375
        NTRK1 and *NTRK3* rearrangements, 374
        RAS mutations, 373
        RET/PTC rearrangements, 374
    papillary carcinoma variants, 376
        cribriform-morular variant, 378
        diffuse sclerosing variant, 377
        encapsulated variant, 377
        follicular variant, 376
        hereditary syndromes, 378
        microcarcinoma, 376
        oncocytic variant, 378
        solid trabecular variant, 377
        tall and columnar cell variants, 378
        Warthin-like variant, 378
    poorly differentiated carcinoma, 379
    undifferentiated carcinoma, 381
Mucin-producing microfollicular adenoma, 226
Mucinous carcinoma, **234**, 258
    differentiation from medullary carcinoma, 258
Mucinous tumors, 233
    mucinous carcinoma, 234
    mucoepidermoid carcinoma, 233

oncocytic carcinoma, 235
papillary carcinoma, 234
signet ring follicular adenoma/carcinoma, 234
Mucoepidermoid carcinoma, **230**, 233, 441
mucinous type, 234
squamous type, 234
Mucoepidermoid mucinous carcinoma, 233
Mucoepidermoid squamous cell carcinoma, 234, 441
Mucosa-associated lymphoid tissue (MALT) lymphoma, 300, 445
Multifocal fibrosing (sclerosing) thyroiditis, 345
Multifocal granulomatous folliculitis, 347
Multinodular goiter, 331
Multiple endocrine neoplasia, parathyroid gland, 568
type 1, 568
type 2, 570
type 4, 571
Multiple endocrine neoplasia type 2, and medullary thyroid carcinoma, 242
Myxoid stromal changes, 235

N

National Cancer Institute (NCI) consensus conference on FNAB classification (Bethesda system), 396
Neonatal severe primary hyperparathyroidism, 571
Neuroendocrine carcinoma of thyroid gland, 241
Nodular goiter, 331
Nodular Hashimoto thyroiditis, **339**, 359
and parasitic nodule, 360
Nodular hyperplasia, 72, **331**, 400
and Hashimoto thyroiditis, 340
cytopathology, 400
differentiation from follicular adenoma, 72, 334; from carcinoma, 334
Nonencapsulated sclerosing tumor, 127
Non-neoplastic goiter, 400
NTRK1 gene, 33, 374
NTRK1 and *NTRK3* rearrangements, in papillary carcinoma, 374

O

Occult papillary carcinoma, 127
Occult sclerosing carcinoma, 127
Oncocytes, 199
Oncocytic adenoma, 203
Oncocytic carcinoma, **209**, 262
angioinvasive, 211

clear cell, 221
clinical features, 209
differentiation from oncocytic hyperplastic nodule, follicular adenoma, follicular carcinoma, papillary carcinoma, 214
follicular type, 214
general features, 209
gross findings, 209
immunohistochemical findings, 212
medullary type, 262
microscopic findings, 210
minimally invasive, 211
molecular genetic findings, 208
papillary type, 143, 214
spread and metastases, 215
treatment and prognosis, 215
widely invasive, 212
Oncocytic cells, 199
Oncocytic clear cell neoplasms, 222
Oncocytic follicular carcinoma, 214
Oncocytic hyperplastic nodule, differentiation from oncocytic carcinoma, 214
Oncocytic medullary carcinoma, 262
papillary oncocytic neoplasms, 215
Oncocytic papillary carcinoma, 143, 216
Oncocytic parathyroid adenoma, 521
Oncocytic thyroid adenoma, 203
Oncocytic tumors, 199, 423
cytopathology, 423
encapsulated papillary oncocytic neoplasm, 216
malignancy, 203
nature of oncocyte, 201
oncocytic adenoma, 203
oncocytic carcinoma, 209
oncocytic cells, 199
oncocytic change, 202
oncocytoma, 202
Oncocytic variant of papillary carcinoma, 216, 433
cytopathology, 433
Oncocytoma, 202
Ontogenous parathyromatosis, 583
Oxyphilic cells, 200

P

Palpation thyroiditis, 347
Papillary carcinoma, 85, **103**, 227, 228, 371, 416
adenoid cystic variant, 431
associated syndromes, 103

clinical features, 103
columnar cell variant, 146
cribriform/morular variant, 149, 378
cytopathology, 416
differentiation from undifferentiated thyroid
    carcinoma, 189; from oncocytic carcinoma,
    214; from medullary carcinoma, 257; from
    parathyroid adenoma, 530
diffuse sclerosing variant, 141, 377
encapsulated follicular variant, 135, 377
encapsulated papillary carcinoma, 130
follicular variant, 85, **131**, 376
    microfollicular variant, 133
general features, 103
grading, 118
gross findings, 104
hereditary syndromes, 378
immunohistochemical findings, 119
macrofollicular variant, 430
medullary carcinoma, papillary variant, 261
metastasis, 121
microscopic findings, 105
    nuclear features, 107
    papillary, 105
    psammoma bodies, 113
    pseudoinclusions, 107
    squamous metaplasia, 111
molecular genetic alterations, 369, 375
mucinous type, 234
oncocytic type, 143, 199
papillary microcarcinoma, 127, 376
prognosis, 125
radiation exposure, 103
solid/trabecular variant, 139, 377
squamous cell, 232
tall cell variant, 146, 378
treatment, 124
variants, 127, 376
ultrastructural findings, 118
Warthin-like variant, 144, 378
with clear cell features, 149, 227
with exuberant nodular fasciitis-like stroma, 430
Papillary medullary carcinoma, 261
Papillary microcarcinoma, 127, 376
Papillary oncocytic neoplasms, 215
Paraganglioma, 259, **311**
    differentiation from medullary carcinoma,
        259, 313

Paraganglioma-like medullary carcinoma, 264
Parasitic nodule, 358
    in nodular Hashimoto thyroiditis, 359
Parastruma, 222
Parathyroid adenoma, **513**, 565
    adenolipoma, 530
    adenoma-associated parathyroid glands, 537
    atypical adenoma, 532, 554
    chief cell adenoma, 517
    clinical features, 514
    cytologic findings, 525
    differentiation from parathyroid carcinoma,
        530, 554; from thyroid neoplasms, 530;
        from chief cell hyperplasia, 565
    general features, 513
    gross findings, 514
    hyalinizing adenoma, 522
    immunohistochemical findings, 526
    lipoadenoma, 532
    microadenomas, 514
    microscopic findings, 517
    molecular genetic findings, 529
    oncocytic adenoma, 531
    treatment and prognosis, 531
    ultrastructural findings, 529
    water clear cell adenoma, 532
Parathyroid carcinoma, 543
    clinical features, 543
    cytologic findings, 552
    differentiation from parathyroid adenoma,
        from parathyromatosis, 554
    general features, 543
    gross findings, 544
    immunohistochemical findings, 552
    microscopic findings, 544
    molecular genetic findings, 553
    staging, 556
    treatment and prognosis, 554
    ultrastructural findings, 553
Parathyroid chief cell adenoma, 517
Parathyroid cysts, 583
Parathyroid microadenoma, 514
Parathyroid gland, normal, 493
    anatomy, 494
    calcium homeostasis, 505
    embryology, 493
    gross and microscopic findings, 494
    immunohistochemical findings, 499

parathyroid hormone, 505
  ultrastructural findings, 501
Parathyroid grafts, 580
Parathyroid hormone, **505**, 591
  intraoperative assay, 591
Parathyroid hormone-related protein, 505
Parathyroid tumors, 311, 589
  diagnosis of, 589
  in thyroid gland, 311
Parathyroiditis, chronic, 565
Parathyromatosis, 498, 554, 562, **583**
  differentiation from parathyroid carcinoma, 554
  primary (ontogenous) parathyromatosis, 583
  secondary (postsurgical) parathyromatosis, 585
Parenchymatous goiter, 331
Pathologic evaluation of thyroid tumors, 467
PAX gene, 41
PAX/PPRG rearrangement, 41
Pediatric tumors, 58
Pendred syndrome, 337
PI3K/PTEN/AKT pathway, **37**, 369
  in follicular carcinoma, 369
Plasma cell granuloma, 307
Plasmacytoma, 307
Pleomorphic adenoma, 320
Pleomorphic carcinoma, 177
Plummer adenoma, 81, 367
Poorly differentiated carcinomas, **165**, 258, 379
  differentiation from medullary carcinoma, 258
  insular carcinoma, 165
  molecular genetic alterations, 377
  mucinous type, 235
  Turin proposal, 173
Postoperative necrotizing granuloma, 347
Postpartum thyroiditis, 347
Postsurgical parathyromatosis, 585
PPARγ rearrangement, **41**, 368
  in follicular carcinoma, 368
Primary chief cell hyperplasia, parathyroid gland, 561
  differentiation from parathyroid adenoma, 565
Primary hyperparathyroidism, 506
Primary parathyromatosis, 583
PRKAR1A gene, 31
Prognostic scoring systems, 125, 474
Pseudolymphoma, 307
PTEN gene, 40

R

Radiologic evaluation of thyroid tumors, 465
Radiation exposure, 57, 103, **348**
  and papillary thyroid carcinoma, 103
  and thyroid tumors, 57
RAS genes, 36
RAS mutations, 367, 373
  in follicular carcinoma, 367
  in papillary carcinoma, 373
Reporting thyroid tumors, 468
  ADASP/CAP protocols, 468
  AJCC/UICC TNM scheme, 468
Riedel thyroiditis, 190, **342**
  differentiation from undifferentiated thyroid carcinoma, 190
RET gene, 31, 243
  and medullary carcinoma, 243
RET/PTC oncogene, 33
RET/PTC rearrangements, in papillary carcinoma, 373
Rosai-Dorfman disease, 347

S

Sanderson polster, 5
Sarcoidosis, 347
Sarcomas, 189, **289**
  angiosarcoma, 291
  differentiation from undifferentiated thyroid carcinoma, 189
  leiomyosarcoma, 289
Sarcomatoid carcinoma, 177
Schwannoma, 315
Sclerosing mucoepidermoid carcinoma with eosinophilia, 230, 233
  mucinous type, 234
  squamous type, 232
Secondary hyperparathyroidism, 506, **575**
Secondary parathyromatosis, 585
Secondary tumors, parathyroid gland, 585
Secondary tumors, thyroid gland, 232, 235, **325**, 447
  cytopathology, 447
  mucinous, 234
  renal cell carcinoma, 327
  squamous cell, 232
Signet ring cell follicular adenoma/carcinoma, 225, 234
  clear cell type, 225
  mucinous type, 234

Signet ring cell mucinous adenoma, 225
Sinus histiocytosis with massive lymphadeno-
    pathy, 347
Small cell medullary carcinoma, 261
Solid carcinoma with amyloid stroma, 241
Solid cell nests, 15
Solid/trabecular variant of papillary carcinoma,
    139, 377, 429
    cytopathology, 429
    molecular genetic alterations, 377
Solitary fibrous tumor, 314
Somatostatin, 13
Spindle cell adenoma, 78
Spindle epithelial tumor with thymus-like differ-
    entiation, 316
Spontaneous silent thyroiditis, 347
Sporadic nodular goiter, 331
Squamous cell carcinoma, 232, *see also* Squamous
    cell tumors
Squamous cell tumors, **228**, 264, 440
    carcinoma with thymus-like differentiation, 232
    follicular tumors, 232
    medullary carcinoma, 232, 264
    mucoepidermoid carcinoma, 230
    non-neoplastic conditions, 233
    papillary carcinoma, 226
    sclerosing mucoepidermoid carcinoma with
        eosinophilia, 230
    secondary tumors, 232
    squamous cell carcinoma, 232
Squamous cell epithelial nests, 233
Squamous cell medullary carcinoma, 233, **264**
Staging, 469, 556
    parathyroid tumors, 556
    thyroid tumors, 469
Stem cell carcinoma, 267
Struma ovarii, 361
Strumal carcinoid, 361
Subacute granulomatous thyroiditis, 342

T

Tall cell papillary carcinoma, **146**, 372, 429
    cytopathology, 429
Teratoma, **313**, 361
    with thyroid tissue, 361
TERT, 369, 375
Tertiary hyperparathyroidism, 506, **579**
Third pharyngeal pouch cysts, 583

Thyroglobulin, 10, 466 , 486
    and clear cell tumors, 221
    in thyroid tumors, 466
Thyroid carcinoma, *see under individual entities*
Thyroid hormones, 10, 11
Thyroid spindle cell tumor with mucous cysts, 316
Thyroid-stimulating hormone, 1, 11
Thyroid-stimulating hormone, 11
Thyroid transcription factor-1, 1, 9, 487
Thyroid tumors, general features, 57, 465, 481,
    530, *see also under individual tumors/
    carcinomas*
    and Hashimoto thyroiditis, 465
    childhood tumors, 58
    classification, 61
    clinical evaluation, 465
    cytopathology, 395
    differentiation from parathyroid adenoma, 530
    frozen section evaluation, 466
    grading, 468
    immunohistochemical markers, 481
    incidence, 57
    iodine deficiency, 57
    molecular genetic alterations, 369
    pathologic evaluation, 467
    prognostic factors, 474
    prognostic score, 474
    radiation exposure, 57
    reporting tumors, 467
    staging, 469
    treatment, 472
Thyroiditis, 339
    fibrosing thyroiditis, 339
    Hashimoto thyroiditis, 339
    malakoplakia, 347
    multifocal fibrosing (sclerosing) thyroiditis, 345
    other forms, 347
    subacute granulomatous thyroiditis, 342
Thyrolipomatosis, 315
Thyrotropin (thyroid-stimulating hormone), 11
Thyrotropin-releasing hormone, 11
Thyroxine, 10
TNM staging scheme, 471
Toxic adenoma, **81**, 367
    molecular genetic alterations, 367
Toxic nodular hyperplasia, 332
TP53 gene, 45
Triiodothyronine, 10

TSH receptor/cAMP gene pathway, 25
TSHR gene, 29
Turin proposal, 173
Tyrosine kinase receptors, 31

U

UICC grading scheme, 468
Undifferentiated (anaplastic) carcinoma, **177**, 227, 380, 433
    anaplastic transformation, 194
    clear cell, 227
    clinical features, 177
    cytopathology, 433
    differentiation from sarcomas, papillary thyroid carcinoma, medullary carcinoma, lymphoma, Riedel thyroiditis, 189
    giant cell pattern, 180
    gross findings, 177
    immunohistochemical findings, 184
    lymphoepithelioma-like carcinoma, 189
    microscopic findings, 177
    microscopic types, 187
    mucinous type, 234
    rhabdoid tumor, 189
    spindle cell pattern, 178
    spread and metastasis, 190
    squamoid pattern, 178
    squamous type, 232
    treatment and prognosis, 192
    ultrastructural findings, 186
Uremic refractory secondary hyperparathyroidism, 579

W

Warthin-like variant of papillary carcinoma, **143**, 378, 429
    cytopathology, 429
Water clear cell adenoma, parathyroid gland, 532
Wegener granulomatosis, 347
Well-differentiated carcinoma, not otherwise specified, 136
Well-differentiated tumor of uncertain malignant potential, 95, 135